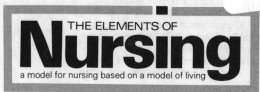

THE ELEMENTS OF Nursing
a model for nursing based on a model of living

NANCY ROPER trained at the General Infirmary, Leeds, UK and later spent 15 years at the Cumberland Infirmary School of Nursing as Principal Tutor. In 1964 she became a self-employed writer. She is the editor of the *Churchill Livingstone Pocket Medical Dictionary, Churchill Livingstone Nurses Dictionary, and New American Pocket Medical Dictionary*; and the author of *Man's Anatomy. Physiology, Health and Environment* and *Principles of Nursing*. In 1970 she was awarded a fellowship from the Commonwealth Nurses' War Memorial Fund and in 1975 she received the MPhil degree for the thesis based on the research project; she also wrote the monograph *Clinical Experience in Nurse Education* (1976). From 1975–1978 she was Nursing Officer (Research) at the Scottish Home and Health Department. Since then she has continued as a self-employed author.

WINIFRED LOGAN, previously head of the Department of Health and Nursing Studies, Glasgow College, Scotland from 1981–1986, was Executive Director of the International Council of Nurses (ICN) from 1978–1980. She had already gained considerable knowledge and experience of nursing internationally, having worked or served as a consultant in Canada, the USA, Malaysia and Iraq. In 1971–1972 she acted as Chief Nursing Officer at the newly created Ministry of Health in Abu Dhabi. Prior to moving to the ICN she worked for 4 years at the Scottish Home and Health Department where she had responsibility for nursing education. She took to that post experience gained from a 12-year term of office, first as lecturer and latterly as senior lecturer, in the Department of Nursing Studies at the University of Edinburgh. She is an arts graduate of that university and did her basic education at the Royal Infirmary of Edinburgh. She has served on various national committees associated with the General Nursing Council of Scotland, the Council for National Academic Awards, and the University Grants Committee.

ALISON TIERNEY is Director of the Nursing Research Unit in the Department of Nursing Studies at the University of Edinburgh, Scotland. From 1973–1980 she was a lecturer in the Department of Nursing Studies, a post which involved her in the development of the foundation nursing course for beginning students and in the clinical supervision of students at various stages of the integrated degree/nursing programme. She herself was one of the early graduates of that same programme. Her PhD degree was awarded for research undertaken in the field of mental handicap nursing while holding a Scottish Home and Health Department nursing research training fellowship (1971–1973). Dr Tierney is the editor of *Nurse and the Mentally Handicapped* (Wiley, 1983) and the author of a number of articles and chapters. She was a member of the course team which developed the Open University teaching package 'A systematic approach to nursing' (1984).

Nancy Roper, Winifred Logan and Alison Tierney are all graduates of the University of Edinburgh. They came together in 1976 to work on the first edition of *The Elements of Nursing* which was published in 1980. Their second book *Learning to Use the Process of Nursing* was published in 1981. They edited a third book *Using a Model for Nursing* and it was published in 1983. In addition they have had published a number of journal articles concerned with the Roper, Logan and Tierney model for nursing.

The authors can be contacted at their publisher's address:
Churchill Livingstone, 1–3 Baxter's Place, Leith Walk, Edinburgh, Scotland, EH1 3AF.
Telex 727511

THE ELEMENTS OF
Nursing

a model for nursing based on a model of living

NANCY ROPER
MPhil RGN RSCN RNT

WINIFRED W. LOGAN
MA DNS (Educ) RGN RNT

ALISON J. TIERNEY
BSc (Soc Sc-Nurs) PhD RGN

THIRD EDITION

Churchill Livingstone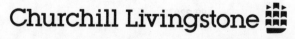

EDINBURGH LONDON MELBOURNE AND NEW YORK 1990

CHURCHILL LIVINGSTONE
Medical Division of Longman Group UK Limited

Distributed in the United States of America by Churchill Livingstone
Inc., 1560 Broadway, New York, N.Y. 10036, and by associated
companies, branches, and representatives throughout the world.

First edition 1980
Second edition 1985
Third edition 1990
  Reprinted 1991

ISBN 0-443-03950-X

British Library Cataloguing in Publication Data
Roper, Nancy
  The elements of nursing.—3rd. ed.
  1. Medicine. Nursing
  I. Title   II. Logan. Winifred W.   III. Tierney,
  Alison J.
  610.73

Library of Congress Cataloging in Publication Data
Roper, Nancy.
  The elements of nursing: a model for nursing based on a model of
  living/Nancy Roper, Winifred W. Logan, Alison J. Tierney. — 3rd ed.
    p. cm.
  Includes bibliographical references.
  ISBN 0-443-03950-X
  1. Nursing.   I. Logan, Winifred W.   II. Tierney, Alison J.
III. title.
  [DNLM: 1. Nursing Process.   WY 100 R784e]
RT41.R724   1990
610'.73—dc20
DNLM/DLC
for Library of Congress   89-22072

Produced by Longman Singapore Publishers (Pte) Ltd.
Printed in Singapore

Preface to the Third Edition

This third edition of the *The Elements of Nursing*, as before, is essentially for beginning nursing students. It is not a comprehensive text in the sense of covering all aspects of nursing knowledge and practice required in the course of a basic education programme; rather, it encourages a logical mode of thinking about nursing in the framework of a model for nursing. An immediately obvious change to the third edition is the title. It has been extended to include, 'a model for nursing based on a model of living'. It would seem that a number of potential readers did not appreciate that *The Elements of Nursing* used the framework of a model for nursing, and the extended title should help to draw attention to this important feature of the book.

The presentation of the book itself has been rearranged and its content substantially revised and updated. Section 1 has been changed. Its introductory chapter emphasises the link between nursing and health — a point which is stressed increasingly by the World Health Organization. The content of the second chapter is new. It includes a discussion, albeit brief, of some of the other internationally well-known models for nursing, in order to provide an understanding of the context in which the Roper, Logan and Tierney model can be considered.

Section 2 has been considerably altered; the objective here being to present the Roper, Logan and Tierney model more clearly, incorporating some of the refinements which have been made since the last edition. It commences with a chronological account of the background to the model showing how it developed from research and a review of the literature.

Subsequently, the model of living and the model for nursing are discussed sequentially — in the previous editions they were separated by three brief chapters introducing some concepts from biology, psychology and sociology. Perhaps this was appropriate when the first edition was published 10 years ago, but increasingly nursing students are expected to study the biological and social sciences as foundation subjects, so these three chapters have been omit-

ted. Instead the third edition emphasises more than previously, the application of such knowledge in the context of 'Factors influencing the ALs', a component of the model. For purposes of clarification too, there are minor alterations in the diagrams of the models, to emphasise the relationships between the components. It is in Section 2 also that we describe how the model relates to the practice of nursing — in 'Individualising nursing' — and proforma are provided as a suggested method for documenting nursing data.

Section 3, as before, consists of 12 chapters, one devoted to each of the 12 Activities of Living (ALs), the main component of the model. All of these chapters have been extensively revised, obviously to update the content but also to reflect the five components of the model more clearly than in the second edition. The first half of each chapter discusses the nature of the AL, mainly in the context of 'healthy living'; the second half provides selected examples of the problems related to the ALs which can be caused by illness.

We have welcomed feedback about the two previous editions of the book, and consider all comments as a means of helping us to refine our thinking; a number of changes in the third edition reflect such feedback. It is appropriate to comment here on two recurring criticisms. A number of readers have been concerned about the apparent lack of provision in the model for consideration of the individual's spiritual needs. Obviously we had not made it sufficiently clear that sociocultural factors (related to each of the 12 ALs) include spiritual, religious and ethical considerations — and this remains the case. We do not see spiritual needs standing on their own (any more than physical needs or sociocultural needs) but firmly related to the individual's ALs because this is how they are manifest. A second area which continues to cause concern is the relevance of the AL of expressing sexuality in a model for nursing. In the first edition, the term was certainly a novel inclusion in a nursing context although it is now used frequently in the mass media, and increasingly in the nursing literature.

However, it is still used too narrowly. We hope we have emphasised its broad application to femininity/masculinity in general and have clarified that, as with any AL, individual circumstances will dictate whether or not it is a relevant subject for consideration.

Also on the subject of feedback, it is appropriate to mention that *The Elements of Nursing* is becoming increasingly well-known in other countries, especially in Europe and more recently in Australia. As a result, a number of translations of the book into other languages has been undertaken.

Of course, no one model can be all-embracing; indeed a challenging feature of any model is that it suggests growing points for further thinking and refinement about the discipline. And no single text can possibly exhaust discussion of something so complex as a conceptual framework for nursing, and its application in practice. We hope this third edition provides a clearer account of the model and a further analysis of those concepts which, we believe, comprise the elements of nursing.

Edinburgh 1990   N.R. W.L. A.T.

Preface to the Second Edition

This second edition of *The Elements of Nursing* retains the format of the original text and, as before, is essentially for beginning nursing students. The fact that the first edition has been positively received, in particular because of its focus on a model for nursing (which incorporates the process of nursing), reassured us that there is still a need for an introductory text of this kind. However, we wish to emphasise that this book is not intended as 'comprehensive'; the expectation is that it will be complemented by other nursing texts and literature from other disciplines such as human biology, psychology and sociology. Our extended use of reference in this edition is intended to encourage students to read widely and, especially, to take account of research as a basis for nursing practice.

The contents of the book are basically as outlined in the preface of the first edition. Section 1, 'Nursing and health care', is still introductory but has been revised, updated and re-arranged.

In Section 2, the chapters on the 'Model of living' (Ch. 2) and the 'Model for nursing' (Ch. 6) have been rewritten for purposes of clarification and to incorporate refinements to the model which are the result of giving considerable further thought to our original ideas in the course of writing *Learning to Use the Process of Nursing* (1981), and of undertaking a project which is described in *Using a Model for Nursing* (1983). The middle chapters of Section 2 — 'Biological aspects of living' (Ch. 3), 'Developmental aspects of living' (Ch. 4) and 'Social aspects of living' (Ch.

5) — have been minimally revised and have been retained to provide beginning students with a brief overview of material which is relevant as a background to Section 3.

Section 3 consists of 12 chapters (Chs 7–18), one devoted to each of the 12 Activities of Living, the main focus of the model. All of these chapters have been substantially rewritten, obviously to update material but also to reflect the components of the model more clearly than in the first edition.

Section 4, consisting of one short chapter (Ch. 19), is new to this edition. One of the current major criticisms about nursing models is that although they may be of theoretical interest, there is difficulty in using them in the real world of nursing. This chapter therefore has been added to help readers to appreciate how the Roper/Logan/Tierney model can be applied in practice. To give some guidance for documentation, we discuss the proforma which developed out of the project of the third book *Using a Model for Nursing* (1983).

No one model can be perfect and no single text can possibly exhaust discussion of something as complex as a conceptual framework for nursing and its application to practice. We hope, however, that this new edition provides a clearer account of our model and a further analysis of those concepts which comprise the elements of nursing.

Edinburgh 1985   N.R. W.L. A.T.

Preface to the First Edition

We planned and wrote this book because of our conviction that the degree of complexity and specialisation of nursing today makes it more necessary than ever for the elements of nursing to be identified and understood. Today's nursing students right from the start of their education programme need to become familiar with those elements common to all branches of nursing and relevant to all patients.

Consequently we examined the core of knowledge required by nurses and we have presented it within a model for nursing which is based on a model of living. The model for nursing incorporates the process of nursing so that together they provide a conceptual framework for the book. It is hoped that this framework will assist learners to develop a way of thinking about nursing which will help them to provide effective and compassionate nursing for people of whatever age who have various problems and who are in different health care settings. In addition, as nursing experience is gained, this way of thinking should facilitate the acquisition of new and specialised knowledge.

In Section 1 the reader is encouraged to think about the meaning of health and illness and how a health care system develops within a country. Nursing's contribution to health care is examined and the section ends with a consideration of the educational preparation needed by today's nurses.

The two models — the model of living and the model for nursing — are described in Section 2. Both models focus on 12 Activities of Living (ALs): maintaining a safe environment; communicating; breathing; eating and drinking; eliminating; personal cleansing and dressing; controlling body temperature; mobilising; working and playing; expressing sexuality; sleeping; and dying. All Activities of Living have biological, developmental and social dimensions and so a chapter is devoted to each of these aspects of living within this section. Finally there is a discussion of the process of nursing, showing how this concept is used as a framework for the analysis of each of the Activities of Living.

This analysis of the 12 ALs makes up the 12 chapters in Section 3 of the book. In the first part of each chapter there is a description of the nature of the activity, the purpose of the activity, factors influencing the activity and body structure and function required for the activity. Guidelines are given on assessing an individual's performance of the activity. The second part of each chapter contains discussion of possible patients' problems associated with that AL. For example, among the problems discussed relating to the AL of eliminating are those arising from lack of privacy in the ward; dependence due to limited mobility or confinement to bed or psychological disturbance; urinary incontinence; urinary catheterisation; and anxiety associated with investigations of the urinary and defaecatory systems. Emphasis is placed on the problems as experienced by the patient, and related nursing activities are therefore presented as assisting the patient to solve, reduce or prevent problems which interfere with everyday living. Each chapter has a summary chart which shows how this problem-orientated approach is used in applying the process of nursing to the AL. Although a chapter has been devoted to each AL, in reality the activities are interrelated and it must be remembered that a problem with one can produce problems with any or all of the other ALs.

At the end of each chapter there are two lists, one of References and the other of Suggested Reading. Relevant research reports are included in both. Most of the listed articles and books contain references which will guide the reader who wishes to gain further information about a particular topic.

In the process of writing this book we were constantly clarifying and extending our thinking about nursing. All three of us feel that we now have a better understanding of the elements of nursing and a greater awareness of their complexity, which we hope we have conveyed to the readers of this book.

Edinburgh 1980   N.R. W.L. A.T.

Foreword to the First Edition

Professional practice is in constant need of review and refinement if it is to adapt to new demands and advances in knowledge. One of the most significant advances in nursing in recent years has been the move towards replacing ritualised and institutionalised approaches with those that are rationally planned and individualised.

The teaching of nursing in the past was often based on body systems, disease entities and procedures. The emphasis is now changing to one that concentrates on the essential nature of nursing action and the principles which underlie practice.

The authors of *The Elements of Nursing* have done a great deal to help us in this direction. They have given a model for nursing based on activities of living and incorporating the process of nursing. Components of the nursing function are analysed and guidelines are given for assessing the patient's functional abilities in each activity of living. A theoretical framework for assessment and nursing care evolves. The result is a unique amalgam of theory drawn from biological and behavioural sciences which should equip a nurse to function on a sound scientific basis.

The book begins with a quotation from Florence Nightingale:
'. . . the very elements of nursing are all but unknown.' The authors have accepted the professional challenge of those words and, 120 years later, they have done much to identify those elements of nursing which should help us towards rational, individualised nursing practice. I believe there is in their work a basis for innovation and improved quality of performance to which we all aspire.

January, 1980   McFarlane of Llandaff

Contents

Contents

SECTION 1

Nursing and health care

1

Nursing in health and illness

It has been said and written scores of times that every woman makes a good nurse. I believe on the contrary that the very elements of nursing are all but unknown.

Florence Nightingale (1859)

These words were written over a century ago but the profession is still refining its ideas about 'the elements' of nursing. This is not surprising. Nursing exists to serve society and as the conditions and needs of society have changed, practices have altered in response to the changes.

WHAT IS NURSING?

History reveals that sick people required and received care long before nursing became an organised occupation; indeed, in the Western world until the end of the last century family members or domestic staff usually nursed the sick in their own homes, and hospitals were used only for paupers or grossly mentally deranged people. The family is the oldest, and still the most used health care service in the world. Even today, patients are discharged from hospital as soon as they can be cared for by the family.

And it is still the custom in some countries to admit the family members to hospital with the patient, complete with bedding and cooking utensils to attend to the sick relative's everyday living activities while the nurses carry out specific treatments associated with the disease condition.

Undoubtedly, however, during the last century nursing has been associated in the eyes of the public with care of the sick, especially in hospital. And as nurses have become increasingly involved with the curative, technical treatments provided by medical staff they have come to occupy a strategic position. Nurses are the link between what are often stressful, complicated technical procedures associated with the disease condition and the maintenance of everyday bodily and mental functions which are so critical to the patient's comfort and so important to him as a person.

Admittedly, looking back at the major professional

developments in nursing in the Western world during the 20th century, it would appear that they have been associated mainly with the 'sickness' services. However, knowledge about disease processes, developments in biological and social sciences, increasing sophistication in technology and a better-educated public have produced a new awareness about health care services in general, and there is increasing public interest in individual, family and community health. The hospital-based, disease-orientated health care system, and nursing within that system, is now being questioned. Nurses along with other health professionals are beginning to see the importance of putting increasing emphasis on maintaining health, preventing sickness, enhancing self-help and promoting maximum independence according to the individual person's capability. It is, therefore, difficult to define 'the elements' of nursing definitively when the needs and demands of society are in a state of flux and when the interface between health and illness is no longer so clearly defined.

But, on analysis, nursing has not only been associated with people who are ill. Over many years, midwives (or the alternative title used in different countries) have monitored the health status of pregnant women, the majority of whom are healthy while undergoing a normal physiological experience; midwives have also facilitated development of the skills required for breast feeding, parenting, inclusion of the new baby into the family and so on. Health visitors (or equivalent title) have provided a service to pre-school children and their families; they have encouraged immunisation, the promotion and maintenance of health as well as the prevention of accident and illness. School nurses have carried out a similar function for children during the period of formal education, and occupational health nurses have provided a comparable service for adults throughout their working lives. In several countries, too, nurses working in the community have been concerned with helping older people to retain an interest in a healthy lifestyle. So, the idea of nurses nursing well people outside hospital is not new. Indeed Florence Nightingale (1859) wrote:

The very elements of what constitutes good nursing are as little understood for the well as for the sick. The same laws of health or of nursing, for they are in reality the same, obtain among the well as among the sick.

Over 100 years later, the World Health Organization has promoted an ambitious worldwide campaign — 'Health for all by the year 2000' in which nurses are involved. To begin to understand this international endeavour, all students of nursing require to examine and develop their concept of 'health ' so that not only will it inform their personal style of living, but will also influence their concept of nursing practice in relation to healthy as well as ill people. So, first of all, can health be defined?

WHAT IS HEALTH?

Perhaps the people of the ancient world were much more aware of maintaining health than we are now. In Ancient Greece, there is little doubt that the pursuit of excellence, encapsulated in the Platonic ideal, required a sound mind in a sound body; both contributing to the good of the soul. In Plato's *The Republic* it is declared that:

. . . in a well-run society each man . . . has no time to spend his life being ill and undergoing cures . . . there's nothing worse than this fussiness about one's health . . . it is tiresome in the home, as well as in the army or in any civilian office.

Perhaps a 'good' state of health was possible in the heyday of the Greek city state. Some time later, Galen (AD 130–201), the celebrated physician, accepted that health in the abstract was an ideal state to which no one attained, yet he found difficulty regarding as unhealthy, all who did not function perfectly. He therefore was prepared to overlook small ailments and to consider health as a state of reasonable functioning and freedom from pain.

These are obviously old ideas about health, but they are being reaffirmed by the World Health Organization, health professionals and members of the lay public in many countries — health is not an absolute quantity but a concept which is continually changing with the acquisition of knowledge and changing cultural expectations. Probably the best known definition of health appears in the Constitution of the World Health Organization (1946), 'a state of complete physical, mental and social well-being, and not merely the absence of disease or infirmity.'

When WHO defined health in this way, however, it was genuinely believed that there was a clear distinction between health and ill-health. For example in the early 1940s when Lord Beveridge, the well-known British economist, was helping to plan the National Health Service in the UK, it was assumed that there was a strictly limited quantity of illness which, if treated, would be reduced; indeed the planners expected that the annual cost of the health service would decrease as treatment reduced the incidence of illness, and people were transferred from the 'ill' category to the 'healthy' category. With the advantage of hindsight, this interpretation of health is too simplistic and in recent years, it has become accepted by most people that there is no such clear-cut distinction between health and ill-health.

In the first place, in strictly scientific terms, it is not possible to demonstrate a cut-off point between an individual's healthy state and diseased state, says the OHE monograph (1971). For a range of biochemical and physical observations which can be made on the individual, there is a continuous distribution curve for the population as a whole, for example for haemoglobin levels or blood pressure readings. The distribution of measurements ranges smoothly from those for the obviously healthy to those for the obviously diseased; and there is a substantial overlap area in the middle where one cannot objectively draw definite conclusions from the measurements. In fact it is probable that for many measurements the optimum varies from person to person so that correcting an abnormality by treatment and bringing the measurement to some average value, would be unnecessary.

In any case, it is a purely subjective judgement on the part of individuals whether they feel well or unwell, and this to some extent is dependent on prevailing attitudes. For example in the UK, disabilities which were tolerated as inevitable in the 1930s are now thought to justify treatment. Formerly, for example, deafness, lack of teeth and failing sight were accepted as part of the ageing process whereas now, corrective treatment is the expectation and considered as a right. Also, sophisticated procedures such as renal dialysis and transplant surgery offer the possibility of treatment to people who, even 10 years ago, were resigned to an incurable affliction and an early demise. There are less dramatic ways in which an increasing number of people are being transferred back to the health category by such treatments as permanent medication for a specific disorder; a special diet for life; a technological implant such as a pacemaker and so on. Perhaps the time is ripe to introduce the concept of 'aided health'.

In essence, health can be conceptualised as a dynamic process with many facets. Currently, there is a move away from visualising health and illness as a continuum, with health at one end, and illness at the other. A growing number of writers and practitioners now consider that the health status of individuals is dependent on their ability to adapt to, and cope with challenges they meet throughout life. In fact, they say that those who feel well and live in a way which they find socially and economically satisfactory may be considered 'healthy' even though they have a significant disability such as a physical or mental handicap or a disease. On the other hand, those with no detectable evidence of physical illness may be judged 'unhealthy' because they feel unwell. It is relatively easy to identify individuals' 'maladaptive' behaviours. It requires a much more subtle understanding of human reactions to detect 'adaptive' behaviours/coping mechanisms and to evaluate whether or not they should be supported and maintained. Coping behaviours resulting in health/wellness, or maladaptive behaviours resulting in illness are often learned within the family, as well as attitudes, values and beliefs about health. It may, in fact, be a false assumption that everyone wants to be healthy.

Although in industrialised countries, the individual has come to be so dependent on the state and in particular, on the health services provided — and all countries in Europe, for example, have some form of health service — it is fascinating to note a resurgence of interest in self-determination in relation to matters of health. In an article on the subject of self-care, Levin (1981) explains that health professionals are having to be educated to reconsider ordinary people as self-providers of health and health care. Self-care is a term that is used increasingly to denote health care activities which include health caring services of the family, extended family, friends, lay volunteer groups, mutual and self-help groups, religious organisations, and in some instances, a whole neighbourhood. Although most published statistics about self-care are confined to the industrialised nations, self-care is the dominant form for most of the world's rural people in developing countries.

Several factors have been suggested as sources of our increasing awareness of self-care and its potential, and have been the subject of various WHO symposia. Levin summarised them as long ago as 1981:

- in the industrialised nations, the massive shift in disease patterns during the last 50 years to almost a trebling of the incidence of chronic diseases when lay caring is a partnership with professional resources
- an erosion of professional mystique; and the public's awareness of rights and of options
- the public's awareness of alternative health care strategies
- a change in public attitudes to disease prevention and health promotion involving personal lifestyle and collective action
- the public's awareness of the economic implications of health care.

Levin ended his discussions claiming that this is an exciting period in the transition of health planning from a professional/industrial to a social model and concluded: 'we shall need a new conceptual vocabulary free of the we/they dichotomy'.

In 1988 the World Health Organization's original definition of health which appears on page 4 was extended. At a nursing conference discussing the 38 targets for the programme 'Health for all by the year 2000', participants were reminded that the targets are based on 'the premise that health is not the mere absence of disease but the opportunity to create well being and realise human potential' (Nath & O'Neill, 1988). The targets take full account of the fact that promoting health and helping to prevent illness are not the prerogative of the 'health care' professionals. There are many other agencies concerned with providing requisites which contribute to health such as housing and sanitation; poor standards in such basic services can provide an unsafe environment (p. 86) which can damage health and cause illness. In the context of change, it is also appropriate to note that as nurses increasingly provide a service to well people to help them maximise their health status, the word 'clients' has become accepted vocabulary to differentiate them from 'patients' who are traditionally perceived to have an illness status.

Yet another language change in relation to the health service in the 1980s is an increasing use of the word 'consumers', conveying the idea used in various politicoeconomic models, that providers of health care are accountable to consumers of that care. Health, and the words used in relation to it, have to be perceived in a very broad and changing context, and the same applies to the concept of illness.

WHAT IS ILLNESS?

From time immemorial, man has sought to explain illness, and his beliefs regarding cause have determined the role of the sick person, the role of the healer and the system of care provided. Primitive man attributed illness to evil spirits and sought to drive them out by practising witchcraft or assuaging their wrath by some sacrificial gift. Centuries later, the ancient civilisations — Egypt, Babylon, India, China, Greece, Rome — still thought of illness as a supernatural phenomenon. The healer might be a magician or a priest-physician or a god, and the care might be offered, for example, in a Greek temple of healing or a Roman military hospital.

With the advent of the Christian era, the sick received care from deaconesses; or from members, male and female, of religious orders; or during the Crusades, from members of the prestigious Order of the Knights Hospitallers of St John of Jerusalem; or under the feudal regime, from the lady of the manor. Care was given with Christian compassion and as illness was sometimes considered to be a just retribution for sinful word or deed, the care included concern for the soul as well as for relief of bodily distress.

In Europe, there was an historical watershed around 1500 and the long period of domination by the feudal system and by the Church was replaced by a great upsurge of new ideas, new discoveries and new inventions. It was during this post-Renaissance period that there were also great advances in man's knowledge about diseases and their treatment. The human body was studied in detail anatomically and physiologically, much of this investigation being made possible by the invention of the microscope.

From the evidence produced by historical researchers, it can be detected that down through the centuries there have been isolated attempts to use a scientific approach in determining the cause of disease but it was not till the 19th century that the caregiver moved away to any extent from magical techniques, religious practices and folk medicine. More reliance began to be placed on methods demanding systematic, objective, verifiable observations about the course of a disease and its treatment. And knowledge acquired was not considered to be static; there was the expectation that observations and conclusions would be constantly re-examined in an attempt to evolve more effective practices.

By the mid-19th century, the experiments of Pasteur were demonstrating the growth of microorganisms but when, in 1843, Holmes published a paper in the USA entitled, 'The Contagiousness of Puerperal Fever', the whole idea of infection was ridiculed by many learned contemporaries and continued to be so, even though objectively corroborated by Semmelweiss in Austria in 1867. This 'germ theory' however was given practical application by Lister in Scotland who started the use of substances called antiseptics, and subsequently used the 'aseptic method' which transformed the course of surgery. More sophisticated surgery became possible after Morton gave the first demonstration of the use of ether as an anaesthetic in Boston, Massachusetts, in 1846, and Simpson employed chloroform the next year in Edinburgh, Scotland. By the early 1900s, many of the microorganisms causing the commonly occurring infectious diseases had been isolated, and this process has continued, a recent example being identification of the human immunodeficiency virus (HIV) which causes AIDS. Each discovery has provided yet another stimulus for the development of agents which inhibit or destroy specific pathogens in the human body, and these advances have contributed to the growth of the pharmaceutical industry.

But not all illness is caused by microorganisms which produce infectious diseases. This idea is introduced here, only at a beginning level. Some pathogenic microorganisms cause other infections which produce inflammation of, for example body organs such as the bronchi (bronchitis). The body response of inflammation can also be produced by allergy, extremes of cold or heat, chemicals and friction; and it can be acute or chronic. Trauma too can remove people from a health to an illness status either temporarily or permanently; it causes many types of wounds involving tissue and even a whole organ: and trauma can also cause sprains, fractures and paralysis, particularly of the limbs. Insects can be carriers of disease; the bites of fleas, lice, mosquitoes and ticks can transmit to man a variety of diseases. Some people of course are in an illness category because of congenital abnormality of body structure or function and this can be hereditary. Such an abnormality can also be acquired and the condition may be familial. There can also be degenerative processes in the tissues thereby changing their structure and function. Organs of the body may respond to adverse body conditions by enlarging (hypertrophy) and this can produce further complications. For all of these illness conditions there is an agreed international classification of medical diagnoses, use of which provides statistical data for investigating patterns of disease throughout the world (epidemiology).

However, it is no longer sufficient to concentrate only on the pathophysiological factors of disease. It is necessary to consider the *social factors* which contribute to the development of health problems including poverty and overcrowding; the *cultural factors* which determine individual lifestyles such as food preferences, and the symbolic significance of critical events such as birth, illness and death; the *environmental factors* including the effects of water and air pollution, poor sanitation and industrial hazards; the *psychological factors* including the manifestation of past experiences in present behaviour.

These sociocultural, economic, environmental and psychological problems are as important as physical disability in creating circumstances which predispose to illness.

Knowledge about these many variables can influence the care provided for the individual and also affect the level of health and illness within social groups and indeed, in the general population of a country. But how can these concepts of health and illness be considered in a nursing context?

HEALTH/ILLNESS IN A NURSING CONTEXT

Taking health first, there are specialised groups of nurses who provide a service for healthy/well people in different environments. Such a service can be rendered to an individual, a family, or a geographically based community of people; or to a group of people centred on a building such as a school, or a workplace. In all these settings the nurses' objectives include supplying clients with the best available up-to-date information in such a way as to motivate them to develop healthy habits of living, thereby promoting and maintaining health, and preventing accident, illness and disease.

As far as illness is concerned, there are two broad categories — acute and chronic. An acute illness is usually relatively transient although it may severely disrupt the person's current mode of living; and often there is little time in which to adapt to the change from a health to an illness status. Nursing support may be required, particularly of a psychological nature, to help the person cope with what can often be a devastating change. But there are also the nursing activities, interventions, procedures, whichever name is used, that are necessary to return the person to a health status. However, from the patient's perspective the psychological support cannot be divorced from the physical nursing procedures. It is not **what** nurses do, but **how** they do it which is so crucial to the patient. Those who have an acute illness will require information and support to help them move gradually into a positive health status which often involves a considerable amount of adaptation. For example people who have suffered a myocardial infarction are encouraged, when it is appropriate, to modify their lifestyle in relation to weight, diet, exercise and management of stress.

For those afflicted with chronic illness the nursing contribution may not be so dramatic but it is just as important from the patient's perspective. It is sometimes difficult for nurses, the majority of whom are in the young adulthood category, to understand what it means to have been ill for many years; or what it means to those who, having been well for many years, gradually or suddenly find themselves in the long-term illness category. Faced with such circumstances nurses require the mental skill of empathy, described by Roper (1989) as: 'identifying oneself with another person or the actions of another person. Putting oneself in another person's shoes.' The nursing contribution in such circumstances is to observe, listen and discuss with these people what nursing help they require to carry out their everyday living activities in such a way as to maximise their quality of living.

Nurses, then, encounter well and ill people in many different clinical settings, and they see well people becoming ill, and ill people becoming well again. How can students of nursing be helped to recognise the 'elements' of nursing which are applicable throughout this diversity? Our model for nursing (pp 35–63) offers a mode of thinking which is relevant to any person in any health care setting, including the home and workplace. However, before discussing models for nursing, it is necessary to mention briefly the current form of health care systems, of which nursing is a part.

Nursing as part of a health care system

In the UK★, three-quarters of the health budget is spent on staff and as over half of the National Health Service staff is on the nursing establishment, nursing manpower is a critical component in terms of numbers and cost. As a professional group, nurses are in great demand not only to carry out direct nursing, but also to teach, to administer and, more recently, to carry out research in nursing. The health care system could not function adequately without nursing personnel.

In any health care system which is constantly short of finance it is difficult to justify the cost of a nursing service if it cannot be demonstrated that it benefits the recipients in some way. Use of the process of nursing, a logical method of carrying out nursing (p. 51) provides data collecting instruments which are being incorporated into several different tools to measure whether or not the overall nursing service is providing 'value for money'. Increasingly, measurement tools such as Monitor, Performance Indicators, Quality Assurance, Quality Circles and Qualpacs are being used in an attempt to measure the quality of the nursing provided, even in relation to apparently simple matters such as the provision of personal clothing systems for long-stay patients.

Of course, an organised health care system (which includes nursing) is not the only service related to health

★ Throughout the text mainly UK statistics are quoted; nurses from elsewhere will need to refer to the relevant sources in their own countries for the equivalent statistics.

which is provided from a country's financial income; others include departments such as welfare, social security, education, housing, law and order, roads and transport and all of these can influence the health/illness status of the people living within the country's borders.

The necessary money is obtained from a variety of sources. Every citizen is aware of various forms of taxes which are levied; it may be a percentage of personal income, tax on certain luxury goods, a flat rate tax on all goods, or a local levy of 'rates' based on the size and location of the house of each citizen. Whatever the source, a country's financial income is finite and the government in power must arrange priorities accordingly. And no matter how desirable it may seem for the health care system to respond to influences in the environment and group pressure for additional services, it can only be done within the constraints of financial allocation.

During this century, even in developing countries, the tendency has been to provide increasingly specialised services, which, at vast expense, have focused on ever more elaborate techniques for diagnosing disease, and on providing hospitals to house the expensive equipment and the people being cured. This method of providing care has been described as a 'disease-based, hospital-based, medical-based model of health care' providing the greatest good, achieved at high expense, for the fewest people.

However, even some of the affluent countries have come to realise the great disparity between the high cost of care in these systems and the low health benefits.

In many countries providers of health services are now recognising that greater emphasis should be given to community-based health care. And with this in mind, the attention of health professionals has been directed more to the desirability of maintaining and promoting health rather than concentrating so much on the individual's isolated episodes of illness which are treated in hospital.

With this change in emphasis, an attempt is being made to shift some of the finance from hospital to community services; from heavy concentration on physical aspects to social, behavioural and economic aspects of care; from the paternal dictates of health staff to a situation where patients are participating in the decisions regarding their own health care.

Accordingly the World Health Organization promoted the concept of Primary Health Care (PHC) (WHO, 1978) whereby the greatest good can be achieved at low expense for the greatest number of people. WHO suggests that the following should be considered:

promotion of proper nutrition and an adequate supply of safe water; basic sanitation; maternal and child care, including family planning; immunisation against the major infectious diseases; prevention and control of local endemic diseases;

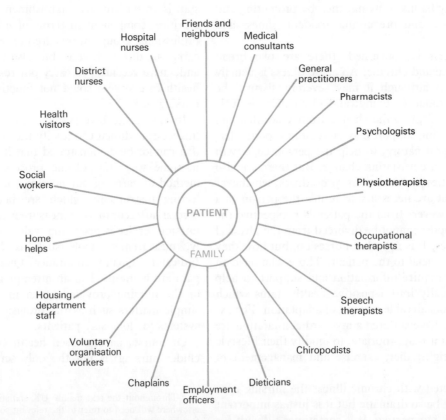

Fig. 1.1 Some members of the health team who assist the patient and family

education concerning prevailing health problems and the methods of preventing and controlling them; appropriate treatment for common diseases and injuries.

Such services must be easily accessible to individual families in the community, by means available to them, and at a cost which that community and country can afford. PHC is presented as a practical approach to achieving an acceptable level of health throughout the world and 'for developing countries it is a burning necessity'.

Discussing PHC nearly a decade later, Powell (1986) writes that, despite some success, there are formidable obstacles in the form of politicomedical controversy when trying to redistribute power from the top, to rural power and he maintains that 80% of health problems can be solved at primary (non-hospital) level.

So important is the concept of Primary Health Care for nurses, that the International Council of Nurses in collaboration with the World Health Organization published a booklet, 'The role of the nurse in PHC' (1979), which describes how nurses can contribute in practice to the promotion of PHC.

Nurses do not practise in isolation of course and even a brief survey of nursing as part of a health care service has to acknowledge that it functions only in relation to a health care team. In this relationship the nurse has an interdependent role and the many disciplines involved are summarised in Figure 1.1.

However, increasingly in the West, account is being taken of the fact that in both health and illness, people have to be assessed in their individual physical, psychological, sociocultural, environmental and politicoeconomic context. Acknowledgement is given to this by phrases such as 'holistic medicine' and 'holistic nursing' and sometimes instead of (or as well as) using the recognised health care service, people are turning to what is termed 'complementary medicine' which includes practices such as acupuncture, homeopathy, hypnosis, meditation and relaxation, osteopathy and yoga. And some nurses are beginning to practise therapies such as touch, distraction, reminiscence and relaxation to complement their traditional skills.

With so many variables to be considered regarding the concepts of health and illness, and regarding the role of nursing within a health care system, it is not easy to define the elements of nursing. While attempting to explore the meaning of nursing and its contribution to health, a number of nurse authors have developed their particular conceptual framework or model for nursing.

Describing a framework or model for nursing can assist nursing students to understand the theory and practice of nursing. The next chapter provides a brief introduction to the use of models for nursing which have become well-known internationally.

REFERENCES

Levin L 1981 Self-care in health: potentials and pitfalls. World Health Forum 2(2): 177–184

Nath U R, O'Neill P 1988 International networks: report from the first Pan-European Nursing Conference. Nursing Times 84 (28) July 13: 21

Nightingale F 1952 (original 1859) Notes on nursing. Duckworth, London, p 15, 16

Powell D 1986 Hospitals for health. Nursing Times 82 (49) December 3: 30–32

Roper N 1989 Churchill Livingstone Nurses' Dictionary, 16th edn. Churchill Livingstone, Edinburgh, p 155

World Health Organization 1946 Constitution. World Health Organization Geneva (Definition of health)

World Health Organization/UNICEF 1978 Primary health care. World Health Organization, Geneva, p 7

ADDITIONAL READING

Senior Nurse 1987 Targets for health for all. Senior Nurse 6 (3) March: 18–20, 36

Office of Health Economics 1988 Health services in Europe. OHE, London

2

Models for nursing

MODELS: THEIR USEFULNESS IN THEORY DEVELOPMENT

Although interest in models is relatively recent, thinking about the nature of nursing is not new. As long ago as 1859, Florence Nightingale was writing *Notes on Nursing* and was deploring the fact that nursing was considered to be little more than the administration of medicines and the application of poultices! It is curious that, even today, many people consider nursing to be simply a series of tasks carried out by the nurse. Undoubtedly observable tasks are a very important aspect of nursing, but this restrictive interpretation does not take account of the thinking processes which are involved before, during and after any observable task. Nor does it take into account the knowledge and attitudes which must be acquired to accompany the dextrous performance of a nursing task which is only a part — albeit an important part — of a deliberate plan of nursing.

So, despite Nightingale's early recognition of the need for a combination of intellectual skills and practical skills, nursing has seemed to retain the attitude of task orientation. As a consequence, to a large extent, nursing has remained at a practical level only, rather than developing simultaneously, a theoretical level on which to base its practice.

Nevertheless, over the years, an increasing number of nurses have considered that 'thinking' and 'doing' were not mutually exclusive; especially during the last three decades, many nurse writers and nurse practitioners have published such ideas. In the process of clarifying their ideas, some of these writers have devised conceptual models for nursing — or conceptual frameworks — in an attempt to identify the main concepts which they consider to be unique to nursing.

The advantage of using models in general is perhaps more obvious if one uses the analogy of a physical model which depicts a concrete reality such as a car, or the plan for a new housing development; or in anatomy, a model of the lungs or an ear. They are made up of three-dimensional parts and can be handled, taken apart and reassembled. Models of a discipline are more abstract and although they cannot be touched as such, they can be seen diagrammatically and can be mentally arranged and re-arranged. They are also made up of parts although in this instance, symbolised by a word or a set of words which can stand for a wide variety of activities — a concept. And just as importantly, a model indicates the relationships between the parts. Of course, models are not peculiar to nursing; they can be, and are, used in any discipline. However, two nurse authors (Riehl & Roy, 1980) provide a useful working definition of a model as:

> . . . a systematically constructed, scientifically based and logically related set of concepts which identify the essential components of nursing practice, together with the theoretical bases of these concepts and the values required for their use by the practitioner . . .

It is important to realise that conceptual models are not made up of a few transient thoughts, hastily put together; they are developed carefully and systematically, sometimes as a result of research, and may involve months or years of observing nursing practices, and thinking about why, as well as how they are performed.

Models are not set in marble, however; indeed they are constructed in the knowledge that they are essentially a basis for further thinking about the discipline. And as new, scientifically acceptable theories are produced to explain observed practice, the model may be modified, or improved, or enlarged or even discarded — as it should be if it is no longer useful. In fact, if one looks at the writings of some model-builders in nursing, over a period of years, the developments in their thinking can be identified both as alterations in the diagrams they present of their model, and from explanations in the accompanying text.

In any discussion about the usefulness of models, it is helpful to appreciate that although a discipline will identify some knowledge which is unique to itself, theories from other disciplines are sometimes included in a model, albeit applied in a specific context. Stevens (1979) makes the point that all disciplines have areas '. . . where the inquiries and answers of one field overlap with another'. Speaking of nursing, she writes:

> . . . borrowed theories remain borrowed so long as they are not adapted to the nursing milieu and the nursing image of man. Once such theories have been adapted to the nursing milieu, it is logical to refer to these boundary overlaps as shared knowledge rather than as borrowed theories . . .

If one shares Stevens' premise, it is possible to accept that already established theories in, for example, biology, psychology, sociology, and economics can be applied to nursing and considered as shared knowledge. In fact, most of the model-builders in nursing acknowledge the use of such theories from other disciplines and this is noted by Fawcett (1984), an American writer, who analyses most of the main nursing models in 'Analysis and evaluation of conceptual models'.

Fawcett (1984) considers that the development of conceptual models, and labelling them as such, was an important advance for the discipline of nursing. To make her point she quotes Reilly (1975):

> We all have a *private image* (concept) of nursing practice. In turn, this private image influences our interpretation of data, our decisions and our actions. But can a discipline continue to develop when its members hold so many differing private images? The proponents of conceptual models of practice are seeking to make us aware of private images, so that we can begin to identify commonalities in our perception of the nature of practice . . .

Conceptual models for nursing, then, are the formal presentations of some nurses' private images of nursing. They consist of the main concepts which identify the essential components of the discipline; show the relationships between the concepts; and may introduce already established theories from other disciplines which are applied in a nursing setting — Stevens' shared knowledge.

Discussion about models is certainly topical. There is considerable debate about the merits or otherwise of models which various nurses have created; models which they have found to be useful in their own thinking about the discipline of nursing — their own 'private image'. In fact several authors have constructively analysed the apparently different approaches used by these various model-builders and, in the process, have identified commonalities and differences (Aggleton & Chalmers, 1986; Fawcett, 1984; Meleis, 1985; Pearson & Vaughan, 1986).

However, despite the apparent differences, there is now considerable agreement that the global concepts common to most models for nursing [Kuhn (1977) coined the phrase 'metaparadigm' to describe the global concepts of a discipline] are person; environment; health; and nursing (Bush, 1979; Fawcett, 1978; Flaskarud & Halloran, 1980; Yura & Torres, 1975). The various models for nursing therefore can be seen as variations on the amalgamation of these four global concepts. The Roper, Logan and Tierney model was not deliberately constructed around this metaparadigm but does, in fact, contain all four of the concepts.

Before going on to consider in detail the Roper, Logan and Tierney model for nursing, which is central to this book, it is useful to have a brief outline of some of the now well-known models so that it can be placed in context. Five models have been selected — Orem, Roy, Neuman, King and Henderson — and they will be outlined in that order.

SELECTED MODELS FOR NURSING

Orem started developing her model as long ago as 1959, essentially in relation to a curriculum for a nursing programme; she was concerned about the absence of an organising framework for nursing knowledge (Orem, 1980). She was a pioneer in the development of distinctive nursing knowledge.

Orem's model assumes that man has an innate ability to be a self-care agent, to make a personal continuous contribution to his own health and well-being. Her model places emphasis on individual responsibility and argues for prevention and health education as key aspects of nursing intervention. When the individual is unable to be a self-care agent (a self-care deficit) nursing compensates by means of a nursing system (a dependent-care agent). Self-care or dependent-care is undertaken to meet three types of self-care requisites:

- universal — focusing on life processes and the maintenance of human structure and function
- developmental — focusing on events during the life cycle, for example pregnancy and the death of family members and friends
- health deviation — focusing on disability, deviations or defects in human structure and function; and on medical diagnosis and treatment of pathological conditions.

Nursing can be seen as having three levels of prevention — primary, secondary and tertiary — and has as its special concern the 'individual's need for self-care action and the provision and management of it on a continuous basis in order to sustain life and health; recover from disease or injury; and cope with their effects'. The goal of nursing is the patient's optimal level of self-care and when this is not maintained, illness, disease or death will occur. So the nurse must determine the need, design the system, plan the implementation and control the system of self-care. It is 'the nurse's mastery of key organising concepts that influences his or her selection and use of knowledge in a wide range of nursing situations'.

Roy first published the basic ideas of her model in 1970 and updated her writings in 1984. She acknowledged the influences of her clinical experience; she was impressed by the coping potential of human beings and recognised that nursing should increase that potential. She acknowledges also the use of concepts from other disciplines.

The focus of nursing is the person — a biopsychosocial being — who is identified as an adaptive system with two major internal processor systems: the regulator and the cognator. These mechanisms are explained by Roy:

The regulator mechanism works mainly through the autonomic nervous system to set up a reflex action which readies the person for coping with the stimulus by approach, attack, or flight. The cognator identifies, stores and relates stimuli so that symbolic responses can be made. It acts consciously by means of thought and decision and unconsciously through the defence mechanisms.

Regulator and cognator activities (i.e. coping mechanisms) are manifest in four adaptive modes:

- physiologic needs: focuses on physiological integrity as manifest in exercise and rest; nutrition; elimination; fluid and electrolytes; oxygen and circulation; regulation of temperature; senses; endocrine activity
- self concept: focuses on psychic integrity including perception of the physical and personal self
- role function: focuses on social integrity and role function and she differentiates three types of role — primary, secondary and tertiary
- interdependence: also emphasises social integrity and is defined as 'the comfortable balance between dependence and independence in relationship with others'

Roy identifies three sets of stimuli — focal are immediately present for the person; contextual are those in the environment; and residual stimuli are those from past learning and its effects.

The goal of nursing is to assist man towards health by promoting and supporting the patient's adaptation to stimuli in one or more of the four adaptive modes. It is accomplished using six steps: assessment of client behaviour; assessment of influencing factors; problem identification; goal setting; selection of intervention approaches; and evaluation. And this is done within the overall goal of the health team.

Neuman's model was first presented in 1972 and there have been several refinements (Neuman, 1982). Initially, it was developed for the use of graduate students: for course content which would present the *breadth* of nursing prior to content emphasising *specific* nursing problem areas. The model, she claims, owes much to observations made during clinical experience in mental health nursing, as well as from a synthesis of knowledge from several other disciplines.

The model focuses on the total person, a composite of four variables — physiological, psychological, sociocultural and developmental — defined as a client system. The client system has:

- a central core of survival factors unique to the individual such as temperature range, genetic response pattern, ego structure, strengths and weaknesses of body organs
- an outer, flexible line of defence which is a protective buffer preventing stressors from breaking through the inner line of defence
- an inner normal line of defence which 'represents the state of wellness of the particular individual, i.e. a state of adaptation the individual has maintained over time'

• lines of resistance (internal factors) within the inner line of defence which attempt to stabilise the person when the inner line of defence is broken

Reaction to a stressor is determined partly by natural and learned resistance, manifest by the strength of the two lines of defence and the lines of resistance. The amount of resistance is determined by the interrelationship of the four variables comprising the client system. Reaction is also determined by the time, nature and intensity of the stressor; by the idiosyncrasies of the central core; by past and present conditions of the individual; available energy resources; the amount of energy required for adaptation; and the person's perception of the stressor.

Reactions to stressors can be intrapersonal (forces occurring within the person); interpersonal (occurring between two or more individuals); and extrapersonal (occurring outside the person). They can be noxious or beneficial.

Neuman considers that the goal of nursing is:

. . . to assist individuals, families and groups to attain and maintain a maximum level of total wellness by purposeful interventions . . . aimed at the reduction of stress factors and adverse conditions which either affect or could affect optimal functioning in a given client situation.

She gives details of three major steps for intervention — nursing diagnosis, nursing goals and nursing outcomes — and intervention can occur at any point at which a stressor is either suspected or identified.

King first wrote about the foundations for her model in 1964, partly arising out of her concern regarding the 'antitheoretical' bias in nursing, and since then has made several refinements (King, 1981). She used information and data from 25 years of active nursing research, practice and teaching to formulate her conceptual framework, and draws considerably from established theories in other disciplines.

King views man as the centre of three general systems: the social system or society; the interpersonal system or groups; the personal system or individual. Man is seen as functioning in social systems through interpersonal relationships in terms of his perceptions which influence his life and health.

The personal system is seen as processing selective inputs from the environment through the senses. Related concepts are perception, self, growth and development, body image, time and space. The interpersonal system is composed of two, three or more individuals interacting in a given situation. Related concepts are interaction, communication, transaction, role and stress. The social system is defined by King as 'an organised boundary system of social roles, behaviours and practices developed to maintain values and the mechanisms to regulate the practices and rules.' These social systems describe units of analysis in a society in which individuals form groups to carry on activities of daily living to maintain life and health, and

hopefully happiness. Related concepts are organisation, authority, power, status and decision-making.

King maintains that nursing is:

perceiving, thinking, relating, judging and reacting vis-à-vis the behaviour of individuals who come to a nursing situation . . . in which nurse and client establish a relationship to cope with health states and adjust to changes in activities of daily living if the situation demands adjustment.

The goal of nursing is perceived as helping individuals to maintain their health so that they can function in their roles and is accomplished by:

. . . a process of action, reaction and interaction whereby nurse and client share information about their perceptions in the nursing situation. Through purposeful communication they identify specific goals, problems or concerns. They explore means to achieve a goal, and agree to the means to a goal. When clients participate in goal setting with professionals, they interact with nurses to move toward goal attainment in most situations.

Henderson was one of the early writers who, in 1955, attempted to clarify the nature of nursing, and her definition of nursing is probably the best known internationally:

The unique function of the nurse is to assist the individual, sick or well, in the performance of those activities contributing to health, or its recovery (or to a peaceful death) that he would perform unaided if he had the necessary strength, will or knowledge. And to do this in such a way as to help him gain independence as rapidly as possible.

(Henderson, 1969)

She goes on to say that this aspect of the nurse's work she initiates and controls; of this she is master although in addition she helps the patient carry out the therapeutic plan as initiated by the physician. Henderson also takes account of the team approach:

the nurse . . . as a member of the medical team helps other members, as they in turn help her, to plan and carry out the total program whether it be for the improvement of health, or the recovery from illness, or support in death.

Henderson was asked by the International Council of Nurses to prepare a booklet incorporating her ideas as *The Basic Principles of Nursing Care* (1969). It was eventually translated into over 20 languages, so along with her other publications undoubtedly Henderson influenced nurses and nursing throughout the world and continues to do so. In the ICN publication, she described 14 'components of basic nursing care' which she derived from the notion of 'universal human needs' and the components were formulated as 'helping the patient to . . .'. Henderson maintained that the primary responsibility of the nurse is 'to help the patient with daily patterns of living or with those activities that he ordinarily performs without assistance'. Some nursing scholars do not agree with using a concept of basic human needs when attempting to describe nursing but in a personal letter to Adam (1980) Henderson emphasised that she used the word 'need' in the positive sense as a 'requirement' rather than in the negative sense as 'a lack'.

Henderson did not use the phrase 'model for nursing' in her writings and did not present a model as such, but undoubtedly she was a pioneer in clarifying the concepts which are basic to nursing. Current model builders inevitably stand on the shoulders of those who have gone before, and the writings of Henderson certainly were influential to the thinking behind the Roper, Logan and Tierney model for nursing.

These are merely outlines of models which have been developed by their originators over many years, and when discussing or using these models it is imperative to go back to the original text in order to understand some of the terms which, on superficial glance, may sometimes seem obscure or esoteric. An outline is no substitute for the model-builder's detailed explanation.

Of course devising a model is not just an intellectual exercise, fascinating though that may be; it can be useful for nursing practice, education, management and research. In practice terms, a model can provide a framework for what the nurse does and how she does it; in education, it can provide a framework which organises the curriculum — the knowledge, skills and approach which are necessary for learning to practise; in management, it can outline the common goals to be achieved; in research, a model can provide guidance about what should be studied in order to extend nursing knowledge and thus improve practice.

Almost all of the creators of models for nursing have incorporated in their models the concept of the process of nursing, in order to help practising nurses to adopt a logical approach to assessing, planning, implementing and evaluating nursing practice.

PROCESS OF NURSING

Most nurses now are familiar with the term 'nursing process'. Universally, it is recognised as describing a systematic approach to nursing which comprises a series (or cycle) of steps (or stages) which, most commonly, are referred to as assessing, planning, implementing and evaluating.

It is interesting to note that, although commonplace nowadays, the term 'nursing process' had only recently been introduced into the UK when the first edition of this book (published in 1980) was in early stages of preparation in the mid-1970s. Some 15 years or so earlier, however, the idea of the nursing process had been introduced into the North American literature by nurse theorists writing about the development of conceptual frameworks for nursing. Perhaps because of its origins and attendant jargon, the notion of the nursing process was greeted with

suspicion by British nurses and when first introduced, it met with considerable resistance. Perhaps a more sympathetic view might have been taken had the nursing process been seen less as an American import and an apparent threat, and more as a vehicle for advancing the expression of interest in reviving individualised nursing and in developing nursing theory which, anyway, was a developing interest at the time in Britain as, indeed, it was worldwide. In the intervening years, much has been written about the introduction of the nursing process and interested readers are referred to Walton's (1986) comprehensive review of nursing process literature published over the period in question.

In spite of the initial resistance, the nursing process gained remarkably rapid recognition at a formal level for, in 1977, the professional registering body of the UK (then the General Nursing Council, now the United Kingdom Central Council) decreed that 'the nursing care of patients should be studied and practised in the sequence of the nursing process' (Dickinson, 1982). Development of the nursing process in terms of practice was given enormous impetus when the Regional Office of the World Health Organization decided to incorporate it into the European Medium Term Programme for Nursing/Midwifery and a number of countries within the WHO European Region, including the UK, collaborated in this multinational study which commenced in 1983. Reports arising from that venture have been published in the form of an overall summary from WHO with separate accounts of the work undertaken in specific countries (e.g. Farmer's 1985 report pertaining to Scotland). This ambitious programme did much to encourage discussion and a sharing of ideas about the nursing process at an international level; and, although aspects of its implementation are peculiar to local practice circumstances, the essential ideas which are encapsulated in the term 'nursing process' are universal, as is the case so often in nursing.

The essential ideas are, in fact, not new in nursing even if the term 'nursing process' is considered as such; the 'good nurse' has always used it. Often, however, nurses did not analyse or explicate what they were doing in terms of a process or steps within it, nor did they document information in an ordered and comprehensive manner. Because nurses had not explained or recorded the nursing, there was no tangible evidence of the intellectual aspect of the process to the onlooker who saw only the observable behaviour of the nurse. Thus, for the onlooking learner in particular, no wonder it was difficult to appreciate and understand the often rapidly executed mental activity which determined the experienced nurse's actions. The process involved was neither explained nor documented and, frequently, the results of the nurse's actions were neither evident nor systematically evaluated. The value, then, in envisaging the nursing process as something new — even recognising that the 'good nurse' has always endeavoured to provide individualised and systematic nursing — lies in its emphasis on strengthening evaluation and on making explicit the intellectual as well as the behavioural component of nursing.

Attention to the intellectual or 'thinking' aspects of nursing has been much neglected and, in a sense, this failing is perpetuated when nurses view the nursing process essentially in 'doing' terms (notably the activity of documentation) rather than in terms which emphasise the process as simply a logical mode of thinking. Viewed in these terms, it becomes easier to accept that 'the process' is not peculiar to nursing; a systematic approach through assessing, planning, implementing and evaluating could be (and is) applied equally in doctoring, in teaching and in studying, irrespective of the discipline. Perhaps if the nursing process initially had been understood essentially as a mode of thinking rather than a method of doing (. . . 'doing assessments' . . . 'doing care plans' . . . and so on), then many of the problems encountered and misunderstandings perpetuated might have been avoided.

Problems and misunderstandings there have been and still continue to be over the nursing process; letters and articles in the nursing press over the years attest to that. Concern has not been confined only within nursing circles either; the scepticism and hostility felt by some doctors towards the nursing process was voiced publicly at one stage in the debate, most notably in a prominent journal paper by a medical professor (Mitchell, 1984) although many of those criticisms could be contested (Tierney, 1984). But, even within nursing and among those who are proponents of the nursing process, it is generally accepted that the way in which this concept was introduced, at least into the UK — in haste and adopting a 'top-down' or 'power-coercive' change strategy (Walton, 1986) — led to many of the prevailing misunderstandings and difficulties. The presence of difficulties, in spite of a more general acceptance in principle, is noted in a report by the UK Nursing Process Evaluation Working Group (Hayward, 1987) which concluded:

It is hard to avoid the conclusion that the problems we are seeing have been brought about by lack of understanding of and negative perceptions towards the nursing process on the part of some nurse managers, educators and staff of other disciplines, coupled with too speedy introduction to an unprepared workforce.

Certainly, with the benefit of hindsight, the introduction of the nursing process approach could have been better managed. It should have been realised more quickly that it would be impossible to introduce a truly individualised system of nursing into practice settings which still operated an essentially 'task-oriented' rather than 'patient-centred' approach. It is now recognised that the nursing process is only wholly feasible in the context of practice which is organised on a basis of patient allocation, team nursing or, best of all, primary nursing.

Very little research has been undertaken with the explicit purpose of evaluating the impact of the nursing process on practice. Work done, such as Miller's (1985) study in the context of the care of elderly patients, requires to be extended if valuable evidence is to be accumulated.

And, in terms of education, more also might have been done to ensure that nurses were adequately prepared to implement the nursing process properly. Although nursing students were learning about the nursing process, already qualified nurses had fewer opportunities for preparation. In an effort to remedy this situation, a teaching package on 'systematic nursing' was prepared for qualified staff and this was widely distributed under the auspices of the Open University. This package (OU, 1984) has proved to be so popular that an updated version is now in the process of preparation.

In recent years, a prominent concern has been to promote understanding of the nursing process as it relates to nursing models. Mistakenly, sometimes the nursing process is described as a nursing model in its own right. But, of course, the process on its own is in vacuo; it has to be used in the context of a conceptual framework. The relationship between the nursing process and various nursing models is the subject of a number of texts published in recent years (such as Aggleton & Chalmers, 1986 and Pearson & Vaughan, 1986). In *this* text, the relationship is examined in the particular circumstances of the Roper, Logan and Tierney model for nursing. And so this introductory discussion about the process of nursing (our preferred term) turns full circle, having begun by explaining how we incorporated it into out model for nursing right from the start.

It must be emphasised again, however, that models are only tools; tools to enhance the analysis of the concepts which contribute to an understanding of the knowledge base required for nursing practice. It is in this context that the Roper, Logan and Tierney model for nursing is presented.

REFERENCES

Aggleton P, Chalmers H 1986 Nursing models and the nursing process. Macmillan, London

Bush H 1979 Models for nursing. Advances in Nursing Sciences 1(2): 13–21

Dickinson S 1982 The nursing process and the professional status of nursing. Occasional Paper, Nursing Times 78(16) June 2

Farmer E S 1985 On introducing a systematic method for the practice and study of nursing: A report of the Scottish component of the WHO (Euro) multinational study of needs for nursing care in two selected groups of patients. Nursing Research Unit, Department of Nursing Studies, University of Edinburgh

Fawcett J 1978 The 'what' of theory development. In: Theory Development: what, why how? National League for Nursing, New York

Fawcett J 1984 Analysis and evaluation of conceptual models of nursing. F A Davis, Philadelphia

Flaskarud K, Halloran E 1980 Areas of agreement in nursing theory development. Advances in Nursing Science 3(1): 1–7

Hayward J (Ed) 1987 Report of the Nursing Process Evaluation Group. Nursing Education Research Unit, King's College, London, p 39

Henderson V 1969 The basic principles of nursing care. International Council of Nurses, Geneva

King I 1981 A theory for nursing: systems, concepts, process. Wiley, New York

Kuhn T 1977 Second thoughts on paradigms. In: Suppe F (ed) The structure of scientific theories. University of Illinois Press, Chicago

Meleis A 1985 Theoretical nursing: development and progress. Lippincott, Philadelphia

Miller A 1985 Nursing process and patient care. Occasional Paper, Nursing Times 80(13): 56–58

Mitchell J 1984 Is nursing any business of doctors? A simple guide to the 'nursing process'. Nursing Times 80(19) May 9: 28–32

Neuman B 1982 The Neuman systems model: application to nursing education and practice. Appleton-Century-Crofts, New York

Nightingale F 1859 Notes on nursing. Duckworth, London (reprinted 1952)

Open University 1984 A systematic approach to nursing care. Open University Press (Course P553)

Orem D 1980 Nursing: concepts of practice, 2nd edn. McGraw-Hill, New York

Pearson A, Vaughan B 1986 Nursing models for practice. Heinemann, London

Reilly D 1975 Why a conceptual framework? Nursing Outlook 23: 566–569

Riehl J, Roy C 1980 Conceptual models for nursing practice, 2nd edn. Appleton-Century-Crofts, New York

Roy C 1984 Introduction to nursing: an adaptation model. Prentice Hall, Englewood Cliffs, NJ

Stevens B 1979 Nursing theory: analysis, application, and evaluation. Little, Brown, Boston

Tierney A 1984 Defending the process. Nursing Times 80(2) May 16: 38–41

Walton I 1986 The nursing process in perspective: a literature review. University of York, York

Yura H, Torres G 1975 Today's conceptual frameworks within baccalaureate nursing programs. In Faculty — curriculum development. Part III. Conceptual framework — its meaning and function. National League for Nursing, New York

A model for nursing based on a model of living

3 Background to the models

References

If a model can be said to have a birthplace, then the Roper, Logan and Tierney model is indisputably an Edinburgh model; all three of the trio are graduates of the University of Edinburgh. Although their paths had crossed in various ways prior to 1975, it was around this time that the trio deliberately joined forces to discuss the idea of developing a textbook based on a conceptual framework for nursing. Nancy Roper had just completed a masters degree at the University of Edinburgh, and Winifred Logan and Alison Tierney were both members of staff at the University's Department of Nursing Studies (in 1960 the first European degree programme for nursing was inaugurated here; the chair was established in 1972; and the first Nursing Research Unit was set up in 1971). As a result of the research undertaken for the masters degree, the original Roper model was created, and was described in her monograph *Clinical Experience in Nurse Education* (1976) and in two other articles published that same year. It was an extrapolation from a review of literature related to a core of nursing; and also the project's findings from data collected in a general, a maternity and a psychiatric hospital, and in 12 community districts. By virtue of a coming together of like minds, the trio — with a collective background of nursing practice, education, management, research and considerable overseas experience in different cultural settings — decided in 1976 to combine their thinking about a model for nursing. It became the basis of a framework for *The Elements of Nursing* which was first published in 1980.

This brief historical account illustrates two points. Firstly, it indicates that the discussion of models and theories is not something new in the UK as the Roper, Logan and Tierney model was under construction two decades ago. Secondly, and more importantly, it helps to underscore a statement already made, that models and theories are not developed overnight; in fact they have a long period of construction and refinement. It is, in a sense, their very tentativeness and flexibility which allows models to help extend our understanding of nursing theory and practice.

Even before the actual publication of the 1980 Roper, Logan and Tierney model, the process of refinement had begun and was written up in a second book *Learning to Use the Process of Nursing* (1981), the aim being to illustrate how the model for nursing could be used as a conceptual framework in the practice of nursing.

The exercise led on to a project which involved actually using the model in nine different practice settings in the community and in hospital, namely medical, surgical, psychiatric, geriatric, midwifery and neurosurgical wards; a diabetic clinic; and in health visiting and district nursing. The nine nursing studies were carried out and written up by practising nurses as described in the publication *Using a Model for Nursing* (1983). It was not a systematic evaluation of the application of the model but it did provide, along with feedback from other nursing personnel, a source of new ideas about the model and its use; and about some of the difficulties encountered when applying it in the real world of nursing practice. Subsequently, the model has been used as the framework for a curriculum in a nursing degree programme in the UK (Kilgour & Logan, 1985), and in India (Logan, 1986); there is a frequent feedback from nurses in the UK and overseas about its application in nursing practice, education, management and research; and there is an increasing number of articles in nursing journals about its application in a variety of settings. The trio have used all this feedback to enhance their own further deliberations and have continued to refine the model, so virtually a fourth generation model is presented in this 3rd edition of *The Elements of Nursing*.

Refinements have been concerned with detail rather than essential characteristics. A constant feature, not always recognised, is that the model for nursing is based on a model of living. Arguments supporting the rationale for linking 'nursing' and 'living' are stronger today than ever before. Ironically this relationship was spelled out in 1859 by Nightingale who identified both nursing's goal and nursing's practice area by declaring that nurses should use what she called '. . . the laws of health, or of nursing for they are in reality the same . . .' It is lamentable that nursing lost sight of this wider vision of nursing and became decidedly disease-oriented. However, nurses, along with others involved in health care, are now increasingly aware that people's health, and the illnesses from which they suffer are inextricably linked with living and lifestyle.

So the Roper, Logan and Tierney model for nursing is based on a model of living. By so doing, nurses should be helped to see the enormous scope they have for health teaching to promote health, maintain health, prevent disease and promote rehabilitation; as well as engaging in the more traditionally recognised nursing interventions related to disease.

REFERENCES

Kilgour D, Logan W 1985 A model for health: its use in an undergraduate programme. Nurse Education Today 5: 215–220

Logan W 1986 Part of the plan (programme for a nursing degree in India). Senior Nurse 6(6) June: 30–32

Nightingale F 1859 Notes on nursing. Duckworth, London (reprinted 1952)

Roper N 1976 Clinical experience in nurse education. Churchill Livingstone, Edinburgh

Roper N, Logan W, Tierney A 1980 The elements of nursing. Churchill Livingstone, Edinburgh

Roper N, Logan W, Tierney A 1981 Learning to use the process of nursing. Churchill Livingstone, Edinburgh

Roper N, Logan W, Tierney A 1983 Using a model for nursing. Churchill Livingstone, Edinburgh

4

Model of living

To encapsulate the complexities of 'living' in a model which is simple enough to be meaningful is, of course, impossible. The model of living presented here is only an attempt to identify the main features of a highly complex phenomenon, and to indicate relationships between the various components of the model (Fig. 4.1). As indicated in Figure 4.1, there are five main components (concepts) in the model, namely:

Activities of Living (ALs)
Lifespan
Dependence/independence continuum
Factors influencing ALs
Individuality in living

In the following text, each of these components will be discussed in turn.

ACTIVITIES OF LIVING

A model of living must offer a way of describing what 'living' means. If asked to describe what everyday living involves, most people— irrespective of their age and circumstances — would mention activities such as eating and drinking, working and playing, and sleeping. If prompted, they would probably agree that breathing, communicating and eliminating are also activities which are an integral part of living, even if at times they may be hardly aware of performing them. All of these activities, and others —such as maintaining a safe environment, and personal cleansing and dressing — collectively contribute to the complex process of living. They are the *activities of living*.

It is this concept which is used as the focus of the model of living; and a set of Activities of Living (ALs), 12 in number (Fig. 4.2), makes up the main component of the model.

The term 'Activity of Living' (AL) is used as an all-embracing one. *Each* 'Activity' has many dimensions;

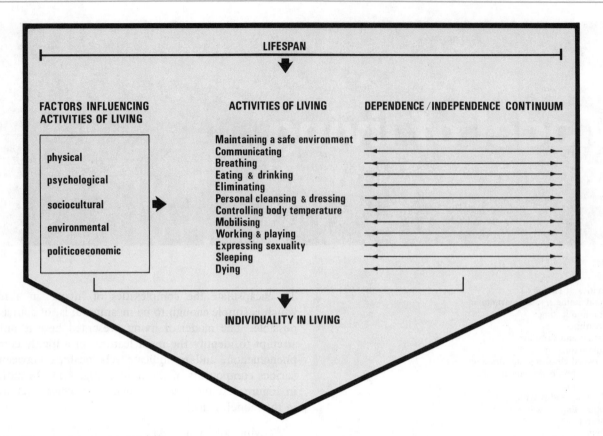

Fig. 4.1 Diagram of the model of living

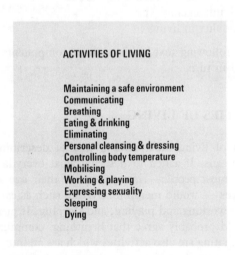

Fig. 4.2 Activities of living

indeed it could be thought of as an overall activity composed of a number of particular activities, rather as a compound is made up of a number of elements. The more one analyses the Activities of Living the more one realises just how complex each one is. Compounding this complexity is the fact that they are so closely related. For example, communicating is related to many of the other

ALs: just imagine eating and drinking, working and playing, and expressing sexuality without communicating! And breathing is essential for all of the ALs. So only for the purpose of description can they be separated, and here only a brief description of each AL is necessary by way of introduction.

Maintaining a safe environment

In order to stay alive and carry out any of the other activities of living, it is imperative that actions are taken to maintain a safe environment. In fact, each day, many activities are carried out with this purpose although, because they are such a routine part of everyday living, they are performed almost without conscious effort. For example, steps are taken to prevent accidents in the home by guarding fires, by keeping poisonous substances in a safe place, and ensuring that carpets are in good condition and trip-free. Every day, too, precautions are taken to prevent accidents when travelling and while working and playing. Maintaining a safe environment on the roads and the workplace is not only a shared responsibility of individuals but also, through action and legislation of the government. Some people, in addition to ensuring their own personal safety, engage in activities — such as campaigning for nuclear disarmament or action to prevent pollution of the environment — which they consider will help to ensure for future generations an environment which is as safe as possible.

Communicating

Human beings are essentially social beings and a major part of living involves communicating with other people in one way or another. Communicating not only involves the use of verbal language as in talking and writing, but also the non-verbal transmission of information by facial expression and body gesture. Communication of this type also provides the vehicle for transmission of emotions: long before a baby has acquired verbal skills, feelings such as pleasure and displeasure can be communicated to others. Communication through touch is equally subtle although less frequently used except in intimate personal relationships and here, as in verbal language, there are distinct cultural differences.

By its very nature, the activity of communicating permeates the whole area of interpersonal interaction and human relationships which are such a fundamental and important dimension of living.

Breathing

The very first activity of a newborn baby is breathing. The ability to do this is vital since by this action the cells of the body will receive from the air, oxygen which was previously supplied from the mother's blood. But, thereafter, breathing becomes an effortless activity and people are not consciously aware of performing it until some abnormal circumstance forces it to their attention. Oxygen is absolutely essential for all body cells; there is irreversible damage to the brain cells when they are deprived of it, even for a few minutes. Consequently all other Activities of Living — and life itself — are entirely dependent on breathing.

Eating and drinking

A baby is born with the ability to suck and swallow so that nourishment can be obtained without which survival and growth are impossible. Human life cannot be sustained for long without eating and drinking so this activity, like breathing, is absolutely essential. Eating and drinking is also a time-consuming activity since apart from the time spent eating meals, food itself has to be procured and prepared. The way meals are taken, and the food and drink selected, reflect the influence of sociocultural factors on this AL. For most people, eating and drinking are pleasurable activities but the fact that great numbers of people in the world die daily from starvation serves as a reminder of the essential nature of this Activity of Living.

Eliminating

We have chosen to describe urinary elimination and faecal elimination together because, although two distinct body systems are involved, there is no good reason to separate them in the context of an Activities of Living framework. The essential nature of this AL is such that in infancy elimination occurs as a reflex response to the collection of urine in the bladder and faeces in the bowel. The acquisition of voluntary control over elimination and independence in this AL are important milestones of development in the early years of life.

Eliminating, like eating and drinking, is a necessary and integral activity of everyday life. However, interestingly, whereas eating and drinking and many other ALs are performed in the company of others, eliminating is regarded as a highly private activity. Throughout the world people are socialised into eliminating in private and this contributes to many strongly held attitudes and taboos which are associated with this Activity of Living.

Personal cleansing and dressing

Cleanliness and good grooming are commended in most cultures, whatever the particular standards and norms. Apart from taking pride in their appearance, people have a social responsibility to ensure cleanliness of body and clothing. The term 'personal cleansing' was deliberately chosen in preference to 'washing' because in addition to handwashing, body washing and bathing, the activities of perineal hygiene and care of the hair, nails, teeth and mouth are also carried out. In relation to dressing it is interesting to appreciate that clothing not only fulfils the function of protection of the body but also reflects important aspects of culture and tradition; has sexual associations; and is a medium of non-verbal communication.

Controlling body temperature

Unlike cold-blooded animals whose body temperature is subject to the temperature of the external environment, man is able to maintain the body temperature at a constant level irrespective of the degree of heat or cold in the surrounding environment. The heat-regulating system is not fully sensitive at birth but, once its function is established, the temperature of the human body is maintained within a fairly narrow range. This is essential for many of the body's biological processes and also ensures personal comfort in continually varying, sometimes dramatically changing, environmental temperatures. Human tissue cannot survive very long when subjected to extremes of heat or cold; trauma and even death can occur from either heatstroke or hypothermia.

Although body temperature is essentially self-regulating, people have to perform certain deliberate activities to avoid the hazards and discomforts of heat or cold. Therefore activities such as adjusting the temperature and ventilation of the surroundings; varying the amount and type of clothing and regulating the amount of physical activity are all carried out with the objective of helping to control body temperature.

Mobilising

Although a rather clumsy word 'mobilising' seemed more explicit than 'moving' to describe the capacity for movement which is one of the essential and highly valued human activities. The devastating effects — physical, psychological, economic and social — of any serious long-term limitation on movement bear witness to this fact.

The AL of mobilising includes the movement produced by groups of large muscles, enabling people to stand, sit, walk and run as well as groups of smaller muscles producing movements such as those involved in manual dexterity or in facial expressions, hand gesticulations and mannerisms; all of which are part of non-verbal communication.

The relationships of mobilising to other ALs should be readily apparent; behaviour associated with the activities of breathing, eating and drinking, eliminating, working and playing and so on, all involve movement and, even in sleeping, the body systems continue their ceaseless activity.

Working and playing

When not sleeping most people are either working or playing; play has been described as the child's work. Usually for most adults working provides an income from which, after essential costs are met, leisure activities are financed. The activities of working and playing can have very different meanings for different individuals. The old adage 'one man's work is another man's play' illustrates this well; for example, one person might earn an income as a market gardener by growing flowers and vegetables whereas, for another, this might be a hobby.

For most people, the sense of belonging to work and leisure groups, the satisfactions from challenge and achievement, and the prevention of boredom, are all important aspects of this AL. Both working and playing can be seen to have positive and negative effects on personal health and well-being. Because both involve physical and mental activity, each can contribute positively to physical and mental health. Conversely, enforced lack of working (as in unemployment or retirement) or insufficient playing may contribute to physical or mental ill-health.

Expressing sexuality

So important is the subject of 'sex' in life today that it cannot be ignored and the publicity associated with the current AIDS epidemic has made it less of a taboo subject . . . but how were we to describe this as an Activity of Living? The specific activity which tends to be directly associated with sex is sexual intercourse. Of course this is an important component of adult relationships — and essential for the continuation of the human race — but there are also many other ways in which human sexuality is expressed.

An individual's sex is determined at conception and throughout the lifespan sexuality is an important dimension of personality and behaviour. Femininity and masculinity are reflected not only in physical appearance and strength but also in style of dress; in many forms of verbal and non-verbal communication; in family and social roles and relationships; and in choices relating to work and play.

Sleeping

It may seem strange to describe sleeping as an 'activity' until it is realised that body processes do not stop being active during sleep. All living organisms have periods of activity alternating with periods of sleep. In human beings this is a 24-hour rhythm of sleeping and waking. Babies spend the major part of the time asleep and even adults spend up to one-third of their entire lives sleeping and so, in terms of time alone, this is an important AL. It is an essential one too; growth and repair of cells take place during sleep and sleep enables people to relax from, and be refreshed to cope with, the stresses and demands of everyday living. Without adequate sleep people suffer discomfort and distress, and a variety of ill-effects result from accrued sleep deprivation.

Dying

The inclusion of 'dying' in our list of ALs has been questioned: for example, it has been pointed out that it seems illogical without also including 'being born'. Death is what marks the end of life just as the event of birth marks its beginning. However, the concern is not solely with the event of death, but rather with the process of dying. It could be said that the process of living is a fatal one and certainly, in the process of dying, all the Activities of Living are affected and eventually cease with death. In describing 'living' it seems essential to acknowledge that death is the only really certain thing in life. The whole of a person's life is lived in the light of the inevitability of death, for some people overshadowing living and for others giving positive meaning to life. And of course people do not live only in anticipation of their own eventual death, but also in the knowledge that loved ones will die. It has been said that 'grief is the cost of commitment' in our lives. Grieving is the activity, inextricably linked with dying, through which a bereaved person comes to term with the death of a loved one and finds the courage to begin living fully once more.

Even from such a brief description of the 12 ALs, it is clear that conceptualising 'living' as an amalgam of 'activities' is a helpful way of beginning to think simply yet constructively about the complex process of living. All of the ALs are important, although obviously some have greater priority than others; the AL of breathing is of prime importance. The order in which the ALs are listed does not reflect an order of priority because, according to circumstances, the priorities change. Also, as previously mentioned, although the 12 ALs are described separately, they are very closely related to each other. Indeed, although the ALs are presented as one component of the model, they should not be thought of in isolation since they are affected by the other components and these too are closely related to each other. However, in their own right, each of the components contributes another dimension of 'living', as the following discussion will show.

LIFESPAN

It is easy to appreciate why a lifespan is included as one component of the model of living. 'Living' is concerned with the whole of a person's life and each person has a *lifespan*, from conception to death.

The lifespan is represented in the diagram of the model by a line, arrowed to indicate the direction of movement along it from birth to death (Fig. 4.3).

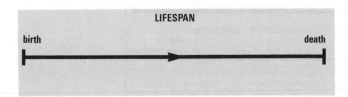

Fig. 4.3 The lifespan

As a person moves along the lifespan there is continuous change and every aspect of living is influenced by the physical, psychological, sociocultural, environmental and politicoeconomic circumstances encountered throughout life.

DEPENDENCE/INDEPENDENCE CONTINUUM

This component of the model is closely related to the lifespan and to the ALs. It is included to acknowledge that there are stages of the lifespan when a person cannot yet (or for various reasons, can no longer) perform certain activities of living independently. Each person could be said to have a *dependence/independence continuum* for each AL. As shown below (Fig. 4.4A), the term 'total dependence'

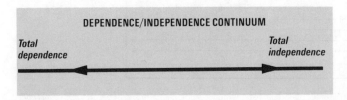

Fig. 4.4A Dependence/independence continuum

Fig. 4.4B Dependence/independence continuum related to the ALs

and 'total independence' are used to describe the poles of the continuum and the arrows indicate that movement can take place in either direction according to circumstances.

To emphasise that the dependence/independence continuum relates to each of the ALs — for on its own the concept is too global to be meaningful — the continuum appears in the diagrammatic representation of the model of living alongside each of the 12 activities (Fig. 4.4B).

A person's position could be plotted on each continuum (at either pole or somewhere between) to provide an impression of the degree of dependence/independence in respect of the 12 Activities of Living. If repeated at intervals of time, any obvious change in direction or movement along the continua would become apparent.

Comparing the dependence/independence status of people at different stages of the lifespan illustrates the close links between these two components of the model. Newborn babies are dependent on others for help with almost every Activity of Living. From this state of almost total dependence, each child according to his capacity can be visualised as gradually moving along the continuum towards the independent pole for each AL. At 5 years old the picture might look like Figure 4.4C: independence has been acquired in the ALs of breathing, eliminating, controlling body temperature, mobilising and sleeping, whereas the child is far from independent in the ALs of communicating and maintaining a safe environment, for example. However, by the time the child is 10 years old, a greater degree of independence has developed and the picture could look like Figure 4.4D. Often in the declining years there is some loss of the independence attained, and Figure 4.4E could apply to an infirm elderly person.

The pattern which has been outlined of links between dependence/independence in the ALs and stage on the lifespan is, of course, only the norm and there are always exceptions to even the most general of rules. By no means everyone has the capacity or opportunity to achieve or retain independence in all of the Activities of Living. Not

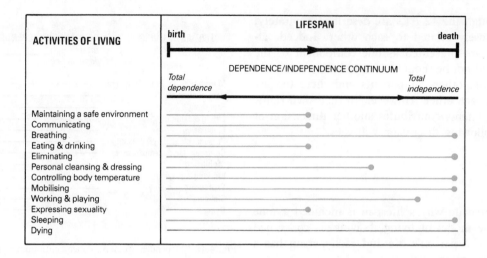

Fig. 4.4C   Dependence/independence at 5 years old

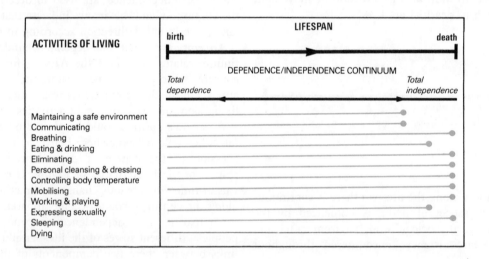

Fig. 4.4D   Dependence/independence at 10 years old

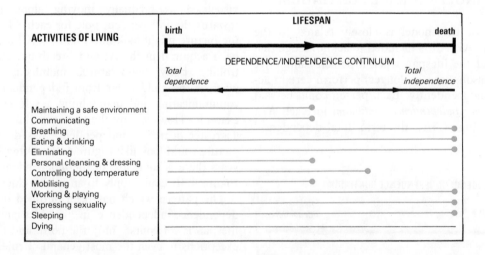

Fig. 4.4E   Dependence/independence in declining years

all children are born with the potential for 'total independence', whether as a result of severe physical or mental handicap or both. In such circumstances, progress during infancy and childhood cannot be measured against normal developmental milestones and the goal is maximum independence in the ALs according to the capacity of the individual child.

Even in adulthood, there are circumstances which can result in dependence in one or more of the ALs: obvious examples are illness and accident. Dependence may be on help from other people or on special aids and equipment: for example, a wheelchair which provides 'aided independence' for the AL of mobilising. Indeed, even healthy able-bodied adults are dependent on others and on aids for their so-called 'independence' in many of the Activities of Living: for example, for the AL of eating and drinking there is dependence on people such as the farmer, fisherman, factory worker and shopkeeper and on various types of equipment which aid preparation, cooking, serving and consumption of food and drink.

There is, therefore, no absolute statement of 'independence' in the Activities of Living. The concepts of 'dependence' and 'independence' are really only meaningful when considered as relative to one another, hence the reason for presenting these ideas in the model of living by means of a dependence/independence *continuum*. Change in dependence/independence status for one AL can, because the ALs are so closely related, cause change in status for one or more of the other activities.

The dependence/independence status of an individual in relation to ALs is not linked only to lifespan, it is also closely associated with the factors which influence ALs.

FACTORS INFLUENCING THE ALs

So far, three components of the model have been described — the Activities of Living, the lifespan, and the dependence/independence continuum. However although everyone carries out Activities of Living (at whatever stage of the lifespan and with varying degrees of independence) each individual does so differently. To a large extent these differences arise because a variety of factors influence the way a person carries out ALs, and these 'factors' form the fourth component of the model.

It would be possible to devise a long list of the different factors: for example, physical, intellectual, emotional, social, cultural, spiritual, religious, ethical, philosophical, political, economic and legal factors.

However, one of the intentions when creating a model is that it should not seem excessively complicated, so the factors influencing the ALs are described in five main groups — physical, psychological, sociocultural, environmental, and politicoeconomic factors (Fig. 4.5). It must be noted, however, that intellectual and emotional are subsumed under psychological factors; that spiritual, religious,

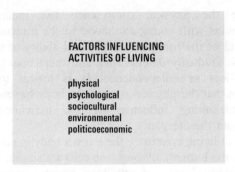

FACTORS INFLUENCING ACTIVITIES OF LIVING

physical
psychological
sociocultural
environmental
politicoeconomic

Fig. 4.5 Factors influencing the ALs

and ethical are subsumed under sociocultural factors because for this model of living it is considered that such values and beliefs often find expression within a particular cultural view; and legal are subsumed under politicoeconomic factors.

The factors are deliberately focused on the Activities of Living. It would be possible to focus them on the individual as a total entity discussing in general terms the effects of the five groups of factors on lifestyle, but this is too global. In preference, discussing them as they influence each of the 12 ALs highlights the individuality in living.

The factors, the ALs, the lifespan, the dependence/independence continuum are interlinked, and the five factors themselves are interlinked. At this stage, however, for the purposes of discussion, a few general points will be made about each factor separately.

Physical factors

For the purposes of this model of living, the term physical is more or less synonymous with biological, in so far as it relates to the human body's anatomical and physiological performance. The body's structure and function have a major influence on how the body functions. Partly this is determined by the individual's genetic inheritance and although the influence of heredity is usually more obvious in facial appearance and physique, it also affects each person's overall physical performance. The individual's physical endowment is important in its own right but it is inextricably linked with other factors — psychological, sociocultural, environmental and politicoeconomic.

Not only are the physical factors interlinked with these others; as a group, the factors are related to the other components of the model. Even in a healthy person for example, the body's physical ability varies according to age (i.e. the lifespan component of the model), and influences the degree of dependence possible to the individual (i.e. the dependence/independence continuum), so inevitably the factors influence the person's individuality in living and affect the way each person carries out the ALs. Despite the phenomenal physical growth of the fetus in utero, a newborn baby is far from physical maturity and unlike most animals, there are many years of further growth before reaching the physical competence and independence synonymous with young adulthood in the human. At the other end of the lifespan, the physical ability of the older person is gradually deteriorating and there may be an insidious loss of independence. It is logical to expect therefore that the physical state of the body has an important contributing influence on the individual's ALs throughout the lifespan.

Like all living creatures, the human body is made up of cells. In the human, although the cells are similar in structure, certain clusters of cells have become specialised to deal with specific activities, for example, those dealing with gaseous exchange of oxygen and carbon dioxide in the lungs; and the cells secreting hydrochloric acid in the stomach to assist with the digestion of foods. Knowledge about these clusters of cells, or tissues as they are called, has grown enormously during this century partly because of increasing technical and technological sophistication in monitoring and measuring cellular activity.

At one stage in the development of such knowledge, the anatomists and physiologists categorised body tissues which seemed to interact structurally or functionally into body systems and labelled them separately, for example, the skeletal, muscular, respiratory and circulatory systems. As knowledge developed, the interrelationship of these systems became even more obvious and terms came to be used such as musculoskeletal, genitourinary and cardiopulmonary systems. More recently, certain tissues with highly specialised functions have been identified which previously had not been considered as systems and reference is made in the literature to, for example, the immunological system; the temperature-controlling system; the reticuloendothelial system; and the biorhythm system related to sleep control.

Obviously the human body is a highly complex organisation of cells and tissues, and there are various classifications which assist discussion. Therefore to assist students to see the relationship of physical factors (human biology) to ALs, the authors have matched a body system with an AL when relevant, for example, the cardiopulmonary system with the AL of breathing; the lower alimentary and urinary systems with the AL of eliminating; the musculoskeletal system with the AL of mobilising; and this is illustrated in later chapters when each AL is discussed separately. This juxtaposition of system and AL provides guidance for the logical consideration and recording of nursing interventions, whether nurse-initiated or derived from medical prescription. However, it must be emphasised that it is only for the purposes of discussion that physical factors are singled out; it is the overall consideration of the whole person which is central to nursing.

Psychological factors

Psychological factors cannot be considered in isolation; they are related to physical, and also to sociocultural, environmental and politicoeconomic factors. As well as being related to the other four factors, psychological factors are related to the other components of the model. They influence living throughout the lifespan, especially intellectual and emotional development, and have a bearing on the person's level of independence; so inevitably they influence the person's individuality in living, and affect the way each person carries out the ALs. In Chapters 6–17 specific examples are given to indicate the influence which psychological factors can have on individual ALs; here, to provide a background to Chapters 6–17, a few general points are made about their influence on a number of ALs.

Intellectual aspects

The term 'cognitive development' is often used to refer to the process of acquiring intellectual skills — thinking, reasoning and problem-solving — which are essential for physical survival and affect all Activities of Living. The process by which people obtain information about themselves and their environment begins as a baby. Via the sense organs, the baby perceives stimuli such as pressure, pain, warmth, cold, taste, sound, changes in light intensity and various visual images. At first, the response to many of these stimuli may be simply a reflex action, because highly differentiated responses are not possible until the cerebral cortex grows and conceptual processes begin to develop. It is important to remember that sensory deprivation, for example, blindness or deafness may result in delayed intellectual development and that this can affect almost every AL. It is just as important to remember that lack of stimulation during the early years of life at home and at school, can retard intellectual development. Indeed the neglected child, even with a genetic inheritance which would promise high potential, has less opportunity to develop intellectually and emotionally thereby affecting ALs such as maintaining a safe environment, communicating, and working and playing.

Intellectual development continues in childhood and early adolescence, by means of formal education and the pursuit of personal interests and leisure. In late adolescence, there is usually a more marked differentiation between individuals, and this can affect decisions about advanced studies and choice of job or career. Establishment in an occupation is one of the major tasks during adulthood and the significance of the AL, working and playing is paramount.

During the ageing process, overall intellectual functioning becomes gradually less efficient and may cause problems with Activities of Living, for example, there may be difficulty with communicating because the senses are less acute; maintaining a safe environment in the home may be less easy as memory fails; opportunities for fulfilling the AL of working and playing may be reduced, and boredom or loneliness may result. However, an enhancing environment can help to sustain even an elderly person's intellectual status making it possible to remain independent for the majority of ALs, thus facilitating residence in the community rather than resorting to care in an institutional setting.

Emotional aspects

Like intellectual development, emotional development is closely related to lifespan and the growth of independence in the relevant ALs. The need for love and belonging is crucial in young children; and from a stable and close relationship in infancy; the child can grow with self-confidence and a feeling of worth. The development of personality is one of the outcomes of emotional development which influences, for example, the AL of communicating in the model of living. Early sex-related behaviour patterns tend to be strengthened and the child often models on the parent of the same sex, sometimes through the AL of playing. Parents are significant in influencing emotional development, and the acquisition of norms and moral standards are part of communicating in the model of living.

Emotional development during the teens is closely related to the physical changes of puberty. Emotional relationships with parents undergo change and adolescents begin to assert their individuality and independence, at first for the 'playing' part of the AL of working and playing and eventually for working; and they may resist adult authority and advice.

During young adulthood, there are usually important emotional relationships associated with courtship and setting up house with a partner (usually of the opposite sex) and the rearing of children, all associated with the AL of expressing sexuality. Consequently late adulthood may bring with it major emotional readjustments when grown-up children leave home; often an experience of tremendous loss although there may also be a new sense of freedom to enjoy the 'playing' part of the AL, working and playing.

For the older person there may have to be many emotional adaptations related to the physical effects of ageing and sometimes declining intellectual ability which can influence ALs such as maintaining a safe environment, communicating and expressing sexuality. There are reduced opportunities for emotional and social relationships as family and friends in their peer group die, which influences the bereavement and grieving part of the AL of dying in the model.

There are individual differences. There are marked variations in the capacity for intellectual development; and enormous differences related to the general ability to cope with the emotional demands of life events. And, of course, this intellectual and emotional development takes place not only within the family; it develops in the context of the society and culture where the individual lives.

Sociocultural factors

For the purposes of the model of living, the term sociocultural subsumes spiritual, religious and ethical aspects of living. Sociocultural factors are closely related to the physical and psychological factors already discussed, and also to the environmental and politicoeconomic factors which will be introduced subsequently.

As well as being related to the other four factors, sociocultural factors are related to the other components of the model. They influence living throughout the lifespan and have a bearing on the person's level of independence, so inevitably they influence the person's individuality in living and affect the way each person carries out the ALs. In Chapters 6–17 specific examples are given to indicate the influence which sociocultural factors can have on individual ALs; here, to provide a background to Chapters 6–17, a few general points are made about their influence on a number of ALs.

Within every society there is some kind of organisation of people into groups and of activities into institutions. The social organisation may be simple, as in a nomadic tribe or it may involve a highly elaborate network of groups and specialised structures, as in technologically advanced countries. *Culture* is the word used in sociology to refer to the way of life of a particular society, and cultural differences exist in even the most basic of everyday living activities. Such cultural idiosyncrasies are highlighted for each AL in later chapters.

An aspect of living which is a reflection of culture, and which is sometimes overlooked, is *spirituality*. It is defined broadly as 'that which inspires in one the desire to transcend the realm of the material' (O'Brien, 1982). Discussing this definition, Labun (1988) maintains that it could refer to religion as well as more philosophical orientations to belief and meaning in life. The characteristics of the spiritual self, she goes on, in combination with those of the emotional and physical self respond to situations as a totality. As far as orientation to belief and meaning in life are concerned, these are reflected in *ethical* standards and manifest themselves in 'being true to oneself' as well as in behaviour to other people.

Organised *religions* can be considered as specific manifestations of spirituality, and are often closely linked to culture. A religion's influence on group and individual behaviour can be considerable; indeed, where there is religious unity in a society, the culture and religion are almost inseparable. Religion can influence ALs such as eating and drinking, eliminating, personal cleansing and dressing, and expressing sexuality. However, secular groups such as humanists or the Greenpeace movement facilitate their members' expression of spirituality in a number of ways which can affect an adherent's Activities of Living just as forcibly as a recognised religion.

As well as belonging to a society and sharing its culture, every person is a member of a *community*. The kind of community in which people live greatly affects the quality of their lives; even their personal safety is to a large extent dependent on the maintenance of safety in the community at large; for example, in its schools and transport systems, at work, and in the provision made for the observance of law and order.

The concept of *role* is helpful in describing the part an individual plays in society. There are many different social roles and each carries very specific expectations and makes specific demands on the individual. From birth, a male baby may occupy the roles of son, brother and grandson and these differ from the daughter, sister and granddaughter roles of a female baby. These are examples of 'ascribed' roles, i.e. those allocated to people at birth according to their sex and existing kinship network. Others are 'achieved' as a result of personal choice and endeavour, for example occupational roles.

Even such fundamental roles as man or woman and child or parent have to be learnt. One of the important functions of the family is the socialisation of children, the process whereby they are taught and learn about the characteristics, expectations and responsibilities attached to the whole range of social roles. In general, there are differences in the degree of *status* attached to particular roles, and in the importance attributed to ascribed as compared to achieved roles.

In any society, each individual has his own unique network of *relationships*. Initially, this emerges from the kinship network into which the person is born, and it comprises relationships with members of the nuclear family and the extended family, then in adulthood to relationships arising from marriage, childbearing and an occupation. During adult life, a person's network continually changes and expands; in old age, there is a gradual retraction in the number and variety of social relationships.

However, an individual does not interact only with another individual. Cooperation plays an important role in a complex society and to this end a great deal of social interaction takes place within *social groups*. An individual begins life as a member of the most generic social group, his family. Thereafter, he spends his entire life joining and leaving various groups which exist in society to serve a multitude of functions: social, occupational, recreational, educational, political and religious. In general, membership of groups is extremely important for the fulfilment of love and belonging needs and the development and enhancement of self-esteem. Those individuals not strongly integrated with social groups may suffer from social isolation and become lonely and depressed, even sometimes suicidal.

Almost every society, in addition to a set of social institutions, has some form of *social stratification* which delineates the role and status of its various groups. Social stratification results from a layering process which creates units described as *social classes*. A social class is a group of people who have in common certain social, economic and occupational characteristics which determine their relative social status within society. There are different systems of class used throughout the world. In industrialised countries, the class system is often based on occupational grouping and in the UK the Registrar General's Social Class Scale is used to categorise social class according to occupation (p. 272). In general, people tend to think of three social classes — 'upper', 'middle' and 'working' class — and to attribute to each a stereotyped set of characteristics.

The concept of social class is useful in order to understand the variations in lifestyles of different social groups. For example, it is known that methods of child-rearing and the value placed on education vary between social classes. Power and status in society are also related to social class, those of the higher classes usually having greater political power and social influence. Whether or not there is the opportunity for social mobility later in life, the social class of a child is determined at birth according to the father's social position. In this and many other matters, it is the social institution of the family which determines and shapes an individual's personal process of socialisation, and therefore influences most of the ALs which interact to produce individuality in living. However, although sociocultural factors have a considerable influence on ALs, individuals in a society are also influenced by the physical environment in which they live.

Environmental factors

Environmental factors cannot be considered in isolation; they are related to physical, psychological and sociocultural, as already mentioned, and also to politicoeconomic factors which will be discussed later. As well as being related to the other four factors, environmental factors are related to the other components of the model. They influence living throughout the lifespan and have a bearing on the person's level of independence; so inevitably they influence the person's individuality in living, and affect the way each person carries out the ALs. In Chapters 6–17 specific examples are given to indicate the influence which environmental factors can have on individual ALs; here to provide a background to Chapters 6–17, a few general points are made about their influence on a number of ALs. In this text the environment is conceptualised in a broad dimension and includes all that is physically external to people.

The atmosphere is the immediate environmental factor as it is in contact with exposed skin and outer garments on which it deposits inorganic matter such as particles which are the products of combustion. Removal of these substances relates this factor to personal cleansing and dressing. Such particles can be inhaled thereby relating it to breathing. The atmosphere also contains organic matter in the form of, for example pollen, pathogenic microorganisms, and vectors such as flies and lice. Pollen can influence breathing by causing hay fever; microorganisms can settle on to food and cause food poisoning thus affecting eliminating and possibly controlling body temperature should there be a fever. Vectors, particularly flies, can also cause food poisoning by depositing pathogenic organisms directly on food; and lice can infest skin and clothes, providing another aspect of the atmospheric factors which relates to personal cleansing and dressing.

Sunrays are transmitted through the atmosphere and some of them can burn exposed skin; most people require to take preventive action by applying screening lotion or wearing garments which cover the skin.

Light rays are transmitted via the atmosphere; they can be from the sun providing daylight; from an electrically- or gas-operated apparatus which provides light when natural lighting is inadequate or absent; from technological apparatus such as batteries, and from burning candles. Light rays not only stimulate the sense of sight in normal eyes, but also provide the ambience for such varied ALs as communicating, when, for example, adequate lighting is essential during interviews; for deaf people to maximise the visual input to a conversation: or for eating and drinking when soft lighting can be relaxing and even romantic; or for working in mines which depend on artificial lighting; or for 'playing' in places such as discos to enhance the excitement of dancing; or for expressing spirituality in cathedrals and churches were candles are lit to meet various spiritual objectives.

Sound waves are also transmitted by the atmosphere and in various ways can influence different ALs. For example those produced by speech are an essential part of communicating for most people. Those produced by singing means that for professional singers they influence working, while for the majority of people, playing will be influenced. They can be an emergency warning such as a fire alarm which will certainly influence the ALs of mobilising and maintaining a safe environment.

Atmospheric components and characteristics can influence several ALs, the obvious one being breathing. The temperature and humidity may well relate to other ALs such as controlling body temperature, working and playing, and sleeping. Atmospheric turbulence in the form of gale force winds, thunder storms and hurricanes are likely to modify the ALs of maintaining a safe environment, and working and playing. The rarefied atmosphere at high altitudes, particularly reduced oxygen content, not only affects breathing, but, because it lowers metabolism, less energy is available for mobilising and working and playing.

Clothing can be considered as an environmental factor which is in immediate contact with non-exposed skin and it provides a further association with personal cleansing and dressing. People modify clothing in relation to controlling body temperature which can be influenced by atmospheric temperature. Clothing is also a part of the non-verbal dimension of communicating and is an aspect of expressing sexuality.

Solid objects are part of the environment and they range from utility items such as eating and cooking utensils to cooking apparatus, refrigerators and washing machines. Each country has its organisations, consumer councils, and some even have laws relating to the quality and safety of these objects so that they are congruent with 'healthy living' while carrying out relevant ALs. Even the decorative items with which we adorn our homes should facilitate this objective. And so should those necessary objects needed for a working and/or playing activity such as gardening. Then there are the crops, trees and foliage which are part of the environment and they too should facilitate healthy living and should not be contaminated with, for example, toxic herbicides.

Buildings are an essential part of the environment and they can influence several ALs. They need for example to be free from hazard so that the people in them can continue maintaining a safe environment. Another example is that they need to be adequately ventilated so that inside atmospheric conditions do not unduly influence controlling body temperature by causing it to rise or fall outwith the range of normal. Housing as part of the concept of buildings can influence so many of the ALs, maintaining a safe environment being particularly important where there are young children and older people. Unreliability of communal lifts in high-rise flats can deter people who experience difficulty when walking or climbing stairs from venturing outside. Space in which to walk about can therefore be important, particularly for those who are more or less housebound. Adequate playing space is obviously an advantage for children's optimal development, especially in inclement weather. Lack of facilities within a house can influence the way in which ALs such as personal cleansing and dressing and eliminating are attended to.

In this section a concept of environmental factors as they influence ALs has been developed. Often, however, they are considerably influenced by politicoeconomic factors.

Politicoeconomic factors

For the purposes of this model of living, the term politicoeconomic factors subsumes aspects of living which have a legal connection; frequently political and/or economic pressure and action is reflected in legislation. Of course politicoeconomic factors do not stand alone. They are closely related to the physical, psychological, sociocultural and environmental factors already discussed.

As well as being related to the other four factors, politicoeconomic factors are related to the other components of the model. They influence living throughout the lifespan and have a bearing on the person's level of independence, so inevitably they influence the person's individuality in living, and affect the way each person carries out the ALs. In Chapters 6–17 specific examples are given to indicate the influence which politicoeconomic factors can have on individual ALs; here, to provide background to Chapters 6–17 a few general points are made about their influence on some selected ALs.

In the modern world, every citizen is the subject of a state. The citizen is legally bound to obey the orders of the state and to a large extent, the individual's activities of living are influenced by its norms. These norms are the laws, and the state has the power to enforce the law on all who live within its frontiers. The state is the apex of the modern social pyramid and has supremacy over other forms of social groupings, so, in general terms, the state regulates human activities of living. For example in relation to the AL of mobilising, traffic regulations are enforced by the state; and in relation to the AL of eating and drinking, there are laws controlling the type and amount of food additives permitted in food processing, and also regarding the cleanliness of premises where food is prepared which, in addition, involves the AL of maintaining a safe environment. However, the state is dependent on the economic system which underlies the legal order; only limited social progress is possible when a state has a precarious economic base.

The state has involvement, in varying degrees, with an enormous range of interests, some personal, for example, the statutory requirement to register births, marriages and deaths; and others corporate, for example, the provision of national and local parklands for the leisure and enjoyment of all.

The power of the state is considerable. But if individuals are sufficiently outraged, they can register disapproval and examples of disapproval can be found in, for example, the suffragette movement, the pacifist movement, and opposition to the use of nuclear power; the contention being that when individuals suspect their rights are being threatened, they will question the state. In a modern democratic society, individuals consider that, for example, they have rights associated with their Activities of Living: the right to a safe environment; the right to work in order to earn a livelihood; the right to leisure; the right to health; the right to education; the right to freedom of speech, freedom of association and so on. But while making such demands, citizens have to accept that rights and freedoms carry with them social responsibilities. They do not have licence to do what they like; they have freedom to act responsibly within the law and appreciate that other people have equal rights to carry out their various Activities of Living.

Of course the individual may not always be immediately conscious of personal political power vis-á-vis the state, but the combined efforts of individuals working as a group can have a profound effect. In the vast modern state, associations have come to assume considerable importance; indeed some focus on their ability to translate the results of their efforts into legislation, for example, employers' associations and trades unions. And many small voluntary groups, pioneering minority causes, may highlight issues which are precursors to legislation. All associations are not directly

relevant to the state; they may be formed for the purposes of sport or for aesthetic pursuits, and add considerably to the variety and quality of daily life.

In varying degrees, the modern state is a welfare state, virtually ensuring for all citizens a minimum level of protection against social risks. The interpretation of 'minimum' is a political decision and is influenced by the country's economic status and level of affluence. Gradually, however, claims against the national budget have come to cover the entire lifespan, for example, for maternity grants at birth; for general education and higher education; during unemployment; for pensions at retirement; and finally for death grants. All groups in society have come to have considerable dependence on the state. However, in periods of economic recession, it becomes more immediately apparent that a national budget is finite, that competing claims have to be arranged in some order of priority, and that in the process, certain demands, albeit worthy, will be unmet.

In the modern world, the state is not concerned only with its own citizens. Each state is one among many and some of the most important current issues are problems which are external to the individual state. It has come to be realised that it is necessary to have regulations between states in the form of international laws; rapid economic and political changes make it unsatisfactory to leave individual states to make decisions in isolation on matters which are really of international concern. The world is now interdependent in a large array of matters related to, for example frontiers, tariffs, marketing, labour laws, monetary markets, shipping channels and flight paths, as well as for health regulations; and in varying degrees these affect each state and eventually the individual's ALs. Indeed some of the politicoeconomic issues have ethical considerations such as the unequal distribution of food — a basic necessity for living; in many wealthy countries there is a superabundance, and in others the economic level of the state is so fragile that its citizens are undernourished and sometimes starving. This vast interdependence has, in fact, created a world community in political, economic and, to some extent, legal terms, operating alongside the national and local structures which have a more obvious influence on the individual's Activities of Living.

INDIVIDUALITY IN LIVING

The model of living attempts to provide a simple conceptualisation of the complex process of 'living'. However, the concern of the model is with living as it is experienced by each individual and this fifth and final component — *individuality in living* (Fig. 4.6) — serves to emphasise this point.

The Activities of Living were selected as the main component of the model and, although every person carries out

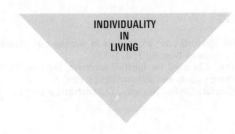

INDIVIDUALITY
IN
LIVING

Fig. 4.6   Individuality in living

all of the ALs, each individual does so differently. In terms of the model, this individuality can be seen to be a product of the influence on the ALs of all the other components of the model, and the complex interaction among them. Each person's individuality in carrying out the ALs is, in part, determined by stage on the *lifespan* and degree of *dependence/independence*; and is further fashioned by the influence of various physical, psychological, sociocultural, environmental and politicoeconomic *factors*.

A person's individuality can manifest itself in many different ways, for example in:

- *how* a person carries out the AL

- *how often* the person carries out the AL
- *where* the person carries out the AL
- *when* the person carries out the AL
- *why* the person carries out the AL in a particular way
- what the person *knows* about the AL
- what the person *believes* about the AL
- the *attitude* the person has to the AL

The idea that this component of the model — individuality in living — is a product of the other components, is conveyed in the way it is depicted in the diagram of the model of living (Fig. 4.7). The other four components combine to produce the unique mix which determines individuality.

Again, it must be emphasised that the diagram of a model is merely an aide-memoire and, indeed, has little meaning without explanation. Although each of the five components was described separately, the fact that they are closely related was emphasised; the relationships are portrayed in the diagram both by position and the addition of arrows. In other words, the whole model is more than simply the sum of its parts.

It must be stressed, too, that although the model is depicted as referring to the individual, individuality in living could be used to discuss the individual, or the family

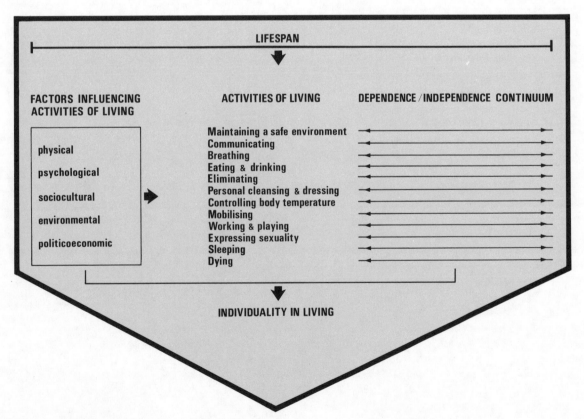

Fig. 4.7   Diagram of the model of living

unit, or a larger grouping, or the community. A conceptual model is not intended to be rigid and restrictive; it is only a tool to assist understanding. The model uses broad concepts which can have wide application.

The Roper, Logan, and Tierney model for nursing is based on this model of living.

REFERENCES

Labun E 1988 Spiritual care: an element in nursing care planning. Journal of Advanced Nursing 3: 314–320
O'Brien M 1982 The need for spiritual integrity. In: Yura H, Walsh M (eds) Human needs and the nursing process. Appleton-Century-Crofts, Norwalk, Connecticut, p 85–95

5

Model for nursing

THE MODEL FOR NURSING

The purpose of the model for nursing is to provide a framework for nurses to plan individualised nursing for those interventions which are nurse-initiated and related to the patient's ALs. A nursing plan also includes interventions which are derived from medical prescription, and from other members of the health care team; and carrying out the associated nursing interventions is an important function of the nurse. However, the model is essentially concerned with the nurse-initiated aspects of nursing. This is an important point to appreciate in relation to the model for nursing and, indeed, to the whole of this book.

A model for nursing which is based on a model of living may seem to be a rather broad and somewhat simplistic view of nursing. In fact, this is deliberate on both counts. While acknowledging the importance and necessity of specialisation within nursing, we believe that, underlying this, there is — and should be — a consensus among nurses as to the beliefs, goals and practices which are common to nursing, whatever the particular setting or circumstances, disease condition or patient/client group involved. Certainly for nurse learners we consider it essential that they are helped to see some connecting thread or theme to provide continuity and cohesiveness in the practice they observe and carry out in various settings, and in the various components of their theoretical instruction. This model for nursing is, we believe, sufficiently broad and flexible to be used as a framework for the process of nursing in any area of professional practice, and as a means of appreciating the underlying unity of the various branches of the profession.

And, certainly, the model appears simple — as simple as the model of living on which it is based. This is not to suggest that either 'living' or 'nursing' are simple processes because, of course, they are not. However, we believe that to be useful, a model should be readily understood, and in the case of nursing, directly relevant and applicable to practice. There is no necessity for a model to exhaust every aspect of the subject and, indeed if its presentation is excessively complicated by detail, its application to practice is unlikely to be readily apparent, however interesting and academically respectable it may be. This model is deliberately uncomplicated: it is offered as an overall framework to assist learners to develop a way of thinking about nursing in general terms, which then can be utilised in practice as a means of developing individualised nursing.

ASSUMPTIONS ON WHICH THE MODEL IS BASED

As already said, the selected concepts and their relationships in a nursing model are a means of interpreting the discipline of nursing. It is not surprising, therefore, that creators of models give considerable attention to the assumptions which underlie their approach to the discipline; Fawcett (1984) considered that creators of models for nursing should make their assumptions explicit because they are indicative of the authors' values and their special points of emphasis. The authors of the Roper, Logan and Tierney model make the following assumptions:

- Living can be described as an amalgam of Activities of Living (ALs)

- the way ALs are carried out by each person contributes to individuality in living
- the individual is valued at all stages of the lifespan
- throughout the lifespan until adulthood, the individual tends to become increasingly independent in the ALs
- while independence in the ALs is valued, dependence should not diminish the dignity of the individual
- an individual's knowledge, attitudes and behaviour related to the ALs are influenced by a variety of factors which can be categorised broadly as physical, psychological, sociocultural, environmental and politicoeconomic factors
- the way in which an individual carries out the ALs can fluctuate within a range of normal for that person
- when the individual is 'ill', there may be problems (actual or potential) with the ALs
- during the lifespan, most individuals experience significant life events which can affect the way they carry out ALs, and may lead to problems, actual or potential
- the concept of potential problems incorporates the

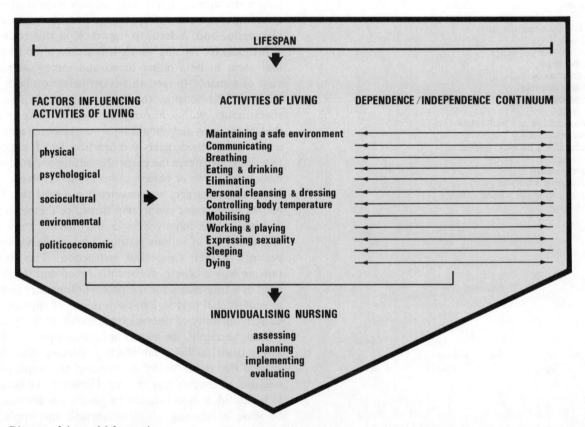

Fig. 5.1 Diagram of the model for nursing

promotion and maintenance of health, and the prevention of disease; and identifies the role of the nurse as a health teacher, even in illness settings

- within a health care context, nurses work in partnership with the client/patient who, except for special circumstances, is an autonomous, decision-making person
- nurses are part of a multiprofessional health care team who work in partnership for the benefit of the client/patient, and for the health of the community
- the specific function of nursing is to assist the individual to prevent, alleviate or solve, or cope with problems (actual or potential) related to the ALs

The language of the assumptions is reflected in the model for nursing (Fig. 5.1) and, as has been said, it is based on the model of living. Indeed the components of the models are exactly the same with one exception: 'individualising nursing' takes the place of 'individuality in living'. The other four components — the Activities of Living, the lifespan, the dependence/independence continuum, and the factors influencing the ALs — are all transferred directly from the model of living to the model for nursing. The similarities can be seen clearly in Figure 5.2.

MODEL OF LIVING	MODEL FOR NURSING
12 Activities of living (ALs) Lifespan Dependence/independence continuum Factors influencing the ALs Individuality in living	12 Activities of Living (ALs) Lifespan Dependence/independence continuum Factors influencing the ALs Individualising nursing

Fig. 5.2 The main concepts in the model of living and the model for nursing

The way of thinking about 'living' generated by the model of living will now be transferred to nursing in the following discussion of each of the five components of the model for nursing. Only an outline is provided in this chapter because the next section of the book comprises 12 chapters (Chs 6–17), one devoted to each of the ALs, in which detailed discussion of the five components of the model is presented in the context of nursing.

ACTIVITIES OF LIVING (ALs)

As in the model of living, the Activities of Living (Fig. 5.3) are considered as the main component of the model for nursing.

ACTIVITIES OF LIVING

Maintaining a safe environment
Communicating
Breathing
Eating & drinking
Eliminating
Personal cleansing & dressing
Controlling body temperature
Mobilising
Working & playing
Expressing sexuality
Sleeping
Dying

Fig. 5.3 The Activities of Living

The ALs are the focus of the model because they are central to our view of nursing. Nursing is viewed as helping patients to prevent, alleviate or solve, or cope with problems (actual or potential) related to the Activities of Living. Recognition of the fact that patients' problems may be actual or potential means that nursing not only responds to existing problems but is also concerned with preventing problems, whenever possible.

In Chapters 6–17 of the book, groups of potential and actual problems are discussed in relation to each of the 12 ALs. The first half of each chapter opens with an analysis of the AL mainly in the context of healthy living: how health can be maintained and promoted, and disease prevented; and how potential problems can be identified and averted before they become actual problems. The second half of each chapter deals with some of the problems which people may experience with the AL when their usual way of carrying out the AL is disrupted — and this may occur in response to various causes and circumstances. Some problems result simply from the *change of environment and routine* which is an inevitable consequence of admission to hospital; others occur when illness or disability experienced either at home or in hospital causes a *change in usual habit or mode of carrying out an AL*; others are a consequence of *change in dependence/independence status*.

So far, only a brief outline of the ALs has been provided in the context of the model of living (pp. 22–24). In the context of the model for nursing, the remainder of this section offers some comments on the ALs collectively.

Use of the concept of ALs
There is, of course, nothing highly original about using the concept of Activities of Living within a nursing model. Virginia Henderson's definition of nursing was quoted earlier (p. 13); she wrote about 14 components expressed as

'Helping the patient to . . . .' and although she did not use the actual term, they are, in fact, Activities of Living. More recently, the term 'Activities of Living' has become a familiar one in nursing and for that reason, it is pertinent to make a few comments about how we came to use the concept of ALs as we did, for the purposes of the model.

We deliberately chose to use the concept of Activities of Living in preference to 'basic human needs', a concept which has been widely used in nursing, based on Maslow's analysis of human needs. He categorised needs and then arranged them in order of priority, creating a 'hierarchy' — and it must be remembered that he was talking about healthy people (Duldt & Griffin, 1985). The hierarchy is frequently illustrated in the form of a pyramid — the physiological needs at the bottom; safety and security needs next, followed by needs for love and belonging, and self-esteem needs; and, at the top, the need for self-actualisation — inferring that those in the lowest category need to be at least minimally fulfilled before motivation is established to seek fulfilment of needs in the next category, and so on to the top. To some extent, this thinking is relevant to the concept of activities of living but, unlike needs, ALs have an advantage for a nursing model in that they are observable and can be explicitly described, and, in some instances, objectively measured. It is not easy for the nurse to assess needs as such; it is less difficult (although still not easy) to describe a patient's behaviour in relation to ALs.

The terms we chose to name the ALs also merit comment. Although anxious to avoid jargon, finding suitable names for some of the activities was difficult. The names of the 12 ALs were selected in an attempt to be consistent in emphasising their active nature (therefore, 'elimina*ting*' rather than 'elimination') and their comprehensiveness (for example, though 'washing and dressing' is the more common term, we decided on 'personal cleansing and dressing' because it is all-embracing of the various activities subsumed within that AL). As a consequence, some of the names may seem rather strange at first but we believe that familiarity with the 12 ALs should result in acceptability of our deliberately and carefully chosen terms.

The set of 12 ALs is unique to our model. Many of the activities are contained in other lists, but in addition, our list contains some activities (such as 'expressing sexuality') which have not always been included alongside the more obvious activities (such as 'eating and drinking') despite the fact that they are integral to the process of living and, therefore, relevant in the context of nursing.

Complexity of the ALs

The fact that each AL is highly complex because it subsumes a variety of activities was a point mentioned in discussion of the AL component of the model of living (p. 22). The point is worth reiterating here because it explains why, in the context of nursing, there is such diversity in the patients' problems and related nursing activities associated with each of the 12 ALs. This will become apparent from discussion of nursing and the ALs in Section 3 of the book (Chs 6–17).

Relatedness of the ALs

The relatedness of the 12 ALs was also commented on (p. 22) and this too is an important consideration in the context of nursing. In the course of obtaining information (by assessment) about any one AL, the nurse is likely to find out a great deal about other closely related ALs. For example, discussion of eating and drinking habits leads naturally to description of eliminating habits. A problem with one AL may well cause problems with one or more of the others: for example, mobilising difficulties are likely to cause problems with other ALs, such as 'personal cleansing and dressing' and 'working and playing'. On the other hand, when applying the model in practice, the identified problem of, for example, pain, could be placed on the Nursing Plan (p. 125) in more than one AL. If the pain can be identified as being specific to the AL of eating and drinking, or eliminating, or mobilising, it would be recorded with that specific AL. If it were generalised pain, it would be recorded under the AL of communicating. To repeat, a model is not a rigid straitjacket; it is intended merely as a tool which can be useful to the nurse in practice.

Priorities among the ALs

Although every AL is important in the process of living, some are more vital than others. The AL of breathing must be considered as of prime importance because it is essential for all the other ALs and, indeed, for life itself. The notion of priorities among the ALs were briefly mentioned in discussion of the model of living (p. 24) and in the context of nursing is an extremely important consideration.

With the exception of the AL of breathing, there is no fixed order of priority among the ALs because, depending on the prevailing circumstances and individual choice, priorities among the ALs alter. Although eating and drinking are activities which are usually carried out regularly at fixed times there are occasions when other activities, such as working and playing, are afforded a higher priority. On the whole, however, those activities which are vital to survival and safety take precedence over others and, in nursing, this principle certainly applies in circumstances of acute illness and any condition which is considered to be life-threatening.

Relevance of the ALs

Closely associated with the order of priority among ALs is the notion of relevance. Although the 12 ALs all have relevance to nursing, not all of them are necessarily relevant to all patients or to any one patient all of the time. For example, although it takes up much time in ordinary life, consideration of the AL of working and playing will not be relevant during a period of critical illness. For a patient who has suffered a myocardial infarction, the AL of expressing sexuality may only seem important again when the person is recovering and, looking ahead, may wish information about whether and when it will be safe to resume sexual relations again. However, for a woman having a mastectomy many aspects of that same AL may assume great importance, both pre- and post-operatively and in the longer term too. What is important is for nurses to be aware that different circumstances create different priorities and, therefore, to apply common sense and professional judgement (which comes from knowledge and experience) in making decisions about the relevance of the ALs for any particular patient: any one, or indeed several, may not merit consideration at all; or may merit consideration only at certain points in a patient's nursing plan.

LIFESPAN

The reason for including a lifespan as one component of the model of living has previously been explained (p. 25). Of course, all people do not live through all stages of the lifespan; some die before birth or at birth, and some otherwise healthy people die prematurely, for example as a result of accident, disease, natural disaster or war. So although each individual has a lifespan from birth to death, its length is variable. Collection of statistics, usually at national level, allows life expectancy to be predicted according to the average age of death, and in most countries of the Western world, the majority of people have an expected lifespan of 70 years or more.

In the model of living, the various stages of the lifespan were described. In the model for nursing, the lifespan (Fig. 5.4) serves as a reminder that nursing is concerned with people of all ages: that an individual may require nursing at any stage of the lifespan, from birth to death.

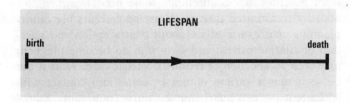

Fig. 5.4 The lifespan

So relevant is the concept of the lifespan to nursing that some branches of the profession, and some professional qualifications, are linked specifically to certain stages of the lifespan: for example, midwives are concerned with the prenatal stage, birth and the immediate postnatal period; paediatric nurses and health visitors with the stages of infancy and childhood; and nursing care of the elderly is the special concerned with old age. Their special knowledge and understanding of the processes of normal growth and development in a particular stage of the lifespan enables them to monitor development and to detect any delay or deviation from the parameters of 'normal'.

Taking account of a patient's age — the fact which identifies the stage of the lifespan involved — has always been recognised as important in nursing. It influences all phases of the process of nursing — assessing, planning, implementing and evaluating — and is an important consideration in individualising nursing.

The following brief comments on each of the main stages of the lifespan help to illustrate the relevance of this component of the model for nursing.

Prenatal stage

Midwives, and in some instances other nurses such as health visitors, work in close collaboration with obstetricians and others to provide what is referred to as 'prenatal care'. A detailed knowledge of growth and development in the prenatal stage of the lifespan is utilised to monitor fetal growth, allowing for early detection of problems which can occur in pregnancy and for appropriate treatment to be initiated.

Another important nursing function in prenatal care is health education: for example, teaching expectant mothers about the dangers of smoking, taking alcohol and drugs and the importance of a balanced diet, exercise and adequate rest. There is knowledge about all the Activities of Living which can be imparted so that the parents-to-be can adapt their lifestyle during the pregnancy with the aim of maximising the mother's health and that of the baby.

Attending a woman in labour is universally the role of the midwife, the word meaning 'with woman'. The great advances in obstetric care which have taken place in this century have markedly reduced both maternal and fetal mortality, and birth is now safer than ever before. It is the event of birth which marks the beginning of the lifespan and the midwife shares with the parents this profoundly important experience. By cutting the umbilical cord, the midwife separates the newborn baby from the mother to begin existence as an independent human being. It is interesting to reflect that in industrialised countries, almost every person is literally brought into the world by a member of the nursing profession.

Infancy

The first moments of life after birth are crucial and, here too, midwives play a vital role. They ensure, for example, that the AL of breathing is satisfactorily established; that there is immediate opportunity for communication between mother and baby; that the baby is dried and kept warm to prevent problems with the AL of controlling body temperature; and so essential to life is the AL of eating and drinking, that the midwife may encourage the mother to suckle her baby at the breast very soon after the birth. Helping the mother to learn to feed and care for her baby is a major concern of postnatal nursing, for after all the baby is totally dependent on the mother in respect of almost all the Activities of Living.

Throughout the first year of life, even the most healthy babies remain vulnerable to the hazards of infection and injury and susceptible to a variety of problems with the ALs, for example, hypothermia, malnutrition and dehydration. In all countries with a developed health care system, child health services are afforded a high priority and nursing makes an important contribution to efforts aimed at achieving ever lower rates of infant mortality and morbidity.

There are of course some babies and young children who, for a variety of reasons, require nursing in a neonatal unit or children's hospital. Their nursing care is provided by specially qualified nurses who, in addition to knowing about treatment of disease, require an in-depth understanding of the normal processes of development in the early years of the lifespan. This is essential for nursing to be tailored to the very different needs and abilities of children of different ages; and to prevent the experience of hospitalisation from adversely affecting the child. There is now widespread acceptance of the need to avoid the adverse effects of separation and for this reason parents are encouraged to visit freely (p. 279) and take an active part in nursing their baby or young child.

Some children have the misfortune to suffer from chronic illness or a fatal disease or a condition which results in long-term physical and/or mental handicap. Frequent readmission to hospital and, in some cases, long-term hospitalisation or community nursing support may be necessary. In such cases nurses play a very significant part in the child's early years of the lifespan.

Childhood
Childhood tends to be a period of relatively good health for the majority, with death an unusual occurrence. In the Western world the single most important cause of death in this age group is accidents (p. 68).

Serious illness is rare too. Apart from transient illness, such as respiratory infections or the infectious diseases of childhood, the majority of children have little need for medical treatment or nursing care. The exceptions are those children with a chronic illness or long-term physical or mental handicap. For nurses involved in their care, whether in hospital or the community, one of the important considerations is to provide nursing in such a way that there is minimal interference with normal development in this stage of the lifespan, such as progress at school; involvement in family life and friendships; and increasing independence in all of the Activities of Living.

However, even 'well' children come into contact with nursing through the school health service. Like health visitors with the younger age group, school nurses are primarily concerned with the monitoring of growth and development, and the early identification of problems: for example, defects of hearing and sight, speech difficulties, dental caries, malnutrition, obesity, inadequate hygiene, poor posture, foot malformation, urinary incontinence or infection, and conditions underlying excessive incontinence or infection, and conditions underlying excessive fatigue or anxiety. In some cases, the nurse may provide treatment but equally important is her ability to refer the child and parents to the appropriate source of help.

Many of the problems mentioned can be considered essentially as potential problems of childhood and preventing them from becoming actual problems through health education is another important aspect of the work of school nurses. Increasingly, health education is viewed as more than simply information giving, and through discussion, debate and experimentation, children are being encouraged to appraise their personal health practices and to develop positive health values at an early age.

Adolescence
During this stage of the lifespan, the dominant feature is puberty. Sex education in school and at home during the years of childhood helps to prepare the adolescent to anticipate and cope with the associated physical and emotional changes. Sadly, a few children at any age from infancy to adolescence, are physically and/or sexually abused and may be scarred for life.

Many of the problems which can arise in adolescence are related to physical and psychological aspects of sexual development. Some adolescents experience severe emotional or psychological problems, such as depression or anxiety, which require psychiatric treatment; some require treatment for drug dependence (p. 284); some may benefit from psychosexual counselling; some need treatment for sexually transmitted disease. Many adolescents use family planning centres for advice about contraception and selection of contraceptives; and girls who do become pregnant may seek an abortion or require obstetric care. Thus it can be seen that a variety of nurses come into contact with adolescents — psychiatric nurses, nurse counsellors, school nurses, nurses who work in genitourinary clinics, and those in family planning services, gynaecology and midwifery.

For all of these nurses, an understanding of adolescence is essential. They are unlikely to deal effectively and sympathetically with an adolescent's problems, whatever they may be, in the absence of an appreciation of the emotional turbulence of this stage of the lifespan and of other features, such as a teenager's changing relationship with parents, the pressures of school and worries about future employment.

Appreciating these difficulties and remembering that adolescence is a period of transition, with fluctuation between the desire for adult independence and regression to child-like dependence, is certainly essential for nurses involved with adolescents who require hospital or home care, whether short- or long-term. Adolescence is, like childhood, a stage of the lifespan when illness is uncommon. For those affected that fact must make illness or incapacity harder to accept when it occurs; for example, an adolescent who becomes physically disabled following an accident or an adolescent with diabetes mellitus.

Even short-term hospital care of an adolescent presents the nurses with a considerable challenge. On the one hand there may be the desire to be talked to and treated as an adult but, on the other hand, the circumstances may well precipitate some regression to child-like behaviour. This may be manifest in signs of fear and anxiety, or in a desire for parental closeness; or perhaps in a reluctance to accept responsibility for self-care and independent decision-making.

The swings of mood common in adolescence may make for difficulties in the nurse-patient relationship and ambivalent feelings towards authority may be projected on to nurses and doctors. Self-consciousness about physical development and relationships with members of the opposite (or same) sex may cause the adolescent patient to experience considerable embarrassment in some physically intimate nursing activities; for example, those related to the ALs of personal cleansing and dressing, and eliminating.

The nursing of adolescents, whatever the circumstances, requires sensitivity and knowledge of 'normal' developments in this stage of the lifespan.

Adulthood

In discussion of development during the lifespan, adulthood is sometimes decribed as comprising three stages — young adulthood, the middle years and late adulthood. Here, all three stages are discussed together.

It is easy to appreciate the necessity of adapting nursing to the very specific needs and abilities of children of different ages. Adults of different ages do have special requirements too but, because of their independence in the Activities of Living and their ability to communicate their needs and desires, there is not the same need to adapt nursing so specifically to age as there is with children. It is also the case that the parameters of 'normal' are very much wider in adulthood, resulting in much greater diversity in lifestyle, abilities and attitudes than among children of a certain age. Appreciating the diversity though is helpful because it warns against making assumptions, pointing to the need to collect relevant information about each adult patient as an individual.

However, there are two dominant areas of concern for all adults, namely, work and family life. Both are directly affected by illness and hospitalisation and, therefore, individualised nursing must take account of the adult patient's work and family circumstances. In some instances these circumstances may be directly related to the patient's need for nursing: for example, a patient who has suffered an accident at work or, in relation to family life, nursing services which are concerned with family planning, pregnancy and childbirth, and parenthood.

Therefore, work and family life not only bring adults into direct contact with nursing but are directly affected, often disrupted, by illness and hospitalisation. There are, too, direct links between work and family life and health and ill-health.

Early adulthood is considered to be a stage of relative stability, with both physical fitness and intellectual ability at their peak. Apart from those young adults who are continuing to cope with a life-long physical or mental handicap, serious ill-health is uncommon and the death rate is low although the AIDS epidemic currently affects this group most severely. Apart from AIDS, the more common conditions include bronchitis, peptic ulceration, gall bladder disease, alcoholism, back injury and psychiatric illness, particularly depression. With advancing age into the middle years of life, ill-health becomes more common. There is a sharp increase in the death rate in late adulthood with three conditions responsible — heart disease, cancer and stroke.

Knowing the causes of morbidity and mortality in the various stages of adulthood gives some idea of the reasons why adults come into contact with the health care system, and with nurses. But there is a more important reason: if the causes of ill-health are understood, then appropriate preventive measures can be directed at people of a particular age. Many of the diseases of adulthood are, to some extent at least, preventable. It might seem trite to point it out, but it is true that much ill-health and injury would be avoided if adults did not smoke cigarettes, drank less alcohol, avoided becoming obese, took more frequent and more vigorous exercise, and learned to avoid or cope more effectively with stress. Health education is one means of encouraging adults to adopt a more healthy life-style, and there are many ways in which nurses can contribute to this effort.

Old age

Nowadays many more people are living longer. Especially in the Western world, elderly people now make up a larger proportion of the total population than ever before; in the UK, it is estimated that by the year 2000 there will be a million more people aged 85 or over (Craig, 1989). With proportionately fewer people to look after them (Craig predicts that by the year 2000, there will be a million fewer in the 16–24 age group) the needs of the elderly are now a matter of concern to many groups, not least to nursing. Despite the legitimately increasing concern, however, it should be kept in perspective because the majority of people in this last stage of the lifespan do manage to remain in their own homes, often totally independent (sometimes referred to as the healthy elderly). Contrary to the somewhat gloomy predictions about the ageing West, the marketing men see a flourishing market where 'maturity sells'; the increasingly affluent and healthy older person, they predict, will alter not only money markets but also fashion and taste. Much can be done, for example by the health visitor, to promote and maintain health in this group of citizens (Drennan, 1988) although there will, inevitably, be some in need of assistance with some of the Activities of Living.

The fact that ill-health is more common in this stage of the lifespan than in any other is reflected in the numbers of elderly patients in the wards of general hospitals. To some nurses this comes as something of a surprise and it certainly would seem to contradict the belief that old people are the concern only of the specialist services for care of the elderly. All nurses, (with certain obvious exceptions such as paediatric nurses) nowadays require extensive knowledge of the process of ageing; a sympathetic understanding of the needs of old people; and a positive attitude towards their care and rehabilitation. Individualised nursing is as necessary for an old person as for a child or a young adult — even more so it might be argued, for there is a longer established individuality in living!

When physical or mental disability is such that an elderly person can no longer stay at home, or cope within a community care setting, placement in a 'continuing care unit' may be the only solution. In such a setting, the primary aim is to help the person to maintain what independence there still is in the Activities of Living and, of course, to provide an atmosphere and environment which is like 'home' as far as is humanly possible. Long-stay care of the elderly wards have not enjoyed a good reputation on the whole and, while inadequate conditions are certainly to blame, staff attitudes probably contributed to the unnecessary routinisation and institutionalisation which prevailed. The emphasis nowadays on individualised nursing, through the process of nursing method (which is incorporated in this model) offers a way of enabling long-stay patients in such a unit to continue their individuality in living.

The inevitable preoccupation of old people with death is something which should always be borne in mind by nurses who are involved with the elderly. In Western society most people die in old age and skilled and sensitive nursing may help a person to come to the very end of the lifespan, to the event of death, in comfort and with the greatest possible dignity.

In this overview of the relationship between stages of the lifespan and nursing, various Activities of Living have been

mentioned. The specific effects of the lifespan on each of the 12 ALs are described in Chapters 6–17; and from that it will be apparent how a patient's age is a relevant consideration in all phases of the process of nursing. Therefore, the lifespan component of the model for nursing is closely related to the AL component, as it is to the dependence/independence continuum which will now be discussed.

DEPENDENCE/INDEPENDENCE CONTINUUM

The reason for including the dependence/independence continuum in the model of living was described (p. 25). The concept of dependence/independence has been widely utilised in nursing and, as a component of the model for nursing, is related directly to the 12 Activities of Living (Fig. 5.5).

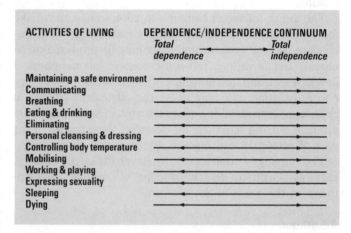

Fig. 5.5 Dependence/independence continuum related to the ALs

There is also a close link between this component of the model and the lifespan. Nursing care for newborn babies acknowledges their total dependence in respect of almost every Activity of Living whereas children's nursing must take account of the fact that the early years of the lifespan are associated with increasing independence in the ALs. Some children do not have the capacity to acquire this independence, to the same extent or at the 'normal' rate, either due to physical or mental handicap. Where nurses are involved in care of such children, whether at home or in an institutional setting, the objective is an individualised programme for the acquisition of maximum independence for each AL. For any child, an episode of illness or injury as a result of accident will not only affect the level of independence already achieved in the ALs but may also require a stay in hospital. Young children are very easily upset by any change in environment or alteration to their daily routine. For example, a child who has recently achieved independence in certain personal cleansing activities, or who is able to dress without help, is likely to be confused if the nurse washes or dresses him. On the other hand, children may be very distressed if expected by the nurses to exercise a degree of independence in the ALs which has not yet been acquired: for example, being expected to use the toilet when still at the stage of using a potty; or being given a game to play with or books to read which are beyond their level of comprehension. It is obvious that nurses require to have detailed information about what each child can and cannot do independently in relation to each AL so that the nursing plan is tailored to the individual child, as well as to the circumstances of his illness or injury.

For the majority of people, independence is a central feature of adulthood. When for any reason there is enforced dependence, for example as a result of illness or injury, many people find this hard to cope with. If the period of dependence in relation to any or all of the ALs is to be only temporary, for example following a surgical operation, it is likely to be more easily tolerated. However if the circumstances mean that there will be some residual dependence in some of the ALs, the patient needs time and support to adjust and to begin to cope with the changed dependence/independence status.

And, of course, handicapped adults are just as likely to suffer from the many conditions which bring the non-handicapped into hospital. So, when nursing adult patients who are physically or mentally handicapped (or who have loss or impairment of sight, hearing or speech), nurses need to have detailed information about their dependence/independence status for each AL. It should not be automatically assumed that because patients have, for example, a physical handicap, they will necessarily be dependent on the nurse. They may well wish to continue to use the coping mechanisms, aids or equipment — 'aided' independence — which have enabled them to remain independent in the ALs outwith the hospital, and nurses should ensure that this is made possible and that relevant information is provided on the patient's nursing plan.

Even for the most able people, independence in the ALs is generally acquired over a long period of time. In old age the loss of independence can be equally gradual and it is seldom for all of the ALs. The AL of mobilising is often one of the first affected and because movement is required to perform many other activities, this may result in loss of independence in some of the other ALs. The elderly patient may be reluctant to bath and careful questioning may elicit that it is due to fear of falling. Difficulties with personal cleansing and dressing activities may in fact be due to problems with mobilising. There are now many gadgets available to help elderly people with such difficulties and provision of these may permit a patient to retain independence, albeit 'aided' independence in these activities. It is worth repeating a point made in the context of the model of living that old age does not necessarily bring about loss of independence, and there is seldom dependence for all ALs.

Because of the recent relative increase in the number in our population of people over 65 years and the even more significant relative increase of those in their 80s and 90s, more provision is being made in the community for assisting elderly people to remain healthy and active, and retain optimal independence. Clubs are available to encourage exercise, recreational games and handicrafts which, as well as encouraging physical and mental activity, also provide a social reason for meeting, and help to reduce the loneliness which often accompanies living alone. Especially in Western cultures with a nuclear family structure, more and more elderly people do live alone and currently there is a trend to provide what is termed 'sheltered housing', often purpose-built, where elderly individuals or couples, who are becoming less able physically, can retain their own home; however each is connected via an intercom system to a warden's flat where someone is constantly on call. Usually these are small developments, organised by local authorities, or by voluntary agencies or sometimes as private enterprise; and as far as possible they are integrated into other local housing so that they do not form ghettos. They are a form of 'sheltered independence'.

An important skill in nursing is developing professional judgement in relation to patients' abilities and never depriving people, however old, of independence in those ALs for which they are capable. There is, of course, a fine line between this and misjudgement in demanding independence when a patient is incapable of so being.

It is, equally, a skill in nursing to know when a patient is in a state of dependence, or should be helped to accept that this is necessary. Although the emphasis in nursing is generally on encouraging patients to achieve or regain maximum independence in the ALs, there are circumstances (for example, unconsciousness or severe illness) when patients are totally dependent on nurses. There are other circumstances when, although patients may desire to be independent, this is not in their best interests. At certain times (for example, immediately postoperatively), in certain illnesses (for example, severe respiratory conditions) and for other reasons (for example, immobilisation in traction), it is important for the patient to move as little as possible and for energy to be conserved. Such patients may need to be helped to accept that their dependence is necessary and their distress is likely to be lessened if nurses carry out activities on their behalf in a willing manner and in a way which does not offend the patient's dignity and self-esteem.

Therefore, sometimes nurses help patients towards independence in the ALs and, at other times help them to accept dependence. The dependence/independence continuum in the model for nursing, as in the model of living, is arrowed to indicate that movement can take place along it in either direction — an important dimension of the concept of dependence/independence in the context of nursing. A very important aspect of nursing is assessing a patient's level of independence in each of the Activities of Living and judging in which direction, and by what amount, they should be assisted to move along the dependence/independence continuum; what nursing assistance they need to achieve the goals set; and how progress in relation to these goals will be evaluated.

This discussion of the dependence/independence continuum as one component of the model has been presented in general terms. In later chapters of the book (Chs 6–17) the concept is discussed more specifically in relation to each of the 12 ALs. In each case there is a section which identifies causes of change in patients' dependence/identifies causes of change in patients' dependence/independence status, and some of the related nurse-initiated

FACTORS INFLUENCING THE ALs

In the model of living (p. 27), this component was introduced to explain why there are many individual differences in the way the ALs are carried out. As described there, the various 'factors' which influence the ALs were categorised into five main groups and in the model for nursing this component is similarly presented (Fig. 5.6).

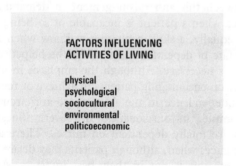

FACTORS INFLUENCING
ACTIVITIES OF LIVING

physical
psychological
sociocultural
environmental
politicoeconomic

Fig. 5.6 Factors influencing the ALs

As already indicated, the five factors influence each of the ALs and are related to the other components of the model — the lifespan and the dependence/independence continuum. The five factors themselves are interrelated, and, when assessing a patient it may be difficult to make a clear cut distinction between the influence of physical as against psychological factors; or between sociocultural and politicoeconomic factors. Despite the overlap, however, the five factors are mentioned separately at this stage, highlighting some general points which are related to health and illness in a nursing context.

Physical factors

It is essential that nurses should have knowledge of physical (biological) factors and how they influence ALs. In the model for nursing therefore, the physical status of the individual, in anatomical and physiological terms, is introduced to indicate how this helps nurses to understand, assess, plan and implement relevant nursing interventions and evaluate the effects. There is no attempt to cover biology comprehensively in this textbook; human biology must be studied as a separate subject which contributes (along with other subjects in the nursing curriculum) to an understanding of human beings in health and illness. More specific examples of the application of physical concepts to each AL are made in Chapters 6–17.

In the context of this discussion of physical factors, it should be mentioned that many members of the public seem to have the impression that nursing is concerned only with physical dysfunction and disease. This is partly true, particularly in emergencies, but nurses are also concerned with the promotion and maintenance of health, and the prevention of disease; and of course, nursing extends beyond a focus on things 'physical', as the range of factors in this model emphasises.

Irrespective of the setting — home, clinic, hospital — the nurse has innumerable opportunities for introducing aspects of health teaching which aim to maintain the body in a physically healthy state. In fact currently, in many industrialised societies, considerable amounts of money are used by governments via the mass media to extol physical health and fitness as a way of life, and the nurse as a health professional should not find it too difficult to reinforce the message. The physical state of the body is not static of course; it is constantly changing. Even during sleep, the cells are perpetually active, and hormonal and chemical substances are regulating the body's internal environment to maintain homeostasis. It is not difficult to appreciate that for various biological functions there is a range of normal in terms of individual differences; and this is corroborated using physiological measurements although even these vary with age, for example, at rest a newborn baby has a pulse rate of 140 beats per minute and the normal rate for a young adult would be 70 beats per minute. It is within the range of normal that the baby functions physically to its optimum.

Of course nurses are also involved in the process of preventing physical disease when, for example, explaining or participating in immunisation programmes and it is important for students to understand the physiological changes which occur in the body in the process of acquiring immunity so that people do not succumb to physical diseases which have the potential to cause dysfunction in one or more ALs.

The individual may, however, succumb to physical disease or trauma and this may necessitate nursing the person at home or in hospital during a brief episode of illness, or perhaps during the course of a long-term dysfunction or perhaps during the process of dying. Some of the causes of physical dysfunction are genetic in origin and some seem to start in a manner, not always understood, within the body's own internal environment, for example, autoimmune disease and idiopathic (no known cause) disease. As would be expected, when there is physical dysfunction in any tissue, the body does not remain passive; it reacts physiologically in a number of ways in an attempt to maintain equilibrium, via reactions collectively referred to as defence mechanisms (p. 83). It is particularly in relation to disease and medical diagnosis that nurses collaborate closely with medical staff; and some nursing interventions, for example the administration of medications, are doctor-initiated. Many diseases have been identified and rigorously researched and there is an internationally agreed Classification of Diseases which provides a yardstick, nationally and internationally, for the collection of epidemiological data about the incidence of disease and causes of death.

In all these instances — for the maintenance of health, prevention of disease, care during episodes of disease and during the process of dying — it is crucial for nurses to have a knowledge base of human biology so that they can understand normal structure and function, and so that they can comprehend the cause of dysfunction (in so far as it can be identified) and how it affects the individual's activities of living.

However, as already indicated, Activities of Living entail infinitely more than the body's physical structure and function; even basic survival would not be possible without intellectual and emotional abilities — the psychological factors.

Psychological factors

It is essential that nurses should have knowledge of psychological factors and how they influence ALs. In the model for nursing, therefore, psychological factors are introduced to indicate how this knowledge helps nurses to understand, assess, plan and implement nursing interventions, and evaluate the effects. There is no attempt to cover the discipline of psychology comprehensively in this textbook. General points only are made at this stage to show how this type of knowledge (along with other subjects in the nursing curriculum) contributes to an understanding of human beings as manifest in their various Activities of Living. More specific examples of the application of psychological concepts to each AL are made in Chapters 6–17.

In relation to impaired *intellectual* development, nurses may come in contact with children or adults who are mentally handicapped because of a genetic disorder such as Down syndrome or brain damage during birth such as cerebral palsy. It is important, therefore, for nurses to know about genetics in order to be able to understand the principles of genetic counselling and the significance of diagnosis in utero via amniocentesis. Knowledge is also required in order to ensure that a person who has a mental handicap is treated essentially as a healthy person, although pathologically slow in developing intellectual skills and the many other skills which are dependent on intellect. And if a suitably stimulating environment is provided based on what such people *can* do rather than what they cannot do, it is usually possible to provide an optimum level of intellectual and emotional growth for each individual. Deprived of stimulation, the mentally handicapped person may be grossly impaired and the effect on ALs is readily observable, for example in poor communication skills; difficulty with eating and drinking in a socially acceptable manner; problems with toileting; and incapacity for work and leisure activities. Carefully staged education and stimulation of the intellect using an individualised plan is of major importance in mental handicap nursing.

Impaired *emotional* development is perhaps less easy to identify. The crucial mother-infant relationship was mentioned earlier: how it nurtures the growth of self-worth and how it influences the way in which the individual will eventually deal with emotions such as happiness, anger, fear, anxiety, stress; all of which can influence the AL of communicating. Each individual learns to adopt coping mechanisms and for some people even apparently large amounts of stress are viewed as challenging, exciting and stimulating rather than predisposing to avoidance tactics.

Psychological stressors are often associated with major life events and for some people may cause extreme anxiety. These significant life events may occur at various points on the lifespan; they may be developmental in nature such as weaning, toilet training, puberty or they may be associated with incidents in living such as changing school, job or house; marriage and divorce; child-bearing; death of family members and friends. The anxiety may affect the performance of several ALs. In any of these situations the nurse may be asked for advice, and through counselling may help to prevent exacerbation of the cause, or assist the person to develop/maintain coping mechanisms until the cause of anxiety is removed or alleviated — and the person returns to a pattern of ALs which is acceptable to the individual.

It is sometimes said that psychological stressors involve the 'fight or flight' mechanism. For the purposes of survival, man is capable of an extreme response to perceived danger — an identifiable cause of fear. Activated by the autonomic nervous system and the secretion of certain hormones, there is an increase in heart rate and flow of blood to the muscles; a rise in blood pressure; an increase in depth and rate of respiration. The body is physiologically prepared for fight or flight. There are many life experiences which are less dramatic, however, and the physiological response is less intense, yet the person will describe a feeling of anxiety which may not have an identifiable cause.

Because it is unpleasant, the individual may try consciously, or sometimes subconsciously, to avoid it. A range of coping mechanisms to reduce anxiety to a tolerable level can be manifest in observable behaviour and are important aspects of living; in psychological and psychiatric literature they are recognised as denial, fantasy, projection, rationalisation, regression, and withdrawal to name but a few.

When, however, the stress is of great intensity and long duration, especially in a susceptible person who has not developed effective coping mechanisms, general systemic changes may occur and cause what are sometimes called psychosomatic disorders such as coronary heart disease, asthma, and ulcerative colitis. Apart from adverse physical sequelae, some studies have shown that when an individual feels unable to alter the stressful circumstances, it leads to a feeling of hopelessness, and eventually pathological depression, categorised as a psychiatric disorder.

The effect on ALs can be far-reaching. For example in a person who is pathologically depressed, there may be withdrawal from communicating unless pressed to respond; disinterest in eating and drinking; difficulty with eliminating such as constipation; disinclination for work or leisure activities; disruption of the sleeping rhythm and so on depending on the severity of the depressed state.

It is important, therefore, for nurses to have knowledge of psychological factors which influence ALs. It is important when dealing with a healthy person because even coming in contact with a nurse for advice on health, or for immunisation to prevent illness, may induce anxiety. How much more so when the person comes into hospital. Not only is the individual anxious about the cause of admission; the strange environment also requires psychological adaptation to the disruption of normal patterns of living such as eating and drinking, eliminating, and sleeping.

The nurse must be sensitive to individual differences in the speed of adaptation to anxiety-producing circumstances. The speed of adaptation is probably more evident at the extreme ends of the lifespan, and will require especially careful handling if the person belongs to a sociocultural group with which the nurse is less familiar.

Sociocultural factors

It is essential that nurses should have knowledge of sociocultural factors and how they influence ALs. In the model for nursing, therefore, social, cultural, spiritual, religious and ethical factors are introduced to indicate how this knowledge helps the nurse to understand, assess, plan and implement nursing interventions, and evaluate the effects. There is no attempt to cover the disciplines of sociology and anthropology in this textbook. General points only are made at this stage to show how this type of knowledge (along with other subjects in the curriculum) contributes to an understanding of human beings as manifest in their various Activities of Living. More specific examples of the application of sociocultural concepts to each AL are provided in Chapters 6–17.

Different systems of health care throughout the world show that culture influences the way societies deal with health and illness. Deep-rooted cultural beliefs and traditions affect an individual's behaviour when ill — for example, responses to pain vary according to ethnic origin. Also cultural factors influence the way people treat others who are ill so that some types of handicap and certain diseases carry a degree of stigma in some societies. The mentally handicapped may be shunned or feared even today because of the legacy of the view once held that idiocy was inflicted on people as punishment for their sins. Sociocultural factors are therefore important in understanding an individual's health behaviour and people's varied responses to illness and hospitalisation.

Of particular interest to those involved in the delivery of health care is what happens to an individual's *role and status* when he becomes ill. Talcott Parsons, a sociologist, described this phenomenon in what he termed the '*sick role*' (Parsons, 1966). He pointed out that most societies exempt a sick person from some of his usual obligations and responsibilities as long as he fulfils a corresponding obligation to seek medical care and cooperate in the process of getting well. In many parts of the world there is in fact legislation to ensure that the sick are given special entitlements; for example, there are government schemes which provide the employee with sickness leave along with protection from financial hardship caused by loss of earnings (p. 273).

However, as more recent writers have pointed out, there are many social implications of illness not considered in Parsons' analysis. It does not acknowledge the subjectivity involved in defining 'health' and 'illness' or take account of the fact that some sick people will never get 'well' (Bond & Bond, 1986) and others may not wish to co-operate in attempts to restore them to health.

Certainly, assuming the role of 'patient' involves many role changes: for example, a young mother is expected to receive rather than give care; the managing director usually responsible for many employees becomes the responsibility of others; and the lawyer and the miner are treated as equals despite occupying quite different social positions in real life.

It is not just roles which change during illness or hospitalisation, but also *relationships*. For example, the doctors' high social status is still reflected in the way some patients tend to behave subserviently to them, submitting to their authority and accepting their advice unquestioningly. Such behaviour also serves to reinforce the traditional asymmetrical doctor-patient relationship. In fact, throughout the whole health care system there is an elaborate set of expectations and rules about the kinds of interaction considered to be appropriate between members of different health care professions and between professionals and patients, although this is changing.

There is also an important correlation between *social class* and health status. Infant mortality tends to be higher in the lower social classes; a baby born into a working-class home being more likely to have a lower birth weight and more likely to die in the first week of life. In general there are differences in the types of illnesses that affect members of high and low social classes. For example, statistics show that heart disease is more prevalent among professional people and respiratory conditions are more common among working-class groups. Not only are there differences in morbidity, there are also differences in mortality rates and interest in such data has re-emerged in the past decade both nationally and internationally (Fox, 1988).

There is also an apparent correlation between social class and response to illness. The best possible use of health services tends to be made by members of the higher social classes; others often fail to take advantage of provisions such as child health or family planning clinics. Sociologists have made a considerable contribution to for example, the analysis of inequalities in health, thus assisting health professionals to understand certain aspects of the aetiology of illness and some determinants of health.

The influence of *religion* on individual behaviour in relation to health and illness is a particularly fascinating aspect of the sociocultural factors, religious doctrines often dictating a very circumscribed lifestyle (Neuberger, 1987). Nurses must be aware of these practices so that every patient's religious and spiritual needs may be appreciated.

Many religions have regulations affecting eating and drinking habits which will affect nursing activities. Orthodox Jews, for instance, consider every meal a religious rite and must eat specially prepared 'kosher' food at all times. Muslims consider the pig an unclean animal and observe total fasting throughout the daylight hours in the month of Ramadan. Of great importance to Hindus is cleanliness as bathing renders one not only physically, but spiritually clean; traditionally the right hand is used for clean tasks only, the mouth is rinsed out after each meal and the anal region is washed after defaecation. Expressing sexuality is yet another activity of living sometimes influenced by religious beliefs and customs: limitations on birth control are imposed on Roman Catholics and Jews, and the Muslim religion prohibits free mixing socially of the sexes.

A person's religious beliefs may also influence his attitudes to health and health care and sometimes may present an obstacle to care and recovery. It is well-known that Jehovah's Witnesses are not allowed to accept a blood transfusion and that Christian Scientists believe in the healing of illness by spiritual means.

For many people, however, religion provides a source of hope and comfort during illness. Sometimes, as in the Roman Catholic church, special sacraments may be offered to the sick and the dying. Baptism, thought by some to be necessary for a person's salvation, is carried out for any infant in danger of death or for a stillborn child (or fetus). The Sacrament of the Anointing of the Sick (formerly known as Extreme Unction or Last Rites) is often performed for a Roman Catholic during illness to aid healing and give moral strength or as a preparation for death. In general, for the dying and the bereaved, religion often assumes a role of great importance, and this subject is returned to in Chapter 17. In fact religion, as a social institution, plays a key role in determining attitudes and customs on matters of life and death in nearly every existing society, regardless of whether the members actively practise the religion.

A concept which is more encompassing than organised religion is *spirituality*, interpreted as a 'search for meaning' in one's life; it involves theistic and non-theistic approaches which can apply to agnostics and atheists as well as to followers of recognised religious persuasions. People who declare themselves agnostics or atheists may still require what Labun (1987) calls spiritual care. Discussing 'Spiritual care: an element of nursing care planning', Labun maintains that during illness, a person with no defined religious belief may wish to explore feelings, values and life with another person; perhaps a close friend, family member or a religious person, or perhaps with the nurse as the person most available, and most aware of the patient's thoughts and feelings. Labun concludes, however, that further exploration of the topic of spirituality is needed before nurses will be able to utilise this potential in a nursing plan.

Inevitably, as it is dealing with human beings, health care has *ethical* aspects. Since the compilation of the Hippocratic Oath in 420 BC, doctors have attempted to arrive at common principles of ethics in health care, but nurses and other health professional groups have also sought common principles to guide their practice, for example the Code for Nurses (ICN, 1973). In essence, such codes concern themselves with, for example, duty to do good and no harm; respect for life and human dignity; justice to individuals such as non-discrimination on the basis of race, sex, religion, political affiliation, social standing, handicap and mental disorder; equal opportunity in terms of access to resources including preventive and treatment services; duty to protect the vulnerable. Discussing fundamental ethical principles in health care, Thompson (1987) acknowledges the primacy of such principles and maintains that the way they are put into practice will depend on the individual's culture and type of experience, and the kinds of criteria used for interpreting, applying and justifying them. One instance of such a dilemma relates to the controversy over emergency resuscitation. Should this technique be used in every instance when breathing and heart rate appear to have ceased? Or are there some instances when the individual should be allowed to die with dignity instead of attempting to prolong an existence where there is no longer any quality of life? To provide guidance for nursing practice, the Royal College of Nursing has produced a Code on Resuscitation and Thom (1988) quotes the Code in a well referenced article which discusses this moral dilemma.

In this section, some of the concepts associated with sociocultural aspects of nursing have been mentioned in order to provide background to the discussion of their influence on each of the ALs in Chapters 6–17.

Environmental factors

As in the model of living, environmental factors cannot be considered in isolation in the model for nursing. They are related to physical, psychological and sociocultural factors which have already been described, and also to politicoeconomic factors which will be discussed later. They are necessarily related to the other components of the model for nursing; for instance a person's stage on the lifespan will influence the type of relevant environmental information required when assessing, planning, implementing and individualising a nursing plan. The same applies regarding a person's status on the dependence/independence continuum. Knowledge from other parts of the curriculum needs to be synthesised into a nursing context so that the environment can be manipulated to achieve people's optimal level of independence for carrying out their ALs. Chapters 6–17 provide specific examples of how environmental factors can influence a particular AL; here, to provide a background to Chapters 6–17, a few general points are made about their influence on a composite of ALs.

Atmospheric pollutants can be both particulate inorganic and organic matter as, for example, in dust, and the minimisation of dust is an important contribution to the prevention of infection, whether people are in their own home, or a health clinic, or in hospital. The organic matter can be in the form of pathogenic microorganisms, some of which cause specific infectious diseases. To give just one example of how they can influence ALs — in the case of mumps, painful swallowing will affect eating and drinking, whereas the accompanying fever will affect controlling body temperature. Other pathogenic microorganisms cause inflammation, for instance in the intestinal tract as happens in food poisoning; they can settle directly from the atmosphere onto food, or they can be transferred to food by vectors (particularly flies), or by unclean hands. The three ALs which are most likely to be influenced are eating and drinking, eliminating and controlling body temperature. There are many nursing implications but one prime example is the importance of handwashing (to remove both resident and transient flora) before handling food, after visiting the toilet and after handling excreta.

Light has many positive uses in a health context, for example to assist in the examination of body orifices. Light from an auroscope is used to examine the external auditory canal which can reveal conditions interfering with hearing, and thereby communicating. Similarly, an ophthalmoscope is used to examine the eye, with the objective of identifying conditions which interfere with sight; also associated with communicating. Yet another example is the bronchoscope for investigating the bronchi when a person is experiencing problems related to breathing. Light can now be transmitted through flexible glass fibres (fibreoptics) and these have been incorporated into the modern bronchoscopes (and other endoscopes) enabling the viewer to 'see round corners'.

In any environment excessive light can be tiring for ill people and can prevent them from resting and relaxing or even sleeping, and can be particularly disturbing for dying patients.

Noise needs special consideration in a nursing context. A research report quoted on page 90 shows clearly that noise in hospital wards interferes with sleeping and ipso facto with resting and relaxing. But noise can also be intrusive and interfere with communicating when, for example, a nurse and a patient are discussing sensitive information. And it can lessen the concentration (a dimension of communicating) necessary to relearn, for example, mobilising skills.

Characteristics of the atmosphere relevant in the model for nursing are temperature and humidity which can not only influence several ALs, but also may need to be therapeutically manipulated in, for example, returning the body temperature to normal after it has been raised (hyperthermia) or lowered (hypothermia) to an unacceptable level.

Clothing in a nursing setting influences the same ALs as in the model of living (p. 31) and it is gradually being realised that once patients are ambulant for several hours, the donning of daytime attire has a rehabilitative effect. Personally-marked clothing systems have been introduced in some long-stay wards, and particular emphasis is placed on the use of personal underwear to maintain patients' self-respect and self-esteem. And the concept of bedclothes is important in nursing; they can influence controlling body temperature. Microorganisms adhere to the scales of the skin's outer layer which is continually being shed on to the sheets and when disseminated into the atmosphere may cause hospital-acquired infections, so bedmaking is associated with the AL of maintaining a safe environment.

Objects in many forms are legion in a nursing environment. They include all those mentioned under environmental factors in a model of living (p. 31), and also those referred to in this section in relation to special lighting, not to mention the furniture, furnishings, equipment and the many aids to mobilising: collectively they give some idea of the many ALs which can be influenced by them. With regard to those in more immediate contact with people, modified clothing and bedclothes have been mentioned. Another example is the presence of flowers and plants brought by visitors, communicating to patients, emotions such as love and affection, belongingness, being valued as a person and so on. They are also aesthetically pleasing and may promote a response which, for some people, borders on spirituality.

The buildings which are relevant in a nursing context are the patient's home, clinics, health centres and hospitals. People's homes are relevant on two scores; firstly, should a member of the family require nursing services at home because of illness, the suitability of the physical layout of the rooms in relation to the problematic ALs needs consideration, as well as the availability of lay helpers, usually family members. If the person is very breathless and the house is on two floors, it may be advisable to put the bed in a room which is on the same floor as the toilet/bath room. Discussion with the family will help them to make appropriate decisions about how ALs such as personal cleansing and dressing, and eliminating will be carried out. Secondly, if ill in hospital, it is appropriate to discuss with patients, before discharge, relevant details about the physical layout of their home related to the affected ALs, for example, the availability of the toilet if the patient has been prescribed diuretics.

Environmental facilities available at clinics and health centres can certainly influence several ALs. Clients with an increased frequency of micturition will need to have easily accessible toilets, clearly labelled. Inaccessibility for people with mobilising problems may deter them from seeking help, which may be related to a problem with another AL. Inadequate provision for pushchairs, cycles and cars can deter a wide range of people, for example, parents with young children, as well as disabled drivers of cars, and they may be seeking help with a variety of ALs.

Hospitals just like other buildings reflect the period in which they were built. One hundred years ago, many patients remained in bed for most of their stay, consequently bathing and toilet facilities seem inadequate to cater for the needs of today's mobile patients. And the same applies regarding storage space for clothes. Yet the relearning of dressing skills is especially important for post-stroke patients, and they need to practise with various fastenings. Having several sets of daytime clothes provides for decision-making and matching clothes to mood helps to prevent such conditions as boredom and institutionalisation. Adequate and pleasant surroundings for ambulant patients' leisure activities, and for eating and drinking are often at a premium; and these environmental factors can influence, for example, the ALs of communicating, eating and drinking, and working and playing.

As many hospital buildings were built last century, money is now needed to upgrade them so that they provide occupants with maximum facilities for attending to the ALs. Environmental factors are therefore closely related to politicoeconomic factors.

Politicoeconomic factors

It is essential that the nurse should have some knowledge of politicoeconomic (including legal) factors and how they influence ALs. In the model for nursing, therefore, political, economic and legal factors are introduced to indicate how this helps nurses to understand, assess, plan and implement nursing interventions, and evaluate the effects. There is no attempt to cover these disciplines in this textbook. General points only are made at this stage to show how this type of knowledge (along with other subjects in the nursing curriculum) contributes to an understanding of human beings as manifest in their various activities of living. More specific examples of the application of politicoeconomic concepts to each AL are provided in Chapters 6–17.

Conventionally, health is considered to be the responsibility of the health professions and they are credited with improvements in health and the fight against disease. They deserve some of the accolade. It is often overlooked, however, that the major determinants of health are firmly rooted in prevailing political, economic and social realities. The economic status of the mass of the population in a country undoubtedly affects living conditions and activities of living, which in turn influence health and the incidence of illness.

It is difficult to appreciate just how precarious life could be for the masses in the Western world only 100 years ago. For example, in the 1880s life expectancy (one indicator of health status) for a male child in the UK at birth was 41 years, and for the female was 45 years (HMSO, 1976). As the result of continuing industrialisation, the population was still adapting to the new urban way of life and experiencing new economic problems created by the growth of industry and decline in agriculture. The hastily built towns with poor planning, overcrowding, unsafe water supplies (AL of eating and drinking) and inadequate sanitation (AL of eliminating) were not conducive to the maintenance of health, and the long hours of work (AL of working) for low wages in poorly ventilated factories and mines, with unguarded machinery, accounted for crippling disabilities due to accidents (AL of maintaining a safe environment) and a lowered resistance to many of the prevalent infections.

In the late 19th century there was an enormous sanitary reform movement which, with political support, culminated in the UK in the 1875 Public Health Act. The UK was not alone in the field of health reform. Around this time most other industrialised countries were taking similar legal action, indeed there was beginning to be international cooperation in an attempt to control the various pandemics; national boundaries were no barrier to the spread of infection.

Around the same period, too, in a number of industrialised countries, there was considerable political activity, which, along with the wealth which accompanied the economic industrial boom was focused to improve housing; provide safer food; create facilities for better education. As a result of these better living conditions there was a decline in the incidence of several killer infections and the health status of the masses began to improve even before the discovery of specific preventive and curative measures in the form of immunisation and pharmaceutical products. In factories, working conditions were also improved.

Much of the industrialised world's economic success which was reflected in environmental reform and improved health was associated with acts of parliament. National parliamentary action, however, was sometimes precipitated by the work of voluntary organisations, often working at a local level, not on a nationwide basis. Voluntary organisations did a considerable amount to improve health and well-being, for example by providing free milk for children (the AL of eating and drinking) or warm clothes (the AL of personal cleansing and dressing); or free contraceptives (the AL of expressing sexuality) to mothers who did not have the finance to support yet more children. When responsibility for making basic provision for such activities of everyday living was taken over by the government, it was possible to contribute to the promotion of health on a national scale. It is fascinating to compare the current position in the so-called developing countries.

When the United Nations Organization was established in 1945, many of the developing countries had the same major objectives as the industrialised countries cherished a century before — to develop the economic and social status of their peoples. The major emphasis was on economic development and investment in modern science and technology. An important economic asset in any country of course, is the health of the work force, but during the 1970s, the World Health Organization (WHO) — the health agency of the United Nations Organization — was showing increasing concern about the lack of improvement in the health status of the world's poorer, mainly rural, population. It began to be realised that not only the conventional health professionals were involved in health; it required an integrated approach at government level from, for example, housing, public works, agriculture and education. Even more significantly, the community-based preventive and health promotive services needed the active participation of the people; and to achieve this, political will and cooperation were needed at national and local levels. It is worthwhile to note WHO's 12 indicators for monitoring and evaluating its Global Strategy for Health for All by the year 2000 (World Health Assembly, 1981). It is remarkable how these minimal requirements reflect the state of affairs in industrialised countries about a century ago; and there is a strong politicoeconomic flavour to the indicators.

Of course it is a rare nation that is economically self-sufficient nowadays. Countries and governments are economically interdependent and inexorably intertwined politically. The economic interdependence of richer and poorer nations was graphically described in 'North-South; a programme for survival' (Brandt Report, 1980). Even the best political plans are constantly being overtaken, and the fragile world economy is not helped by the fact that the West is moving out of an industrial economy to a bio-technological economy where robots are already doing the routine, manual chores at the work place and even in the home.

Clearly the economic and social circumstances of an individual's community and the political will of the state exert a considerable influence on the lifestyle and health status of the individual and the family unit; and this will vary from country to country. As an example, in the UK, in the formal health service as such, political and economic circumstances influence the legal provision. Parliamentary Acts enforce the registration of qualified practitioners such as nurses and doctors; for example, the Nurses, Midwives and Health Visitors Act of 1979 regulates the nursing profession and the preparation of its future practitioners. The UK Central Council for Nurses, Midwives and Health Visitors (UKCC), funded by the government, issued in 1983 for example, the Code of Professional Conduct for a Nurse, Midwife or Health Visitor (UKCC, 1983). This is a directive, not a guideline. Parliamentary Acts and legal requirements do not influence only the practitioners in the health service; patients are also involved. Patients with certain types of disorders are protected by the law, for example the Mental Health Act 1983 focuses on the rights of mentally ill people especially regarding consent to treatment (McFadyen, 1989).

In the UK, too, as well as having government regulations related to the practice of the professional groups employed, and to certain groups of patients, the health service itself is a nationalised institution, funded by government and influenced by the economics of the national budget. From costing £450 million in 1949, the health budget is now over £23½ billion (Moore, 1989). Of necessity, the financial allocation to health is finite, yet with technological advances making cure possible for increasingly esoteric disorders, the demand for the relevant expensive treatment is prodigious and cannot always be met; thereby creating considerable ethical dilemmas for both professionals and politicians. Most industrialised countries have similar regulations for similarly organised health services, and for the professional staff who work in them.

So to understand the patient's circumstances, and the nurse's legal duties and responsibilities, the nurse must have background knowledge of the political and economic factors which can, potentially, influence the individual's Activities of Living; and also influence the nurse's professional interventions in helping individuals to practise their Activities of Living in a manner acceptable to the individual and the community.

Although dealt with separately for the purposes of discussion, the five factors and the manner in which they influence ALs are interlinked, to the extent that it can be difficult to make clearcut distinctions between physical, psychological, sociocultural (including spiritual, religious, ethical), environmental, and politicoeconomic (including legal) factors. The five factors are not only linked to each other, they are linked to the ALs, the lifespan, and the dependence/independence continuum; together they combine to influence the fifth component of the model for nursing — individualising nursing.

INDIVIDUALISING NURSING

Individualising nursing is accomplished by using the process of nursing. As indicated earlier (p. 14), this process involves four phases — assessing, planning, implementing and evaluating (see Fig. 5.7) — and these follow on one from another in a constant cycle of activities and feedback. 'The process' is neither a 'model' nor a 'philosophy' as it is sometimes described but simply a method of logical thinking and it needs to be used with an explicit nursing model. This is the rationale for incorporating the process of nursing into the model for nursing.

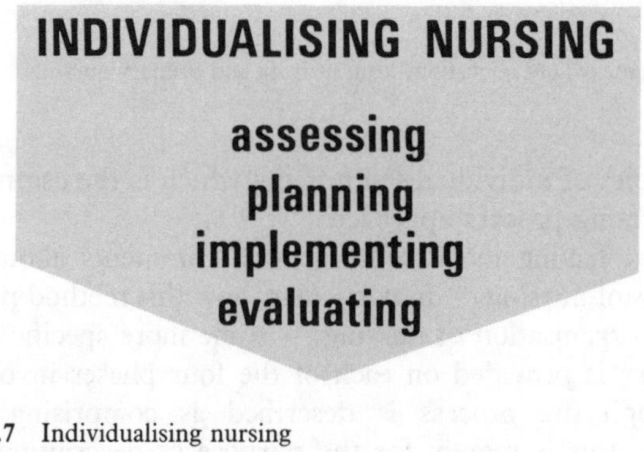

INDIVIDUALISING NURSING

assessing
planning
implementing
evaluating

Fig. 5.7 Individualising nursing

It will be readily apparent that, in the model for nursing, 'Individualising nursing' is developed from its equivalent component in the model of living; namely, 'Individuality in living'. In both models this fifth component takes account of the interaction of the others. We have already stated the rationale for using the model of living as a base for the model for nursing, and the patient's individuality in living should be borne in mind in all four phases of the process of nursing.

Throughout the process the patient should wherever possible be an active participant: for example, making decisions about continuing to carry out certain activities of living and perhaps agreeing to modify others in the interests of health and recovery from illness. Encouraging a sense of personal responsibility for health, and protecting

autonomy even in illness, increasingly are seen as important principles in modern health care, hence the emphasis on viewing the patient as an active participant. Of course participation may not be possible in the case, for example, of a child, a confused or an unconscious person. In these instances family members or significant others may participate in decision-making on behalf of the patient, possibly carrying out some of the activities, as is usually the case when patients are nursed in their own homes.

Patient participation demands a somewhat radical approach to nursing by both patients and nurses. To take patients first — in the past the majority accepted what happened to them while they were in the health care system, assuming that the doctors and nurses 'knew best'. With social changes which have occurred in the last few decades, particularly the influence of the mass media, more and more patients are knowledgeable about what is happening to them and wish to be involved in discussions and decisions about their health and treatment. However, there are still people who are not sufficiently assertive to indicate their desire to be so involved and others who do not wish to be so, and these variations need to be recognised and acted on accordingly by the nurse.

Patient participation has repercussions in nursing which also require recognition. For example, the introduction of a policy allowing self-medication has obvious advantages for patients in terms of independence and preparation for discharge home; but, at the same time, this policy alters the nurse's role to one of teacher and supervisor rather than administrator of drugs and it reduces her control, thereby increasing the risk of errors and mishap.

In a more general sense, use of the process of nursing demands an overall change in approach, not just to individual patients but to the organisation of nursing. The nursing process approach is incompatible with organisation solely in the mode of 'task allocation' or 'job assignment'. This method, based on the industrial concept of 'division of labour', meant that the care of patients was fragmented into a series of jobs, these assigned to different nurses of different grades and thus creating a hierarchy of staff and jobs with no continuity for individual patients; indeed, patients were subordinated to the system rather than central to it.

Dissatisfaction with this method of organising patient care led to the introduction of more patient-centred systems, such as 'patient allocation' (in which each nurse is allocated a small number of patients to look after during a shift) and 'team nursing' (in which a small team of nurses is responsible for a small group of patients). More recently, there has been a growing interest in perhaps the ultimate of patient-centred nursing systems — an approach called 'primary nursing'. The key feature here is that one nurse (the 'primary' nurse) assumes total responsibility for an individual patient and this responsibility theoretically extends over the entire period during which the patient requires

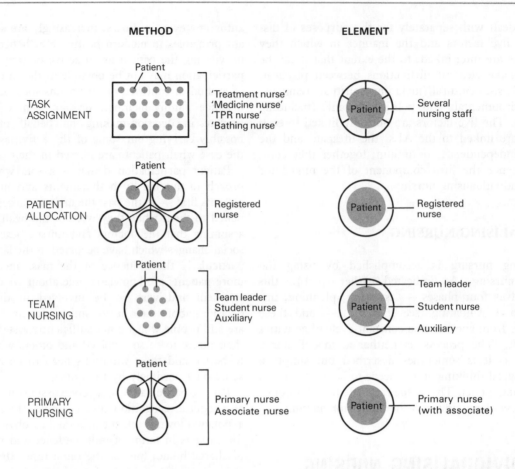

METHOD   **ELEMENT**

TASK ASSIGNMENT — 'Treatment nurse' / 'Medicine nurse' / 'TPR nurse' / 'Bathing nurse'   Several nursing staff

PATIENT ALLOCATION — Registered nurse   Registered nurse

TEAM NURSING — Team leader / Student nurse / Auxiliary   Team leader / Student nurse / Auxiliary

PRIMARY NURSING — Primary nurse / Associate nurse   Primary nurse (with associate)

Fig. 5.8   The organisational method and the element of organisation in task assignment, patient allocation, team nursing and primary nursing

nursing although, in practice, in that nurse's absence the nursing is delegated to others (the 'associate' nurses).

The key features of these various methods of organising nursing are encapsulated in Figure 5.8 in the chronological order described. Although it is true to say, in the UK at least, that 'task assignment' was almost exclusively practised in the 1960s in the context of hospital nursing, it should not be forgotten that nurses in the community inevitably have always operated some form of individualised, patient-centred system. Nor should it be forgotten that 'task assignment' has by no means disappeared, for in some circumstances it may be the only feasible way of ensuring adequate nursing within the limits of available staff numbers. The most stringent staffing requirements of 'primary nursing' are, of course, an important issue but not the main one; much can be learned about the philosophical imperatives of this approach from the writings of nurses such as Zander (1980) in North America who have been developing primary nursing for a considerable number of years prior to the first initiatives in the UK (see Pearson, 1988). There is no doubt that primary nursing fits well with all of the contemporary issues (perhaps especially accountability in nursing) which are being discussed by nurses worldwide. Certainly, primary nursing embodies all of the

principles of individualised nursing which is the essence of the nursing process approach.

Now, having made some general comments about the process of nursing — in particular, how this method relates to the organisation of nursing — some more specific commentary is provided on each of the four phases involved. Although the process is described as comprising four phases, this is merely for the purpose of description and discussion. The implication in describing four phases is that they are carried out sequentially but in reality all four phases are connected. It is important for nurses to realise this from the outset so that thinking will not be rigid and compartmentalised because, in practice, the process operates naturally and flexibly with continuous feedback.

Assessing

The word 'assessment' has been adopted for the first phase of the process of nursing by the majority of nurses. However, we think that over-use of the word assessment encourages the idea that it is a once-only activity and we prefer to use 'assessing' to encourage recognition of the ongoing nature of the activity. There is some dubiety about what assessment includes, so it is necessary to clarify our use of the word; it includes:

- collecting information from/about the patient
- reviewing the collected information
- identifying the patient's problems
- identifying priorities among problems

The information will be gained by observing, interviewing, examining, measuring and testing as appropriate: data gained at the initial assessment form a baseline against which further information can be compared. It is likely that as rapport with the patient is established, more information will be volunteered and, indeed, new and supplementary information becomes available to the nurse in the course of each contact with the patient.

The primary source of information about the patient is the patient. However, secondary sources such as health records and family members are important and especially so in the case of children and disoriented, unconscious or severely mentally ill or handicapped patients. Information volunteered by the patient is classified as subjective, whereas other types of information, such as data from measurement, are objective. The use of objective measures is becoming more common in nursing, partly an outcome of nursing research, and some of the available tools are mentioned in the later chapters of this book; such as Norton's scale for assessing patients' risk of developing pressure sores (p. 222).

In building up a data base for each patient, the initial assessment is of great importance although, as has been said, this is only the beginning and not the end of assessment. The first meeting of nurse and patient may be during admission (whether as an emergency or from the waiting list), or at home, or at a health centre. In hospital, it may well be that after greeting the patient, he is shown his bed, introduced to nearby patients and shown the toilet and bathroom facilities. The rationale for this is that it gives the patient time to settle and become composed before the nurse returns at a suitable time to carry out the 'initial assessment'. However, the patient may be so ill that such civilities become irrelevant and only absolutely essential information is ascertained before the nurses proceed to carry out essential treatment.

Assessing as part of individualising nursing should ideally be carried out as early as possible in the patient's stay. In reality it is often not possible to collect extensive information within a few hours of admission, and McFarlane & Castledine (1982) illustrate a 'first stage history format' which they say 'provides enough information for the nurses to start looking after the patient', then it is followed as soon as possible by using a more detailed second stage format. There are however some topics about which information must be collected early. Any bleeding or injury would of course be assessed immediately; information about pressure sores or any bruises is essential; it is cus-

tomary to record the temperature, pulse and respiration, blood pressure and the result of testing a specimen of urine. It is also necessary for the staff to know of any sensitivities, allergies and any medicines which are currently being taken. All of this information is important to record. Many wards now provide specific stationery on which the information from nursing assessment is written. Beginning nurses may be confused by the various names which are used for it — nursing assessment form, patient assessment form, nursing Kardex, nursing history and patient profile. Whatever the name and format, the objective is to record two different sorts of information: for our purposes, one we call the patient's 'biographical and health data', and the other is 'Activities of Living data' which are concerned with the individual's usual routines and current problems. We designed suitable forms for recording these two different sorts of data; they are illustrated in Figure 5.9 and how they are used for assessing patients is explained below.

Biographical and health data
The patient's biographical and health details include such obvious items as name, sex, age; next of kin and usual place of residence. This list is deceptively simple! But even these apparently straightforward items must be carefully collected. For example, take the name; the custom in Western countries is to use the surname of the family, or in the case of a married woman, the husband's family name; but this is not so in all cultures and nurses may need to seek expert help so that the 'correct' surname is recorded. Likewise it used to be customary to talk about 'Christian' names but with changing social mores the word 'Forename' is now widely used. Increasingly nurses are directed to ask patients what form of address they prefer as some people use a name other than the one on their birth certificate, and use of the familiar one can help them to retain their sense of personal identity. Another sometimes complicated item is the patient's marital status and nurses should be sensitive to the fact that there may be embarrassment over mentioning separation or divorce.

Beneath that item, the form asks for the patient's address and it is becoming more common to record the type of living accommodation — information which is particularly relevant to community nurses on relief duty when visiting patients in their own homes, and indeed for hospital nurses so that they know for instance whether the patient will need to climb stairs at home. Noting the 'mode of entry' to the home may be necessary information for the community nurse who needs to know how to gain entry when, for example, the patient is unable to go to the door. Knowing who else resides with the patient may also be relevant information in certain circumstances.

'Next of kin' requires to be known for legal purposes and, usually, as the person to be contacted if the patient's condition is giving rise to concern. However, a patient who is separated from a spouse may wish to name a partner or, perhaps, an alternative contact as may be necessary if the next of kin is abroad. In contrast, 'Significant others' are important to know in terms of the patient's social network and sources of support. It is usual to record any specific support services being used such as meals-on-wheels or visiting by community nurses as on discharge, arrangements for their resumption may have to be made.

Occupation is a useful piece of information. From a health point of view it may have contributed to the patient's health problem, for example an injury sustained at work, or in other instances there may be implications for return to former employment, for example when an accident causes paraplegia. Recording of key information about religious beliefs and practices is essential if they have implications for care, such as the provision of a special diet. The recording of recent significant life events may sometimes be relevant because illness can follow a life crisis such as bereavement which may impede recovery. In any event it will be important for the nurse to be aware of, and sympathetic to, any major recent events in the life of the patient.

It is useful, too, to know the patient's and the family's perception of the patient's current health problem. Asking the patient about the reason for admission/referral can give an indication of the patient's level of understanding or it can reveal a lack of knowledge; for example, that an 'operation' is scheduled, when in fact it is an investigation. Alongside this the actual reason for admission/referral can be stated and some additional medical information recorded about the patient's diagnosis, past history and any allergies. It is usual to record the address and telephone number of the patient's own doctor and consultant. Finally, the form directs the admitting nurse's thoughts to 'plans for discharge', acknowledging the importance of health teaching, rehabilitation and discharge planning even from the beginning.

So, this outline gives an idea of the sort of information which might be collected at the initial assessment. These biographical and health data are unlikely to change and will be useful and, therefore, should be available to all nursing staff whether the patient's stay is long or short.

Assessing ALs

The second part of assessment focuses on the patient's Activities of Living — the individual's usual routines and current problems. Use of the ALs for assessment is central to our model for nursing. Those who will nurse the patient need to know about usual routines — importantly what the patient can and cannot do independently — and whether or not there are any problems or discomforts associated with any AL; if so, whether these have been experienced previously and if this is the case, how they have been coped with. The following outline provides only an introduction to assessing the ALs because each is developed more comprehensively in its particular chapter in Section 3. The form on which AL assessment information is recorded is deliberately without ruled spaces for each AL so that the nurse can use the space to best advantage for each particular patient, ordering the data in terms of the most problematic ALs first or whatever seems the most appropriate order in the circumstances. A few other general comments about the documentation of AL data and related patients' problems will be made following a brief comment on assessing each of the 12 ALs.

Assessing ability to maintain a safe environment is of particular importance if the patient is physically or mentally handicapped. The nurse needs to know whether or not the patient appreciates the dangers in the environment and knows how to prevent accidents. Assessing the level of safety in the home is an important responsibility of the nurse who visits elderly people or families with young children.

Assessing communicating skills is necessary in order to discover the patient's level of communication and this is important whether in the home, health centre or hospital. It is very important for nurses who have an extensive technical vocabulary to remember that not all patients will be familiar with nursing and medical terms, however ordinary or straightforward they seem to staff. The nurse should observe whether the patient is reticent or forthcoming when talking about home and health problems. It is sometimes possible to discern from the conversation whether the person is gregarious by nature or shy. It may be necessary to gather specific information about one of the sensory organs if the nurse suspects a deficiency or dysfunction which is affecting the patient's AL of communicating. Finally, when assessing this AL, any general information about the patient's pain should be sought and recorded. The rationale for linking pain with the AL of communicating is based on the fact that pain is a subjective experience, its presence and degree is communicated to us by the patient (p. 121). Additional data about pain which affects specific ALs (e.g. abdominal pain affecting the AL of eating and drinking) should be recorded at that AL.

Assessment of breathing may involve counting the number of respirations per minute. For the majority of patients, however, it is simply a case of the nurse noting whether there is an apparent breathing difficulty and asking whether there is the problem of a cough or breathlessness. In turn, this may offer an opportunity to discover whether or not the person smokes and if so how much. The nurse should attempt to discover the patient's perception of the multiple ill-effects of smoking and whether or not help with giving up or reducing smoking would be welcomed. More detailed assessment of breathing is necessary when a patient is unconscious, still under the effects of an anaesthetic or suffering from a disease affecting the cardiopulmonary system. It should be noted that information about haemorrhage (other than bleeding related to a specific AL; e.g. vaginal bleeding would pertain to the AL

Patient Assessment Form : Biographical and health data

Date of admission   Date of assessment   Nurse's signature

Surname   Forenames

Male ☐   Age ☐

Female ☐   Date of birth _____

Single/Married/Widowed/Other

Prefers to be addressed as

Address of usual residence

Type of accommodation
(incl. mode of entry
if relevant)

Family/Others at this residence

Next of kin   Name   Address

Relationship   Tel. no.

Significant others
(incl. relatives/dependants
visitors/helpers
neighbours)

Support services

Occupation

Religious beliefs and relevant practices

Recent significant life events/crises

Patient's perception of current health status

Family's perception of patient's health status

Reason for admission/referral

Medical information (e.g. diagnosis, past history, allergies)

GP Address Tel. no.   Consultant Address Tel. no.

Plans for discharge

Fig. 5.9

Page one   *Roper, Logan, Tierney*   © Longman Group UK Limited 1990

Patient Assessment Form: Assessment of ALs

Date

Activity of living AL	Usual routines: what can/cannot be done independently previous coping mechanisms	Patient's problems: actual / potential (p)

Reminder of the 12 ALs

Maintaining a safe
   environment
Communicating
Breathing
Eating and drinking
Eliminating
Personal cleansing
   and dressing
Controlling body
   temperature
Mobilising
Working and playing
Expressing sexuality
Sleeping
Dying

Fig. 5.9

Page two   *Roper, Logan, Tierney*   © Longman Group UK Limited 1990

Nursing Plan: Related to ALs

Goals	Nursing interventions related to ALs	Evaluation

Roper, Logan, Tierney © Longman Group UK Limited 1990

Nursing Plan: Derived from medical/other prescription

Nursing interventions derived from medical/other prescription	Goals	Evaluation

Other Notes

Fig. 5.9

Roper, Logan, Tierney © Longman Group UK Limited 1990

of expressing sexuality) should be recorded under the AL of breathing on the basis that the cardiopulmonary system is related to this AL.

Assessing eating and drinking routines is relatively easy because most people enjoy talking about this AL. When nursing underweight and overweight patients it is especially important to talk with them about what they eat, as well as when and how much. Nurses will need information about how handicapped people manage this activity. When the patient complains of discomfort associated with eating or drinking, more specific assessment will be required.

Assessing a patient's eliminating habits is a nursing function even though admission to the health care system may not have been associated with bowel or urinary dysfunction. But there may well be a persistent problem with, for example, constipation and this may be elicited from the assessment. Many people find it embarrassing to talk about elimination and the nurse needs to broach the topic with sensitivity and phrase the questions carefully and clearly to avoid embarrassment yet elicit information.

Initial *assessment of personal cleansing habits and dressing* is possible by observing the result of these activities; ill-cared-for clothes may be an indication of financial hardship or a lack of self-esteem which can characterise exhaustion or mental illness. The nurse may discover unhygienic practices, for example related to cleaning teeth or lack of handwashing after visiting the toilet. With this knowledge the nurse can plan to include relevant teaching in the nursing plan. It should be noted that assessment of the AL of personal cleansing and dressing should include an assessment of the patient's skin status (including signs of bruising which could be from abuse) and an assessment of the person's risk of developing pressure sores. The rationale for including this here is on the basis of the link between the integumentary system and the AL.

Assessing control of body temperature usually involves taking the temperature with a thermometer on admission and regular measurement may become necessary if the patient is suffering from pyrexia or hypothermia. There are other ways of assessing this AL — observation may reveal flushing of the skin, excessive perspiration, the presence of goose flesh, shivering, and excessively hot or cold hands and/or feet.

When *assessing mobilising*, initially it may only be necessary to observe that the patient does not appear to have any problems. But later observation might reveal, for example, stiffness of the joints on rising after sleep, a common occurrence for the older person. People who have persistent back pain often adopt a posture to minimise low back movement which is noticeable. Other mobilising problems are usually self-evident and nurses need to know how the patient copes with them and detailed information should be obtained on this from physically handicapped patients so that nursing can be planned to enable maximum independence to be retained.

Assessing working and playing routines is an essential part of an initial assessment. By the way the patient talks about these activities, the nurse will gather what is considered challenging and what boring. The physical conditions at the patient's place of work may have contributed to the accident or illness which has necessitated admission to hospital. On the other hand, difficulty in social relationships because of personality problems or mental illness may be revealed or suspected, and difficulties inherent in enforced unemployment would be important to know about for patients in that situation.

Assessing the AL of expressing sexuality involves observing how people express their gender in a general way, for example, in mode of dress, use of cosmetics and so on. Specific assessment is not usually necessary or appropriate unless the patient's problems or potential problems are somehow associated with sex and reproduction; most people find it embarrassing to talk with strangers about this private AL. However, the observant nurse will perceive cues which are expressions of sexuality, or indicators of anxieties related to the AL of expressing sexuality. With sensitivity the nurse can create an atmosphere in which patients feel able to discuss sex-related problems and diseases and a detailed assessment may become necessary in certain circumstances.

Assessing sleeping routines at an early stage is important so that nurses have information on which to base nursing activities aimed at promoting sleep. Patients are not usually admitted to hospital because of a sleep problem as such, but adequate sleep is important for progress towards recovery, whatever the reason for admission and promotion of sleep requires knowledge of the patient's usual routines and use of medication, if any.

Assessing the needs of the dying is a very important role of the nurse in hospital and in the community. Constant sensitivity and acute observation are necessary to recognise whether or not the patient wants to talk about the many aspects associated with death, dying and bereavement. Much more is discussed about assessing the needs and problems of the dying in the chapter on the AL of dying (Ch. 17).

Assessing is not a once-only activity and additional data will be collected as the nurses have further opportunity to observe patients and talk with them in the course of their nursing. Whether additional data is obtained and recorded on a daily basis or less frequently will depend on factors such as the patient's condition, length of stay in hospital, or frequency of visits in the case of a patient at home. And, equally, the amount and type of information collected about the ALs will vary according to different circumstances and, in some, information about all of the ALs may not be relevant. Assessing therefore is not a rigid routine carried out at a particular time and in a set pattern; it is an ongoing activity and one which requires to be tailored to the circumstances of the individual patient.

Assessing is just as applicable to patients who are in the health care system for surveillance or maintenance of health as for those who are in hospital for investigation and/or treatment of illness. Some nurses think that the identification of patients' problems is not applicable to health maintenance and promotion, but in healthy living the aim is to avoid potential problems from becoming actual ones and the process of identifying potential problems with the ALs is the same as that involved in the identification of actual problems.

Whatever the person's health/illness status, while collecting information about the patient's ALs the nurse will necessarily take account of the stage on the lifespan, one of the components of the model. There is a reminder to consider the patient's 'Previous routines' and it is necessary to remember that these will have been fashioned by physical, psychological, sociocultural, environmental and politicoeconomic factors — another component of the model. The nurse is reminded of the dependence/independence continuum of the model by the heading 'what can/cannot be done independently'. And there is a prompt 'previous coping mechanisms' for the nurse to remember that if there are problems or discomforts with any of the ALs, enquiry should be made about how these have been coped with.

In summary, then, the objective in collecting information about the ALs is to discover:

- previous routines
- what the patient can do independently
- what the patient cannot do independently
- what problems the patient has, both actual and potential, with the ALs.

Identifying patients' problems

Identifying the patient's problems is the final activity of the assessing phase of the process of nursing. In many cases, the presence of *actual* problems (such as pain, bleeding, anorexia, pyrexia) will be obvious to the patient and to the nurse. But it has to be remembered that there can be a 'nurse-perceived problem' of which the patient is not aware (raised blood pressure being an obvious example); and, also possible, a 'patient-perceived problem' (such as a particular worry) of which the nurse is not immediately aware. Being alert to these possibilities will ensure that they are explored in the course of assessment.

When it comes to identifying *potential* problems, the nurse's greater knowledge of factors which predispose to ill-health, and are complications of illness and treatment, make it possible to collect information which the patient may not volunteer without prompting. It is the concept of potential problems which also highlights the aspects of nursing which are concerned with the maintenance and promotion of health.

A statement of the patient's problems, as ascertained from the nursing assessment, is increasingly being referred to as 'a nursing diagnosis'. In an article entitled 'Can nurses diagnose?' Marks-Maran (1983) says that the garage mechanic tells her that he has 'diagnosed' what is wrong with her car; he is not afraid of the word 'diagnosis'. A reluctance to use this term in nursing, at least in the UK, may be for the reason that 'diagnosis' is traditionally the doctor's role. But, in fact, a nursing diagnosis is a description of the problems which patients experience with ALs, whereas the medical diagnosis is usually concerned with pathological changes. Returning to Marks-Maran's article, she states that a patient with one medical diagnosis may have several nursing diagnoses. The development and classification of nursing diagnoses has advanced in recent years, particularly in North America where there is an extensive literature and Gordon (1979) is regarded as a classic reference.

In this model, however, the term nursing diagnosis is not used and we prefer the simpler idea of 'patient's problems with the ALs'. The proforma (p. 56) provides space for each problem identified from assessment to be listed, alongside the related AL, and specified as 'actual' or 'potential' (by noting 'p' against the latter). Having reached this stage, all that remains before proceeding with planning is to decide on the relative priority among the problems. It hardly needs to be said that life-threatening and health-threatening problems take precedence over other less immediate or less important problems and, among these, the priority will be decided in collaboration with the patient and maybe with the family. The patient's priority may not always be the same as the nurse's, and this must be taken into account for it will affect motivation and cooperation. The priority of problems can be indicated on the form by arranging the problems in order or, alternatively, numbering their priority.

Planning

The second phase of the process of nursing is planning — the objective of the plan being *to prevent* the identified potential problems from becoming actual ones; *to solve* actual problems; where possible *to alleviate* those which cannot be solved; and *to help the patient cope with* those problems which cannot be alleviated or solved.

Setting goals

To achieve this, a goal has to be set for each actual and potential problem (in collaboration with the patient whenever possible and maybe with the family) with a distinction made between short-term and long-term goals. Instead of the word 'goals' some nurses prefer the term 'patient outcomes'; it is a matter of preference.

Goals should be achievable within a patient's individual limits otherwise there is the danger of disheartenment. Whenever possible, goals should be stated in terms of outcomes which are able to be observed, measured or tested so that their subsequent evaluation can be accomplished. Whenever feasible, a time/date should be specified alongside a goal to indicate when evaluation should be undertaken. So the nurse (along with the patient when relevant) sets a goal and estimates when it might be achieved just as the traveller decides on a destination and, according to the mode of travel, estimates the time of arrival. But, it needs to be said, such travelling is considerably less complicated and more certain than nursing!

Preparing a nursing plan

Before nursing plans can be written, account has to be taken of existing resources which in a nursing context may be equipment, personnel and physical environment: and available support services may have to be considered when a patient is being nursed at home. Possible alternative nursing interventions may be determined by the availability of resources and influenced by the patient's expressed preferences. *A plan* is then made of all the proposed nursing interventions to achieve the goals, stated in sufficient detail so that any other nurse, on reading it, would be aware of the plan of nursing. There is no argument against a written plan being essential since no one nurse can be on duty throughout the 24 hours. Social changes such as decreased working hours, and an increase in both annual leave and use of part-time staff, have made it essential for nurses to develop the skill of communicating by writing adequate nursing plans. If such social trends continue, it may well be that the nursing plan will assume even greater importance as a means of communication between nurses. And furthermore, assessing a patient and writing a nursing plan helps the nurse to know the patient which aids the establishment of a satisfactory nurse/patient relationship, the unique basis of the nursing contribution to a patient's health care.

The Nursing Plan which is part of the proforma for use with the model is shown on pages three and four of Figure 5.9. There is a section for noting nurse-initiated interventions (i.e. those derived from problems with ALs) and another section which is for medically-prescribed interventions (e.g. prescriptions for wound or pain management). Explanation of these sections of the Nursing Plan is provided below.

Nursing Plan related to ALs. The Nursing Plan on page three of our document (Fig. 5.9) is related to the ALs and it forms the right side of the double fold. This positioning is deliberate so that the problems, both actual and potential, identified at the initial assessment, do not need to be written again. Opposite the problems the goals are written, together with the 'Nursing interventions' to achieve these; and there is a column in which to record the result of 'Evaluation'.

The Nursing Plan may have nursing interventions at an AL even although there is not a specific problem stated.

An example is when the patient does not have a problem with the AL of personal cleansing and dressing but has a particular preference for a shower rather than a bath. Noting this fact will alert nurses reading the Plan to the patient's preference and deter them from initiating an alternative form of intervention. Similarly, a disabled patient may not have a problem as such with the AL of mobilising as long as aids which are relied on remain available; noting details of the patient's requirements for aided independence will avoid unnecessary dependence on the nursing staff as well as frustration for the patient.

The Nursing Plan is just that — a *plan* which tells nurses what to do and when. Extra information should only be written on it when a goal has been achieved; when the nursing intervention has to be changed to achieve the already set goal; when for any reason the goal has to be modified; when the date for evaluation is changed; or if the patient develops other problems. Other day-to-day information about the patient should be recorded in the Patient's Nursing Notes.

Nursing Plan derived from medical/ other prescription. We have discussed so far the nurse-initiated nursing interventions related to ALs but clearly there are nursing interventions which are derived directly from medical prescription and, increasingly, from the prescriptions of other members of the health care team such as the dietitian or physiotherapist. Although some such prescriptions may be charted separately (e.g. prescribed drugs on the patient's medicine chart), others are not, and it was for this reason that we decided to add this fourth page to the nursing proforma.

At the bottom of this part of the Nursing Plan is a space for 'Other Notes'. The information which could be recorded here might be about the time and place of clinic appointments; arrangements for transport to and from these clinics; and particulars about the loan of equipment, such as a walking frame for the patient to use at home. These examples alert the nurse to the fact that planning is necessary for the patient's discharge. However, there is no constraint on the type of relevant information which nurses may record in this space.

Summarising the planning phase of the process — it involves writing a nursing plan which contains the following information: stated goals for each problem; a date on which the goals are expected to be achieved; and the nursing interventions (and patient participation) to achieve the goals. The objective of the nursing plan is to provide the information on which systematic, individualised nursing can be based.

Implementing the nursing plan

Implementing the plan of nursing is the third phase of the process of nursing. Traditionally, nursing has been associated with 'doing', so nurses have little difficulty in knowing how to go about this phase of the process. It is, however, being recognised increasingly that it is both help-ful and necessary for nurses to make explicit the thinking and decision-making which underlie and explain the nurs-ing interventions which they carry out.

Activities which could be described as 'nursing interventions' are many and varied. For any one patient it is likely that the number and range of nursing interventions carried out will far exceed those specifically listed in the Nursing Plan. It is likely that the Plan will include all the essential and important 'main' interventions but, alongside carrying out these particular, specified activities, the nurse will be doing many other things as well. In carrying out nursing interventions, the nurse draws on an amalgam of skills — from listening, talking and observing to helping and, perhaps, deliberately not helping — in her contact with the patient over time. It may be that some of the 'unplanned' or apparently 'unimportant' interventions of this kind seem to merit recording. Such a record can be made alongside the 'daily report' on the patient. The proforma for use with the model does not contain a section for these purposes and we suggest the use of a separate sheet or document which could be called 'Patient's Nursing Notes'. These would contain information supplementary to the Patient Assessment Form and Nursing Plan. Such in-formation could be helpful for purposes of evaluating nursing intervention.

Evaluating

It is difficult to justify planning and implementing nursing interventions if the outcome cannot be shown to have benefited the patient in some way. Hence, the fourth phase of the process of nursing — evaluating — is crucial and, in turn, it provides a basis for ongoing assessment and planning as the patient's circumstances and problems change.

The evaluating phase of the process has caused difficult-ies for nurses. This is not surprising because evaluation is an extremely difficult and complex matter and this is true not only in respect of nursing. Put simply, the objective of evaluating is to find out whether or not (or to what extent) the goals which were set have been (or are being) achieved. In this sense, evaluation is of the type known as 'outcome evaluation'. The skills which are used in evaluating are es-sentially similar to those used in assessing — observing, questioning, examining, testing and measuring. Whereas they are used in assessing to provide baseline data, in evaluating they are used to discover whether or not the set goals are being or have been achieved: in other words evaluating involves comparison against an objective.

Goal achievement in effect cancels the nursing interven-tion. However, it may be necessary to ask the question 'Was the goal set too low?' and a reconsideration of the original goal setting might answer this question. In the ab-

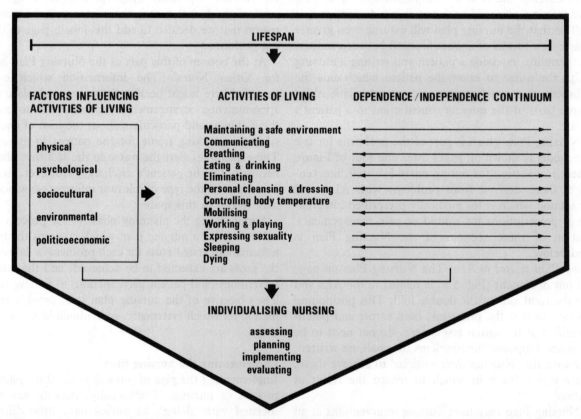

Fig. 5.10 Diagram of the model for nursing

sence of complete goal achievement the nurse might ask:

- is it partially achieved and is more information needed before reconsidering whether or not to continue the intervention?
- is the problem unchanged/static and should the nursing intervention be changed or stopped?
- is there a worsening of the problem and should the goal and the planned nursing intervention be reviewed?
- was the goal incorrectly stated or inappropriate?

All of these possibilities rest on the assumption that the goal was achieved or not, solely by the nursing intervention and, in many instances, this cannot be assumed. Nurses need to recognise that the contribution by other health workers in a multidisciplinary team inevitably influences and interacts with their own intervention and, indeed, it is seldom possible to isolate out the nursing intervention and, therefore, directly and unequivocally link the 'outcome' with 'input'. Thus, the evaluating phase of the nursing process is beset with complexities and an important challenge for the future in nursing will be to improve and extend our evaluation skills.

In this chapter it has been shown how the model for nursing (Fig. 5.10) is developed from the model of living which was discussed in Chapter 4. The 12 ALs are the main component of the model for nursing and are influenced by the others — lifespan, dependence/independence continuum and the factors influencing ALs: physical, psychological, sociocultural, environmental and politicoeconomic factors. All these components interact and have to be considered when individualising nursing, which in our model is synonymous with the process of nursing.

Because the 12 ALs are the main focus of the model, each AL will be discussed in a separate chapter in Section 3. Of course it is only for the purpose of discussion that each AL is considered separately; in reality they are closely related.

REFERENCES

Bond J, Bond S 1986 Sociology and health care. Churchill Livingstone, Edinburgh

Craig A 1989 Why old means gold to the marketing men. Sunday Telegraph March 19: 11

Departments of Health and Social Security 1976 Prevention and health: everybody's business: a re-assessment of public and personal health. HMSO, London

Drennan V 1988 Celebrating age. Nursing Times (Community Outlook) June: 4–6

Duldt T, Griffin K 1985 Theoretical perspectives for nursing. Little, Brown, Boston, p 5

Fawcett J 1984 Analysis and evaluation of conceptual models of nursing. F A Davis, Philadelphia

Fox J 1988 Social network reaction; new jargon in health inequalities. British Medical Journal 297(6645) August 6: 373–374

Gordon M 1979 The concept of nursing diagnosis. Nursing Clinics of North America 14: 487–496

Independent Commission on International Development Issues 1980 North-South: a programme for survival. Pan Books, London (Brandt Report)

International Council of Nurses 1973 Code for nurses: ethical concepts applied to nursing. ICN, Geneva

Labun E 1987 Spiritual care: an element in nursing care planning. Journal of Advanced Nursing 13: 314–320

Marks-Maran D 1983 Can nurses diagnose? Nursing Times 79(4) January 26: 68–69

McFadyen J 1989 Who will speak for me? Nursing Times 85(6) February 8: 45–48 (Mental Health Act 1983)

McFarlane J, Castledine G 1982 A guide to the practice of nursing using the process of nursing. Mosby, St Louis, ch 4

Mitchell J 1984 Is nursing any business of the doctors? A simple guide to the 'nursing process'. Nursing Times 80(19) May 9: 28–32

Moore J 1989 A health service for people. In: People as patients and patients as people. Office of Health Economics, London

Neuberger J 1987 Caring for people of different religions. Lisa Sainsbury Foundation, London

O'Brien M 1982 The need for spiritual integrity. In: Yura H, Walsh M (eds) Human needs and the nursing process. Appleton-Century-Crofts, Norwalk, Connecticut, p 85–95

Parsons T 1966 On becoming a patient. In: Fola J, Deck E (eds) A sociological framework for patient care. Wiley, New York

Pearson A (ed) 1988 Primary nursing: Nursing in the Burford and Oxford Nursing Development Units. Croom Helm, London

Thom A 1988 Who decides? Nursing Times 85(2) January 11: 35–37

Thompson I 1987 Fundamental ethical principles in health care. British Medical Journal 295(6611) December 5: 1461–1465

Tierney A 1984 Defending the process. Nursing Times 80(20) May 16: 38–41

United Kingdom Central Council for Nurses, Midwives and Health Visitors 1983 Code of Professional Conduct for a Nurse, Midwife or Health Visitor. UKCC, London

World Health Assembly (34th) adopts global strategy for Health for All 1981 WHO Chronicle 35(4): 118–142

Zander K S 1980 Primary nursing: development and management. An Aspen Publication

Nursing and the Activities of Living

6

Maintaining a safe environment

The activity of maintaining a safe environment

Every day people are engaged in many activities with the specific purpose of maintaining a safe environment, whether at home or at work or at play or travelling. In order to maintain health, both personal and public, much energy has to be directed at maintaining an external environment which is as safe as possible, not only for the present but for future generations to inherit.

THE NATURE OF MAINTAINING A SAFE ENVIRONMENT

Throughout history man has been concerned with controlling the external environment or adapting to its vagaries. To an amazing degree man has conquered the dangers inherent in the physical environment and has devised methods of protecting his family, his dwelling, his crops and his livestock. Most humans no longer live in constant threat of danger, although there are powerful natural forces such as earthquakes, floods and drought which man is impotent to control. The fact that this is the case is illustrated by events in recent history, such as devastating forest fires in the USA in 1988, the virtually annual floods in the Indian subcontinent in the wake of the monsoon rains, and the continuing drought in parts of the African continent which have taken the lives and livelihood of countless people. It should not be forgotten either that in this so-called era of peace, there are wars going on in many parts of the world which means that some people are living in an unsafe environment and in constant danger.

Even under normal circumstances, however, people

throughout the world are still exposed to a variety of environmental hazards which jeopardise their safety, health, happiness and, indeed, survival. Increasingly too, in this age of technological and scientific advancement, there are yet new hazards to contend with — such as the risks associated with radiation, chemical waste, the illicit use of drugs and modern war weaponry — and these, in contrast to natural forces, have been created by man himself.

There are many dimensions to the AL of maintaining a safe environment and, obviously not all can be discussed in this chapter. Many different kinds of activities contribute to maintaining a safe physical environment and, because most are essentially *preventive* in nature, the remainder of this section considers the following topics:

- preventing accidents
- preventing fire
- preventing infection
- preventing pollution

Preventing accidents

Accidents can occur anywhere and at any time. Frequently, though not always, they are avoidable. Preventing accidents — in the home, at work, at play and while travelling — can and should be everyone's concern, both for their own personal safety and for others. The human suffering which results from an accident can be severe and can result in some form of life-long disablement or disfigurement for the victim, not forgetting the stress and guilt which is borne by the person who may have had some responsibility for the accident occurring.

In recent years the problem of accidents and accident prevention has come very much to the fore because the huge scale of the problem is now recognised. In Europe, accidents are now the third most important cause of death, and yet fatalities represent only the tip of the iceberg.

Accidents in childhood are of particular concern. They are currently the single most common cause of death in England and Wales accounting for about one-third of all child deaths. Accident injuries are also a major cause of morbidity in childhood, and the reason for a substantial proportion of hospital admissions among children in the 1–14 age groups (Constantinides, 1987). Constantinides went on to discuss the permanent disability rate of 18.6–20 per 100 000 children per annum following accidents (road accidents, recreational accidents, and burns and scalds), and the type of disability included brain damage; deformity; loss of mobility; scarring; and sensory loss mainly due to eye injuries. Discussing the aftermath of accidents involving burns, Forshaw (1987) maintains that the psychological damage, and indeed the necessary treatment, are as traumatic as the injury itself.

Injuries due to accidents are not random events. They show clear regional, age, sex and social class variation; boys consistently show more accident injuries than girls and there is a steep social class gradient in child accident fatalities. In a study in London carried out by Constantinides & Walker (1986) to look at all types of accidents in under-5s, there was a statistical correlation between more serious child accidents and unemployment, overcrowding, and lack of parental education beyond secondary school. Injuries due to accidents they say, even if minor, are distressing events for children, parents and carers and great skill and tact are required during the follow-up period because parents often continue to feel guilty, anxious and defensive.

Internationally, the scale of the problem is similar. The WHO (1986) reported that in industrialised countries, accident injuries rank fifth among the leading causes of death in children and young people. It is now generally realised that unless something is done to reduce accidents, other measures taken for the good of a nation's health are being undermined. Health care professionals have a vital role to play in accident prevention, though the problem needs to be tackled by multidisciplinary effort, organised at national and international levels. Health education is an important aspect of prevention but that is unlikely to be effective in the absence of increased safety measures and legislation. Individual effort is also vital. Accident prevention cannot be viewed only in terms of the elimination of hazards. The potential for accidents will always exist, so each individual must become skilled at maintaining safety in the face of hazards inherent in the environment. Some of the ways in which this can be achieved are described in the discussion which follows of preventing accidents *in the home; at work; at play; and while travelling.*

Preventing accidents in the home

Most people probably think of their home as a 'safe' place but, in reality, the average home is potentially a very dangerous environment. Even in countries where housing standards have improved immeasurably, and the promotion of safety in the home has been of long-standing concern, the problem of accidents is one of some magnitude.

The Royal Society for the Prevention of Accidents Annual Report (1986) in the UK quotes that there are 5700 deaths and 3 million people injured each year in home accidents at an annual cost to the NHS of about £350 million. As has already been mentioned, young children are particularly at risk, and they are dependent on adults to protect them from the potential dangers in their home environment.

What then are some of the hazards in the home environment which can cause accidents? Some different groups of hazards are described below, along with related preventive measures.

There are *fire* hazards. Open fires are increasingly less common in homes today but, where they do exist, the crawling child and toddler need to be protected. A large safety guard securely fixed to the wall will prevent a child coming into contact with a fire, and children's nightwear should be flame resistant. Unfortunately, much modern household furniture is a fire hazard, and burning cigarette ends in chairs, settees, or beds can cause serious accidents not only because of the flames, but due to suffocation caused by noxious fumes from materials used in the manufacture of modern upholstery.

In recent years, so great has been evidence of the death toll due to noxious fumes, that legislation about furniture was enacted in the UK in 1988 — the Furniture and Furnishings (Fire) (Safety) Regulations (Statutory Instrument No. 1324). The regulations are phased. From November 1988, among other things, manufacturers must use foam which passes the ignitability test, and foam-filled furniture must carry permanent labelling; from March 1989, all furniture must pass the cigarette test; from March 1990, all furniture must have match-resistant covers; and from March 1993, all secondhand furniture must comply with 1988 regulations. Not only manufacturers are involved; retailers must ensure that appropriate labels are displayed, and records of furniture supplied must be retained for 5 years and be available for inspection by the Trading Standards Office.

There are *electrical* hazards. No matter how new and safe the wiring in a home, there is always the danger of injury and electrocution. Faulty electrical appliances should be repaired by an electrician and even simple procedures, such as fixing a new plug or renewing a light bulb, can be hazardous if a mistake is made. In any home where there is a young child, socket guards should be fitted to prevent a finger or pencil being poked into a potentially dangerous electrical socket.

There are *chemical* hazards. Poisoning comes high on the list of accident cases, especially to children, and all toxic substances should be kept labelled and carefully stored in a safe place, preferably a specific cupboard in the kitchen, bathroom, garage or garden shed. Wherever they are kept, they should be out of reach of children and, where appropriate, under lock and key. The increasing use of child-proof containers for medicines is helpful, but vigilence is still necessary. It is unwise to keep medications in a handbag which could be lost or might be explored by a child, with disastrous results. Apart from medicines, there are many other potentially dangerous chemicals, solid or liquid, which may be in any ordinary home: for example, substances for cleaning and decorating, and killing weeds and rodents. One particularly toxic cleaner found in the kitchen is dish-washer powder. One should not forget other commonly used substances, such as bleach and hair dye or nail polish and perfumes, which may well be left out in the bathroom or bedroom.

There are *thermal* hazards. If tapwater is very hot, it can easily scald sensitive skin and one precaution is to run the cold water into the bath before turning on the hot tap. Hot liquids, whether in a kettle or pot on the cooker, or in cups on the table or in the hand, should always be dealt with carefully, especially when there are young children because even an apparently small volume of liquid can cause severe scalding.

Hot food and drinks should not be placed on a table where there is an overhanging tablecloth; in a second, a scalding accident can occur if a child pulls on the overhanging end of the cloth. Another potentially lethal hazard has been identified when baby-walkers are used (Gray, 1987); it is easy for the child to reach out and pull on a kettle flex or iron flex which perhaps seemed safely tucked away and despite the apparent pleasure derived from baby-walkers, there is enough evidence of related accidents to recommend that they should not be used. Other hazards in the kitchen include the hot cooker and hot baking utensils although protecting the hands and wrists with heat-resistant gloves helps to avoid burns.

There are hazards associated with *sharp equipment*. In the home, there are scissors, pins and needles used for sewing; razor blades in the bathroom; sharp knives and, possibly, a food processor with sharp blades in the kitchen; nails and other sharp instruments in the toolbox; and shears and other tools in the garden shed. All need to be used and stored with forethought and care, especially in the interests of children.

There are hazards associated with *house design*. Safety should be considered in relation to positioning of lighting in the house and access areas, particularly where there are steps or stairs. Provision of a stair guard, and secure door and window locks, are sensible precautions with children. For elderly people, grab rails at strategic places (including the bathroom/toilet) and use of a non-slip bath mat are devices likely to prevent accidents. Similarly, use of non-slip polish and non-skid pads under rugs, and prompt repair or replacement of frayed carpets, will help to keep the floor trip-free. Glass is another danger and modern house design tends to favour large areas of glazing — glass doors and full length glass panels, either fixed or sliding — to allow for maximum natural lighting. Safety glazing is effective but the high cost sometimes prohibits its use in private dwellings. However, one inexpensive precaution is to apply self-adhesive warning stickers on the glass at eye level: for example, on a patio door which someone might inadvertently walk or run into while their attention is fixed on the garden beyond.

Whatever precautions are taken to minimise the hazards mentioned, accidents still can and do happen. At the risk of repetition, it is worth mentioning again that children (especially those of preschool age) are particularly vulnerable to home accidents. Kendall (1986) reminds us that accidents in infancy are related to what the child can do, so are related to stage of development, and quotes the relative incidence:

0–3 months   — suffocation, smothering, choking, strangulation by clothing

3–6 months   — burns, scalds, falls (causes of most head injuries), choking

6–12 months — falls, cuts and bruises, burns and scalds, choking, poisoning, drowning

As the child's mobility increases, accidents are often related to play, and when constant adult surveillance cannot be assured, young children can at least be protected by being put in a playpen or securely fastened in a bouncing cradle (placed on the floor), highchair or pram. However, physical restraint is not a solution to accident prevention and, indeed, excessive over protection will only deny a child the opportunity to explore and learn about the environment. All children have to develop a concept of safety and an ability to cope with the hazards which exist in that environment. Parents and, depending on the circumstances, grandparents and childminders too, have a vital role to play in preventing accidents in the home.

Because they go into homes, health visitors have a unique opportunity to assess levels of safety and to offer appropriate guidance and help to parents. However, to accomplish this, nurses need to be well informed about the subject of home accidents. Articles by Moore, Ray and Ahamed are collected together, along with a fact sheet, in an issue of 'Community Outlook' (1982) which is devoted to the subject of home accidents and clearly shows that there are many ways in which the nursing profession can contribute to their prevention; although these articles are not recent, they contain useful information which is still relevant. But others, too, must accept their share of responsibility for safety in the home. They include house designers and manufacturers, especially those concerned with the production of child safety equipment (CAPT, 1986), children's furniture and toys; and household products, especially commonly used chemicals and other potentially dangerous substances and articles.

Apart from children, the other groups most vulnerable to accidents in the home are those at the other end of the lifespan, the elderly, particularly those in the over 75 age group. Falls are of particular concern. There is a high mortality associated with old people who lie undetected for a long time, both related to the injury sustained and to complications; such as hypothermia, dehydration, bronchopneumonia and breakdown of pressure areas (Wild et al, 1981). Fear of this happening may cause old people to be admitted to residential homes though, as Blake & Morfit (1986) show, falls are by no means uncommon in that setting either.

In the community, the fact that many simple, preventive measures are possible is well illustrated in an article by Mitchell (1984) and these range from encouraging elderly people to wear well-fitting shoes rather than slippers, to the use of alarm systems, and the involvement of neighbours and regular callers to an old person's house. Again, as in childhood accidents, prevention of accidents in the home to the elderly requires a variety of approaches. Everything possible needs to be tried if, as the numbers of elderly people increase by the year, the sought-after goal of independent life at home in the community is to be achieved. The organisation, Age Concern, designated 1989 as the year for a Focus on Falls Campaign in order to attract support from orthopaedic surgeons, health authority general managers, and social work directors (Women's Herald, 1989).

Preventing accidents at work
Even when at work the AL of maintaining a safe environment cannot be forgotten. Carelessness when cigarette- or pipe-smoking is a well documented cause of accidents and in many work places, smoking is now forbidden in designated areas because of the fire hazard (quite apart from public concern about smoking-related diseases p. 131). In certain industries, indeed, smoking is a major hazard and employees are prohibited from taking matches, lighters and cigarettes into the work area. But associated with the prohibition is the education and training of workers so that they are aware of the dangers and understand the reason for preventive action.

What has already been said about thermal hazards can also apply at work. Where automatic stoking equipment is not in use, furnace workers wear heat-resistant clothing, especially gloves; and also goggles to protect eyes from glare and sparks. This also applies where substances like molten steel, glass and tar are poured. In some climates, outdoor workers have to be trained to take protective measures against exposure to long periods of sunlight leading to dehydration because of perspiration loss; or to heat stroke; or after long exposure, to an increasing rise in the incidence of skin cancer (Nichols, 1988).

At the other end of the scale, there are industries where excessive cold is used such as refrigeration in the fishing industry, and cold storage rooms in the catering business. Workers need to understand how quickly human tissue freezes, and the necessary precautions to prevent its occurrence. Workers who can be exposed to excessively cold weather conditions have not only to know about survival measures during over-exposure, but be able and willing to carry them out.

Workers in the pharmaceutical industry and in laboratories obviously have to be knowledgeable and skilled to avoid the many chemical hazards which can threaten the safety of their environment. When the chemicals could damage the skin or the eyes, adequate protection is essential. And in establishments where workers handle infected material, for example in laboratories or in hospital laundries, strict contamination control measures and protective clothing are obligatory.

Where workers make sharp equipment, or use machines

with cutting edges and moving parts, use of adequate guarding is essential to maintain safety in their environment. Wherever possible automatic safety factors are built into the machines, for instance by making them unworkable unless the guards are in place. If this is not the case, it is imperative that workers build safety factors into their work pattern from the beginning and there is usually work training to underscore this.

Some groups of health care workers are subject to certain types of injury and accident. For example, back injury is common among nurses and there is growing concern about the need to instruct nurses in proper lifting techniques (p. 252) and to encourage them to use mechanical lifting devices as much as possible. Exposure to radiation is another area of concern, affecting radiologists, doctors, dentists and nurses who are involved in the use of X-ray procedures and care of patients undergoing treatment with radioactive substances. Female staff of childbearing age, particularly women who are known to be pregnant, require special protection from radiation hazards and there are codes of practice which apply to radiotherapy and X-ray procedures.

Quite apart from radiation hazards in the health care sector, there is concern about the magnitude of the risk of cancer for workers in the nuclear industry itself. In an attempt to quantify the risk, the Ministry of Defence in the UK commissioned a study of staff engaged in atomic weapons research at Aldermaston and associated establishments who had had repeated exposure to low levels of ionising radiation. A total of 22 552 workers were followed up on an average of 18.6 years. Overall mortality was 23% lower than the national average for all causes of death and 18% lower for cancer. For a small group of workers, however, who had experienced above average external exposure and had also been monitored for internal contamination by radionuclides, the mortality from cancer of the prostate gland and the lung was raised (Beral et al, 1988). In workforces in the USA, excess mortality from prostatic cancer has also been reported in the Oak Ridge National Laboratory and in a weapon plant but, Beral et al continue, recent data from the Japanese atomic bomb survivors show no association between a single acute exposure to high levels of radiation and mortality from prostatic cancer. The authors indicate therefore that excesses of prostatic cancer in industrial workforces are unlikely to be due to external radiation. Cancers in other specific body sites were also monitored and compared with surveys from other countries but more research requires to be done.

Certainly following the far-flung effects of the disaster at the Chernobyl nuclear power station in 1986, the health hazards associated with nuclear products have been highlighted, not only for employees and people in the immediate environs of a nuclear plant but also for people and terrain far distant from the scene of the nuclear leak. Considerable public pressure is being put on governments and large companies to utilise energy sources other than nuclear power for industry and commerce, and there are strident demands for stricter supervision to prevent accidents and to monitor the disposal of nuclear waste products. According to the International Herald Tribune (Keller, 1988) there are reports from Moscow that five planned Soviet nuclear power stations have been cancelled since the 1986 disaster in the Ukraine.

So important is the subject of a safe work environment that most countries have legislation requiring protective practices at all places of employment. Standards are set for ventilation, heating, lighting, hygiene, safety features of tools and equipment, fire precautions, first aid facilities and provision is made for occupational health services. In the UK, the Health and Safety at Work Act 1974 is an important piece of legislation in this respect. It imposes statutory obligations on employers to set down and implement policy to safeguard the health and safety of their employees. However, the employees also have responsibilities and are required both to exercise reasonable care, and to cooperate with their employers' health and safety policies. More is said about the subject of safety in the ALs of working and playing.

At international level, the International Labour Organization (ILO) and the World Health Organization (WHO) collaborate to produce various recommendations which seek to establish worldwide standards of safety with the purpose of preventing avoidable accidents at work.

Preventing accidents at play

It seems paradoxical that man must attend to the AL of maintaining a safe environment even during leisure activities. But for those who choose arduous outdoor recreations like climbing, water sports and ski-ing this is particularly so. Suitable attire is essential; careful attention should be paid to the weather and its forecast; and extra rations and a heat-reflective sheet for warmth must be carried if there is any possibility of encountering adverse environmental conditions.

Those who pursue water-related sports should learn to respect natural events like tides and floods. For safety they should cooperate when local authorities display signs, warning that the seashore is dangerous. Becoming a competent swimmer is obviously sensible and for those who sail a knowledge of seamanship is essential. Sailing is becoming much more popular in the UK and from the USA comes a warning about personal standards of responsibility while enjoying water-related recreation. Williams & Gonzalez (1987) highlight the increasing problem in the number of accidents caused by drinking and driving afloat. According to the National Safety Council boating accidents are the second leading cause of transport injuries, and the US Coastguard estimates that at least half of those accidents are alcohol-related. Discussing the ever mounting toll, they maintain that 'combined with the effects of all the sun, wind, spray, vibration and happy fatigue which go with boating, even moderate amounts of alcohol can be dangerous'.

Even at festive times like Christmas, extra safety precautions need to be taken with Christmas trees, fairy lights and decorations. Extra precautions are necessary on other occasions when bonfires and fireworks form part of the festivities. An increasing number of countries are moving towards a policy of prohibiting the sale of fireworks to the public and instead, having organised displays operated by experts; ensuring that there is careful segregation of spectators from staff who are igniting the fireworks.

In spite of knowledge of precautions, injuries from accidents during sport and leisure activities are common-place and account for a significant proportion of emergency admission to hospitals. This may reflect the fact that many people today have more leisure and money to spend on such pursuits than in the past. Certainly sports such as motor-cycling, hang-gliding, ski-ing, skating, yachting, diving, skate-boarding, marathon running and squash have become popular among a broad cross-section of the community. All of these, some more than others, carry the risk of injury from accidents and even the safety of some long-standing sports — notably rugby — has become the focus of attention. It has been roundly criticised because of the risk of cervical spinal cord injury, and there has been a plea for changes in the rules to make it safer (Burry & Calcinai, 1988). Boxing has been the subject of adverse criticism for some time (Corsellis, 1989).

It is not only players of a sport who risk injury, but in some cases the spectators too, and for example the problem of 'football hooliganism' has become a matter of concern in the UK. In an attempt to prevent violence and injury, steps have been taken to combat drunkenness at football matches and to improve crowd control. Of course even in a well-controlled crowd there are bound to be accidents when many thousands of spectators are gathered together, and Sadler (1983) describes the medical problems which commonly occur and how they are managed on such a large scale, with particular reference to the nurse's role.

In the main, sporting accidents affect young adults; the more challenging and potentially dangerous sports inevitably appeal to people in that age group. However, accidents do happen to school-age children in the course of play, and consistent with the activities of this age group, they suffer fewer accidents in the home (compared with pre-school age children) but more accidents outdoors and in the school playground. The results of a study undertaken in Cardiff (Wales, UK) of 10 000 school children injured by accident are reported by Maddocks (1981). In the 5–9 year age group, 15% of injuries happened in school and 24% out of doors (compared with 23% at home); and for 10–15- year-olds, 29% occurred in school and 26% out of doors (compared with 11% at home). The comment is made that the proportion of accidents in school is high,

considering the relatively small part of total time spent there. It is also relevant to note that 55% of injuries which occurred at school happened in the playground. Some schools have attempted to increase playground safety but here again, as in the home, preventing accidents needs to balance the necessity of supervision and restriction in the interests of safety, against the need for children to enjoy themselves and to develop a sense of personal responsibility for their own safety.

Preventing accidents while travelling
Every person has a responsibility for maintaining safety while travelling. Laws and regulations can lay down safety standards but individuals have to comply with those standards. Ignorance is no plea in law, so people have to be taught about safety while travelling, and encouraged to develop a positive attitude and strict self-discipline in relation to prevention of accidents.

This is said to be the 'age of travel'. Certainly this century has seen incredible advances in the speed of travel, both inter-city and international, and in the distances people travel — indeed as far as the moon. Holidays and business trips abroad are now commonplace occurrences and an elaborate network of international communication attempts to ensure the safety of travellers by land, sea and air. There are also carefully planned strategies to cope with emergencies and the victims of major travel accidents, wherever they may occur in the world.

At national level, the major concern is with preventing accidents on the roads. According to Central Statistical Office data (1988) the largest number of road casualties per hour coincide with the times of day when traffic is at its heaviest, reaching a peak between 5 and 6 p.m. and with a secondary peak between 8 and 9 a.m. Child casualties peak between 3 and 4 p.m. with a secondary peak at lunchtime. Making international comparisons between seven EEC countries, Japan and USA, the data shows that the UK had the lowest death rate of these nine (9.4 per 100 000 population) and Portugal the highest in the EEC countries with 30.2 per 100 000 population.

Safe road surfaces, adequate street lighting and sign posting, compulsory driving tests, road use regulations, compulsory speed limits and minimum mechanical safety standards for vehicles are all examples of measures taken by national governments to maintain a safe environment on the roads and to prevent accidents. In addition, many governments have extended legislation to other areas, for example, laws which permit police to use a breathalyser test to detect and detain drivers who have been drinking in excess of the alcohol limit.

It is obviously still a necessary preventive measure because in a recent survey reported by Eason (1989) involving 1576 motorists, when asked whether they obeyed speed limits and other road laws, 5% admitted driving while over the alcohol limit. Extrapolated, this figure means that as many as 1.5 million British drivers regularly drive after drinking too much. The UK government is concerned about the number of deaths caused by careless driving while unfit because of excessive alcohol consumption, and a recent White Paper, *The Road User and the Law*, recommends among other things, that this offence should carry obligatory disqualification from driving for at least 2 years, an unlimited fine and a maximum penalty of 5 years' imprisonment (Lowry, 1989).

In an increasing number of countries, use of seat belts in cars is now obligatory. Even in the short time since the introduction of seat belt legislation in January 1983 in the UK, there has been a demonstrable reduction (of approximately 25%) in the number of deaths and serious injuries (e.g. internal chest injuries and fractured skull) among front seat car occupants. Pressure groups are now campaigning for the law to be extended to cover back seat passengers too, principally with the safety of children in mind but also to protect front seat occupants who can be injured in a crash if an unrestrained person in the back is thrown forward. Pending such legislation, improved baby carriers are constantly being produced, and many manufacturers now fit back seat belts into new cars. It is interesting to see how a law has so rapidly effected a dramatic and important change in people's behaviour concerning safety while travelling where even aggressive publicity campaigns apparently failed to make the necessary impact.

In a number of countries for some years, the wearing of crash helmets by motor cyclists has been obligatory. Currently, in an endeavour to reduce serious injury and fatalities, especially among children and teenagers, brightly-coloured helmets for pedal cyclists are becoming popular. Most pedal cycle deaths are caused by severe head injuries and a recent Australian study suggests that head injuries can be substantially reduced by wearing helmets, indeed certain schools insist on their use by children who cycle to school (Doyle, 1988).

Apart from the risks to car drivers, passengers, and cyclists themselves however, *pedestrian* casualty figures are also alarming. Safety campaigns aimed solely at pedestrians are not sufficient in view of the fact that a substantial proportion of pedestrians are struck by vehicles and killed or injured, not on the road but on the pavement.

Preventing accidents while travelling is an enormously complex issue. Legislation has a part to play in maintaining safety but individuals have a responsibility to control personal behaviour for their own benefit as well as for the survival and well-being of others.

Preventing fire

Any activity which aims at preventing fire is a component of the AL of maintaining a safe environment. These activities are an essential part of living and in many countries there are educational pamphlets and programmes from several sources to spread knowledge about fire hazards and to encourage self-discipline in carrying out precautions.

At a domestic level, fire can be prevented by maintaining equipment in a safe working condition, for example repairing frayed flexes, avoiding trailing flexes, ensuring that electrical circuits are not overloaded, having fires adequately guarded, and using self-extinguishing devices for movable articles which can be knocked over with relative ease such as oil lamps and oil-heaters. In the kitchen, a major contribution to safety is carefulness when using fat for cooking purposes; if it ignites, the most effective way of controlling the blaze is to cover the pan with a lid or metal tray and turn off the heat supply to the cooking apparatus. Individuals are responsible for fire safety in their own homes but most householders insure against the possibility of accidental fire damage to the fabric of their home and to the contents.

For public buildings — shops, hotels, warehouses — proprietors have the responsibility to take adequate precautions against fire and there is legislation which permits inspection of premises to ensure that the necessary safety measures are enforced. Despite precautions human carelessness can precipitate the utter devastation caused by fire. Unsafe disposal of lighted cigarette ends has been thought to cause many fires involving buildings used by the public, for example the football stadium disaster in Bradford, England in1985 and the King's Cross Underground station fire in London in 1987. Similar tragedies can occur even in rather unusual settings and caused by a different train of events, for example the North Sea Piper Alpha episode 1988, where staff died either on the blazing oil installation or drowned in the surrounding sea of fire. Such disasters with heavy loss of life and the untold misery of injury and scarring for survivors, highlight the need for closer supervision of existing preventive strategies; greater staff awareness of alarm and rescue measures; and increasing vigilance on the part of companies and individuals to reduce human error.

When fire does occur, detecting, containing and extinguishing the flames are the three main principles of immediate action. Smoke detectors may give the first alarm but detection is often by smell and by seeing smoke and flames. Combustion cannot continue in the absence of oxygen and certain commercially produced fire extinguishers work on this principle. If sufficiently limited in extent, however, merely smothering the fire with thick material will cut off the atmospheric oxygen supply and extinguish the flames. Closed windows and doors help to contain smoke and flames for about 20 minutes, and as inhaled smoke can immobilise people who are attempting to escape, these vital minutes may permit a more orderly evacuation from other parts of the building, and simultaneously allow time for professional help to arrive. Most countries have a paid, professional fire brigade who are expert in fire fighting. They also, however, contribute to fire prevention and play a considerable part in educating the public, especially school children, to become more fire prevention conscious.

Apart from conflagrations in buildings, environmental fires can occur. For example in hot dry weather, carelessly attended picnic fires and inadequate disposal of lighted cigarette ends can start a forest fire, although ignition can occur spontaneously from the heat produced by sun shining through glass carelessly left lying on the ground especially near dry shrubland and trees. Obviously knowledge as well as self-discipline is necessary to prevent accidents and maintain a safe environment.

Preventing infection
An essential dimension of the AL of maintaining a safe environment is preventing infection. Infection results from the successful invasion of the body by pathogenic microorganisms and, because these are ever-present in the environment, preventing infection is a fundamental issue in disease prevention and health promotion. Much is now known about the biological characteristics of pathogens and the epidemiology of infection, and successful methods have been developed which can inhibit the growth and spread, and harmful effects of these organisms. However, while public health measures at national and international levels can do much to prevent and control infection, the participation of individuals is vital because of the continuing importance of many basic personal and domestic hygiene activities. Therefore, everyone requires to understand about the sources of infection, the modes of transmission of pathogenic microorganisms, human portals of entry, susceptibility to infection and principles basic to the control of infection. These topics are discussed in detail in textbooks dealing with microbiology but are outlined briefly in the remainder of this section and the main points of the first three subjects are summarised in Figure 6.1.

Sources of infection. The source of infection is the site where the pathogenic organism grows and multiplies. The natural warmth of the human body encourages microorganisms to multiply rapidly. However for pathogens to establish themselves in the human body they must be in the right place, in sufficient numbers and be sufficiently virulent. The body's defence mechanisms against infection — immunity (p. 82) — can usually cope with small numbers and the body only succumbs to infection when the invading numbers are large or when, for various reasons, resistance is lowered.

Pathogens are usually species specific and, therefore, the most common sources of infection in man are human beings themselves. The skin and all body orifices are colonised with microorganisms shortly after birth; indeed, the body acts as 'host' to these microorganisms which are called commensals, and are referred to as the body's natural or *resident flora*. They are not usually pathogenic but can become so under certain circumstances, for example when the body's immune system is not functioning

SOURCES OF INFECTION: EXAMPLES

● human sources	– auto-infection: a person who contaminates himself at a site other than the original infected source
	– other humans: person who is incubating an infection
	: person who is suffering from an infection
	: person who is recovering from an infection
	: a carrier – person who is not affected but is harbouring pathogens
● animal sources	– e.g. dogs, cows, monkeys
	– e.g. birds, insects
● inanimate sources	– soil

MODES OF TRANSMISSION: EXAMPLES

● by direct contact	– direct transmission from an infected person to another person as in certain skin diseases, sexually-transmitted diseases and some respiratory infections
● by fomites	– indirect transmission from infected person to another via inanimate objects in the environment
● by airborne droplets and dust	– infected person sprays pathogens into the air when breathing/coughing/sneezing/talking/laughing: pathogens fall to the floor and mix with dust
● by contaminated food and drink	– infection (e.g. from infected food handler) transmitted in food and drink
● by animals/insects	– mechanical transmission (e.g. pathogens carried on the body/legs) or spread of pathogens by blood-sucking insects

HUMAN PORTALS OF ENTRY: EXAMPLES

● by the placenta	– to the fetus from the mother's blood supply, e.g. syphilis, rubella
● by inhalation	– entry of airborne pathogens, e.g. common cold, measles, whooping cough, diphtheria, respiratory tuberculosis
● by ingestion	– pathogens in food and drink are ingested and digested, e.g. dysentery, typhoid, gastroenteritis, brucellosis, and bacterial food poisoning
● by the skin	– infection of skin and mucous membrane by direct contact, e.g. certain skin diseases, conjunctivitis, infective foot disorders, sexually-transmitted diseases
● by invasion of tissue	– via a cut in the skin or surgical wound (e.g. staphylococcal infection)
	– via the bite of an animal or insect

Fig. 6.1 Infection: summary of sources of infection, modes of transmission and human portals of entry

adequately, or when they are transferred to another part of the body, usually by the hands. A good example of the latter is the transference of commensals such as *E. coli*, from the anal area, to the entrance of the female urethra, leading to infection of the urinary tract. When tissue begins to react to the commensals causing inflammation, the process of colonisation has given way to infection. Therefore people can infect themselves and auto-infection, as it is called, is important to recognise as a source of infection.

Quite apart from resident flora, *transient flora* may cause infection. They can be acquired from other people and any form of interpersonal contact may allow microorganisms to be transmitted from one person to another. The source of infection may be a person who is incubating an infectious disease, or actually suffering from an infection, or recovering from one, or a carrier who is personally not affected but is harbouring pathogens which can infect others.

Animals provide another source of infection in the environment and, like humans, animals can harbour and spread pathogenic microorganisms. The common house fly can carry many different pathogens; the mosquito carries malaria and yellow fever; brucellosis can be contracted from milk cows; and rabies in man results from a bite by an infected dog. These are just a few examples of animal-borne infection to which humans are susceptible.

A few infections arise from inanimate sources: for example, pathogens that cause tetanus are harboured in the soil.

Modes of transmission. In order to understand how infection is spread, it is necessary to know about the various modes of transmission.

These are noted in Figure 6.1 and are briefly discussed below.

Direct contact is most likely to lead to infection of the skin, conjunctiva or mucous membrane. Skin diseases, such as impetigo or scabies, are transmitted by direct contact. The sexually-transmitted diseases (e.g. syphilis, gonorrhoea, AIDS and non-specific urethritis) are so-called because they occur as a result of direct sexual contact with an infected partner. Some oral and respiratory infections follow direct contact: for example, infectious mononucleosis (glandular fever) is frequently described as the 'kissing disease'. Direct hand contact can transmit infection from one person to another or, in the same person, from one location to another. For this reason, *handwashing is the single most important personal activity in preventing infection,* so it is essential that people wash their hands after going to the toilet and before touching food.

Indirect contact involves transmission by fomites (inanimate objects in the environment such as clothing, bedclothes, crockery and cutlery, instruments and furniture) and these can act as reservoirs for infection. Fomites with smooth hard surfaces e.g. glass, are easier to clean than those made of fabric. Disinfection by physical and chemical means is important in preventing the spread of infection by fomites.

To prevent the spread of infection by airborne droplets, people should cough and sneeze into a handkerchief, preferably a paper one which can be disposed of by burning or flushing down the toilet. Even during breathing and talking, organisms present in the nasopharynx, throat and mouth are expelled in droplets of secretion. For this reason, masks may be worn by personnel in operating theatres and on other occasions e.g wound dressing, when the patient is likely to be at risk of succumbing to infection. [It should be noted, however, that there is still considerable controversy about the wearing of masks. Ingleston (1986), discussing an updated surgical dressings technique, declares that masks are not needed, while Ayton (1985) questions the use of masks even in theatre and says, 'if there is good ventilation, the levels of airborne contamination may not be altered whether masks are used or not'.]

Droplets also fall to the floor and contribute to the dust and its microbial flora and this mode of transmission is especially important in streptococcal and staphylococcal infection in hospitals, hence the emphasis on reducing dust by damp dusting and vacuum cleaning in this environment. Adequate spacing of beds also helps to prevent direct droplet spread of infection in hospital, as does good ventilation. A person known to have an infectious disease is usually nursed in an isolation cubicle; and barrier nursing is another means of isolation. Many of the common infectious diseases of childhood are transmitted by airborne droplets (e.g. chickenpox) and, therefore, isolation from other children during the period of incubation and infection is a means of preventing spread of these diseases.

Protection of food and drink from contamination, for example by flies, and handwashing before touching food are basic measures to prevent the transmission of infection in food and drink. People who have infected sores, such as boils or styes, or who have diarrhoeal conditions, should not prepare food, especially when it is to be distributed to large numbers. Contaminated food, water or milk can result in an epidemic outbreak and these infections, such as the salmonelloses and bacillary dysentery, are further spread by unwashed hands contaminated with faeces. Milk and food can also be contaminated by infection in the animals which provide them and preventing the transmission of such disease (e.g. brucellosis) involves strict control over the source and supply of animal food products for human consumption. Animals can also transmit infection on their bodies, as can insects (e.g. flies becoming contaminated with faeces) and many widespread epidemic infections are transmitted by blood-sucking insects such as the mosquito which causes malaria.

Human portals of entry. The microorganism must invade the body tissues before infection results and, following invasion, infection will develop only if the body defence mechanisms fail to prevent multiplication of the pathogen. There are various portals of entry. Even before birth, the fetus can be infected from the mother's blood via the placenta, and for this reason, pregnant women have their blood tested to detect, e.g. syphilis so that treatment can be provided to ensure that the baby is not infected. Rubella (German measles) can cause devastating damage to the fetus in early pregnancy and girls who have not had an attack of this disease by the age of puberty are offered immunisation against this virus so that any baby conceived would be protected, although this should soon be rare in the UK because from 1988, MMR (measles, mumps, rubella) protection has been available to all infants.

Many microorganisms enter the body via the respiratory tract and those who have colds, for example, should minimise the spray from their sneezing and coughing by the use of a paper tissue which can be disposed of safely after one use.

Ingestion is another means by which microorganisms gain entry to the body. The pathogens which cause dysentery, typhoid and some forms of gastroenteritis are excreted in the faeces, so hands contaminated with faeces, if inadvertently put near the mouth, can re-infect the person himself or infect food which may be consumed by others. Strict handwashing routines are imperative to prevent this. Fortunately the technology of the food processing industry is now so sophisticated that infection from this source has been virtually eliminated. However, fresh food, and food consumed which has been prepared and cooked by others, must always be regarded as a potential source of infection. Whether in a large institution, a small restaurant, a bakery, a take-away food shop or the kitchen at home, those who handle and cook food must adhere strictly to the rules of food hygiene. Food poisoning (p. 159) is increasing; in fact, in the UK it is agreed that the published figures grossly underestimate the true incidence (Holmes, 1988). The main types of bacteria responsible are salmonella (mainly in meat and poultry); *Staphylococcus aureus* (the skin and nose of human carriers is the main source); *Clostridium perfringens* (which contaminates raw meat, poultry and some dried products) and listeria, especially associated with cook-chill food products. Raw foodstuffs are the most likely source of food poisoning and foods which encourage bacterial growth are meats and poultry (raw and cooked), foods with a meat base (e.g. soups), eggs, milk and milk products (e.g. cream) A national scare about salmonella in eggs/hens during December 1988 cost the UK government millions of pounds in compensation to farmers, and the increasing incidence of food contamination has given rise to concern about gaps in the UK food hygiene laws. The government plans to announce shortly what it describes as the most far-reaching legislation since 1938 (Editorial, Glasgow Herald 1989). There are three main principles involved in the prevention of food poisoning. Firstly, the spread of contamination is prevented by separating foodstuffs (to avoid cross-contamination); by cleanliness on the part of the foodhandler; and by cleanliness of cooking equipment. Secondly, pathogens already in food can be prevented from multiplying by adequate

refrigeration of perishable foods and avoiding delay between preparation and serving of food. Thirdly, thorough cooking and rapid cooking will usually destroy pathogens although it cannot be relied on to destroy spores or preformed toxins. Holmes provides practical information about the hidden dangers of food and how to overcome them.

The intact skin, usually a barrier to infection, can sometimes be successfully invaded by pathogenic microorganisms, as can the body's mucous membranes (e.g. the conjunctiva). Common examples of infective foot disorders are athlete's foot and verruca, notoriously picked up from public swimming pools and communal bathrooms.

A cut in the skin does potentially allow the entry of pathogens and for this reason even minor cuts and grazes should be attended to properly and observed for signs of infection. Prevention of infection is the objective whenever surgical wounds are cleaned and covered with a sterile dressing or spray. The number of microorganisms on the skin at the time it is cut will depend on how recently the skin was washed or, in the case of surgery, how adequately skin preparation was undertaken.

Invasion of tissue by pathogens may result from the bite of an animal or insect, e.g. rabies is caused by the bite of an infected dog; Marburg disease by the bite of a green monkey; and malaria is caused by the bite of a mosquito.

Susceptibility to infection. People will be less susceptible and more resistant to infection if they have an adequate diet and sufficient exercise, sleep and rest. Tired, malnourished people are prone to infection.

When a person is ill, the body's natural defence mechanisms are already under stress, and therefore, less able than usual to resist the invasion of pathogenic microorganisms. An unfavourable environment may also decrease resistance to infection: for example, prolonged exposure to cold and damp may increase susceptibility to infection. Resistance to specific infectious diseases can be acquired in several ways (p. 82), and, of course, infants during the first few months of life are relatively unsusceptible to many infections because of transplacentally derived immunity.

Prevention of infection. In any scheme aimed at preventing infection, destruction of the pathogenic microorganisms plays a large part. Agents which destroy organisms are called disinfectants or antimicrobial agents, and they are physical or chemical in nature. Physical disinfectants include the natural elements like sunlight and freezing as well as generated heat and cold: chemical disinfectants include liquids and gases. A success story of the 20th century is the discovery of antibiotics, substances which can be introduced into the human body to combat pathogenic microorganisms.

Another approach in preventing infection is based on the principle of isolation. Isolating an infected person has long been used as a means of preventing the spread of infection and has been very effective in campaigns against the more serious and highly infectious diseases, such as smallpox (now eradicated from the world), Lassa fever and tuberculosis. As well as isolating the person suffering from the disease it is, of course, important to locate people who have been in contact with the sufferer and, if necessary, they too must be isolated, treated or kept under surveillance. For this reason, 'contact tracing' has become an integral part of the control of infectious disease. Galbraith (1983) outlines the aims and methods of contact tracing which has been used in recent years in the UK in relation to sexually transmitted disease and tuberculosis, and during limited outbreaks of typhoid fever, diphtheria and Lassa fever; and Brookbanks & Hampstead (1987) describe contact tracing related to hepatitis B.

Measures to increase people's resistance to infection are also important in prevention, and it is in this context that immunisation has played such a major role (p. 82). In the United Kingdom, parents are advised to have their children immunised against diphtheria, tetanus, poliomyelitis, whooping cough, measles mumps and rubella (Renn, 1987). Immunisation against tuberculosis is given to non-reactors to tuberculin in adolescence (the BCG test). Nurses, particularly health visitors, have an important role to play in encouraging parents to take up immunisation and there is concern about falling rates of acceptance. This may be partly due to the fact that in the UK, young parents of today are less aware of the seriousness of some of the diseases as Sieving (1988) points out in her discussion of the ravages of measles in developing countries. There is no doubt too that parents have become more aware that immunisation can carry a risk of adverse reaction and this has been most publicised in relation to the whooping cough vaccine. On the one hand there have been reports suggesting that the vaccine can cause brain damage, albeit in a tiny minority of children and, on the other, the whooping cough epidemics in recent years have re-awakened fears of the damage the disease itself can inflict.

Discussing infectious diseases on an international scale, Rogers (1987) quotes the UNICEF State of the World's Children Report (1987) which indicates that 3.5 million children under the age of 5 die each year from preventable childhood diseases and a further 3.5 million are disabled, mainly in the developing world. Although the numbers have fallen in the last decade, a high proportion of the world's children do not even have the opportunity of having protection from some of the major childhood killers, diseases for which vaccines are available — measles for example is a major cause of childhood mortality. However, an increasing number of countries are committing themselves to the goal of immunising 80% of their children by 1990 under the World Health Organization's Extended Programme on Immunisation (EPI). Of course vaccines alone will not prevent child mortality caused by infectious diseases; better social and economic conditions, and better education about prevention play a major part, as they did in industrialised countries about a century ago.

Apart from immunisation of young children, pregnant women are considered to be a priority group because certain infectious diseases can cause serious damage to the developing fetus. In the UK the rubella vaccine has been offered to all girls in early adolescence and to non-pregnant women of child-bearing age who are found to be serologically negative for this antigen but with the use of the new measles/mumps/rubella (MMR) vaccine to small children (1988), this will eventually become unnecessary. Cytomegalovirus is a less well-known infection which affects considerably greater numbers of babies than rubella. However, although only a minority affected by it develop microcephaly and other conditions associated with mental handicap, it is common and attempts have been made to develop a vaccine which would prevent potential damage.

Indications for vaccination against other infectious diseases (e.g. enteric fevers, cholera, typhus, yellow fever and rabies) depend on individual risk of exposure and international travel regulations. The nature of immunisation programmes as a means of preventing infection is determined according to the prevailing circumstances of a particular country and readers in countries other than the UK should supplement this section with relevant local information.

Nobody now needs to be, nor should be, vaccinated against smallpox. This disease has been eradicated from the world, an achievement which must rank as one of WHO's greatest successes, although some vaccine is being kept in a limited number of centres in case of resurgence of smallpox.

Control of epidemics. Controlling epidemics is important in preventing infection and, in this age of travel, is a concern which extends beyond the boundaries of any one nation; it requires international collaboration. Incidence of infection in each country is notified to the World Health Organization so that necessary strategies can be implemented to prevent spread to other countries by travellers, cargoes and animals. An account of the spread of cholera through Asia and Europe in the 1830s is given by Swan (1983) and makes interesting reading even today.

A current threat which exercises considerable concern in the UK is rabies, and it has recently been highlighted by the decision to build a Channel tunnel. Rabies was indigenous to the UK before successful eradication at the turn of the century. However, the threat of importation of the disease has returned, not only on a small scale relating to violation of quarantine regulations by dog owners but because the rabies virus has been spread throughout Europe into France (UK's nearest continental neighbour) by the red fox and concern is rising too about rabies-infected bats in Europe. If the rabies virus were to take root in the wild life of the UK, domesticated pets would be at risk and so, in turn, would the population. Apparently, however, the European Commission is planning a rabies eradication campaign within the next 4 years; a new vaccine for animals, it is hoped, will enable rabies to be eradicated in Europe (International News, 1988). Concern about rabies may seem a somewhat trivial issue in a discussion of the huge topic of preventing infection, but it serves as a reminder that prevention is a subject which will always be fundamental to maintaining a safe environment, though the precise nature of the concern will vary among countries and over time.

As one disease is conquered or controlled, others appear, particularly those caused by viruses, and finding cures or methods of immunisation is a lengthy exercise. Throughout the world, the virus hepatitis B has recently become a major health problem. Acute and persistent infection is common and the incidence increasing. The carrier state may lead to chronic liver disease including chronic active hepatitis, cirrhosis and hepatocellular carcinoma (Brookbanks & Hampstead, 1987). High rates of infection have been found in neonates of carrier mothers, sexual contacts of carriers especially among homosexual men, intravenous drug abusers, and health care workers exposed to blood and blood products. In 'Controlling an epidemic' Brookbanks & Hampstead describe how they contacted intravenous drug users and their contacts to help stop the spread of an outbreak, and WHO recommend that all health care workers receive vaccination against hepatitis B.

An even more alarming threat throughout the world is the growth in the incidence, and the accompanying high death rate associated with AIDS (acquired immune deficiency syndrome). Essentially it is a sexually-transmitted disease but it is also carried in infected blood and blood products so 'at risk' are intravenous drug users; recipients of blood transfusions, for example haemophiliacs; and anyone who is in contact with the blood of infected individuals. The WHO Special Programme on AIDS (SPA) predicts that by 1991, 1 million new cases of AIDS could develop in people infected with HIV, the human immunodeficiency virus which causes AIDS. A global effort to combat its spread has been mounted by health care staff, international groups, governments and top-level policymakers and in January 1988, health ministers and/or colleagues from 148 countries (representing 95% of the world's population) attended the World Summit of Ministers of Health on Programmes for AIDS Prevention in London, organised jointly by WHO and the UK Health Ministry.

Kay (1988), writing about WHO's strategy, describes recent developments, current preventive programmes and recommended policies, and highlights not only the epidemics of HIV infection and of AIDS, but also the 'global epidemic of social, economic, political and cultural reaction and response to AIDS and HIV infection'. Kay gives an example of the *economic* implications by quoting the statistic that some 20–35% of patients in medical wards of some African hospitals have AIDS or AIDS-related diseases, so the impact on already slender health care resources is obvious. In *socioeconomic* terms, AIDS affects the 20–49 age group, the most vital segment of the population when considering social and economic development. Any social debate about AIDS acquires a *political* dimension with associated prejudice about race, religion, social class and nationality; in fact, it has become a direct threat to free travel between countries and to open international exchange and communication. Kay mentions ideas posited by various groups such as promoting 'sex cards' certifying alleged freedom from HIV infection; stamps or tattoos to identify HIV-infected people; or a type of quarantine in which HIV-infected persons may live in society yet could not marry, be employed or travel; but these have all been rejected as unenforceable or unethical or unacceptable.

It is not surprising that health care staff seek guidance about a syndrome where there is still considerable uncertainty, and the International Council of Nurses issued a Joint Statement with WHO in April 1987, regarding the rights and responsibilities of nurses worldwide in caring for HIV-infected people (ICN/WHO, 1987). This was followed up by joint guidelines on the nursing management of people infected with HIV (ICN/WHO 1988), and WHO declared December 1, 1988, a World AIDS Day to heighten awareness about the disease, and to provide information, as opposed to myth and rumour, about its spread and means of containment. The United Nations Development Programme, the World Medical Association, and the Council of Europe are other examples of transnational organisations which are providing guidelines for controlling the spread of AIDS and offering strategies for collaboration in caring for people who are infected. Further discussion about AIDS and how it affects the individual is included in Chapter 15 dealing with the AL of expressing sexuality.

Preventing pollution

One dimension of maintaining a safe environment is the prevention of pollution. Preventing the pollution of drinking water by untreated human excrement, for example, has long been recognised as a basic health concern. Nowadays, in most industrialised countries, national measures to ensure safe water are taken for granted but in several developing countries, polluted water is a major cause of diarrhoeal disease, often with a high mortality rate. Unfortunately, industrialisation and urbanisation have brought a different set of problems, for example, in relation to air pollution. Admittedly, air pollution has been brought under control over many populous areas as a result of smoke control measures and legislation associated with Clean Air Acts. However, in the USA, the chemical fallout from industry and agriculture has prompted an environmental expert to warn of the many unseen air pollutants which are not covered by the Clean Air Act and are damaging not only to human health — linked to ills from leukaemia to heart disease — but are implicated in the formation of 'acid rain' which has devastated vast tracts of forest (Begley, 1988). Increasingly acid rain is a problem in Europe too.

Not only the air we breathe but the natural waterways of the world are endangered. Disposal of industrial waste into rivers and seas is a major source of water pollution, and a recent article in Newsweek (Hewitt et al, 1988) maintains that we have managed to clog the seas of the world with 20 billion tons of garbage. Coastal waters have suffered most, yet they play the most important role in the chain of life as that is where the majority of marine species spend at least part of their lives, for example in the North Sea many fish have been found to suffer from skin infections, deformed skeletons and tumours. Not only that, sea birds are often the victims of oil spills. Human bathers, too, risk viral hepatitis, skin reactions and oral thrush. However, the article goes on, during the last decade, a United Nations Organization programme has been coordinating the work of environmentalists to halt the scale of pollution, although political will by individual governments is also essential if the fragile ecosystem is to be preserved.

One pollutant which has attracted considerable concern in recent years is lead. Lead occurs widely in nature, in the soil and in the water. In compound form it has come to be used in paint as a pigment, in plastics as a stabiliser and in petrol as an anti-knock agent. Lead has long been used by man and its toxic properties have long been recognised. Severe lead poisoning is a cause of intellectual impairment. It is widely known that there are harmful effects from inhalation of outfall from a lead works; for children who ingest it by licking lead-painted toys; and for families whose drinking water is supplied through lead pipes. Some local authorities have removed lead pipes from the water supply system; and others have provided financial grants to enable house owners to do likewise. However, more recently, concern has shifted to the more insidious problem which affects the entire population — pollution of roadside areas by leaded petrol. Fall-out from exhaust emissions is not only directly inhaled but can be ingested because lead settles on the hands and on vegetables, crops and fruit growing near roadsides. In many countries there has been a phased reduction in the lead content of petrol and in the UK, for example, lead-free petrol is on sale at a lower price, at selected petrol stations (the engine requires a minor adjustment to use it) and there are indications of a move towards the obligatory use of lead-free petrol for all vehicles.

Another concern which has been raised recently in the UK is the excessive amount of aluminium present in some baby milk powders, and this is exacerbated in certain areas of the country where the tap water used in reconstituting the milk also shows a relatively high aluminium content. Excessive aluminium content is conducive to brain and bone damage and is said to contribute to the onset of Alzheimer's disease, a form of dementia, at an older age (Hodgkinson, 1988). Research is in progress to seek further evidence.

An entirely different kind of problem in modern living is 'noise pollution' and that term is increasingly being used to describe the problem of excessive noise. Everyone does not regard noise in the same way. Latin and Anglo-Saxon temperaments are at variance about what would constitute an acceptable noise level; and young people do not seem to be so intolerant of noise as their elders. However, an environment in which people cannot sleep adequately because of excessive noise cannot be considered a safe environment. People who live near noisy factories, close to flight paths near airports, and in the proximity of busy motorways, all suffer from excessive noise by night and day. During the day, other city dwellers can be disturbed by the noise of traffic, especially heavy lorries going past their homes. People who work in heavy industry are subjected to the noise of machines and measures to minimise the effects include the use of noise-abating apparatus and the wearing of ear muffs. As well as affecting sleep, noise is thought to create tension and fatigue, both of which can contribute to accidents and mental ill-health. One of the most serious consequences of excessive noise exposure is partial deafness which may progress to a substantial hearing loss and constitute a severe social handicap.

Preventing pollution is one dimension of maintaining a safe environment which is largely a public rather than a personal responsibility. However, there are many ways in which individuals can protect themselves and others from the potentially dangerous effects of pollutants.

Obviously, the first and foremost purpose in all of the activities discussed — preventing accidents, fire, infection and pollution — is human survival. However, in circumstances when life itself is not threatened, the purpose becomes one of preventing, or at least minimising, injury and ill-health. An accident can result in some form of disablement or disfigurement and, even if its effects are only temporary, the human suffering involved can be intense. The effects of fire can be devastating: the pain of burned tissue, the stigma of visible scars and the loss of property and personal possessions. Infection too can involve discomfort and absence from work; and it can mean isolation. Pollution, though often more insidious in its effects, can cause ill-health and even permanent intellectual impairment.

To sum up, it seems logical to prevent rather than cure but of course prevention as well as being a politicoeconomic consideration, demands knowledge and self-discipline, and for these to be applied, individuals must develop an understanding of the nature and purpose of maintaining a safe environment.

LIFESPAN: EFFECT ON MAINTAINING A SAFE ENVIRONMENT

The inclusion of the lifespan as one component of the model serves as a reminder that living is a lifelong process, from birth to death. Safety is a basic human requirement for survival, development, health and self-fulfilment at every stage of the lifespan.

During prenatal existence, a safe environment is provided by the mother's uterus but, from the moment of birth, a baby becomes instantly exposed to all the hazards in the external environment and is totally dependent on adults for the provision of a safe environment in which to thrive and survive. For young babies, choking and suffocation are major death risks; and protection from accident, infection, and excessive heat or cold is of vital importance. When they become more active and curious, crawling babies and toddlers are increasingly vulnerable to accidents in the home and, as has already been described, falls, burns, scalds and accidental poisoning are major causes of injury and death at this stage of the lifespan.

In contrast, school-age children are most at risk to hazards in the outdoors environment, particularly in the roads and in the school playground. Once at school, children cannot be under constant adult surveillance and learning about safety and personal responsibility for maintaining a safe environment is an important dimension of their education.

During adolescence bicycle accidents and sporting injuries become more common and, although more aware of danger, rebelliousness or over-confidence may result in lack of consideration for personal safety and the safety of others.

For young adults, hazards in the work environment become an added area of responsibility in the AL of maintaining a safe environment and the degree and type of danger vary according to the nature of the work. Adults, especially when they become parents, seem to develop an increasing sense of responsibility concerning safety and may become involved politically over issues of personal, local or national safety, for example, safe road crossings outside schools, and local dumping of nuclear waste.

The process of ageing, which involves a gradual deterioration of physical and intellectual ability and loss of acuity of the senses, inevitably results in lessened ability to carry out the many activities involved in the AL of maintaining a safe environment. Elderly people become more prone to falls often because of arthritic joints or dizziness, are vulnerable to pedestrian accidents perhaps due to lessened acuity in sight and hearing and at risk to the hazards of fire. Maintaining a safe environment during the final stage of the life-span may involve dependence on others

and on safety aids and require renewed awareness of the hazards which are ever-present in the external environment. Cave (1988), editor of the safety magazine of the Royal Society for the Prevention of Accidents (ROSPA), describes how to avoid some of the most common accidents which occur in this age group, and in conjunction with Age Concern, ROSPA had a Home Safety Campaign in 1989.

DEPENDENCE/INDEPENDENCE IN MAINTAINING A SAFE ENVIRONMENT

There are several different aspects of the concept of dependence/independence which is incorporated in the model, and can be considered in relation to the AL of maintaining a safe environment.

The general principle that dependence/independence status is closely linked with an individual's point on the lifespan was outlined in the discussion of the model of living, and is certainly applicable to this AL. Broadly speaking, there is dependence in the early stages of the lifespan; independence during adulthood; and the likelihood of at least some degree of dependence again in old age.

Without question, babies are totally dependent on others for the maintenance of a safe environment and require to be protected from accidents, fire, infection and pollution. Young children are also to a very great extent dependent on adults for their safety. They do not have either the mental or physical equipment to be able to carry out the many complex activities involved in the AL of maintaining a safe environment. Neither do they have any real appreciation of the hazards in the environment or a well-developed understanding of the concepts of safety and personal responsibility for maintaining safety.

Throughout adolescence, such attributes develop but, although more independent, people of this age-group are still dependent on adult guidance and surveillance. In contrast, adults are expected to assume independence for maintaining a safe environment and are involved in doing so in the home, at work, at play and while travelling. In old age, there may be the will to retain independence in this AL but circumstances and the effects of the process of ageing may force an elderly person to be dependent on others, at least to some degree. Financial constraints may limit maintenance of safety in the home: for example, an old person may not be able to afford to replace worn carpets or an ageing electricity system and both are potential causes of accident. In addition, loss of acuity of the senses — particularly impaired sight and hearing — will reduce an elderly person's awareness of danger, for example when crossing roads or when cooking in the kitchen. Even if the senses are acute, physical frailty reduces the ability to take the necessary quick action to avoid accidental injuries, such as by falls or burns.

Although independence in the AL of maintaining a safe environment is the norm during adulthood, the fact that by no means all adults have this capacity is important to recognise. People who are mentally handicapped cannot be expected to cope with many aspects of this AL independently. As they may be engaged in a wide range of adult activities, such as cooking, shopping and so on, their dependence on others for safety is especially important to recognise. Similarly, although many physically handicapped adults are extremely independent in their everyday lives, the AL of maintaining a safe environment is one aspect of living with which they may need considerable help. In addition to dependence on people, a person who is physically handicapped will almost certainly be dependent on aids and equipment; for example, a specially equipped bathroom to minimise the risk of falling while bathing and going to the toilet, and special safety gadgets in the kitchen to ensure that cooking can be accomplished without the risk of being cut or burned.

Another group of people who are unlikely to achieve full independence for maintaining a safe environment in adulthood are those who are visually handicapped. To a remarkable extent, blind people do cope with the many hazards to personal safety which exist but they are likely to be more vulnerable in an unfamiliar environment. Therefore, while they may be independent in their own homes, dependence on others may be necessary in other settings, for example when out of doors or when travelling by public transport. It is interesting to reflect on the value of a guide dog to a blind person as an aid to independence in the AL of maintaining a safe environment.

People who are mentally, physically and visually handicapped have been described in terms of their 'dependence' and this has been compared with the 'independence' enjoyed by intelligent, able-bodied adults in relation to the AL of maintaining a safe environment. However, it is worth pausing to question whether 'independence' in this AL is actually attainable by any adult person, irrespective of mental and physical ability. The fact is that no individual has complete independence in this AL. Irrespective of personal efforts to maintain safety, all people are exposed to dangers — natural forces as well as man-made hazards — which are inherent in the environment and which the individual is impotent to control or eliminate. Equally important, the safety of any individual is dependent on the safe behaviour of others. People can take every precaution to avoid accidents while travelling but cannot guarantee their safety because there are others who drive dangerously, or there are conditions such as poor visibility and icy roads, and these factors are outside their control. Similarly, a person can attempt to avoid infection by washing hands before handling and eating food, but nevertheless, is dependent on others as to whether or not the food itself was free of pathogenic microorganisms when it was purchased. Numerous other examples are easy to think of supporting the idea that complete independence in the AL of maintaining a safe environment is just impossible. Every individual is dependent on others — other ordinary individuals as well as people with special responsibilities for maintaining a safe environment who include, for example, politicians, town planners, public transport personnel, employers and manufacturers, firemen, safety officers and police.

FACTORS INFLUENCING MAINTAINING A SAFE ENVIRONMENT

The AL of maintaining a safe environment is, by nature, multidimensional and therefore, not surprisingly, many different factors play a part in influencing the way individuals carry out the activities involved. In keeping with the relevant component of the model, the factors involved are discussed under the following headings — physical, psychological, sociocultural, environmental and politico-economic factors.

Physical factors

If a person is to carry out the AL of maintaining a safe environment, many of the recognised biological systems are involved. No one system is readily aligned as in the case of the AL of eating and drinking, for example, which is readily associated with the upper alimentary system. However, for maintaining a safe environment, acuity in all of the five senses is obviously important because external safety hazards are identified by means of vision, hearing, touch, smell and taste. Any impairment associated with the senses, therefore, will make a person less able to identify hazards in the environment and, consequently, more likely to have an accident. For example, impaired vision and impaired hearing are obvious limitations on safety as a pedestrian, making such simple tasks as crossing a road a hazardous undertaking. Impairment can be of the sensory receptor, or of the pathway carrying the impulse to the brain, or of the brain's interpreting ability. Even if there is no impairment in an individual's ability to become aware of a hazard to safety, there may be some reason why he is prevented from taking the necessary avoiding action. A physically disabled or ill person or a frail elderly person are obvious examples of people who may be physically unable to avoid accidental injury in certain circumstances.

Apart from specific anatomical and physiological disabilities which may make it less easy for the individual to maintain safety, there are many external agents in the environment which can cause injury and disease. However the body has several physical internal mechanisms for combating the adverse external conditions which are an inevitable part of living. For instance, the body has many reserve capacities which ensure that vital functions can continue even when an organ is injured or diseased: there is more lung tissue than is normally required, there is reserve liver tissue, there are two kidneys, eyes and ears. Apart from this 'over-provision' there are other mechanisms.

Physical barriers and secretions. The skeleton acts as an internal physical barrier and is protective; the hard bony skull protects the brain; the vertebral column protects the spinal cord; and the ribs protect the lungs and heart. The intact skin acts as a barrier between the internal and the external environment which contains many potentially harmful agents. The filtering function of lymphatic tissue enables the tonsils and adenoids to trap pathogens. The cilia in the respiratory tract hasten the exit from the body of possibly harmful foreign material. By reflex action — a mechanism of the nervous system — the threatened hand is instantly withdrawn and the threatened eye closed. The eye is further protected by the constant secretion of tears.

The inflammatory process. Inflammation is another internal defence mechanism and is a reaction of living tissue to infection, injury and irritants. Regardless of the cause, the reaction is similar. A substance, histamine, is produced by injured cells; it causes capillaries in the area to dilate thus bringing greatly increased amounts of blood to the site of injury. If this occurs on or close to the skin, it can be observed as redness and it feels warm to the touch. As well as dilating, the capillaries become more permeable and allow fluid to escape into the tissues, which produces swelling. In many instances, this swelling is enough to produce pressure on sensory nerves causing pain; to minimise the pain, the patient usually keeps the part as still as possible. The cardinal features of inflammation are therefore redness, heat, swelling, pain and loss of function. But these features are protective since they usually induce rest and aid healing. Furthermore inflammation is frequently accompanied by fever and an increased temperature is unfavourable to survival of some microorganisms.

The process of tissue repair. As inflammation subsides and damaged tissue cells are cleared away in the blood, repair begins in one of two ways:

- *repair by first intention* occurs when there is replacement by cells identical to those which were damaged. The best example is a surgical incision, which is sutured and heals without complication of infection. Only a small amount of new tissue is required to fill the gap.
- *repair by second intention* occurs when a considerable amount of tissue has been lost and the wound edges cannot be approximated; a mass of new tissue is required to fill the gap. First, the damaged tissues are sealed with tissue fluid and blood, which clots. Then blood vessels invade the clot and connective tissue cells from the blood enter the clot and form fibroblasts. At this stage the healing area is reddish in appearance and is referred to as

granulation tissue. The fibroblasts are then converted to fibres which, when they contract, draw the wound edges together. As the process proceeds many blood vessels become nipped and the scar tissue changes in colour from red to white which can take many years.

The healing process is completed when epithelium grows in from the edge and covers the granulation tissue. The skin and the tissue in the digestive tract heal quite rapidly; bone takes longer and the cells of the brain and spinal cord, once damaged, cannot be replaced.

The rate of healing is influenced by several factors:

- *degree of injury* is pertinent; the repair process takes longer when extensive areas of tissue have been damaged
- *nutritional state* of the tissues is important; substances such as protein and vitamin C are essential for rapid healing. Protein is needed for the formation of new tissue and vitamin C for the maturation of fibrous tissue
- *blood circulation*, particularly any occlusion of blood flow, delays healing by depriving the cells of nutrients and oxygen, so vital to tissue repair
- *age* can affect the rate of healing which is usually more rapid in younger than in older people. This is partly due to the decreased circulatory effectiveness in the elderly
- *infection* inevitably delays wound healing because the pathogenic microorganisms destroy tissue

The process of immunity. Immunity is another type of internal defence mechanism usually arising in response to an infection. The basic response to infection is inflammation (see above); another response is related to immunity. The body reacts to the entry of any foreign materials (antigens) by developing substances called immune bodies. Immune bodies which destroy microorganisms are called antibodies and those which destroy toxins produced by microorganisms are called antitoxins. For purposes of description, the process of immunity can be classified into four main types (Fig. 6.2).

Natural passive immunity. Antibodies and antitoxins circulating in the pregnant woman's blood are passed via the placenta to the fetus. This inherited, natural, passive (the baby has not produced it) immunity to, for example, measles and whooping cough usually lasts only for a few months after birth. Thereafter, the baby is vulnerable to such infections and this is borne in mind when organising immunisation programmes for the child.

Natural active immunity. This type of immunity can be naturally acquired in two ways both of which involve the production of antibodies:

- By having an attack of the infectious disease the body is stimulated to produce appropriate

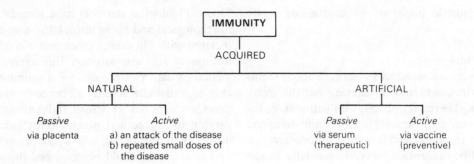

Fig. 6.2 Types of immunity

antibodies not only to assist recovery but also to provide a sufficient quantity to remain in the blood for a longer period, sometimes throughout life, for example after an attack of rubella
● By being exposed to repeated small doses of the infecting agent. The amount is insufficient to cause the classical signs and symptoms of the disease but is sufficient to stimulate the body to produce antibodies which remain in the blood throughout life. Many adults have developed an immunity to tuberculosis in this manner.

Artificially initiated active immunity. This is produced by injecting a small dose of the antigen into the body and allowing time for the person to produce antibodies himself, which then remain in the body for a variable time. It may be short-term, for example as a protection against influenza, or almost life-long, for example against diphtheria. The antigen can be a modified toxin called toxoid and it stimulates the body to make antitoxins.

Artificially initiated passive immunity. This is produced by injecting ready-made antibodies (usually developed in the blood of another human or in a horse serum and suitably treated for injection purposes). This technique is only used when a person is dangerously ill and his own blood would not have time to develop the antibodies. It can be life-saving.

The phenomenon of shock
The body responds to both physical and emotional trauma by a phenomenon known as shock. When it occurs, the body defences immediately try to compensate.

Basically shock is a state of circulatory failure. The average adult body contains about 6 litres of blood and if all the innumerable blood vessels were widely open simultaneously, there would be insufficient blood to fill them. The body functions with this relatively small volume of blood by controlling the muscle tissue in the walls of the small arteries (arterioles), thereby narrowing (vasoconstricting) or widening (vasodilating) the lumen. The control is very exact and normally it is a state of vasoconstriction. However, when the control is disturbed

and the lumen of many arterioles are simultaneously vasodilated, the volume of blood is insufficient to maintain effective circulation and there is some degree of shock.

In shock, the body defences immediately try to compensate by permitting the vessels supplying blood to vital organs such as the brain, heart and kidneys to continue to do so, while the supply to muscles, skin and intestines is severely restricted. In a severe form of shock, the body temperature falls; the blood pressure falls; the pulse increases; the person complains of feeling cold; the skin is grey, cold and moist; and there is generalised prostration. If the cause of shock is treated satisfactorily, these adverse changes will be reversed but if not, the blood pressure falls further and death will ensue.

The most common causes of shock are the inhibition of vasoconstriction due to:

● loss of blood, as in haemorrhage
● loss of plasma, as in severe burns
● loss of electrolytes, as in continued vomiting and/or diarrhoea, and heat exhaustion
● alteration in permeability of blood vessel walls, as in injured tissue
● severe pain
● severe fright, as when hearing bad news or seeing horrifying sights

When there is, for example, loss of blood or plasma (sometimes called oligaemic shock) the reason for circulatory failure is more readily understood and expected because there is actual loss of circulatory volume. But in instances of severe pain or severe fright there is no loss of fluid; shock (sometimes called neurogenic shock) is due to reduced vasoconstriction. It is just as important to expect and recognise the body's warning signals of neurogenic shock so that it can be effectively treated.

All of these mechanisms — the inflammatory process, the process of tissue repair, the process of immunity and the phenomenon of shock — are anatomical and physiological body defence mechanisms against injury and disease which are protective, and are an attempt to prevent further damage. However, there are other non-physical factors which are just as important in maintaining a safe environment.

Psychological factors

Intellectual processes are involved in learning about maintaining a safe environment and in carrying out the many activities involved. Therefore, people who suffer from intellectual impairment may be unable to acquire adequate knowledge and to respond quickly and appropriately to a threat to safety. For this reason, severely mentally handicapped people depend on others for protection and surveillance and, similarly, parents and teachers accept responsibility for the safety of children in their care.

Attitude to safety and prevention is important and it is desirable that people develop a concept of safety and an awareness of their personal responsibility in maintaining a safe environment, for themselves and for others. Undesirable attitudes do not help such as thinking that accidents, fires and infection happen only to others and hoping that someone else will do the campaigning about pollution issues.

Personality and temperament play a part in the attitudes people hold about maintaining a safe environment and affect their efficiency in carrying out the activities involved. Mood is also an important factor. Angry people may become aggressive and violent, possibly causing injury to themselves or to others, and 'non-accidental injury to children' and also to the spouse and to the elderly are increasingly recognised as serious current social problems. Depressed people may endanger their own safety because tiredness, lethargy and loss of motivation and self-confidence result in a lack of attention to maintaining a safe environment. Worried and preoccupied people are also vulnerable to accidents, perhaps especially on the roads either as drivers or pedestrians.

Confidence also plays a part in maintaining safety. The over-confident driver or motorcyclist may overtake without due caution, thus increasing the risk of causing a road traffic accident. Conversely the under-confident person may be hesitant to predict danger or to react to it with sufficient purpose or determination. Therefore, both over-confidence and under-confidence may play a part in creating an environment in which accidents happen more readily.

The individual's level of stress is known to be important in relation to maintaining a safe environment. Some writers use an engineering analogy and point out that the words 'stress', 'strain', 'tension' and 'pressure' are used when the load becomes too great and a breaking point is reached; it is the point where the strain is so great that metal ceases to bend and it snaps. Hans Selye, who pioneered the stress concept in the 1950s, concluded that stress was the wear and tear on the body in response to stressful agents. These he called 'stressors' and said that they could be physical, physiological, psychological or sociocultural.

Physical/biological stressors have already been mentioned. Psychological and sociocultural stressors are frequently associated with life events/crises and can often cause intense feelings of fear and anxiety. Life events can be developmental in nature: weaning, toilet training and puberty are examples that characterise all people's lives. Others are the periods of inevitable stress and anxiety which although varying in degree and pleasurability/sadness do surround incidents like changing school, job or house; getting married or divorced; child bearing, and death of loved ones.

Psychological stressors are known to be important contributory factors in relation to accidents. For example, research findings suggest that children of families under stress are more vulnerable to accidents, such as ingestion of poisons. Stress factors include circumstances such as serious illness in a family, pregnancy, recent house move, one parent away from home and anxiety or depression in one or both parents (OHE, 1981). And the potentially harmful effects of psychological stressors at work are discussed by Rogers & Salvage (1988).

The complexity of psychological factors involved in the AL of maintaining a safe environment means that publicity campaigns and health education programmes must go beyond simply imparting information about safety, realising that people often know what they should and could do, and yet do not act on their knowledge. Health education programmes in schools can contribute towards the development of a concept of safety and a responsible attitude towards maintaining a safe environment. In the same way, publicity campaigns and advertising and television documentaries can disseminate knowledge about safety, and attempt to change attitudes and behaviour in a positive way.

Injury, however, is not always accidental, and it is not only physical. The emotionally devastating effects of non-accidental injury, especially to children, has been receiving dramatic mass media coverage recently. The latest reports from Britain's two main protection agencies give a measure of the size of the problem. The National Society for the Prevention of Cruelty to Children (NSPCC) helped almost 51 000 children in 1986/87 and the National Children's Home campaign Children in Danger showed that 30 000 children are now on the local authority 'at risk' register, an increase of 22% in the last year (Pope, 1988). The plight of abused (physically, emotionally and sexually) children is a tragic and sensitive story which apparently often goes undetected because the mother, fearing reprisals or removal of the children, does not report abuse by her husband/partner or visiting relative (who often is the perpetrator); in many cases having suffered violence herself from him (Jones, 1988).

In an NSPCC Report (Vousden, 1987) workers involved with families were asked to indicate the factors they thought precipitated child abuse and, as in previous years, the one recorded most frequently was 'marital problems', particularly in cases of emotional and sexual abuse. Other factors were 'inability to deal with normal child behaviour' and 'inability to respond to the maturational needs of the child'. External stress caused by unemployment, debts and poor housing were also mentioned but not with the same frequency as issues concerned with the parent/child relationship. The Butler-Sloss Report (Cleveland Report, 1988) highlighted the problems in the UK and makes recommendations, and the Children's Legal Centre has published a booklet (1988) which concentrates on the procedures professionals should follow when dealing with suspected child abuse. The specific problem of sexual abuse in children and rape in women will be mentioned in more detail under the AL of expressing sexuality.

While the problems of child abuse and violence against women have been much publicised, abuse of the elderly — sometimes called 'granny bashing' (Eastman, 1988) — has been given less consideration. Garrett (1986) quotes Hocking who called the syndrome 'miscare' and considers that many families begin their caring commitment with genuine concern and sympathy but become overwhelmed by the task, so the relationship sours, resulting in harm to the old person. Garrett goes on to indicate that the harm may not ohly be physical, but may include mental and social suffering such as neglect (withholding, e.g. food, fluid, washing facilities, or overmedicating); exploitation (often financial — misappropriation of pension, savings, jewellery); psychological abuse (ridicule, humiliation, removal of decision-making); and even sexual abuse including rape, and not always against female elderly. Such treatment could not be condoned but it must also be borne in mind that an increasingly dependent elderly person may be a heavy burden on a carer who has other family commitments including children, or who also may be obliged to continue paid employment; and the stress on the carer is considerable (Tyler, 1987). And such circumstances of course, are not helped by low income and poor, overcrowded housing. When indications of abuse are identified, says Garrett (1986), a supportive programme to relieve the pressure on the family may be appropriate such as counselling, home care assistance, the provision of incontinence supplies, and the organisation of respite care. It is occasionally necessary to remove the elderly person to hospital, temporarily or permanently, and in certain circumstances this is the only possible action.

The issue of non-accidental injury, although mentioned under psychological factors, obviously also has physical, sociocultural, environmental and politicoeconomic aspects and is another reminder that although in this textbook, the five factors are dealt with separately for the purposes of discussion, in reality they are closely related.

Sociocultural factors

Each culture has a unique interpretation of the concept of 'safety' and what is deemed to be responsible, 'safe' behaviour by individuals. This is true largely because the problems associated with maintaining a safe environment are different in different parts of the world. The most obvious differences are apparent when comparing problems in so-called developing societies with those which confront the industralised societies. There are obviously wide differences in the provision of social amenities and social services. The structure of the society, too, may vary from a large extended family system where care for all dependants — the young, the elderly, the mentally handicapped, the ill — is shared, to the small nuclear family, typical of the Western world, where often the state has taken over many of the traditional caring activities of the family, with their attendant safety aspects.

Within any one society also, there are internal differences in relation to the problems of maintaining a safe environment and the particular kinds of hazards to which certain groups of people are exposed. There are social class differences as is apparent, for example, in statistics concerning accidents. Analysis of such statistics pertaining to the UK (OHE, 1981), showed that there is a substantial social class difference in childhood mortality from accidents and violence, the overall rate for children of parents in unskilled occupations being nearly five times that for children of parents in the professions. The differential is even greater when pedestrian fatalities are singled out for analysis; and significant class discrepancies have also been observed for specific types of non-fatal accident, such as burns and scalds. Such social class disparities have been linked to a variety of factors, for example, the deficiency of safe play areas for children of the lower social class groups is offered as one explanation for the high rate among them of pedestrian fatalities. Social class inequalities are always difficult to explain precisely but there is no doubt that they exist in relation to the AL of maintaining a safe environment (Whitehead, 1987).

Currently, especially in the Western world, the mass media provide a constant reminder that personal safety is threatened not only by the elements, and objects and events in the environment, but also by the humans who make up the society. Social disorder is not new but throughout history, it has had varying degrees of prominence as a problem. During the last few decades, despite the distress of individuals who are the victims of such social disorder, the problem has seemed relatively 'containable' in social terms. Now, however, there is mounting anxiety about the rising tide of crime, social disorder, purposeless thuggery and vandalism, much of it accompanied by violence. According to an article in the Telegraph Sunday Magazine (Hall, 1987) some large housing estates, known to have violent inhabitants, have even been singled out as 'no-go' areas, where milk floats, postmen and repair men venture at their peril. On the other hand, upmarket housing developments are now heavily protected by high gates, guards and video cameras, although even modest householders, in city and quiet rural areas alike, are resorting to burglar alarms on their homes and cars, or organising Neighbourhood Watch schemes. In various ways, legally and illegally, more people are arming themselves against potential attackers at home, in the street, and even in recreational settings. Some football hooligans, the article goes on, are now so organised that they have the audacity to leave professionally printed calling cards in the pockets of their battered victims.

In the international sporting context, there is also grave concern about the safety of competitors and viewers at meetings such as the Olympic Games because terrorists, sometimes representing minority and almost unknown groups, stage an attack to wreak revenge or to gain publicity for their cause. For similar reasons, hijackings involving aircraft, ships and cars are not uncommon.

In the work setting, too, incidents involving violence are becoming increasingly common; assault and even murder are now occupational hazards. It is perhaps not too surprising that staff in the diplomatic corps and in government intelligence agencies are targets for violence while engaged in their daily work, but it is relatively recent in the UK, for example, to have an estate agent, a social worker, and a health visitor murdered while at work (Smith, 1988). And there is an increasing number of instances of assault at work targeted at community nurses and staff on accident and emergency units in hospital (Finney, 1988), a circumstance which would have been almost unthinkable even a decade ago.

Recently in an attempt to reduce the current wave of social violence, projects have been piloted in the UK and 20 'safer cities' will be set up in selected areas which have high rates of crime and violence, and other social and community problems (Delamothe, 1988). There is now much more public demand for support to the victims of violent crime. In addition to medical prescription, victims require emotional support and reassurance which is not available from sources such as the family. They also require information about compensation; help with approaches to the Criminal Injuries Compensation Board, social services, crime prevention officers, and legal advice centres; and practical help to repair or recover property following robbery (Shepherd, 1988).

Environmental factors
It is obvious that environmental factors exert a far-reaching influence on this particular AL and, indeed, the concept of 'safety' has no real meaning unless it is considered in relation to 'the environment'.

In many developing societies the lack of basic amenities, such as clean water and proper sanitation, produces an inherently unsafe environment. Infectious diseases, particularly the diarrhoeal diseases, are both difficult to prevent and control in such circumstances and they are largely responsible for the high morbidity and mortality rates in many areas of the world. In industralised countries, such rudimentary amenities as piped water and sanitation have long been taken for granted and there has been a virtual elimination of major infectious diseases over the past century. However, affluence and technological advances have created new kinds of safety hazards for people who live in Western society. There are all the industrial hazards such as excessive noise, polluted air and contamination of water by industrial waste and, as has already been described in detail, a large-scale problem in the form of accidents.

In an earlier section of this chapter, a great range of activities which individuals carry out in maintaining a safe environment were mentioned in relation to preventing accidents in the home, at work, at play and while travelling. Houses, factories and offices, sports grounds and playgrounds, and roads are also 'environments'. In each of these environments there are numerous 'factors', many of which constitute a threat to the safety of individuals and numerous such hazards have been mentioned.

Taking a broader view of the term 'environment', other kinds of factors can be seen to influence this AL: for example, climate and geographical location. It does not take much imagination to appreciate that maintaining a safe environment in high latitudes and high altitudes with the long months of snow, ice and subzero temperatures will differ from maintaining a safe environment in the humid heat of a tropical forest.

Even conditions beyond the earth's immediate environment can affect human beings and currently there is concern about the effect on health of an appreciable hole in the springtime ozone layer over Antarctica (McKie & Rycroft, 1988). Apparently it has been recognised for over a decade that chlorine from chlorofluorocarbons may deplete the stratospheric ozone layer. It matters because this layer absorbs all ultraviolet C and a proportion of ultraviolet B from sunlight before it reaches the earth's surface. Concern for humans is raised because increased exposure to ultraviolet B is closely linked to skin cancer which is an increasingly common problem. The Montreal Convention 1987 aims at reducing the production of chlorofluorocarbons by half by the end of the 1990s but the scientists maintain that a drastic reduction is needed soon 'to prevent an environmental problem from becoming an environmental catastrophe'. One response to that plea was the convening in London, in March 1989, of the Saving the Ozone Conference, attended by 124 nations; among other topics, the delegates discussed possible international cooperation which would strengthen the Montreal Protocol (Cramb, 1989) — a matter obviously requiring political will.

Politicoeconomic factors
Both political and economic factors influence the AL of maintaining a safe environment to a very great degree. Although many of the activities involved are carried out by individuals, and there is much scope for personal decision-

making and responsibility, the business of maintaining a safe environment is very much a political concern and responsibility — at local, regional, national and international levels. As has been described, many aspects of maintaining a safe environment are controlled by legislation. Laws exist which ensure that as far as possible, accidents, fire, infection and pollution are prevented. Governments also accept a responsibility to increase public awareness of hazards and safety measures and desirable standards of safety through publicity campaigns and education. All such activity is in the interests of both personal and national safety, but also is based on an economic argument.

An unsafe environment will result in accident and ill-health, and both are a burden on a nation's economy. Of course, preventing accidents and promoting safety also costs a great deal of money. Safe houses, roads, vehicles, workplaces and play areas all cost money. So too does the provision of emergency services (such as the fire service) which are sufficiently well-equipped and manned to respond promptly and effectively when required.

The economics of maintaining a safe environment are not just the concern of government for, through taxation, individuals contribute to the national purse. For example, a substantial proportion of the road tax levied on vehicle owners goes towards paying for road maintenance and improvements. For individuals, the costs of maintaining a safe environment are, however, by no means all in the category of indirect taxation. Maintaining safety in the home is an expensive business and, for families with children, the purchase of recommended safety equipment — such as car safety seats, stair gates, a playpen and a cooker guard — adds up to a considerable sum. For families of low income such items are almost certainly prohibitively expensive. At other stages of the lifespan, maintaining a safe environment in the home for elderly or disabled people may also be expensive. Families caring for elderly or disabled relatives save the state up to £24 million a year, according to a report by the Family Policy Studies Centre (Glasgow Herald, 1989). It follows publication of a report by the Office of Population Censuses and Surveys in 1988 which maintained that there were 6 million people in Britain providing informal care for a sick, elderly or disabled relative or dependant, i.e. one adult in seven. Most carers were aged 45–64; and six out of ten were committed to looking after the dependant for at least 50 hours a week.

People do not need to be politicians to engage in politics. Individuals and pressure groups can exert a considerable influence on government and have indeed done so very effectively in relation to many aspects of the AL of maintaining a safe environment. For example, the recent introduction of seat belt legislation in the UK was at least in part due to persistent lobbying by sections of the community, including the medical profession. Frequently too, people who live in a particular geographic location combine together to form a pressure group if their neighbourhood has been earmarked by government for the siting of, for example, a new motorway or nuclear power station or the dumping of nuclear waste which is considered to constitute a substantial threat to their safety and health. All citizens have a responsibility to be involved in the politicoeconomic decisions which influence the AL of maintaining a safe environment — not necessarily for their own safety, but for the safety of others and especially for their children and, indeed, their children's children.

It is perhaps that long-term perspective which is at the root of present-day concern over the nuclear arsenal held by the superpowers. Knowledge of the devastating effect which even a limited nuclear attack would have on the environment and the people in it has motivated increasing numbers to campaign vociferously for nuclear disarmament, either multilateral or unilateral. It is interesting that doctors and nurses, who on the whole prefer to remain apolitical, have become actively engaged in this campaign. Some are members of the CND, others of the Medical Campaign Against Nuclear Weapons. In 1983 the Royal College of Nursing, the professional organisation for British nurses, issued a report on the nursing implications of planning for nuclear war. The report outlines what would happen in the event of nuclear war and maintains that talk of planning for, and training in triage and mass casualty techniques is meaningless, because surviving nurses would be able to do little other than help to provide limited care for casualties and comfort the dying.

Opinion on the nuclear issue is divided and other arguments are involved too, for example economic considerations. Some people think that the vast amounts of money spent by governments on nuclear weapons would be better spent on other needs, such as health care. Protagonists argue that the nation's defence is more important and that the mere possession of nuclear weapons prevents attack by other nuclear powers. However, there is no disagreement that preventing nuclear war is vital to maintaining a safe environment for people now, and for future generations.

INDIVIDUALITY IN MAINTAINING A SAFE ENVIRONMENT

The purpose of the model is to describe how a particular person develops *individuality* in carrying out the Activities of Living. The following list is a résumé of the topics which have been discussed under the headings of the components of the model in relation to the AL of maintaining a safe environment.

Lifespan: effect on maintaining a safe environment
- Babies   — vulnerable to accidents, infections, excessive heat/cold

- Preschool children — vulnerable to accidents in the home
- Schoolchildren — vulnerable to accidents on the roads and in the playground
- Adolescents — vulnerable to road, bicycle and sporting accidents
- Adults — vulnerable to hazards in the work environment; vulnerable to road traffic accidents; responsible for safety of children
- Elderly people — vulnerable to falls in the home, hazards of infection and fire, pedestrian accidents

Dependence/independence in maintaining a safe environment

- Dependence in infancy/childhood/old age
- Constraints on independence in adulthood (e.g. mental/physical/sensory handicap)
- Dependence on others
- Dependence on aids

Factors influencing maintaining a safe environment

- Physical
  - — acuity of the senses
  - — physical ability/disability
  - — susceptibility to infection
  - — state of physical health/ill-health, anatomical and physiological responses to infection and trauma
- Psychological
  - — intellectual ability/impairment
  - — attitude to safety (home, work, play, travel)
  - — personality and temperament
  - — mood and motivation
  - — level of confidence
  - — level of stress
  - — level of knowledge about safety precautions
  - — responsiveness to safety legislation/health education
  - — non-accidental injury
- Sociocultural
  - — cultural factors (e.g. concept of safety)
  - — social factors (e.g. prevalence of infectious diseases)
  - — social class (e.g. risk of accident)
  - — social unrest and violence
- Environmental
  - — housing
  - — standard of safety in the home

- — exposure to hazards in work settings
- — hazards in play settings
- — risk of accident on the roads
- — exposure to environmental pollution
- — climatic and geographical factors
- — extraterrestrial factors
- Politicoeconomic
  - — knowledge and attitude to safety legislation
  - — awareness of local environmental hazards
  - — personal spending on safety measures
  - — political awareness/involvement (e.g. pollution, nuclear products)

Maintaining a safe environment: patients' problems and related nursing

Each day, throughout the day, although not always aware of it, people are engaged in carrying out numerous activities which have the specific purpose of maintaining a safe environment. As with all of the Activities of Living, there are many similarities in the way different people carry out this AL. However, as the preceding section shows, a variety of circumstances determine an individual's vulnerability to certain hazards in the environment, and result in individuality in the way necessary preventive activities are carried out. The concept of individuality provides the link between the model of living and the model for nursing.

Individualised nursing is based on knowledge of a patient's individuality. Therefore, in relation to the AL of maintaining a safe environment, the nurses need to know about the patient's individual habits and any actual or potential problems. While observing and discussing relevant topics with the patient (along the lines suggested in the résumé above), the nurse might bear in mind the following questions:

- what kind of activities does the individual usually engage in with the purpose of maintaining a safe environment?
- what factors influence the way in which the

individual carries out the AL of maintaining a safe environment?

- what is the individual's level of knowledge regarding maintaining a safe environment?
- what is the individual's attitude to maintaining a safe environment?
- has the individual experienced any difficulties in the past with maintaining a safe environment and, if so, how have these been coped with?
- does the individual have any actual problems or perceive any potential problems with maintaining a safe environment?

The objective in collecting this sort of information is to discover the patient's usual routines; what can and cannot be done independently; what previous coping mechanisms have been employed; and what problems exist or may develop in relation to this AL. By its very nature it is likely that most will be potential problems relevant to the circumstances (though there may be actual problems too), and, therefore, the goals set and the mutually agreed nursing interventions will be mainly preventive in nature. Accordingly, evaluation will be undertaken to ascertain that the preventive measures implemented have been effective. The goal of individualised nursing for this AL will be achieved if assessing, planning, implementing and evaluating all take account of the patient's individuality in maintaining a safe environment.

That, in the most general of terms, describes how the nursing process method is applied. However, in different circumstances, nursing assessment of the AL of maintaining a safe environment would differ in approach, scope and content. For example, assessment by a health visitor of a mother's knowledge about maintaining a safe environment for her young child in the home would obviously be quite different from an occupational health nurse's assessment of an employee's risk of accident at work. Therefore, in different nursing contexts there will be different kinds of problems identified and, accordingly, different types of nursing activities will be implemented. Teaching is one type of nursing activity which is always relevant in relation to the AL of maintaining a safe environment. Exploiting opportunities for education of people of all ages and in various settings (home, school and workplace) is probably the main way in which nurses can contribute to the collective effort to prevent injury and ill-health which is caused by accident, fire, infection and pollution. These subjects were dealt with in detail in the first part of the chapter and should be recognised as background knowledge relevant to nursing in relation to the AL of maintaining a safe environment, so are not discussed further.

The remainder of the chapter deals with some circumstances in which nurses are directly involved with assisting patients who have problems in maintaining a safe environment. There are two sections. The first of these is concerned with patients in hospital. Florence Nightingale said 'the hospital shall do the patient no harm'. Yet in most countries there is continuing concern about the number of patients who develop a hospital-acquired infection quite unrelated to the reason for their admission; about the accidents which happen to patients while they are in hospital; about the perennial danger of fire in hospitals; and about the dangers associated with the use of prescribed drugs in hospital. In a way this is not surprising when one considers the size and function of a hospital, and the fact that hospitals are busy places: 'busyness' increases stress and tension, and errors and accidents are more likely to occur in such an atmosphere. From the patient's point of view, admission to hospital involves a change of environment and routine and that, in itself, creates problems with the AL of maintaining a safe environment.

The second section, with which the chapter ends, may be relevant to the nursing of patients in hospital but is not confined to that context. It considers, in very broad terms, the variety of circumstances which can cause a change of dependence/independence status for the AL of maintaining a safe environment. This section, therefore, provides a direct link between the model of living and the model for nursing.

CHANGE OF ENVIRONMENT AND ROUTINE

Most human beings are conservative and dislike change, particularly enforced change as when a patient is admitted to hospital. Patients can feel insecure and frightened in this new environment and anxiety increases the risk of accident. A patient in an anxious state is more likely to bump into, or trip over, objects; shaking or tense hands are more likely to drop things, spill things and so on. Some patients become disoriented, a more likely reaction if the patient is elderly or has already shown signs of mental confusion (Clarke, 1987; Ford et al, 1986). Nurses can help all patients by talking with them, keeping in mind the objective of orienting them to the new environment and routine. The sooner this is done the better.

Unfamiliar environment
Familiarity with an environment makes it less hazardous; for example people adjust spatially to avoid objects in their immediate vicinity. Just on admission, a patient has not had time to make any necessary spatial adjustments. This could well relate to the design of the hospital bed which may not be at the same height as the one with which the patient is familiar. For some patients more than others, it is important for the nurses to know that familiar height.

Where mechanically-operated height-adjustment beds are provided and the patient is capable with instruction, of operating the mechanism, independence in this respect can be maintained. When the patient is not capable, then the nurse is responsible for operating the mechanism to maintain the patient's safety. Several surveys conducted in hospitals have shown that the majority of accidents occur at the bedside (Moorat, 1983). As long ago as 1978, the Scottish Hospital Advisory Service reported from observation visits to long-stay hospitals throughout Scotland that even when adjustable beds were provided, they were frequently found at a height too high for the patients' safety and unfortunately, this is often still true.

Patients may have to be nursed on a bed with a ripple mattress or an air bed. While providing greater safety from the pressure hazard, they can create spatial problems for the patient. The increased height relative to the bedside locker and bed table may require spatial adjustment. Over-reaching for an article on nearby furniture is a frequent cause of accidents. Patients can be helped by nurses who, before leaving the bedside, test whether or not the patient can comfortably reach articles on the locker.

Disabled and older patients who experience difficulty when rising from a chair will like most people, have their 'special' chair at home, out of which they can rise relatively easily, and on which they may hang a walking stick to help with safe rising. These patients can experience many kinds of problems when in a different environment such as increased stiffening of the back and limbs due to lack of exercise because they find it so difficult to get out of the hospital chair; and incontinence for the same reason. Actual shearing injury to the sacral tissues and the heels may even be caused by patients sliding forward on vinyl-covered chairs. Nurses can help, within the constraints of the type of chairs provided, by 'matching' the chair to the patient, not just helping the patient to any chair.

Noisy environment

Quite justifiably, hospitals have been labelled as noisy environments. One study of noise in hospital by Bentley et al (1977), and still considered a classic reference, used the dB(A) scale, from among several decibel scales, because of its close relationship to noise which damages human hearing. Measurements were taken in an open Florence Nightingale ward, a cubicle in a cul-de-sac of this ward and a general intensive therapy unit (ITU). A profile based on pooled data of all observations is shown in Figure 6.3 and it should be studied in conjunction with the yardstick provided by The International Proposal for Noise Abatement with Respect to Community Response which suggests the following basic noise limits:

day time	45 dB(A)
evening	40 dB(A)
night time	30 dB(A)

Figure 6.4 shows that the noise level in the Nightingale ward and in the cubicle during the night was above the figure suggested for the usual bedroom; and during the day, the level in the ITU was above the 'annoying' level.

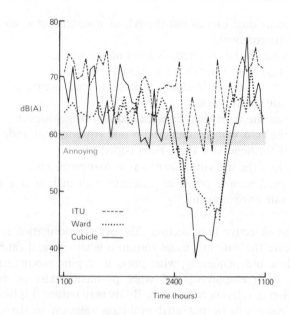

Fig. 6.3 Noise: profile based on pooled data (from Bentley et al 1977 Perceived noise in surgical wards and an intensive care area. British Medical Journal 2: 1503–1506)

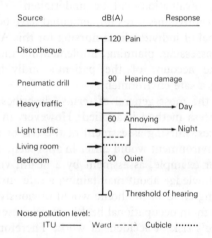

Fig. 6.4 Comparison of noise levels (from Bentley et al 1977 British Medical Journal 2: 1503–1506. Figures 6.3 and 6.4 reproduced by kind permission of the authors and editor of the British Medical Journal)

A more recent study by Soutar & Wilson (1986) in the UK does not show much improvement. They measured night-time noise, from 22.30 to 06.36, in the area next to the nurses' station in three different types of wards and found that night-time noise over 8 hours in the psychiatric ward was 49 dB(A); in the general medical ward was 68 dB(A); and in the acute admitting general ward was 66 dB(A) — the general wards being well above the Bentley et al 'annoying' level. The 91 patients in Soutar & Wilson's study were asked their opinion about the effect of noise on sleep and of the 28 who admitted that sleep was more difficult in hospital than at home, only 9 said it was because of the noise. These results led the authors to assume that patients were unwilling to complain about noise levels.

The noise levels in hospitals in the USA seem to be similar. A study reported by Hilton (1987) starts by providing references to show how excessive noise can provoke detrimental physiological responses — it can startle; damage hearing; stimulate epinephrine production; induce sensory disturbance; constrict peripheral and coronary arteries; reduce digestive secretions; and slow gastrointestinal motility. Psychological disturbances have also been cited including annoyance and irritation; heightened arousal; impaired judgement; altered perception; interference with thinking; and reduced ability to hear. It is considered, too, that at 50 dB(A), pain perception is enhanced. Hilton's study carried out in four ITUs and two medical/surgical wards showed the noise level above the recommended figure at night. In the recovery room, more than half the talking exceeded 67 dB(A), although considerable noise was also created by oxygen administration equipment, ventilators and alarms on monitors, as well as toilet flushing sounds and telephones ringing. Hilton did a similar study in Canada with similar results.

Improvements are recommended in all of these studies such as shutting doors quietly (and oiling them when necessary); handling equipment carefully to reduce noise; muting the alarm systems and telephones; wearing soft-soled shoes; providing soundproof covers for computer printout machines; reducing conversations between staff and talking quietly; providing earplugs if requested; isolating 'noisy' patients from general wards when practicable so that they create the least possible disturbance to other patients — and, as Soutar & Wilson point out, most of these suggestions are simple and inexpensive remedies. It has been suggested that from time to time, sound engineers should show staff how much they pollute the environment and by means of this simple measurement, educate staff to prevent noise pollution. Discussing the patient's 'auditory environment' Gough (1986) provides vignettes showing how noise means different things to different people and reminds nurses that it is possible to be upset by silence, for example a child in an isolation unit — a salutary reminder of the importance of individualising nursing according to the circumstances.

Risk of accident

Some mention of accidents has already been made but further, more specific comment is relevant. If nurses are to attempt to prevent avoidable accidents to patients, they need to be aware of what and where the hazards are; when accidents are most likely to occur; and which patients are most at risk. For patients who are identified from assessment as being at particular risk, relevant preventive activities should be included in the list of interventions written on the patient's nursing plan. Some of the nursing activities which might be relevant can be deduced from the

following discussion, which is based on the reports of two studies of accidents in hospital.

The study reported by Moorat (1983) involved an analysis of accident reports from 1979 to 1981 in an English general hospital. The following information was collected: patient's age and gender; time and place of accident; activity being undertaken at the time; and type of accident and injury sustained. The questions asked and the main results of the study are summarised below:

- How many patients have accidents while in hospital, and is the number increasing?
  Over the 3 years in question, the number of accidents rose from 406 in 1979, representing 3.8% of patients, to 605 in 1981 (5.1%).
- Where in the ward do accidents most frequently occur?
  The findings were in keeping with what is known: that accidents most frequently occur at the bedside. Other main locations were the toilet, dayroom, shower/bathroom and corridor.
- What is the most dangerous time of the in-patient's day?
  Contrary to popular belief that night-time is most dangerous, results dispelled this. Early morning was shown to be the peak period, with most accidents taking place between 0600 and 1100 hours. Afternoon was a relatively safe time, but a peak occurred in late evening (1900–2100 hours) when patients go to the toilet or commode and get into bed.
- During which activities are accidents most likely to happen?
  The two activities of using the toilet or commode and getting out of bed were responsible for 49% of all accidents. Other main activities related to accidents were getting up from a chair, walking unaided and getting into bed. It is interesting to note that getting out of bed is much more hazardous than getting in; even when 65% of the beds were of the adjustable height variety.
- What kind of patients are particularly at risk?
  Of all the accidents reported, 68% involved patients between the ages of 56 and 86 years. Patients over the age of 70 are particularly at risk (44% of accidents involved that age group). Female patients who had accidents were older than the male patients: those at risk being 76 years old or over.

While Moorat's study shows that older patients are especially prone to accidents in a general hospital, Blake & Morfitt (1986) carried out a study in a residential home. Over a 16-month period, 296 accidents were reported and of these, 285 were falls (3 were scalds, and 8 were abrasions caused by wheelchairs) and the falls were most likely to occur among those who had suffered previous falls indoors, frequently because of impaired gait and balance, associated usually with a pathological condition. Of course, it is the active, more independent person who is most at risk of falling, and it has to be borne in mind that the prevention of all falls is not an appropriate objective in the care of elderly people. Instead the primary aim should be the promotion of patient activity within acceptable limits of safety. This does not, of course, imply that nurses should not be concerned with the prevention of unnecessary accidents. Earlier in this chapter (p. 70) striking a realistic balance between protection and freedom was discussed in the context of preventing accidents in relation to children. It is equally relevant when providing a nursing service for people at the other end of the lifespan — the elderly. One of the themes in developing a mode of thinking about nursing and its practice must surely be preventing the potential problem of accident from becoming an actual one.

Risk of fire

Fire is a potential problem in all NHS premises and every year in the UK at least 2000 hospital fires are reported (Rogers & Salvage, 1988). The consequences of fire in hospitals and other health care premises can be especially serious because of the difficulties and dangers associated with the emergency evacuation of patients, many of whom may be highly dependent. The aim therefore, according to the government document 'Firecode: Policy & Principles' (DHSS, 1987) is to ensure that outbreaks do not occur; and if they do, that they are rapidly detected, effectively contained and quickly extinguished. Overall fire safety, says the document, depends on physical factors (building design and construction, equipment, furnishings); proper installation and maintenance of detection and alarm systems; local policies for handling emergencies; and staff training in all these matters. The document summarises statutory requirements and policy guidance, and comments on information contained in other Firecode series documents. However, irrespective of specific legislation directly related to fire safety, the Health & Safety at Work Act 1974, places a responsibility on all employers and employees to observe safety in their work premises.

As far as hospital employees are concerned, Dooley (1981) sees nurses as the front line operators when fire does occur:

Fire is a lethal and perennial menace in hospitals . . . It is the nursing staff more than any other category of employee who will bear the burden of the consequences of fire. It is the nurse who will have to decide on whether to evacuate or who to move, how and where. It is a heavy responsibility and the appropriate attitude and degree of awareness should be cultivated.

Dooley, 1981

Dooley suggests that staff training should cover: how to guard against fires; how to react in case of fire; how to raise the alarm; how to help evacuate patients; how to stop fires spreading; and how to help fight the fire. The charge nurse of a ward has a special responsibility to know precisely what action should be taken in the event of a fire; to be aware of any special risks, such as oxygen or cyclopropane cylinders; and to familiarise all new staff to the ward with the routine and the location of fire alarms, exits and fire-fighting equipment. Some patients, perhaps especially those who express anxiety about the risk of fire or who are known to have experienced a fire, may welcome being told about the fire precautions in the ward.

The prevention of fire in hospital has had considerable publicity recently via the mass media and patients are more aware of the potential danger, probably partly because in the UK public buildings have been obliged by law to instal smoke doors in public corridors — and they cannot escape one's notice!

Risk of infection

When patients come to hospital they are living in close contact with more people than usual. The human body is a reservoir of microorganisms as illustrated in Figure 6.5 and they are easily transferred to other things and people via the hands. A potential problem for patients is the risk of infection because they are in contact with greater numbers of pathogenic microorganisms than at home. And this at a time when resistance is likely to be lowered. A large number of organisms and lowered resistance are two of the necessary conditions for infection to become established.

It was to keep down the population of pathogenic microorganisms in hospital that 'damp dusting' of all laying surfaces used to be considered a nursing activity. Nowadays such activities have been designated 'non-nursing' duties, but nurses liaise with domestic management to achieve a safe environment for patients. Dust invariably contains pathogens which have settled out of the atmosphere.

In ordinary breathing droplets are projected 150 to 180 cm into the atmosphere and the distance is increased during talking, coughing and sneezing. There is therefore ample opportunity for all surfaces in a ward to be contaminated, particularly bedclothes, bedcurtains, floors and footwear as illustrated in Figure 6.6. It also shows the methods of spread of infection in hospital, an ever present patient's potential problem. Nurses must be constantly vigilant in every activity so that there is no break in infection control and this is especially necessary because the patient can come into contact with pathogens which have become resistant to one or more of the antibiotics.

From studying Figures 6.5 and 6.6 it will be seen that in hospital there are many potential danger points for contamination by direct contact, for example with infected articles or with hands which have been inadequately washed or not washed at all after dealing with contaminated discharges or materials.

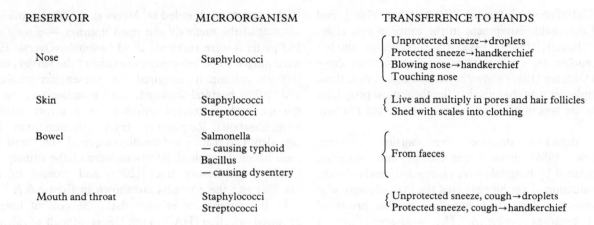

RESERVOIR	MICROORGANISM	TRANSFERENCE TO HANDS
Nose	Staphylococci	{ Unprotected sneeze→droplets Protected sneeze→handkerchief Blowing nose→handkerchief Touching nose
Skin	Staphylococci Streptococci	{ Live and multiply in pores and hair follicles Shed with scales into clothing
Bowel	Salmonella — causing typhoid Bacillus — causing dysentery	{ From faeces
Mouth and throat	Staphylococci Streptococci	{ Unprotected sneeze, cough→droplets Protected sneeze, cough→handkerchief

Fig. 6.5 The human body as a reservoir of microorganisms

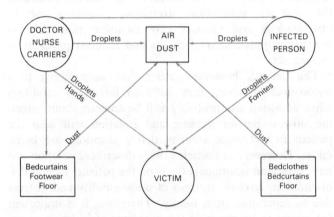

Fig. 6.6 Spread of infection in hospital

Handwashing is undoubtedly the main activity in preventing the spread of infection. The hands harbour the resident flora (p. 74) and also perhaps transient flora (p. 75) particularly between the fingers and under the nails and even immediately after washing, a few colonies of microorganisms can be cultured.

Handwashing seems such a simple task but in fact is a subject of surprising contention among health professionals. Discussing the problem, Blackmore (1987) quotes several sources explaining why handwashing is essential if the transfer of infected material from person to person is to be restricted. The bacterial flora of the hands are similar to other skin sites but hands are of special significance in the transmission of infectious agents and the most important site of contamination. Most *resident skin flora* (p. 74) are not highly virulent and are not normally implicated in infections except when prosthetic surgery or other invasive procedures are performed, or when neonates or immunocompromised patients are involved. In contrast, *transient flora* (p. 75), often found on the hands of hospital personnel can be pathogens acquired from colonised or infected patients and are often involved in cross infection.

Fortunately, these transient flora are more effectively removed by handwashing than the resident flora. Handwashing practices, she goes on, are often based on tradition and ritual, but adequate facilities should be available to do the job effectively. In the study carried out by Blackmore she found that a cotton towel removed bacteria more efficiently than did paper towels but concluded that both types of towel were far superior to warm air drying methods.

Irrespective of facilities, however, Gidley (1987) discovered that handwashing techniques were lamentable. After washing, twist taps were not turned off with the paper towel; and where elbow taps were available, they were used properly only four times; and when disposing of the paper towel in foot-operated pedal bins, nurses used their hands to open and close the bins. The study (admittedly a small one with 33 observations of handwashing) demonstrated that the technique was poor; the time taken was brief; and it was not even carried out after all 'dirty' interventions. Campbell (1988) also found that the technique used by nurses was often questionable. Right handed people washed the left hand more thoroughly and vice versa, and they missed some parts of their hands while washing, eg. the wrists, under finger nails and under rings. Obviously the teaching, or the learning, or the memory span, or the example shown by senior staff was defective. Campbell pointed out that certain factors may influence non-compliance with accepted techniques, e.g. hand paper towels may lead to skin irritation and in turn to skin abrasion and infection; hot air dryers are noisy, slow and also may cause irritation; soap may be irritant and therefore not used; and sinks may be inaccessible. Nevertheless, no amount of sterile packs and antiseptic agents will protect a patient from a staff member who has contaminated hands.

Measures to prevent infection have featured in the literature recently related to issues other than handwashing, e.g. in relation to bedmaking (Overtone, 1988); bed-bathing (Horton, 1988); changing urinary drainage bags (Blenkharn, 1988); giving enteral feeds (Hobbs, 1989); setting up intravenous infusions (Krakowska, 1986); and re-use of disposable equipment in the cause of cost-effectiveness (Baxter, 1987). Even the ubiquitous nurse's scissors bought by every student may not be free from blame as Oldman (1987) shows in her research. From these few examples, it was obvious that the theoretical principles related to the spread of infection were not always put into practice.

These defective practices are causing concern. Grazebrook (1986) gives a résumé of how infection problems faced by hospitals have changed since the 1960s. The introduction of antibiotics saved the lives of many who would previously have died, but their use has produced new and complex problems. The widespread use of prophylactic antibiotics has contributed to the development of a dependence on their effectiveness and less emphasis on the importance of surgical principles, a breakdown of isolation procedures and the establishment of antibiotic-resistant and virulent bacteria in hospital. Moreover, she goes on, these problems are accentuated by the complexities of modern surgery and the large number of high-risk patients being admitted for hitherto inoperable conditions, particularly the very young, the elderly debilitated patient, diabetic, cancer and transplant patients, the severely injured, the burned and those undergoing surgery. Other high-risk patients are those undergoing therapy with immunosuppressive agents, anti-cancer drugs and steroids.

Infection control is only one element in the care of a patient but it is an indicator of standards and there is no disputing how vital it is when one considers the prevalence of nosocomial or hospital-acquired infection (HAI). The National Prevalence Survey conducted in England and Wales and masterminded by Meers et al (1981) provides an account of the methods and main findings — a total of 18 163 patients were surveyed in 43 hospitals. Overall 19.1% were judged to be infected at the time of the survey, namely 9.9% community-acquired, i.e. present on admission, and 9.2% hospital-acquired, i.e. infection-free on admission and contracted infection as a direct result of hospitalisation. Respiratory tract infection was most prevalent and mainly community-acquired. The most common hospital-acquired infections were of the urinary tract (30.3%), respiratory tract (20%) and wound infection (18.9%) and these results are shown in Figure 6.7.

In the absence of reliable data, the cost of hospital-acquired infection (HAI) in the UK is difficult to calculate, but Ayliffe & Collins (1982) suggest that if 5% of patients acquire a nosocomial infection and spend three extra days in hospital, the cost to the country is £30 million excluding the cost of antibiotics, dressings, increased use of microbiology and primary care facilities; plus sickness benefits, supplementary benefits and reduced payment of income tax.

The patient, however, rather than succumbing to a nosocomial infection, may have an infectious condition when admitted and probably will be anxious about infecting others. Barrier nursing and isolation will help the patient to feel some security that precautions are being taken. However, as Barnett (1983) describes, isolation can have profound emotional effects on the patient: such as disorientation, anxiety, feelings of undesirability and distress due to separation from family. Therefore, it is important for nurses to be aware of the problems of isolation as experienced by the patient, and to attempt to alleviate them. It is essential that patients are told why they are being iso-

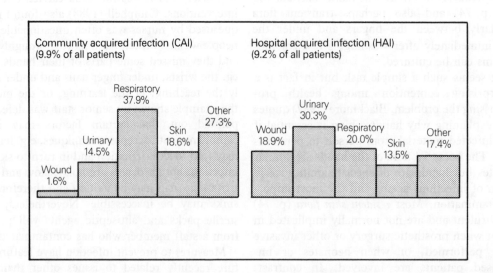

Fig. 6.7 Infection among patients in hospital (Meers, 1981). The prevalence of infection among patients in hospital divided according to the major types of infection concerned, according to a survey of 18 163 patients in 43 hospitals in England and Wales, 1980 (Reproduced from The Times Health Supplement with permission)

lated and the reason for the various precautions should be explained. Information is needed too about the part the patient is expected to play in preventing the spread of infection. Again, patient teaching is a vital nursing activity.

Just as cooperation between nurse and patient is absolutely essential for infection in hospital to be effectively controlled, so too is cooperation among all members of the multidisciplinary health care team. One profession cannot successfully isolate and combat infection. Only by the cooperation and commitment of all hospital personnel can any infection control programme be really successful; therefore a multidisciplinary approach is logical and must be actively encouraged. A collaborative policy is required, for example, in ensuring that there is safe collection of, and provision of storage for hospital waste prior to incineration; quite apart from installing enough incinerators to deal with the growing amount of disposable equipment now used in hospitals.

Not only hospitals require an infection control policy. As more and more people are being discharged early from hospital, pressure increases on community nursing services. Timoney (1987) reports on a study undertaken to examine the current control of infection practices in a community unit of management, and makes some recommendations regarding improved communication with hospital staff, use of protective clothing, wound care, practices related to the use of catheters and drainage systems, disposal of equipment and so on. The problem of waste from the patient's home is highlighted by Archer (1988) who reported the findings of a small study involving the practices of community nursing staff.

Control of infection is a constant challenge. As our defence systems against pathogens improve, so does the adaptability of the pathogens to each new environment we provide, a point which is amply illustrated by the emergence of apparently 'new' diseases such as Legionnaire's disease, myalgic encephalomyelitis, (postviral fatigue syndrome) and acquired immune deficiency syndrome (AIDS). In the absence of an infection control policy these infections can become major outbreaks with enormous cost implications, not to mention the suffering, pain and even death of the patients involved.

Risks associated with medications

At home many people have a personal medication routine such as taking medications orally; inhaling them from a nasal spray; applying them to the skin; putting medicated drops or ointment into the eye; injecting them from a syringe; inserting them in the form of a suppository into the rectum or in the form of a pessary into the vagina. People are responsible in their own homes for maintaining safety in relation to these medications whether they are self-prescribed or doctor-prescribed.

Recently, there has been considerable national publicity and extensive media coverage demonstrating increasing public concern about self-medication, and about the adverse effects of 'multi-prescription'. Elderly people as a group, have received particular attention.

According to McGuire et al (1987) the literature suggests that 80% of elderly people admitted to geriatric hospitals are on medication and 10% are admitted with iatrogenic drug-related problems. The McGuire et al's study looked at the medication regimen of a group of patients on admission and on discharge. The initial interview indicated that they knew little about their drugs and 20% admitted to having a problem, some relying on others to sort them out; some evolving a system which helped them; and others omitting to take the drugs altogether. Knowledge of what they were expected to do on discharge was equally scanty and the elderly people did not seem to connect the pattern of drug-taking in hospital with a possible continuation once they were home.

In order to decrease the risks associated with medications following discharge from hospital, McGuire et al introduced a programme of drug self-administration with selected patients in one ward, in the belief that elderly people can be helped to understand their medications; that compliance can be improved by understanding; and that one of the most effective ways of improving understanding is through teaching and counselling about the process of self-medication prior to discharge from hospital. Evaluating the scheme one year on, the programme of instruction was continuing and indeed, had been extended to other wards.

Maintaining safety in relation to medications is a personal responsibility while at home. In hospital, however, the patient usually forfeits this responsibility and becomes dependent on nursing, medical and pharmaceutical staff. In these circumstances, in the interests of patient safety, nurses become accountable for giving the correct drug, at the correct time, in the correct dose, by the correct route to the correct patient.

Due to the potential danger of drugs, and in the safety interests of all members of society, most countries legislate to control drugs. In the UK the Misuse of Drugs Act 1971 and its various amendments are in force. Very strict rules apply to those drugs which in the Act are called 'controlled drugs'; each dose has to be accounted for in a Controlled Drugs Register, whether the drug is given in hospital or in the home. Different but equally stringent rules apply to the 'scheduled drugs', those on the 'poisons list' and all other 'drugs'. The UK Central Council for Nurses, Midwives and Health Visitors has issued new guidance to nurses (UKCC, 1988) about drug administration which is a follow-up circular to clarify its 1986 'Advisory Paper'. It includes issues such as medicine administration in the community, and management's responsibility when there is any question of penalising a nurse for making a mistake which might have been associated with overwork or poor management. Although rare, medication errors can occur in hospitals too, and there is usually a hospital policy about the action to be taken in such circumstances.

Apart from risks to patients related to medications, nurses themselves may be at risk, for example, when handling cytotoxic drugs which are being used increasingly in the treatment of cancer. It is, therefore, important for staff to adhere strictly to guidelines regarding the use of protective clothing, especially gloves, when administering these drugs, and also when disposing of any spillages; for their own safety and also for the safety of patients and other staff.

CHANGE OF DEPENDENCE/INDEPENDENCE STATUS

The dependence/independence continuum in the model of living serves as a reminder that all people experience change of dependence/independence status for the Activities of Living in the normal course of the lifespan. In the context of nursing, the concept of dependence/ independence is an important one. According to the circumstances, nurses either help patients to cope with enforced dependence (short- or long-term), or help them to regain the level of independence to which they were accustomed prior to the episode of ill-health. There are many different reasons why people can experience difficulty in achieving or maintaining independence for the AL of maintaining a safe environment and, therefore, may require assistance from nurses or others. The main reasons are briefly described under the following headings: physical problems; mental problems; problems due to sensory impairment/loss.

Physical problems
Physical mobility is essential for the many activities aimed at maintaining safety, whether at home, at work, at play or while travelling. Those born with severe deformity of the skeleton, or absence of one or more limbs, usually experience some life-long difficulty in carrying out all the activities for maintaining a safe environment. Some people, on the other hand, are suddenly rendered immobile, for example some of the 'emergency' admissions to hospital and those who suddenly collapse or become ill and are nursed at home. For many of them, their inability to maintain a safe environment is only temporary, but for others it may be permanent.

Certainly, a tetraplegic person will be permanently and totally dependent for this AL. People who are unconscious are also totally dependent. Severely ill people can experience exhaustion and they simply do not have the energy to carry out the necessary preventive activities; they are dependent on nurses and others for maintaining a safe environment.

Even apparently minor problems, such as any enclosure of the hands or restriction of finger mobility, can render a person less independent for this AL. If there is any restriction on movement, however slight, of the spine, hips and lower limbs, the person may be unable to get out of the way of a dangerous moving object with sufficient speed to prevent mishap. Those who are bedfast or chairfast are similarly unable to take avoiding action. Patients with broken bones can be additionally restricted by traction apparatus and they forfeit much of their independence for this AL.

Physical imbalance of any kind can interfere with independence too, for example affecting the patient who has had a limb amputated. Recent anaesthesia and certain medications can cause patients to feel dizzy and unable to maintain their balance. People who take sleeping pills can also be at risk of falling, especially if they rise to void during the night, and the 'hang- over' feeling in the morning can create a safety risk.

Most of the physical problems, therefore, are primarily mobilising problems. These are discussed in detail in Chapter 13 but for each patient, the nurse needs to assess what that particular mobilising problem means in relation to the AL of maintaining a safe environment. She can then identify actual and potential problems and include in the patient's nursing plan whatever precautions are necessary, for example to prevent accidents.

Mental problems
As well as those born mentally handicapped, there are people whose intellect is impaired as a result of infection or injury to the brain. They may not recognise when they are in danger, for example when crossing a busy road, or they may not know how to carry out even the most basic safety precautions necessary for the prevention of fire, accidents and infection. In a hospital for the mentally handicapped much of the nurse's time is devoted to maintaining a safe environment for the patients and also helping them to understand and put into practice essential safety measures.

Certain types of mental illnesses result in a diminished awareness, so that the sufferers are not able to be completely responsible for carrying out the activities to achieve a safe environment. Depressive illness can result in suicidal thoughts and there may or may not be expression of intent. Such people need help in maintaining their environment in a condition which is safe for them until their mood improves.

If this cannot be assured, then the person may require admission to a psychiatric unit. One important role of such units, is that they provide a safe environment for mentally disturbed people, at the same time in severe cases, protecting members of the community from possible harm as a result of violence to persons or property. Nurses are concerned with the AL of maintaining a safe environment in relation to individual patients but, at the same time, must bear in mind the safety of others. The fact that this AL has a collective dimension in addition to the personal one was mentioned in the early part of this chapter.

Problems due to sensory impairment/loss

All five senses are used in activities carried out with the purpose of maintaining a safe environment and, therefore, impairment or loss of any one can result in problems. Some of the problems can occur so gradually, for example the onset of deafness, that the person adjusts gradually and so is able to maintain independence for this AL. Sudden impairment or loss, however, is likely to cause dependence, at least temporarily.

Visual impairment/loss

It is unusual for a person to lose the sight in both eyes at the same time, but loss of sight in one can be followed later by loss of sight in the second eye. One can get some idea about what it means to try to maintain safety by blindfolding even one eye and noting the several changed perspectives. It is important to establish empathy with patients who have visual problems in order to discover what they might find helpful, and what is required for independence to be maintained or regained.

Aural impairment/loss

Again it is unusual for a person suddenly to become deaf in both ears, but for example, a loud nearby explosion can cause sudden deafness, perhaps permanently. The use of earplugs can simulate the effect, and help one to appreciate the implications for safety if a person does not hear the whistle of the boiling kettle, or the sound of a pot of food boiling over, or the noise of approaching traffic.

Sensory impairment/loss

The patient with sensory loss has a problem in that he cannot feel heat, cold, pain and pressure. To help anyone who has sensory loss a nurse should try to imagine maintaining a safe environment with no awareness of heat, cold, pain and pressure. Sensory loss sometimes occurs in large areas such as the lower limbs and lower trunk; in all four limbs and the whole trunk; in the arm and leg on the same side of the body. Sensory loss frequently occurs with motor loss; the patient is paralysed and it compounds the problem of maintaining a safe environment. The different types of paralysis are illustrated in Figure 6.8.

Smelling and tasting impairment/loss

When cooking, many people check the contents of for example bottles and packages by smelling or tasting them. When deprived of these sensations they cannot be used as checks when maintaining a safe environment. Nurses can help these patients by first observing tactfully whether or not they can read and write. If so, they can be advised to pay special attention to labelling containers and paper bags

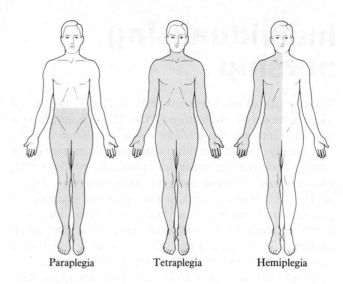

Fig. 6.8 Sensory loss in types of paralysis

Paraplegia   Tetraplegia   Hemiplegia

as to their contents. People who cannot read and write could be advised to use a signing system and could be encouraged to use any available adult literacy programme.

As has been implied from the comments made, the nurse's ability to identify patients' problems with the AL of maintaining a safe environment which result from impairment/loss of the senses, to a great extent depends on an ability to be imaginative and empathetic. Once aware of what the problems are, the nurse can help the patient to develop alternative ways of detecting and responding to hazards in the environment, thereby maintaining maximum independence for this AL.

Perhaps the importance of preventing potential problems from becoming actual problems is more obvious in this AL than in some others. And one of the major ways of emphasising prevention is through health teaching. Health teaching does not necessarily imply an elaborate pre-planned programme of instruction; it does involve being alert to cues from the clients and assessing the appropriate time to discuss issues which they and the nurse consider important to the client's circumstances. A recent research study (News, 1988), for example, showed that patients' smoking habits changed more favourably after nurses' intervention, compared to studies involving other health care professions. There may be numerous opportunities for health teaching in the course of a nurse/patient relationship; on the other hand, the patient/client may be coping adequately, and therein lies a skilled nursing judgement — knowing when to withdraw.

Individualising nursing

The first part of this chapter reflects the Roper, Logan and Tierney model — the nature of the AL of maintaining a safe environment; the relationship of the lifespan to the AL; the effect of an individual's dependence/independence status; and the influence of physical, psychological, sociocultural, environmental and politicoeconomic factors on the AL. Mainly, the first part provides examples of potential problems occurring in everyday living and what might be done to prevent them from becoming actual problems. In the second part of the chapter, a selection of actual problems and discomforts which can be experienced by people in relation to the AL have been described. This provides a background of general knowledge about the AL as such.

While describing the Roper, Logan and Tierney model for nursing, general information was provided about individualising nursing (p. 51) which, in fact, is synonymous with the concept of the process of nursing.

Out of this background of general knowledge about the AL of maintaining a safe environment, and about individualising nursing, it should then be possible to extract the issues which are relevant to one individual's current circumstances (whether in a health or an illness setting) i.e. make an assessment of relevant issues according to the individual's stage on the lifespan; according to current level of dependence/independence; and take into account the relevant physical, psychological, sociocultural, environmental and politicoeconomic factors. Collectively, this information would provide a profile of the person's individuality in living for this AL, and therefore guides the nurse in devising a plan for individualising nursing.

As indicated earlier in the text, this assessment would be achieved by various means such as observing the person; acquiring information about the person's usual habits in relation to this AL partly by asking appropriate questions, partly by listening to the patient and/or relatives; and using relevant information from available records, including medical records. The collected information could then be examined to identify any actual problems being experienced with the AL and these could be arranged in some order of priority. The nurse might also recognise some potential problems — not all possible potential problems but those which are relevant. Realistic goals, mutually agreed with the patient when this is possible, could then be set to prevent potential problems from becoming actual ones; to alleviate or solve the actual problems; or to help the person cope with those which cannot be alleviated or solved. Of course, some of the patient's problems with this AL, although identified from the nurs-

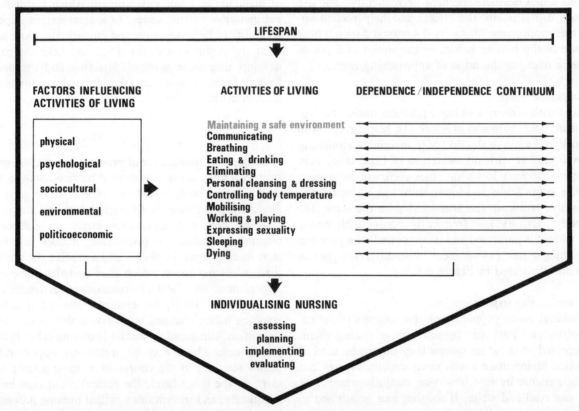

Fig. 6.9 The AL of maintaining a safe environment within the model for nursing

ing assessment, may well be outwith the scope of nursing intervention. In such instances, after discussion with the patient when appropriate, these problems may be referred to other members of the health care team such as medical staff, dieticians, physiotherapists or social workers.

Keeping in mind what the person can and cannot do unaided, the nursing interventions to achieve the mutually set goals could then be selected according to local circumstances and available resources.

Following implementation of the interventions, their effects could be evaluated in relation to the goals set, and if goals were not reached, they could be revised or rescheduled, or even discarded.

It is worth repeating here that although discussed in four phases — assessing, planning, implementing and evaluating — individualising nursing is not a linear progression; it assumes a built-in responsiveness to feedback at any of the phases, giving ample allowance for change within the overall framework. Also, during an illness episode, an important consideration is rehabilitation of the individual, and planning for this could commence as soon as the person enters the health care system. Another important feature is the professional judgement needed to discontinue the nurse/patient relationship when it is no longer relevant.

This chapter has been concerned with the AL of maintaining a safe environment. However, as stated previously, it is only for the purposes of discussion that any AL can be considered on its own; in reality, the various activities are closely related and do not have distinct boundaries. Figure 6.9 is a reminder that the AL of maintaining a safe environment is related to the other ALs and also to the other components of the model for nursing.

Acknowledgement
Thanks are extended to Miss M. Strachan, Senior Nurse, Glasgow University Department of Infectious Diseases, Ruchill Hospital, Glasgow for checking the sections of this chapter which deal with infection.

REFERENCES

Archer H 1988 Waste in the home. Nursing Standard 2 (21) February 27: 26–27

Ayliffe G, Collins B 1982 Infection control in the United Kingdom. Aspects of Infection Control. Imperial Chemical Industries

Ayton M 1985 Infection control: protective clothing. The Add-on Journal of Clinical Nursing 2 (38) June: 1136–1139

Barnett R 1983 Isolated but not alone. In: Infection control in hospital and the community. Supplement to Nursing 20 December: 7

Baxter B 1987 Too good to throw away. Nursing Times 83 (11) March 18: 24–26

Begley S 1988 A summer of smog. Newsweek CX11 (9) August 29: 46–47

Bentley S, Murphy F, Dudley H 1977 Perceived noise in surgical wards and an intensive care area: an objective analysis. British Medical Journal 2 (6101) December 10: 1503–1506

Beral V, Fraser P, Carpenter L, Booth M, Brown A, Rose G 1988 Mortality of employees of the Atomic Weapons Establishment. British Medical Journal 297 (6651) September 24: 757–770

Blackmore M 1987 Hand-drying methods. Nursing Times 83 (37) September 16: 71–74

Blake C, Morfit J 1986 Falls and staffing in a residential home for elderly people. Public Health 100 (6) November: 385–391

Blenkharn I 1988 Urinary drainage systems: a new look. Nursing Times 84 (9) March 2: 72–76

Brookbanks M, Hampstead N 1987 Controlling an epidemic. Nursing Times 83 (38) September 23: 38–39

Burry H, Calcinai C 1988 The need to make rugby safer. British Medical Journal 296 (6616) January 16: 149–150

Butler-Sloss E 1988 (Cleveland Report) Report of the inquiry into child abuse in Cleveland, 1987. HMSO, London

Campbell C 1988 Could do better. Nursing Times 84 (22) June 1: 66–71

Cave J 1988 Growing old dangerously. Community Outlook in Nursing Times 84 (41) October: 18–19

Central Statistical Office 1988 Social Trends 18: 122, HMSO, London

Child Accident Prevention Trust 1986 Keep them safe: a guide to child safety equipment. CAPT, London

Children's Legal Centre 1988 Child abuse procedures — the child's viewpoint. CLC, London

Clarke C 1987 Reaching for reality. Nursing Times 83 (30) July 29: 24–26

Community Outlook 1982 Children and accidents at home. Nursing Times 78 (32) August 11: 212–223

Constantinides P 1987 The management response to childhood accidents. Primary Health Care Group, King's Fund Centre, London

Constantinides P, Walker G 1986 Child accidents and inequality in a London borough. Unpublished Report to NE Thames Health Authority, London

Corsellis J 1989 Boxing and the brain. British Medical Journal 298 (6666) January 14: 105–109

Cramb A 1989 Thatcher in ozone plea to the world. Glasgow Herald 6: 1

Dawson M 1988 Immunology. Nursing Times 84 (17) April: 75–78

Delamothe T 1988 Violence: next on the public health agenda. British Medical Journal 297 (6644) July 30: 314–315

Department of Health and Social Security and Welsh Office 1987 Firecode: policy and principles. HMSO, London

Dooley T 1981 Fire! The nursing response. Nursing Times 77 (43) October 21: 1845–1848

Doyle C 1988 Needs of today's young people. Daily Telegraph April 19: 5

Eason K 1989 1.5 million motorists drink and drive. The Times February 9: 6

Eastman M 1988 Granny abuse. Community Outlook in Nursing Times 84 (41) October 12: 15–16

Editorial 1989 Unscrambling the Min. of Ag. Glasgow Herald January 25: 8

Finney G 1988 One false move. Community Outlook in Nursing Times 84 (15) April 13: 8–9

Ford M, Fox J, Fitch S 1986 Light in the darkness. Nursing Times 83 (1) January 7: 26–29

Forshaw A 1987 Burns and aftercare. Nursing Times 83 (1) January 7: 51–52

Galbraith N 1983 Contact tracing in the control of infectious disease. Nursing Times 79 (23) June 8: 55–56

Garrett G 1986 Old age abuse by carers. The Professional Nurse 1 (11) August: 304–305

Gidley C 1987 Now wash your hands. Nursing Times 83 (29) July 22: 40–42

Glasgow Herald 1989 Carers saving state billions. Glasgow Herald 30: 3

Gough G 1986 The patient's auditory environment. The Professional Nurse 1 (8) May: 217–218

Gray C 1987 Burn-injured children. Nursing Times 83 (21) May 27: 49–51

Grazebrook J 1986 Counting the cost of infection. Nursing Times 82 (6) February 5: 24–26

Hall M 1987 Arms and the suburban man. Telegraph Sunday Magazine 548 (April 26): 22–24

Health and Safety at Work Act 1974

Hewitt B, Marshall R, Hoscheka T, Hager M 1988 Our ailing oceans. Newsweek CX11 (5) August 1: 34–41

Hilton A 1987 The hospital racket: how noisy is your unit? American Journal of Nursing, January: 59–61

Hobbs P 1989 Enteral feeds. Nursing Times 85 (9) March 1: 71–73

Hodgkinson N 1988 Researchers alarmed over danger in baby bottle milk. Sunday Times November 20: 1

Holmes S 1988 Christmas feasting — danger or delight? Community Outlook in Nursing Times 84 (50) December 14: 11–14

Horton R 1988 Linking the chain. Nursing Times 84 (26) June 29: 44–46

Ingleston L 1986 Make haste slowly. Nursing Times 82 (37) September 10: 28–30

International Council of Nurses World Health Organization 1987 Joint Declaration on AIDS. ICN, Geneva

International Council of Nurses/World Health Organization 1988 Joint Guidelines on the nursing management of people infected with HIV. ICN, Geneva

International News 1988 Europe. Nursing Times 84 (41) October 12: 8

Jones I 1988 Home is where the hurt is. Nursing Times 84 (6) February 10: 48–49

Kay K 1988 The global struggle against AIDS: WHO's strategy. International Nursing Review 35 (2) March/April: 35–38

Keller B 1988 Soviet public wary of nuclear power. International Herald Tribune October 14: 1

Kendall S 1986 Home safety and accident prevention. The Add-on Journal of Clinical Nursing 3 (12): 454–457

Krakowska G 1986 Practice versus procedure. Nursing Times 82 (49) December 3: 64–69

Lowry S 1989 Making roads safer. British Medical Journal 298 (6671) February 18: 408

McGuire J, Preston J, Pinches D 1987 Two pink and one blue . . . . . Nursing Times 82 (2) January 14: 32–33

McKie R, Rycroft M 1988 Health and the ozone layer. British Medical Journal 297 (6645) August 6: 369–370

Maddocks G 1981 Accidents in childhood: Growing to independence. Nursing Mirror, Clinical Forum 5, 152 (21) May 20: viii–xiv

Meers P, Ayliffe G, Emmerson E 1981 Report on the National Survey of Infection in Hospitals 1980. Journal of Hospital Infection, December 2 (Supplement)

Mitchell R 1984 Falls in the elderly. Nursing Times 80 (2) January 11: 51–53

Moorat D 1983 Accidents to patients. Nursing Times 79 (20) May 18: 59–61

News 1988 Nurses help change patients' smoking habits. Nursing Times 84 (39) September 28: 6

Nichols S 1988 Beware of the midday sun. Nursing Times 84 (23) June 8: 38–39

Office of Health Economic 1981 Accidents in childhood. OHE, Briefing No. 17 (September) London

Oldman P 1987 An unkind cut? Nursing Times 83 (48) December 2: 71–74

Overtone E 1988 Bed-making and bacteria. Nursing Times 84 (9) March 2: 69–71

Pope N 1988 A cry for help. Nursing Times 84 (14) April 6: 20

Renn M 1987 Prevention in triplicate. Nursing Times 83 (44) November 4: 16–17

Rogers L 1987 Boosting protection. Nursing Times 83 (48) December 2: 34–36

Rogers R, Salvage J 1988 Nurses at risk. Heinemann, London, p 54–66, 37

Royal Society for Prevention of Accidents 1986 Annual Report. RSPA, London

Sadler C 1983 Healing the hordes (how occupational health nurses manage accidents in large crowds). Nursing Mirror 79 (20) May 18: 17–20

Scottish Hospital Advisory Service 1978 New facilities: old practices. Health Bulletin 36 July 4: 152

Shepherd J 1988 Supporting victims of violent crime. British Medical Journal 297 (6660) November 26: 1353

Sieving R 1988 Measles vaccination timing: finding the right age. International Nursing Review 35 (1) January/February: 17–21

Smith S 1988 Take care: be aware. Community Outlook in Nursing Times 84 (15) April 13: 10–12

Soutar R, Wilson J 1986 Does hospital noise disturb the patient? British Medical Journal 292 (6516) February 1: 305

Stannard D 1989 Pressure prevents nausea. Nursing Times 85 (4) January 25: 33–34

Statutory Instrument (1324) 1988 Furniture and Furnishings (Fire) (Safety) Regulation. HMSO, London

Swan P 1983 Cholera: A visitation on Victorian Society. Nursing Mirror 157 (15) October 12: 30–34

Timoney R 1987 A policy for community practice. Nursing Times 83 (9) March 4: 64–71

Tyler J 1987 Give us a break. Nursing Times 83 (50) December 16/23: 32–35

United Kingdom Central Council 1988 The administration of medicines. (Circular PC/88/05). UKCC, London

UNICEF 1987 State of the world's children. UNICEF, London

Vousden M 1987 Behind closed doors. Nursing Times 83 (16) April 22: 24–30

Wild D, Nayak U, Isaacs B 1981 Prognosis of falls in old people at home. Journal of Epidemiology and Community Health 35: 200–204

Williams S, Gonzalez D 1987 A few too many on the water. Newsweek CX (5) August 3: 25

Whitehead M 1987 The health divide: inequalities in health in the 1980s. Health Education Council, London

Women's Herald 1989 Age Concern puts focus on falls. Glasgow Herald January 24: 9

World Health Organization 1986 Accidents in children and young people. WHO Statistics Quarterly 39 (3)

ADDITIONAL READING

Atkinson J 1989 AIDS focus: which care setting for pentamidine? Nursing Standard 26 (3) March 25: 26–28

Brodie E 1987 Legionella: the story of an outbreak. Nursing Times 83 (41) October 14: 52–54

Carr P, Rothburn M 1989 Listeriosis in midwifery. Nursing Times 85 (18) May 3: 73–74

David A, Wessely S, Pelosi A 1988 Postviral fatigue syndrome: time for a new approach. Lancet 296 (March 5): 696–698

Galbraith N 1988 Changes in notifiable infectious diseases. British Medical Journal 297 (6659) November 19: 1291

Goodman C 1985 Cytotoxic drugs: their handling and use. Nursing Times 81 (47) November 20: 36–38

Kay E 1989 Accidents will happen. Nursing Times 85 (3) January 18: 26–29

Pratt R 1988 AIDS: a strategy for nursing care. Edward Arnold, London

Pickersgill F 1988 The case against re-use. Nursing Times 84 (44) November 2: 45–48

7

Communicating

The activity of communicating

Man is essentially a social being and spends the major part of each day communicating with other people in one way or another. The activity of communicating is therefore an integral part of all human behaviour.

There is now considerable knowledge from research in the behavioural sciences about body or non-verbal language, use of which can enrich the AL of communicating. And even in the more familiar mode of verbal language, research has uncovered some interesting and illuminating aspects.

An understanding of the complexities of both components of communicating is likely to help people to carry out this AL in a manner which is effective and brings satisfaction to themselves and others. But what does 'communicating' mean?

THE NATURE OF COMMUNICATING

Most written languages have an alphabet, and in English everyone is familiar with the 26 letters from which many thousands of words can be constructed, each having a dictionary definition to help the process of communicating. Words however are only symbols and they can have different meanings for different people. Even in the English-speaking countries of the UK and North America there are differences as the following pairs of words show: nappies, diapers; lift, elevator; pavement, sidewalk; the bonnet of a car, the hood of a car. So there are occasions when it is important to check the meaning attached to a particular word. Words can also have different meaning according to the context in which they are used. Think of the word 'game' associated with a sports stadium and a butcher's shop; the word 'eye' related to biology and to embroidery.

The arrangement of words can affect meaning. 'Blanket this on child the put' has no meaning, Yet if these six words are rearranged to read 'Put the child on this blanket', the sentence does have meaning. However, if they are rearranged to read 'Put the blanket on this child' the sentence has a different meaning. Choice of words and their arrangement in sentences to convey exact meaning are therefore vital in the activity of communicating.

Some words such as 'older' and 'younger', express relativity; to make them meaningful, further information is needed such as 'older than x'. Words can be emotionally neutral and factual like 'black man' and 'illegitimate', whereas others — 'nigger' and 'bastard' — not only indicate a fact but suggest a derisive attitude. Yet other words denote a value judgement assigned by the user — large, medium, small; good and bad being examples. Consequently, especially when recording and reporting information, the need to use neutral, factual words is necessary.

The use of language involves a number of skills, mainly speaking and listening; reading and writing. When *speaking*, it is not only what is said but equally important how it is said. With practice, the clarity, speed, pitch, inflection and tone of voice can all be used to convey exact meaning. In response to a request, the answer 'I don't mind doing it' can be said in a pleasant positive manner, assuring the listener that the task will be done willingly. On the other hand it can be said in a grudging negative manner leaving the listener uncomfortable and possibly guilty at having made the request.

Listening is much more than hearing; it is an active process whereby the listener attends exclusively to the speaker, not only to the words that he is speaking. There are advantages to listening in a face-to-face conversation which communication links such as the telephone and tape recorder do not offer, although being in the presence of the speaker is not an absolute prerequisite for 'effective listening'. For instance a telephone listening service is offered to people in distress by associations such as the Samaritans and Befrienders. The listeners are trained to hear and interpret silences, sighs, sobs and so on.

Reading is a skill which many people take for granted. Yet even in developed countries there is concern about the extent of illiteracy among adults, and special classes are offered to cope with this problem. Many readers are hindered by inaudibly 'pronouncing' each word rather than scanning a group of words to get the meaning of a sentence and rapid reading classes can be helpful in correcting this deficiency.

Again, the skill of *writing* is often taken for granted, yet there are adults who are handicapped because they cannot write their name. Adult literacy campaigns aim to improve writing as well as reading. But even so-called educated people can have difficulty in writing fluently, especially

when under stress as for example in an examination setting or when emotionally upset.

Individuality, and many of the complexities of human beings are reflected in their speaking, listening, reading and writing, so it is useful to consider the total process of communicating.

The process of communicating

The study of cybernetics has contributed considerable information about the process of communicating. Basically communication is said to occur when a person (the sender) has a message which he sends in a particular medium, so that it is received by a recipient in whom it produces a response, followed by feedback to the sender (Fig. 7.1). This seems a simple process.

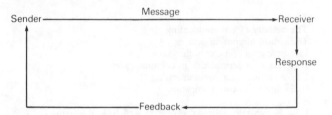

Fig. 7.1 Basic model of communicating

Further thought reveals however that it is not so simple, and that there are several stages, at any one of which error can occur which breaks a link in the chain of communication (Fig. 7.2). At the beginning of a conversation, one person has an idea which is encoded in language symbols and then sent by speaking. The other person (the receiver) hears them, decodes and interprets by attaching meaning to them (interpretation). 'Foreign' words can be heard but meaning cannot be attached to them; they cannot be interpreted. In response to interpretation the sequence is repeated in reverse and so on.

The complexity of the AL of communicating can already be appreciated. Effective communication, of course, is dependent on the communicators' several abilities within the verbal language component, notably those of thinking, speaking, listening, reading and writing (Fig. 7.3). However the necessary skills within the body language component are also of enormous importance.

The study of non-verbal communication or body language is now receiving much more attention and the term 'kine' has been adopted for each 'unit' of body movement which transmits a message. The kine is analogous to a letter in the verbal alphabet. Kinetics is still a young science but it would seem that human ability to exert conscious control over body language is less easy than with verbal communication and most people, at times, are aware of sending contradictory messages. For example, in response to a ring of the door bell the words 'Do come in, I'm pleased to see you' might be spoken while the facial expression might say 'I'm busy, I wish you hadn't called.'

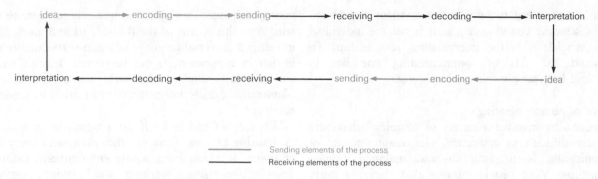

Fig. 7.2 Stages in the two-way process of communicating

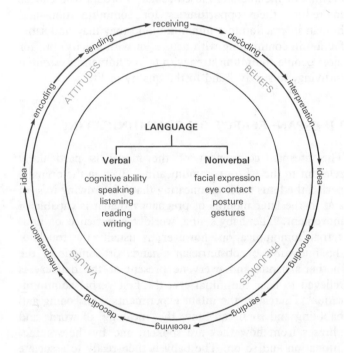

Fig. 7.3 The complexities of communicating

Non-verbal communication serves a number of purposes depending on the context. The whole body may be conveying a message. Humans use their bodies to express themselves in for instance the way they walk. Walking boldly into a room may be indicative of a feeling of well-being; on the other hand it may be conveying a mood of anger, so analysis of further cues is required to differentiate. In contrast walking slowly into a room may indicate reticence or apprehension. The stance people take, too, can transmit an impression as varied as boredom, exhaustion, attentiveness and interest.

Facial expression is a rich source of information regarding the emotional state of the individual and some evidence of this can be found in the amount of space and time authors and playwrights give to describing the facial changes in their characters. One can transmit impressions such as disapproval, disgust, anger, irritation, pleasure, love and

understanding by facial gesture, indeed its effectiveness is recognised in colloquial expressions such as 'a look enough to kill' or 'a sour look'. The eyes can be particularly revealing, and people vary in the amount of eye contact they make and maintain while communicating. The lecturer who stares out of the window, for example, is unlikely to convey to students much personal interest in their learning.

Hands are also important in body language, usually to provide points of emphasis, while shaping with the hands the object being discussed, or an event, or signalling directions. Hands also convey emotion, for example the interviewee attending a selection panel who reflects inner anxiety by restless, wringing movements or fiddling with small objects; or the angry person who shows white knuckles or clenched fists. Feet, too, are used in communicating, for example toe-tapping may express a degree of anxiety, or enjoyment of the rhythm of music.

It is apparent that physical appearance and presence are powerful aspects of non-verbal communication, and the amount and variety of make-up products, jewellery, perfume, aftershave, spectacle frames in department stores is an eloquent reflection of the range of taste. Clothes, too, although essentially intended to protect from the elements, provide a great deal of information about the wearer. They express current mood, state of finance, preparation to take part in sport, or to go to work. Indeed, the term 'language of clothes' is quite commonly used and is discussed in more detail in the chapter dealing with the AL of personal cleansing and dressing (p. 204). Actually some groups in current Western society wear what could almost be termed a uniform, in that it serves to give them a distinct identity, for example skinheads, hippies, and the tinted, spiked hair brigade; in fact these non-verbal cues can influence interaction to such an extent that one has to be careful to avoid stereotyping, sometimes quite erroneously.

Communicating is a highly individual activity. Communicators bring to the conversation their attitudes, beliefs, values and prejudices, these being fashioned by previous experience which must necessarily be affected by social background. The contribution of each person is affected by their current needs: the need to be dominant or submissive; the need to be talkative or silent and so on. Yet in discussing communicating, it is not the individual who is crucial; it is the interpersonal relationship. To understand the AL of communicating one has to understand how people relate to each other.

Purpose of communicating

Communicating involves a variety of complex behaviours which are difficult to categorise. One main purpose of communicating is to establish and maintain human relationships. Most people imagine that they are fairly competent communicators; adults have been doing it all their lives! In fact, it is all too easy to conclude that if one's message is misunderstood, the receiver is at fault; and if the other person's attempt to communicate is not understood, then the other person's mode of expression is deficient in some way. The individual's interpretation of a situation is based on personal beliefs about communication competence — one's own and the other person's — and these beliefs affect how the individual relates to others, and how others relate to the individual. A lot depends on how individuals view themselves. This self-perception is said to start at birth as the infant begins to develop a feeling of trust. With a feeling of trust comes, among other things, the ability to recognise personal strengths and weaknesses, the development of self-respect and faith in oneself, the development of respect and concern for others; all of which are essential for the establishment and maintenance of human relationships, and are basic to the AL of communicating.

The simplest form of communication is dyadic, the individual with one other person such as a parent, a marriage partner, a friend, a colleague, but there are extensions of the dyad in the form of small group communication, as indeed happens even with children when they go to school and find opportunities for communicating with different children and adults, beyond the home setting. Eventually adults become members of more and more dyadic, small and large group communication systems. A term often applied to a large group system is an organisation and these are usually created to accomplish a specific purpose, for example a hospital is organised for the treatment of people with disease; and is perhaps within a yet larger organisation, a national health service, which in addition is responsible for maintenance of health, prevention of disease and rehabilitation.

In an organisation such as a hospital, communicating is a means to an end but in some organisations it is an end in itself. For example in schools and colleges and universities, the purpose is communication in a teaching/learning context. The mass media too are concerned essentially with communicating, usually *giving* information although it may also involve *exchange* in the form of readers' letters to a newspaper or phone-in programmes on radio. Of course the mass media are not concerned only with information

giving/exchange; they also communicate in order to entertain. And this is true of the theatre, art and music. Music in fact is a universal language of a non-verbal nature which is rich in expression. It can be played, listened to, read and written throughout the world, irrespective of mother tongue and usually brings great satisfaction to sender and receiver.

Whether an end in itself, or a means to an end, communicating in some form or other permeates every aspect of living — maintaining a safe environment, eating and drinking, dressing, working and playing, expressing sexuality and so on. There are a few individuals such as hermits or members of closed religious orders who choose to reduce their opportunities for communication and human interaction to a minimum (and they may find satisfaction in communing with nature, or with a deity) but for most people communicating with fellow humans is essential to living, to survival and to the quality of life.

LIFESPAN: EFFECT ON COMMUNICATING

The lifespan component of the model is particularly relevant to the AL of communicating. Even in the prenatal period the fetus is communicating that it is growing in size; and in the later months of pregnancy that it is capable of movement. The baby's first worldly experience of non-verbal communication, however, is usually the touch of the midwife's or obstetrician's hands or sometimes the mother's hands and everyone present at the delivery is relieved to hear the initial cry, the first verbal communication. Thereafter the infant experiments with cooing and babbling and soon can sense the 'meaning' of words and phrases from how they are spoken, and by the volume, intonation and so on. The baby is then ready to associate words with objects or people, and later begins to utter the correct word in response. By a long process the child gradually learns and uses an increasing vocabulary. A vital aspect of this learning is the stimulation from other people in the environment especially the mother or mother substitute who by speaking and singing to the child, and touching and cuddling, provides the basic experiences for interpersonal communication which are so crucial to further development. Indeed, children deprived of such stimulation may grow up to have difficulty with human relationships.

During adolescence, the teenager may develop special meanings for certain words known only to the peer group and not understood by adults. However as well as this private communication channel, most adolescents extend their vocabulary and modes of expression, verbally and non-verbally, as they move away from the constraints of home and school contacts, and explore new environments with different types of relationships.

It is estimated that the majority of adults have a speaking

vocabulary of 3000 to 5000 words although their reading vocabulary may well be more. On the other hand there are those whose speaking vocabulary contains only a few hundred words of not more than three syllables and their reading vocabulary not many more. Often current slang and colloquialisms make up the bulk of such people's language. These factors will naturally have their effect on acquisition of writing skills.

In old age, deterioration of vision and hearing can lessen the ability to communicate effectively by causing distortion of sensory input. Also there is a gradual loss of function of some brain cells which can result in forgetfulness and sometimes confusion. Arthritic finger joints can make writing difficult. Frailty can interfere with body posture and gesture and therefore with body language. All these factors may contribute to problems in the older person's AL of communicating.

DEPENDENCE/INDEPENDENCE IN COMMUNICATING

Communicating is an AL where movement along the dependence/independence continuum has a direct relationship with the lifespan component of the model. Even when a baby is born with the intact body structures required for communicating, it is necessary to learn to use those structures, to perceive, and to attach meaning to discrete sounds. Stimulation from parents enhances the speed of learning, and great patience is required to perceive and decode the communicating done by babies and children, both verbally and non-verbally. On the other hand, adults can be curiously lacking in perception. An extreme example would be an instance when there are signs of child abuse and the cues are not picked up by people outside the home setting. Another example is the puzzling situation when an otherwise bright, healthy child has difficulty mastering reading and spelling — a syndrome labelled as dyslexia — and investigation is required, perhaps to be followed by a special educational programme (Yule, 1988). The young are certainly dependent on others for the AL of communicating and likewise, sometimes, the elderly.

Physical body structure, of course, influences the degree of dependence in communicating. Intact physical structures which enable one to see, hear, taste, smell and touch, and those which permit speech and body language are basic to independence, although some degree of impairment can often be compensated for or coped with. However, mechanical aids can do much to lessen the disability of impaired body structure. The problem of diminished sight can be reduced or corrected by using spectacles or an illuminated magnifying glass: and for those who are severely handicapped the use of specially prepared large-print books or of Braille or of tape-recordings can help considerably in retaining a measure of independence. For those who have impaired auditory structure and function, it is possible now to have quite sophisticated, unobtrusive hearing aids which dramatically improve their quality of living and there are also amplifiers available for telephone conversations and public meetings. For those who are dumb, a sign language is useful and especially for mentally handicapped people who have speech difficulties, there are symbolic languages such as the Bliss Symbolic Communication System and the Makaton Vocabulary Language Programme which have greatly improved their capacity for communicating (Kiernan et al, 1983).

A few years ago, it was quite revolutionary to provide an aid, called Possum, for those who were quadriplegic; it enabled the paralysed person, by blowing on a type of keyboard, to manipulate light switches, radio and television sets, telephone and so on. However, recent technological advances have made possible a robot which can be programmed to carry out a range of services on command. These developments hold great promise for severely disabled people who, although dependent on a machine, can have a feeling of relative independence; their range of control in communicating and getting an appropriate response is increased and they are less dependent on people to carry out a number of everyday living activities.

FACTORS INFLUENCING COMMUNICATING

Like all other ALs, communicating is influenced by a variety of factors. In keeping with the relevant component of the model, these are discussed under the following headings — physical, psychological, sociocultural, environmental and politicoeconomic factors.

Physical factors

Many physical factors influence a person's ability to communicate by means of verbal and non-verbal language, and especially important are adequately functioning body structures in the nervous and endocrine systems. For example, for the acquisition of speech there has to be at least adequate hearing, an adequately functioning speech apparatus and the opportunity to hear others' voices for imitation. The achievement of reading skills requires at least minimal vision, and the accomplishment of writing skills is further dependent on an adequately functioning preferred hand. Communicating by body language is dependent on adequately functioning nervous and musculoskeletal systems.

Hormone production is also related, although less obviously, to communicating. The sex hormones are responsible for the distinguishable difference between the male and female voice. Structurally the male larynx is on average longer anteriorly/posteriorly so that the male voice after puberty is lower in pitch than that of the female. However both males and females differ in the control which they have over the many muscles, including the diaphragm, used in voice production. Thus some people have low, monotonous voices and others can modulate the voice for effective and varied expression. There are also differences related to patterns of physical contact as a means of communicating between males, between females, and between males/females; and these are mentioned in Chapter 15 when expressing sexuality is discussed.

As explained earlier when describing the model of living and the model for nursing, the 12 ALs are interrelated; so too the body systems as categorised by the human biologists are interrelated and it is only for the purposes of description and discussion that they are dealt with separately. In order to show how human biology relates to the model for nursing, the authors suggest that the AL of communicating be particularly associated with the larynx containing the vital vocal cords, and the mouth, tongue and lips; the nervous system including the sense organs; and the endocrine system. This juxtaposition of AL and body system gives guidance for curriculum planning, and also for knowing where to record problems, actual and potential, related to the AL of communicating if the Roper, Logan and Tierney model is used as a guideline for nursing plans.

Psychological factors

Level of intelligence affects communicating in that it influences learning ability. It therefore plays an important part in the extent of the vocabulary acquired for use in everyday living. A person with a limited vocabulary can usually manage well in familiar surroundings but may experience difficulty, for instance when filling in many of the forms which have become a feature of our modern society such as an insurance form. However problems can arise even for intelligent people with an extensive vocabulary, for example when they are communicating with someone on a subject other than their own speciality.

Anxiety affects communicating as people going for an interview know only too well; interviewees may come away feeling annoyed that their ability to respond fluently has been impaired and they have not done themselves justice. For others, in spite of adequate content in their conversation, the non-verbal behaviour of tremulous hands, dilated pupils, perspiration on brow and upper lip, can inform the interviewer of the state of tension.

Current mood also has its effect on communicating. Excitement usually increases the rate of speech, raises the voice pitch and there may be more than usual gesticulation. Anger is usually expressed by raising the voice. Depression flattens the voice almost to monotony; movement is slowed, and a dejected facial expression is characteristic of many people when they are in a low mood. In comparison, cheerfulness lightens the voice, and is likely to be reflected in a smiling expression. Of course communication is two-way, and the mood of the recipients is also important for effective communication. It is not uncommon to refer to a 'hostile audience' or a 'receptive audience'.

Loss of self-respect and faith in self may make communicating a problematic activity. In such circumstances, an event which normally would be considered insignificant might produce a reaction of worthlessness, guilt or shame; or might provoke over-criticism of others, probably a subconscious effort to raise self-esteem. Those who have not experienced some type of long-term, warm, trusting relationship in their early years often lack self-confidence and may find it difficult to communicate effectively with other people.

Some people are aware of their lack of self-confidence. As one of a variety of possible techniques to develop self-confidence, it is sometimes suggested that 'assertiveness training' is helpful, the idea being that stress is reduced if one knows, in appropriate circumstances, how to be assertive rather than aggressive. Fessey (1988) maintains that assertiveness techniques should be used only if a need requires expression or a right is about to be denied. She writes:

. . . assertiveness skills help to focus the emphasis of the request on the specific problem, and prevent the asserted comment from being aggressive or intensely personal. In this way, the respondent's self-esteem is not severely diminished . . . the technique appears simple but requires an examination of the values and attitudes which shape our responses to others. This process can be painful and revealing but it leads to greater self-awareness — the first step to unambiguous communication.

Bond (1988) discusses a self-help scheme of assertiveness training which, although geared to nurses, is really a specific application of general principles which can assist good communication in any context.

Communicating, both verbal and non-verbal, and deliberate or non-planned, is the basis of all activities associated with learning and teaching, and there is a considerable literature about the contribution of psychological principles in the approach to information-giving, teaching, and counselling. These psychological principles are used in everyday living related, for example, to child development, all aspects of organised education, the impact of the mass media, and also in a variety of community services including health care services.

Psychological factors certainly affect both verbal and non-verbal communicating.

Sociocultural factors

Now more than ever, an increasingly mobile and multiracial society demands that consideration be given to sociocultural factors in communicating. Watson (1986) suggests how some of the communication problems can be surmounted when in contact with minority ethnic groups who have difficulty with a second language but even within one language there can be several local vocabularies which strangers cannot understand. Accent or dialect can communicate place of residence during acquisition of language; and it may take time for the listener to become accustomed to a different dialect. Social status can also be conveyed by language. For example in the UK, the range of vocabulary can be indicative of level of education attained; this can influence the type of job procured which determines economic bracket of income and in turn determines the person's social class according to the Registrar-General's classification (p. 272).

Apart from dialect or accent or social class indicators, the specialist vocabulary in certain occupations and professions is almost a 'language culture'. Technical expressions which are in everyday usage within an occupational group, can be totally alien to outsiders. For example, despite the computer revolution, the language of computer users still has to be interpreted to the uninitiated; and for clients in the health care system, the vocabulary of staff is often unintelligible or, when only snatches are overheard and understood, is open to misinterpretation and can cause the client and family great distress.

Other sociocultural differences affect body language. Mode of dress can communicate such diverse information as a person's ethnic origin, religious affiliation, occupation or social group and Helman (1984) cites examples of even self-mutilation to the body to indicate 'group' membership such as the insertion of large ornaments in the lips or earlobes in Brazil, East Africa and Melanesia. The acceptability of touching fellow humans also varies. Although communicating by touch is the most primitive mode, there are culturally determined touching patterns for adults. Some cultures permit a reciprocal hug to signal welcome on arrival, and again on departure to signal appreciation of the visit. The accepted practice in other cultures on these occasions is a kiss on each cheek; yet in others a kiss on the lips: in some it is nose-rubbing; and in others only reciprocal hand-shaking is acceptable. There are also differences regarding the amount of gesticulation and mobility of the lips when communicating which are culturally determined. There are culturally determined practices related to eye contact, for example certain aborigines, to be polite, do not look into each other's eyes as they talk, whereas in the Western world it is polite to maintain eye contact during conversation.

The individual's social and cultural background usually influences the system of values and beliefs which determine behaviour, for example in the expression of spirituality via various ALs, possibly following a formal religion, or in the acquisition of a moral stance on particular issues. In our model, these are subsumed under sociocultural factors and are involved closely with the AL of communicating. Organised religions usually lay considerable stress on group interaction, and the selected places of worship, sometimes enormously costly to build and maintain and often elaborately decorated, provide the focal point for communication, sometimes in groups or sometimes for personal communion with a god or deity. A concept which is more encompassing than organised religion is spirituality (Labun, 1988) interpreted as a 'search for meaning' in one's life and encompassing theistic and non-theistic approaches, which applies to agnostics and atheists as well as followers of a recognised religious persuasion. Irrespective of personal interpretation of spirituality, the related system of values and beliefs can often bring comfort and reassurance during times of stress and when the individual is faced with moral dilemmas which require resolution.

Environmental factors

The appropriateness of the physical environment can certainly contribute to the effectiveness of the AL of communicating. Poor ventilation in a room and extremes of temperature can be conducive to discomfort and interfere with concentration when communicating. Lighting, too, is important. Excessive light and glare can make a person feel too uncomfortable to converse, and poor lighting can mean that important non-verbal cues are missed. Soft lighting is deliberately used for example by restaurateurs to induce a feeling of relaxation, enhance the enjoyment of the meal, and promote pleasurable conversation. Environmental noise can have an effect on communicating. Some people find it easier to speak about personal matters if there is background noise, be it music or the hum of conversation, while others find even the slightest noise distracting. Rooms which afford aural privacy usually help when personal matters need to be discussed, for example, an interview or consultation with a member of health care staff. In such a setting, too, conversation is more likely to be encouraged if the furniture is so arranged that the interviewee and the interviewer are not physically separated by a desk; that the chairs are reasonably comfortable and in a position to allow eye contact; and that there are no unplanned interruptions.

Apart from personal interviews, the physical layout of a room is important for any group work; chairs with desks in serried rows for example are not so conducive to discussion as chairs arranged in a circle or round a central table. This type of arrangement allows all members of the group to see who is speaking, to have eye contact, to observe body language and to maximise the impact of non-verbal cues which are so important to the AL or communicating.

Politicoeconomic factors

The economic status of an individual will almost certainly be communicated to others in a variety of ways, for example by the choice of neighbourhood for purchase of a house, the choice of social circle and the type of occupation — at least in Western cultures.

Communicating can also be influenced by the economic status of the Local Government group which serves a neighbourhood. For example it may influence the availability of such services as play-groups and nursery schools when young children have wider opportunities to practice communicating; new types of activities and different relationships can be explored in these settings which add to the child's capacity to communicate and are critical at this stage of development.

Of course, technological advances have greatly enhanced the individual's capacity to communicate. In industrialised societies, even in lower economic echelons, most people have access to and are influenced by mass media communications in the form of newspapers, radio and television. Then at national and international levels there is an elaborate network of telecommunication, sometimes incorporating the use of satellites, which permits rapid transworld communication.

The availability of telephone, radio and television is often dependent however on services provided by government, so politicoeconomic decisions are involved and some would even maintain that the mass media provide opportunities for political pressure, and for communicating in the form of propaganda.

Nowadays all large organisations — including hospitals or indeed a whole health service — are aware of the need for effective communication within and between different levels and grades of staff in order to achieve efficient management. There is widespread use of informal meetings, circulation of reports, notice board announcements, newsletters, in addition to the communication associated with committee structures and official correspondence. Many organisations in fact are overwhelmed by a super-abundance of communications and some are looking to computerisation to solve some of the problems created by information bombardment.

The rapidly growing use of computers in many areas of everyday living is often referred to as the computer revolution, similar in scale to the 19th century industrial revolution. In the Western world, the use of computers is no longer novel in, for example, industry, commerce and banking, and the need for computer literacy is recognised to the extent that education for the computer age now begins at primary school level.

Currently in the nursing field, computers are being used as a medium for communicating in nursing practice, education, management and research. Koch & Rankin (1987) and Ball et al (1988) describe examples of computer application, and the proceedings from an international nursing conference, held in Dublin (Nursing and Computers, 1988), give some idea of the extent of computer usage in the profession in a number of countries.

Of course, new technologies bring new problems and one cause for anxiety is the ease of retrieval of data. This is especially true of personal data but also of enormous importance when research data or top secret intelligence are stored in computers. One of the concerns is the use of a password for computer security which, it is now found, can be abused with relative ease. So-called biometric security devices such as finger scanners are considered safer; they check finger prints to authenticate a person's identity before it is possible to gain entry to the system (Ernsberger, 1988). The biometric security market also includes voice recognition and hand geometry devices. Concern about the confidentiality of large amounts of personal data has necessitated legal action. In the UK, in 1984 a bill was introduced in parliament seeking legal safeguards to ensure that computerised personal health data about patients is available only to health professionals and not to groups such as the police, tax authorities, industry, and social services personnel. Vousden (1987) looks at the implications for nursing and medical records.

Politicoeconomic and legal factors have enormous potential to influence the AL of communicating.

INDIVIDUALITY IN COMMUNICATING

One of the fascinating things about individuality in communicating is that each person develops a distinctive voice, instantly recognisable, for instance, on a telephone. Given the individuality of voice, it is little wonder that people also vary enormously in their communicating habits. Any description of individual habits in this AL is influenced by the interplay of the four components of the model already discussed and how these focus on the fifth component, individuality in communicating. The following is a résumé.

Lifespan: effect on communication
- Fetal growth and movement/birth cry
- Infancy and childhood — increasing skills/forming relationships
- Adolescence — extension of skills/relationships
- Adulthood — variety in performance
- Old age — gradual loss of activity/reduction in skills and relationships

Dependence/independence in communicating
- Unimpaired body structure and function
- Seeing aids
- Hearing aids
- Speech aids
- Possum/robots

Factors influencing communicating
- Physical
  - intact body structure and function
  - speaking/voice pitch
  - hearing
  - seeing
  - reading
  - writing
  - gesticulating

- Psychological — intelligence/range of vocabulary
  - self-confidence
  - self-respect, perception of self, and effect on perception of others
  - prevailing mood
  - information giving, teaching and counselling

- Sociocultural — mother tongue
  - dialect/accent
  - vocabulary
  - personal appearance/dress
  - patterns of touching
  - eye contact/gesticulation
  - attitudes, values and beliefs

- Environmental — temperature/ventilation
  - light
  - noise
  - type/size of room
  - arrangement of furniture

- Politicoeconomic — income
  - occupation
  - communication channels/mass media
  - computers
  - legislation to protect data/individual

Communicating: patients' problems and related nursing

Unless they are detrimental to health, it is important that, during an episode of illness, the patient's individual habits of living are changed as little as possible. It is therefore important that the nurse should know about these habits and use the knowledge to devise an individualised plan of nursing. In order to discover what the patient can and cannot do, the nurse will be seeking answers to the following questions:

- how does the individual usually communicate?
- what factors influence the way the individual carries out the AL of communicating?
- what does the individual understand about communicating?
- what are the individual's attitudes to communicating?
- has the individual any long-standing difficulties

with communicating and how have these been coped with?
- what problems, if any, does the person have at present with communicating, or seem likely to develop?

The nurse will find answers to these types of questions in the course of conversing with the patient and his family and observing their behaviour; and there may also be relevant information in other records such as medical records to which the nurse has access. The collected information can then be examined, in collaboration with the patient when relevant, to identify any problems being experienced with the AL. The nurse may recognise potential problems and it may be appropriate to discuss them with the patient. Mutual, realistic goals can then be set to prevent potential problems from becoming actual ones; to alleviate or solve the actual problems; or to help the patient cope with those which cannot be alleviated or solved. Bearing in mind what the patient can and cannot do for himself, the nursing interventions to achieve the set goals can then be selected according to local circumstances and available resources. These interventions should be written on the nursing plan along with the date on which evaluation will be carried out in order to decide whether or not the stated goals have been, or are being, achieved. All these actions, reactions and interactions are necessary in order to provide individualised nursing.

These same activities are used whatever the setting — home, clinic or hospital — and communicating is even more important (if that is possible) when a child is involved, or a mentally handicapped person, or when the contact is made for psychiatric problems, as Hardcastle (1988) clearly outlines in 'First impressions'.

Particularly in hospital, communicating is the only means patients have of acquiring information about their illness, telling staff of problems, keeping in contact with relatives and relating to other patients. However effective their communicating skills, it is highly probable that they will experience some problems in the course of adjusting to a new environment such as a hospital.

Many patients have the highest praise for the effectiveness of communication with hospital staff but there is also, undoubtedly, a lot of criticism, and it is useful to outline some of the problems which can arise when a patient is admitted to hospital. Against the background of the general discussion in the first part of this chapter, the remainder of this section highlights some types of patients' problems related to communicating and the relevant nursing activities. They are grouped under headings which indicate how the problem can arise:

Change of environment and routine
Change of dependence/independence status
Experience of pain

CHANGE OF ENVIRONMENT AND ROUTINE

Once the patient is inside the ward several dimensions of his communicating have changed, for example the social dimensions. Members of the group with whom he lives, usually the family, are no longer present; the people with whom he communicates at work are absent; and likewise the people with whom he chooses to spend the leisure part of each day.

Unfamiliar people

The patient's problem is that he has joined a group of unfamiliar people, some of whom, the patients, are present all the time; others, the nurses, are in his vicinity for some of the time; and a whole variety of others appear 'to come and go'. It is little wonder that even the most confident individuals experience some difficulty in trying to make sense of such an environment, one which is alien to most people.

Admission. In some instances the patient is very ill on admission and in these circumstances explanations and introductions have a lower priority than life-sustaining treatment and nursing. So what can the nurse do to help the patient with the AL of communicating? Initially only essential information need be communicated — that he is in hospital, that relatives have been informed, how to summon the nurse and so on. As the condition improves there can be gradual and fuller exchange of information between nurse and patient.

For a patient admitted from the waiting list, the nurse who 'admits' him (that is the initial showing of the patient to the bed and the space which he will occupy) should help with the inevitable quandary of meeting new people in somewhat unusual circumstances. It should be remembered that an anxious person, even an intelligent one, does not retain as much new information as normally. The nurse should therefore attempt to communicate only the information necessary for the patient to manage say, the next 24 hours. In one study, patient anxiety was measured and found to be highest in the first 24 hours of a hospital stay (Wilson-Barnett, 1978). Throughout a hospital stay, communicating is important for all patients but in psychiatric nursing, communicating is the major therapeutic tool and the patient's initial relationship can particularly influence the effectiveness of the subsequent therapy.

Communicating with children (and their parents) requires special skills and Glasper et al (1989) discuss this, as well as the importance of the communication links between hospital and community services when children are ill.

Introduction of nurse and patient. The first nursing activity is introduction of the nurse, by name, to the patient. If name badges are worn, nurses need to remember that people who wear bifocal spectacles have difficulty in reading at that level, and any cues regarding inadequate vision

should be noted. The patient should be told of the mode of address used in that particular hospital for professional staff. It is important to remember that patients need some information about the different members of the health care team so that they can relate satisfactorily to them. If uniforms distinguish the different grades of nursing and domestic staff, then this is useful information for the nurse to communicate to the patient.

Introduction to other patients. For all but the very ill or those admitted as an emergency the nurse can help the patient with his problem of being among unfamiliar people by introducing him to the other patients in his immediate vicinity. These are the people who will be present throughout each day and they help to give the new patient a feeling of 'belonging', indeed other patients can be a great support and source of information to new patients (Rowden & Jones, 1983). Only factual information such as how long each patient has been in the ward should be given. It is important for the nurse to remember the professional responsibility of maintaining confidentiality so the medical diagnosis and any personal details about the other patients must not be divulged.

Communicating staffing patterns. The nurse who admits new patients needs to explain whether or not they have been allocated to her in a patient allocation scheme; if so, for how long she will be on duty; and the staffing arrangements that will be made for the other two shifts. If team nursing is the pattern, then this has to be explained and the other members of the team for that shift can introduce themselves as and when necessary. If the work pattern is neither of these, again patients need to know this. They should be encouraged to express any particular anxieties and queries until the nurse assesses from verbal and nonverbal interaction that they have a reasonable grasp of the staffing pattern as it applies to them and know from whom they can seek any further help. Patients cannot be expected to feel safe and secure without this information.

Nurse/patient relationship. The relationship between nurse and patient is essentially a human one. However each patient is in the health care system for a purpose, seeking help with health problems, actual or potential. The nurse is there to make the nursing contribution to the solution, amelioration or prevention of the patients' actual or potential problems. Nurses therefore are not in the individual patient/nurse relationship from choice, but in the capacity of making a professional contribution. A consideration of what the nurse brings to the relationship is therefore necessary.

The nurse brings to the relationship herself as a unique human being, the culmination of her particular life experiences. She also brings compassion for people and a commitment to nursing, together with nursing knowledge and skills. Her emotional maturity should be such that she does not have to gratify personal needs at the patient's expense. For example a need to be dominant and make decisions may deprive patients of practice which they require in order to deal with, for example, their problem of indecision, common in some mental illnesses. Or again, a strong mothering need may motivate a nurse to dress patients when it would be in their best interest to re-learn dressing skills.

The nurse brings to the relationship a maturity which permits toleration of frustration if, for example, a patient is not at home when she makes a house call; or if a patient does not take the prescribed medication; or removes a dressing or falls out of bed. The trigger points are innumerable but the nurse should have the maturity to deal with the resultant feelings in a constructive way that avoids reflecting any annoyance on to the patient. Nobody expects a paragon of virtue but the nurse is meant to be realistic, is meant to have self-knowledge because the 'self' must be used in the relationship. Personal needs have to be met by other supporting staff, by counsellors or by the significant others in the nurse's life.

The patient is also a unique human being who has been fashioned by life experiences. Something is wrong, so already the image of self has changed. Change is uncomfortable at the best of times and the patient is discomforted. If the diagnosis is uncertain and an array of diagnostic tests is required, then the patient is bound to be anxious both about the tests and the potential results, and inevitably, is worried if surgery is prescribed. Worried people do not concentrate, hear or understand so well as usual. However, if the nurse takes the time to give information to the patient, it has been shown in various studies to be beneficial (Hayward, 1975; Wilson-Barnett, 1978; Boore, 1979; Bond, 1982). By becoming a patient, not only treatment is sought; comfort is also sought from nursing staff, and information-giving seems to be an important component of comfort.

Psychological comfort is inextricably related to physical comfort although some interactions are deliberately planned by staff to contribute to psychological comfort. It may be as fleeting as a look of acknowledgement when passing the patient's bed; or it may be less transient, for example helping the patient through the stages of accepting and coping with chronic illness; or when a patient has a mental illness, it may be the major emphasis for most interactions.

The value of therapeutic touch as a form of psychological comfort is currently receiving considerable attention in the professional literature. Touch is the earliest and most primitive form of communication and is an important form of non-verbal communication throughout life; it can convey a myriad of positive and negative messages between people. However the use and acceptance of touch depends on numerous cultural norms and personal characteristics; each culture has rules about how, when and where to touch another human, and this is related to gender, age and maturity. Pearce (1988), writing about the use of touch in an intensive care unit, differentiates between *instrumental* touch (deliberate, physical contact needed to perform a specific task such as washing a patient or dressing a wound) and *expressive* touch (a relatively spontaneous and affective contact which is not necessarily a component of a physical task, such as holding a patient's hand during a painful procedure). Expressive touch, she quotes, is used to enhance verbal communication in conveying empathy, trust, reassurance, security and the proximity of another person, and she goes on to quote several authors who have examined the effects of tactile language in a variety of health care settings — with the elderly, with the terminally ill, with people in pain, with anxious people and during labour. It must be recognised, however, that for some people, touching would be an unacceptable invasion of personal privacy (Turton, 1989), and skill is required to detect this reservation, especially when the person has reduced personal independence.

Not only touch, but all activities carried out in the vicinity of the patient, offer the nurse an opportunity to show empathy. Empathy is described in various ways and Burnard (1987a) discussing its use in psychiatric nursing quotes Carl Rogers' definition as 'a process of entering into the perceptual world of another person'. Burnard goes on to mention some of the skills involved: the ability to listen (to the words but also noting volume, pitch, eye movements and related body language); ability to offer free attention (to note and accept, not analyse and interpret); to suspend judgement (to refrain from categorising as good/bad, right/wrong); and to control what is said in reply and how it is said, with a facial expression which is genuine, not mechanical. By behaving in this way, the nurse shows respect for the person's individuality, a point reinforced in our model for nursing.

In a later article, Burnard (1988) compares empathy and sympathy:

To empathise is to set aside our own perception of things and attempt to think the way the other person thinks, or feel the way he feels . . . a very different quality to sympathy. Sympathy involves 'feeling sorry' for the other person — or perhaps, it involves our imagining how we would feel if we were experiencing what is happening to him. With empathy, we try to imagine what it is like being the other person and experiencing things as he does.

Empathy of course does have limits. It is not possible to completely enter someone else's frame of reference because other people live different lives but, Burnard goes on, nurses should try to empathise. It does, however, require skill and in the 1988 article, Burnard outlines practical exercises to help develop empathy in a variety of nursing settings, while at the same time citing the problems involved in empathy training.

Every nurse needs to develop psychological and social skills as well as manual skills in order to maintain an effective nurse/patient relationship while the patient requires it; and these skills are also required to relinquish the relationship when appropriate.

Of course it is not only the nurse-patient relationship which contributes to the patient's care and well-being. Inter-professional communication is required and Pearson (1985) enlarges on the importance of information exchange between nurses and other members of the health team. When deficient, there are omissions or repetitions of activities; uncoordinated interruptions to the patient's rest and comfort; failure to meet the patient's psychological needs — in essence poor communication causing a breakdown in the continuity of care.

Discharge. Providing patients with information on admission to hospital and throughout their stay may be acknowledged as an important part of nursing but frequently, discharge is a very rushed affair. All too often patients and their families are not given enough information about planning the convalescent period, about continued medications and treatments, expected rate of progress, and return to employment. But in *Using a Model for Nursing* (Roper et al, 1983), the third year student nurse contributing to the study in a surgical ward, commented that the model approach helped her to appreciate the need for planned discharge goals; even when admitting the patient, she was alerted to consider what the patient required to know on discharge in order to resume her usual Activities of Living.

Staff-to-staff communicating between hospital and community nursing services is another important aspect when considering a patient's discharge and Parnell (1982) highlighted some of the problems in her study. For example available information was not being sent; there was reluctance to put certain items in writing; telephone messages left with a third party could be distorted; there was incomplete information; there was a lack of feedback. She concluded that although her findings showed considerable improvement since previous studies, there were still problems and she made proposals to rectify at least some of them. It would seem that better communication has been introduced in some areas. Chisnell (1988) followed 50 post-surgery patients who required the services of district nurses following discharge from hospital, and communication with community staff certainly had improved for this small sample.

Unfamiliar place

Lack of usual contacts. Patients newly admitted to the hospital environment will naturally be anxious about keeping in touch with family, friends and work associates. Anxiety may be lessened by information about such things as a mobile shop where stationery and newspapers can be bought; ward arrangements for collection and delivery of mail; for making and receiving telephone calls, and for visiting. Gradually the patients' new environment seems less strange and threatening as they become aware of the

possibilities for communication between hospital and their familiar environment.

Disorientation. Information is also needed by the patient to permit the continuance of other everyday activities. It can be communicated by adequate labelling of, for example, toilets and bathrooms. The letters should be sufficiently large and should be placed so as to cater for patients with poor vision. This is especially helpful to older patients who may have difficulty in learning and remembering, and who may require to visit the toilet during the night.

As the days pass in this unfamiliar environment, some patients (particularly those with deficient vision and hearing, and those who for one reason or another do not read a daily newspaper) can lose track of the time of day, the day of the week and the day of the month. The provision of a large calendar and clock in each ward can be useful in preventing this apparent disorientation.

The problem of disorientation has been studied particularly in relation to elderly people and the techniques of reality orientation (RO) seems a promising area for development. It is really a psychological approach to the confused elderly person which aims to improve and maintain their level of functioning by stimulating them and their environment. Ratcliffe (1988) describes it as a technique used in rehabilitating people with memory loss, confusion and time-place-person disorientation which adds a humanistic element to care, and discusses in some detail how it affects communicating.

Environmental factors, too, can affect communicating. Ford et al (1986) carried out a study in a psychiatric setting in the USA arising from their concern that many confused elderly people, particularly those in advanced stages of Alzheimer's disease, did not respond to verbal communication and staff found it difficult to understand their attempts at communicating. They altered the noise levels, and the lighting levels at mealtimes and were surprised themselves at the dramatic effect on behaviour — less agitation, reduced noise from the patients, shorter feeding times, and greater consumption of food. Further studies are required, they say, but in this particular study, elements in the physical environment undoubtedly influenced communication and behaviour.

Unfamiliar language

Lack of understanding. The new patient who probably has the biggest problem with communication is the one who does not speak the national language (Watson, 1986). With increasing multiracial societies in most countries and the speed of modern-day travel such patients are found in hospitals throughout the world. This is recognised as an international problem and voluntary organisations such as the League of Red Cross Societies have produced helpful translations in many languages. At a local level, voluntary help is usually available; there is often a list of people speaking other languages who are willing to act as interpreters. Failing this, nurses can help by using empathy, ingenuity and miming.

Even when the same national language is spoken by patient and nurse, both can experience problems in aural perception when their attention has to be directed to listening because of accent or dialect. The nurse can help to avoid this problem by speaking clearly and slowly, stopping for clarification when this seems necessary.

A problem can also be experienced when there is a difference in the vocabulary used by patient and nurse. This can operate in both ways — the patient might use words which the nurse does not readily understand and vice versa. Take the words used for the place for eliminating: bathroom, convenience, lavatory, loo, toilet, water closet (WC). There are countless other examples but the above should serve to alert nurses so that they can prevent patients' problems in this area. This is accomplished by becoming expert at observing and interpreting non-verbal cues indicating incomprehension, and by exploring with the patient the cause of the break in the chain of communication and correcting it.

Technical terms. Further differences in vocabulary can produce problems for patients when words with a medical definition are used in the process of communicating: insomnia, migraine, obstruction. Nurses should therefore discover from patients what meaning these words have for them, so that they can be sure that they and the patients are talking about the same conditions. This naturally applies also to specific medical words, and when they are used, the nurse may find it necessary to correct inaccuracies and add explanations.

Embarrassing topics. Some patients experience difficulty when talking with nurses about activities such as eliminating and expressing sexuality. They may fear that they are not using the 'right' words. It is therefore helpful if nurses start by saying that people use different words, and asking patients to give the information in their own words. Yet another type of vocabulary can have difference in meaning for patient and nurse and thereby give rise to difficulties — words describing parts of the body, though having a particular anatomical reference, do not necessarily have that reference for lay people, even intelligent lay people. Where appropriate, pointing to the area on one's own body is helpful or using visual aids, which can be as simple as drawing a diagram while explaining the location of the part.

Even the use of ordinary vocabulary can result in problems for patients. An example is given by Lelean (1973). The surgeon instructed a patient not to bend her back after an operation. When she was allowed out of bed the nurses (who presumably had not received the instruction) no longer assisted in washing her and the patient said that she would be glad to get home so that her legs and feet could be washed.

Unfamiliar activities

Giving information to patients. The activities which occur inside hospital and are taken so much for granted by staff can be bewilderingly strange to the patients. Not surprisingly they feel anxious. It is now recognised by staff that much of the apprehension and anxiety can be traced back to lack of communication and Wilson-Barnett (1988) discusses the development of different approaches to rectify the situation, drawing distinctions between information-giving, patient teaching or education, and counselling. The provision of factual information seems to alleviate some of the initial anxiety on immediate arrival at the ward and many hospitals send to those who are being admitted from the waiting list, some type of preparatory material ranging from a leaflet to an illustrated brochure, the latter in particular for children. But this type of information presupposes that the recipients have the necessary vision and can read, and that they are sufficiently orientated to understand what they are reading. When this in not so, they are deprived of this initial preparation as are all those who are admitted as 'emergencies'. Of course, the written word is enhanced when given in conjunction with verbal information.

The value of giving information about specific nursing interventions, too, has been studied and documented (Hayward, 1975; Wilson-Barnett, 1978; Boore, 1979; Bond, 1982). As well as being comforting, it can have other effects. Hayward (1975) illustrated the value of giving preoperative information as a prescription against pain in the postoperative period. Boore (1979) investigated the effect of preoperative information about treatment and care, and teaching exercises to be performed postoperatively; her study showed reduced stress in patients following surgery and also a reduced incidence of infection.

These studies are examples which illustrate the effects of good staff communication but there is also evidence of the results of communication breakdown. Maguire (1985) investigated the reasons for poor nurse-to-patient communication and gave examples of some of the consequences in relation to diagnoses; to treatment; to investigations; and to potential complications which became actual problems. The importance of effective nurse-patient communications cannot be overemphasised.

There is also a considerable amount of evidence to indicate that patients themselves see communication as a crucial part of their care. Cartwright (1964) and Raphael (1969) did some early work on this issue yet in a recent article Macleod Clark (1988) reminds us that studies in the 1970s and early 1980s indicate that patients were more dissatisfied with communication than any other aspect of their care. These studies examined nurse-patient communication in a variety of settings such as intensive care units, geriatric wards, surgical wards and radiotherapy units, and their findings were disturbingly consistent. One of the recurring discussion points was the apparent lack of communication skills teaching for nursing staff.

Giving information to relatives. Relatives, too, seem concerned about lack of communication and the 'unavailability of the nurses'. Information collected about the relatives of cancer patients showed that only a minority have anything more than superficial contact with the staff caring for the patient, and a number of these relatives would have welcomed an opportunity to share their anxiety, not only about the patient but about their own feelings (Bond, 1982). Darbyshire (1987) provides an interesting outline of the approach to relatives down through the ages and quotes the Health Service Ombudsman who highlighted current complaints related to 'failure to give relatives adequate or timely information . . . .'

Teaching and counselling v. information-giving. Having commented on the perceived need for information-giving experienced by staff, patients and relatives, it is interesting to note some recent work which shows that facilitating certain strategies for *coping* during stressful procedures is more effective than information per se for reducing signs of distress. Wilson-Barnett (1988) indicates how information-giving seems to be gravitating towards 'teaching' individuals how to cope. Wilson-Barnett differentiates between teaching (involving a change in behaviour) and information-giving (a process, and having less concern with how it is received . . . and not necessarily involving interaction or assessment of individual need). The didactic emphasis, she continues, is now being questioned and shifting towards a more patient-centred involvement. And as patients have become more involved in identifying and negotiating areas for learning and behavioural change, the field of investigation has come to borrow from the theories and practice of counselling.

Discussing the counselling process, McEvoy (1988) describes counselling as 'an enabling interaction between two people which seeks to support the weaker person as a responsible human being'. Burnard (1987b) commends the use of counselling and although writing specifically about psychiatric nursing, the skills can be used selectively by nurses in any setting. Central to patient-centred counselling, he says, is the idea that individuals are the best arbiters of what is and is not right for them. They may listen to others, but decide on their own course of action. People are free to choose their own future, so the patient knows what is best. Listening is the basis of counselling. In the process of counselling, he goes on, the nurse does not offer interpretations laced with 'oughts' and 'shoulds' — or the exercise degenerates into advice which may not fit the patient's beliefs and value systems. The counsellor's task is to attempt to enter and share the personal world of the patient non-judgmentally, and understand the patient's view of the world at that particular time. Counselling skills can be learned but they do require practice and Burnard warns that counselling techniques should not be overused or they may indeed impede listening and communication.

Essentially counselling is non-directive and without censure. The objective is that the patient gains the insight to make a personal decision from the options available. This approach, he maintains, is different from other aspects of nursing when the nurse uses knowledge and expertise to advise and educate. Counselling is concerned with coping mechanisms which may be related to physical health problems, or may be personal and linked to relationships, or sociocultural issues including spiritual beliefs, or may be linked to economic difficulties. Faulkner (1985) illustrates how counselling techniques can be used in the context of the nursing process.

Patient-centred approaches such as counselling are being evaluated in a research context and most studies, so far, have been with patients who have chronic illnesses. Wilson-Barnett (1988) quotes from work with cancer patients, patients who have had a myocardial infarct, and patients who have rheumatoid arthritis; all examples where long-term contact with health care staff is more likely than in instances of acute and more transient illness. (In realistic terms, there may be less opportunity for the use of counselling techniques during a brief hospital stay.) She concludes that a mix of information-giving, teaching techniques and counselling may be required for any one patient.

Nowadays nurses are faced with complex situations, not only to take account of psychological and sociocultural factors during illness but also as promoters of health, and in helping patients and families to become involved in their own health care. Appropriate knowledge and communication skills (information-giving, teaching, counselling) are required for these activities and skill is needed also to decide which communication approach is relevant to the circumstances. Macleod-Clark (1988) maintains, however, that even in current basic nursing programmes, students are not given adequate preparation to function in this way. If this is so, it is not surprising that so many complaints continue to be made by patients and relatives about poor communication. However, legitimate concern about improvement must be tempered by the countless instances when communication certainly is effective.

Change of role

In the familiar world of the adult patient many parts are played and there is communication with many people: spouse, offspring, other family, friend, acquaintance, co-worker, employer and club-member. There is control over when, how and where they communicate. Now, on admission to hospital, the AL of communicating has to continue while assuming the sick role or patient role discussed on page 46.

Family relationships. In hospital, the spouse's communication with the patient, in a setting that includes nightclothes, bed, single or multiple room/ward, is essentially different. When the visiting spouse is accompanied by offspring or other family members, further modification of the partners' behaviour may be perceived to be necessary. At this sensitive period in these people's lives, such modification can be misinterpreted by any one or more members of this group and may have repercussions in family relationships. Nursing includes 'caring' about the family and what they mean to the patient. Indeed family disruption may have contributed to the illness. After visitors have departed, nurses should pay attention to a patient's non-verbal behaviour as well as to what is said. Nurses should not pry but they need to be sensitive to any cues which indicate a patient's desire to discuss anxieties.

Reversal of roles. The reversal of roles can cause the patient anxiety. Should the patient be the person who had attended to the business and financial side of family life, then there will have to be a reversal of roles; these items will have to be attended to by a responsible other person, usually the spouse. And the previous level of frankness in communication between the spouses about these matters can narrow or widen the possibility of stress between them during these communications in a hospital ward.

Visitors. The reaction of friends to the change of role can be a sensitive matter. Patients may find it difficult to come to terms with which of their friends, co-workers and employers did, or did not, communicate with them during hospitalisation. Some of these people may not have found it convenient to visit but may have phoned; some may have 'visited' but not gained access to the ward. It is therefore important that the patients' lines of communication are kept open by relaying these enquiries to them — they are easily jotted on a memo pad and delivered at a convenient moment. More is said about the importance of visiting on page 279.

Information-giver and confidentiality. Another potential problem for patients is that they find themselves in the role of information-giver, and it is often information of a very personal nature. Patients may not see the relevance of giving information about their social history when their problem is a physical one — and it may not be. When it is relevant, great sensitivity is required in eliciting such information and telling patients how it helps in planning their nursing. For example, if the person is severely incapacitated and has difficulty in mobilising, it can be important to know whether, when at home, it is necessary to go upstairs to the toilet. It is therefore important to understand at the outset that anything communicated to members of the professional staff will be treated as confidential.

The knowledge that confidence will be respected is an important feature of effective nurse/patient communication, and is incorporated in professional codes of practice in a number of countries. The UKCC Code of Professional Conduct (1984) states that registered nurses, midwives and health visitors shall:

respect confidential information obtained in the course of professional practice and refrain from disclosing such information without the consent of the patient/client or a person entitled to act on his/her behalf except where disclosure is required by law or by order of a court, or is necessary in the public interest.

This sounds reasonable but application of the principle may contain inherent conflicts of interest and further guidance was provided in an advisory paper on confidentiality produced by the UKCC in 1987. Moore (1988) discusses the advisory paper and concludes that the UKCC clearly acknowledge the role of the profession, together with the Statutory Bodies, in defining acceptable ethical standards, but it remains the responsibility of the individual nurse to set standards through practice. Melia (1988) comments on the UKCC document also and provides thought-provoking examples of circumstances where the guidelines could be applied.

Related to confidentiality is the collection, storage and retrieval of written records, a permanent form of communication. Information imparted by, and collected about the patient is given in confidence, so the information gatherer has a responsibility to be familiar with the records system in use, know who has access, and be aware of risks associated with the legitimate use of records (Cowan, 1987). Do all health professionals have access? Do students have access? Do research workers have access? Is the system supervised? With the advent of computer storage of records, the topic of confidentiality has received considerable coverage and some of the implications of the Data Protection Act, 1984, are discussed by Keighley (1987). Members of the public in general are concerned about personal information held by computers. Where health information is stored in computers, it is important that the patient understands the safeguards against unauthorised people gaining access.

Information-receiver and informed consent. As already mentioned, an increasing number of research reports shows that a frequent complaint made by patients is lack of information. Sometimes the required information is about what tests are going to be performed and why; the results of tests; the medical diagnosis, particularly if, for example, heart disease or cancer are suspected; how long to expect to be away from work and so on. Whatever the nurse staffing arrangements, each one needs to know what the patient has been told and what currently appears to be understood. Adequacy of communication is an essential part of nursing, not only to reduce patients' complaints but to permit nurses to comply with their professional duty to be accountable. The UKCC Code of Professional Conduct (1984) states:

Each registered nurse, midwife or health visitor is accountable for his or her practice, and in the exercise of professional accountability shall: act always in such a way as to promote and safeguard the well-being and interests of patients/clients.

and a UKCC document published in 1989 'Exercising accountability' provides guidelines for professional practitioners.

Apart from receiving and understanding information, has the patient consented to the various tests and treatments — what has come to be termed 'informed consent'. Discussing informed consent, Foden & Beauchamp (1986) remind us that the nurse/patient and doctor/patient relationship used to be founded on trust but now the trend is for mutual partnership, patient involvement and patient autonomy. The nub of informed consent, they say, is that every human of adult years and sound mind has a right to determine what will be done with his body, and they trace the history of informed consent citing the Nuremberg Code (1949) and the Declaration of Helsinki (1964, amended 1983), which in the aftermath of war atrocities, attempted to ensure the principle of informed consent. In relation to current practice in nursing, Wells (1986) refers to the European Charter on the Rights of the Patient (1983), which enshrines the rights to receive information about diagnosis, therapy and prognosis, and the right to decide whether treatment will be started or continued. He then discusses the legal position in the UK when, if the patient needs diagnostic investigations which involve anaesthesia and surgery, **written** consent must be obtained by the surgeon, but points out that, in fact, the document protects the surgeon and the hospital, not the patient.

Related to informed consent and information exchange is the concept of patient advocacy. Wells (1986) discusses the nurse's role as a patient advocate — not making decisions for the patient but ensuring that no one usurps the needs, rights and humanity of the patient — and in 'Ethics and information' discusses the potential difficulties; he sees a place for the nurse as the patient's advocate in certain circumstances. Melia (1986) sounds a note of caution. She poses the question that if nurses are asked to clarify information provided by the doctor about any procedure, does the nurse have a duty to inform the patient about inherent risks? And how much information does the patient require to make a rational decision? Melia suggests that as far as strictly medical treatment is concerned, it would be prudent to leave doctor's business to doctors!

The informed consent of the patient is also relevant when considering research which involves patient participation. In the UK's National Health Service, ethical issues related to the conduct of research are countenanced in that each Health Authority has an Ethical Committee, and nursing research involving patients must be submitted to its scrutiny before a project can proceed. Informed consent in relation to nursing research is discussed by Macmillan (1987).

CHANGE OF DEPENDENCE/INDEPENDENCE STATUS

It is understandable that with an Activity of Living which has so many dimensions, a number of variables can affect the individual's capacity to be independent. Any change in status can be influenced by the age of onset, perhaps congenital; the type of onset, sudden or gradual; the degree of difficulty, ranging from partial to complete; and whether or not the problem is reversible. Some of the main problems which patients can encounter in relation to the AL of communicating are outlined below.

Problems related to cognition.

Children who are born mentally handicapped frequently do not possess the necessary intellectual ability to communicate verbally so start life with a severe impediment as far as independence in communicating is concerned. However with patient teaching, many can learn to respond to verbal messages such as greetings and simple instructions, and some are able to learn to speak. For children who are mentally handicapped, non-verbal communication assumes greater importance than usual. Through play, physical contact, hand language and body language, mentally handicapped people can be encouraged to achieve their optimal level for communicating, and several studies are reported by Hunter (1987) where mentally handicapped, psychiatric and brain-damaged people have been helped to learn, using computers.

Sometimes there is impaired cognition following an illness or an accident. Prior to the event, communication had not been a problem, and this loss of mental acuity may involve drastic changes in lifestyle related to employment and loss of earning capacity, as well as loss of self-respect and hardship to the family. The nurse needs to know how aware such patients are of the impairment, how they experience the impairment, what they feel about it, and so on. They need to talk about what the change means in their lives; whether or not they will be able to communicate sufficiently to continue at work and carry out their leisure time activities. If the patients do not recognise their assets, it is important that they are helped to do so, and positive comment on whatever they accomplish will help them to regain self-respect.

In declining years some people show signs of diminishing skills in thinking and remembering, for instance by giving inappropriate replies while talking with another person. Nurses should continue to talk to these patients as if there were no deterioration, because they do have unpredictable rational periods and at those times they can be mortified at being spoken to as if they were children. Should these patients be at home there must be surveillance to be sure that they can manage the AL of communicating at a safe level.

Problems related to speech

Independence in verbal communication may be impaired by distortion of the voice caused by a variety of physical dysfunctions. Dryness of the mouth interferes with speech. It may be due to a variety of causes such as reduced fluid intake; or associated with excitement or anxiety; or infection; or it may be caused by the use of drugs for example certain anti-emetics and anti-depressant drugs. Dryness of the mouth, of course, is deliberately caused preoperatively when a drug such as atropine is given to dry up secretions prior to general anaesthesia. Mouth dryness is frequently a feature, too, when parenteral feeding has been prescribed (p. 167) and among other things, can inhibit verbal communication at a time when the patient particularly requires interpersonal contact. Unless contraindicated, a drink will relieve dryness of the mouth, a mouthwash may prove helpful, and something as simple as sucking a sweet or medicated lozenge may stimulate salivation sufficiently to relieve discomfort.

Specific local infections such as laryngitis and swelling such as enlarged tonsils will also cause speaking problems but these conditions are usually temporary in nature and reversible. A distortion of longer duration occurs when a child is born with congenital hare lip or cleft palate. These can be corrected by surgery but a considerable amount of speech therapy is required in the post-surgery period to ensure that such children can communicate in a way which is understandable to others.

There are occasions when one is at a loss for words but most people find it difficult to imagine what it would be like to be unable to speak. Certainly one could still see, listen, read, write and communicate non-verbally. So these are the modes which have to be exploited when a patient suddenly loses the ability to speak, whether it be temporary or permanent in nature.

Temporary loss can be produced when, for instance it is necessary to make a surgical incision of the trachea and insert a metal tracheostomy tube to maintain patency (p. 142). Where possible it is important that the patient understands the nature of the operation, but sometimes it has to be performed in an emergency. The patient will almost certainly be conscious and needs considerable support which the nurse can supply by the manner in which activities are carried out, continuing to talk with the patient even although there is no verbal response. A pad and pencil is an alternative means of communicating, and it is important that some means, such as a bell, is within the patient's reach in order to attract the nurse's attention when help is required.

Permanent loss occurs when there is surgical removal of the larynx, a laryngectomy. In such circumstances the patient needs to understand the permanency of the loss of natural voice production. Usually every encouragement is given to develop oesophageal speech, and effective collaboration between nurse and speech therapist will do much to assist the patient and family during the early stages of learning. Air is swallowed and forced into the oesophagus by locking the tongue to the roof of the mouth. When air is expelled the walls of the oesophagus and pharynx vibrate causing the column of air in the oesophagus to vibrate and produce a low-pitched sound. The sound is formed into words by the patient's tongue, lips, teeth, and palate to form intelligible speech. The nursing contribution involves encouraging the patient to carry out the speech therapist's instructions; not showing impatience as he practises; and not showing embarrassment at the changed voice. The patient can be advised to join one of the self-help groups — Laryngectomee Clubs — which exist to give support and encouragement to people with similar problems and assist them to regain independence in verbal communication, Milne (1988) discusses some of the problems.

Aphasia is loss of ability to speak; it is experienced by some though not all people who have a stroke. Depending on the exact location in the brain of the cerebrovascular accident (CVA), so the patient's problems are different.

Expressive aphasia is the term used when people know what they want to say, yet although able to move the mouth, simply cannot speak. It is the right-handed person's problem when there is a CVA in the left motor speech area, because the speech area is best developed in the left cerebral hemisphere. It is frustrating because intelligence is unimpaired. Also hearing has not changed, although strokes tend to occur in the older age group who may already have some impairment, so it is important in these circumstances to collect information about hearing ability.

It is also important for the nurse to note whether the patient does manage to speak any word or words. With the objective of the patient speaking an increasing number of words, the nurse puts into practice advice given by the speech therapist. This usually consists of encouraging the patient to say particular words, separately at first to ensure success, then short sentences and so on. Nursing time is much better spent on these exercises than on long one-sided conversations, which may only produce frustration when the patient cannot talk. Indeed great distress can be caused when nurses and relatives do not appear to understand the disability and talk as if to a child. It is more emotionally satisfying if the nurse just stays with the patient from time to time during each day, providing company, a way of showing that he is still valued as a person.

Receptive aphasia is the term used when there is impaired comprehension of spoken and written words, although the patient can still say the words aloud. According to the patient's previous reading ability and hearing acuity, (and this information must be collected) the words can still be seen and heard but there is difficulty understanding and remembering. Receptive aphasia is difficult to recognise as the patient's correct responses may result from practice rather than comprehension. Chalmers (1985) gives an account of this complicated disability and a useful comparison of expressive and receptive aphasia. The right-handed person can have receptive aphasia when there is a CVA in the left sensory speech area, again because it is best developed on the left side and the fibres cross over. The ability to think and vocalise words is retained, but the words spoken may be out of context. The patient requires to re-learn association of words with things — the things he needs in everyday living such as toothbrush, toothpaste and so on, and it is useful to keep these articles on a tray near the patient so that the nurse can encourage extra repetition whenever opportunities are available to spend time with the patient.

Of crucial importance is the continuation of encouragement and support in the community once the person is discharged from hospital and a study carried out by Sawyer (1986) emphasises the importance of the nurse who visits such people at home. Family, friends and home helps can collaborate effectively even when progress seems slow and groups such as the Chest & Heart Association, and Action for the Dysphasic Adult group (ADA) produce leaflets containing helpful exercises and useful ideas to assist communicating (ADA, 1987); and local groups organise social trips and activities where dysphasic people can meet others with speaking difficulties, and with whom they can empathise without so much embarrassment.

Problems related to hearing

The congenitally deaf or hearing-impaired baby has difficulty in acquiring vocal communication skills because of the inability to hear. One of the early assessments of all babies is a simple hearing test so that, should any impairment be identified, specialist advice can be sought early (Bax, 1986).

Recurrent middle ear infections can produce a problem for young children who are still acquiring basic communication skills; the resulting reduction in hearing capacity can retard the learning process. Of course at any stage on the lifespan an ear infection or even the presence of excessive wax may interfere with hearing. However these are usually transient impediments. It is a different matter when there is a sudden loss of hearing; the person is now in a silent world, and even in the midst of people, there is intense loneliness. Nevertheless visual cues are still received and sometimes when others glance in the deaf person's direction while talking, the reaction varies. There may be signs of paranoid behaviour; there may be loss of self-respect; the person may become more easily cross and irritable. On the other hand, deaf people may feel so uncomfortable in the company of others that there is physical withdrawal which may well increase the feeling of loneliness.

A discomfort which sometimes accompanies hearing impairments is tinnitus. The intra- and extra-cranial blood vessels in the head and neck, the molecular motion of air within the middle ear, as well as circulating blood in or near the organ of Corti, are all possible explanations of tinnitus (Lindsay, 1983). Almost everyone can hear noises in the ear if in quiet enough surroundings but environmental noise usually masks it. However the tinnitus which accompanies impairment of hearing is said by sufferers to be worse than hearing loss, and the monotonous buzzing or ringing sounds can cause insomnia and depression and total distortion of their living pattern. Drugs do not seem to bring relief; surgery can correct some problems; electrical stimulation of the cochlea may give substantial improvement; but so far, portable masking devices such as an ear-level hearing aid which delivers a continuous masking sound, often closely imitating the distressing tinnitus sound, has proved most successful. Biofeedback techniques have also shown improvements in this distressing condition for some sufferers.

Everything possible must be done by the nurse to convey to the patient that although deaf, he is still valued as a person and the Royal College of Nursing booklet (1985) gives guidance to nurses working with hearing-impaired people. Nurses must use non-verbal language as much as possible paying attention for example to the manner in which they set down a meal tray. The patient has no loss in cognitive ability or speech and can still pass an opinion about the meal, indeed should be asked to do so. If nurses persevere, patients who are deaf will begin to lip-read and can be encouraged to join a class for development of this skill. To help lip readers, the nurse's face should be at the same level as the patient's, at a comfortable distance to accommodate the patient's vision, and in a good light.

Patients and members of their families may decide that use of a hand language would solve their communicating problem. With practice it can be quicker for the other members than writing the input part of conversation with the deaf person who can still speak in reply! With tolerance and good humour the problem of communicating can at least be reduced, if not overcome. Within a group of deaf people, the British Sign Language (BSL) may be used. It has its own rules and grammar and uses finger-spelling instead of words, but is not suitable for deaf people who are mentally handicapped — Makaton (Tompkins, 1988) may be helpful for them. Makaton uses selected words and signs graded in complexity from basic needs to more complex concepts and can be taught to individuals or groups without the need for any sophisticated equipment.

If there is even minimal hearing, to help the patient use it when communicating, it may be possible to augment it with a hearing aid. However the aid magnifies every sound and at first some sounds can be startling until the patient learns to filter them out. It needs a lot of encouragement and support during the learning period to use the aid to best advantage. If it is the 'body-worn' type, most people find it works best if worn near the midline on the chest with the microphone facing outwards. It is clipped on to an article of clothing. Nurses should speak slowly and clearly to the exposed microphone and encourage lip reading. With technological developments it is now possible, however, to have small unobtrusive aids which are effective as well as being aesthetically more acceptable.

Various aids have been devised for the use of deaf people at home, for example a flashing light when the doorbell or telephone rings, and there are special adaptors for radio, television, telephones and even facilities in selected parts of some churches to enable deaf people to enjoy spiritual enrichment in the company of likeminded worshippers. A recent idea is the introduction of a scheme to provide 'Hearing Dogs for the Deaf'. Guide dogs for the blind have been used in the UK since 1931 and this is an extension of the same idea (Haddon, 1987).

Problems related to sight

In contrast to deafness, it is usually possible to notice quite readily that a person is blind. A baby may be congenitally blind and from the outset, the parents require careful specialist advice so that other communication channels are exploited to the optimum. When a person becomes suddenly blind the problem is different.

People who lose the sense of sight suddenly change from a world of light and colour to a world of perpetual darkness. They cannot see their environment or the person to whom they are speaking, so miss all the visual communication cues. They cannot write letters although may still be able to write a signature if the hand is placed exactly where it is required. They cannot read letters and the friendships maintained in this way are no longer 'private' because a nurse or volunteer has to read them to the patient. Of course there are tape recordings, but again they are less 'private'. A phone at home can be modified, but it may be less easy to use the hospital telephone.

When there is a sudden loss of sight the nurse can give more effective help if she understands that people, suffering any form of loss go through similar psychological stages to those of dying (p. 339). The nurse therefore needs to help such patients to deal with, and not deny, the feelings of anger and frustration, and must convey the intended message by voice alone since it is not complemented by visual cues. However the patients still have visual memory of colour, shape, size and so on and can be helped to develop mental images if the nurse describes the environment and what is going on, emphasises landmarks, and encourages others to do likewise. Description is particularly important if any treatment is going to be carried out so that the patient knows what to expect but it is also helpful for the patient to have ordinary activities such as a food tray described while the nurse is helping the newly blind patient with a meal. For anyone whose sight has been suddenly impaired, it is important that nurses indicate their approach before touching the patient and that they speak in a normal voice; sudden loud speech will startle the patient.

Some patients may have sudden loss of sight in only one eye and although the human body is amazingly adaptable, it takes some time to adjust to visual communication when part of the usual visual field has been lost. For those who have undergone certain types of ophthalmic surgery the covering of both eyes in the immediate postoperative period, although transient, can be alarming. If such patients are in the older age group, they are usually less adaptable and inability to see can add to the confusion at being in the strange environment of a hospital; in fact, some can become disoriented. The Royal National Institute for the Blind (1987) have produced an amusing but sensitive booklet suggesting ways of helping visually handicapped people in hospital.

If blindness is permanent, the transition from hospital to the community can be traumatic as the person attempts to adjust to living in the everyday world without the advantage of sight. Donnelly (1987) carried out a study of 71 people who had been recently registered as blind. Major concerns were the loss of independence; anxiety about being a burden on others, in fact some were doubly concerned as they themselves were carers of a disabled spouse; and finance and work opportunities. Blind people have to cope with many disadvantages, one being the inability to learn at the same speed as others; they rely heavily on Braille (invented 1824), talking books and tapes. However, the computer revolution is providing exciting extensions to their options for communicating. An article in Newsweek (Ernsberger & Robinson, 1987) describes a computer, Eureka, which is a word processor, calculator, alarm clock, diary, telephone directory and music composer. It has been used by blind children to take notes at school and prepare written papers, and has increased enormously their capacity for learning. As well as a learning aid, computers can be used by adults to increase their potential for work opportunities and for pleasure activities.

In the community, a number of blind people use specially trained dogs as an aid to their everyday activities, but as well as increasing their capacity for independence, the dog provides them with faithful companionship in a world where social contacts may be diminishing.

Problems related to body sensation

Sensation via the skin is a topic which people do not readily discuss. Only when deprived of skin sensation does the individual realise what an important, and indeed pleasurable, part of communicating it can be (pp. 107, 111). In purely physical terms, however, when someone loses the sensation of touch via the skin, a vital component of communicating is lost. Loss of sensation impairs the person's ability to receive cues which are protective. It is not possible to detect excessive heat, and the skin area may be burned; or the person may bump into sharp objects without realising the damage to skin and underlying tissues. Impaired sensation is often a feature following a cerebrovascular accident and certain spinal injuries, occurring along with impaired movement.

Problems related to body movement

When a patient loses the ability to move, the affected area of the body can no longer be used to convey non-verbal messages. According to the extent of the paralysis (Fig. 6.8, p. 97), so the change in mode of communicating is different as are the compensatory needs to maximise the remaining components of verbal language.

Hemiplegic patients can be deprived of up to 50% of their ability to communicate non-verbally. Hemiplegia is most commonly associated with stroke, a condition caused by a cerebrovascular accident (CVA). When it occurs in the right cerebral hemisphere there is a left hemiplegia because the nerve fibres cross at the base of the brain. A left CVA results in a right hemiplegia, and since the majority of the population is right handed, many people with a left CVA are also deprived of the writing component of communicating.

Furthermore hemiplegia can be accompanied by facial paralysis. The lip lies limp and down-drawn on one side but it may not be conveying the sadness and depression which body language experts associate with down-drawn lips. Facial paralysis may include a drooping eyelid which minimises the eye contact component of body language and the visual input component of verbal language. A left hemiplegia can also interfere with speaking.

Again it is a case of the nurse helping the patient to work through the various emotional stages of coming to terms with lost abilities in the several components of communicating. Nurses need to become skilled at recognising cues (other than down-drawn lips) of sadness and depression and dealing with these as seems appropriate. The nurse when communicating with the patient should be on the same side as the unaffected eye both for the patient's comfort and to maximise visual input.

Whatever the extent of the hemiplegia, nursing activities include provision of emotional support, and encouragement to relearn control of the paralysed muscles — as advised by the physiotherapist — so that there will be improvement in the patient's AL of communicating non-verbally and by writing.

The *paraplegic patient* is also deprived of up to 50% of the ability to communicate non-verbally, but it is a different distribution from the 50% of the hemiplegic patient, so the problems are different. The most common cause of the condition is accident and a preponderance of the victims are young males. They cannot move from the waist downwards so they are deprived of their characteristic walk and the other information conveyed by this portion of the body, one of the greatest anxieties usually being related to the communicating elements of expressing sexuality.

Helping the patient with the AL of communicating includes several of the nursing activities given for the hemiplegic patient. However as soon as possible the paraplegic patient is rehabilitated to a wheelchair life, which in itself can present communicating problems. Just as a small child's eye level when standing is at the adult's leg level, so the wheelchair patient's eye level is at most people's waist level. Nurses can help by offering same level eye contact to prevent a feeling of being talked down to — physically, of course!

The *tetraplegic patient* is deprived of most of the ability to communicate non-verbally; retaining only the function for facial expression and eye contact. It is not possible to use a hand to write; otherwise the function for communicating by verbal language is intact. Some of these patients can be encouraged to write holding a pen in the mouth and sometimes they can be encouraged to use a special typewriter by tapping keys with a rod held in the mouth. They too can be rehabilitated in a wheelchair, and same level eye contact helps.

Problems related to body language

Much of present-day knowledge about body language is the result of research on 'normal' subjects. However, there are people who do not have a 'normal' body either in structure or function, with which to transmit such a language. Not only is there a problem in transmission of body language but there is a problem in interpreting the body language transmitted by these people. For example, a congenital curvature of the spine can result in several types of 'hunch back', sometimes accompanied by a drooped shoulder or shoulders. One of the patients' problems is an inability to assume the 'upright' posture with braced shoulders which is characteristic of a confident, cheerful and optimistic mood. They have therefore to express these emotions and reactions in other ways. Nurses should learn to recognise that the body language of mood and attitude cannot be expressed in the usual way by people who have structural or functional defects which affect posture and gait.

Generalised overactivity is often an expression of anger and frustration. However there are patients who, while not being angry or frustrated, simply cannot relax and sit still; it is characteristic of hyperactive children and some mental illnesses, and can be a problem to the individual and to others in the family. It is usually inadvisable to restrain forcibly such patients as this can make them angry or even violent. Special attention therefore needs to be paid to the environment so that they do not harm themselves or others, as they pace restlessly back and forth or indulge in meaningless movement which distorts the usual cues of body language.

Some patients have a problem with localised overactivity seen as an inability to control one or more muscle groups. For example the arms might swing in purposeless movement, so the patient is unable to communicate by pointing to something that is wanted. Because frequently there is an associated low level of intelligence which precludes acquisition of verbal skills, nurses need to observe these patients' body movements closely, to discover whether or not any message is being transmitted.

Though there may not be structural abnormality, enforced posture such as lying in bed, sitting in a wheelchair or chair can produce body language problems. This is particularly so for eye contact, which is more likely to occur when eyes are at the same level. Nurses can help by being seated when talking with these patients.

Changes in various modes of communicating have been discussed separately in order to give each its importance but in reality, the patient may be adapting to change in several modes simultaneously. For example a patient with a left hemiplegia may have both a sensory and a motor loss; and may have either a receptive or expressive aphasia, or a mixture of both. Because such a patient is likely to be in an older age group, there may also be lessened visual and auditory input, so helping with the AL of communicating is an enormous challenge to the nurse.

Patients in intensive care units also have problems with communicating. Some distressing event has led to their admission; they are surrounded by strange equipment and unusual sights and sounds, including other critically ill patients; and staff carry out frequent investigations and treatments. They may feel too ill or too drained of energy to ask appropriate questions or may get the impression that the staff are much too busy to listen, or may have an injury which impedes conversation or makes it difficult to receive a communication. When patients have difficulty in responding, research has shown that they often receive limited deliberate communication (Ashworth, 1985; Alderman 1988).

For a patient in coma (p. 328) there is no communication by any mode. However any gradual return to consciousness is often observed as a response to touch. The manner in which a nurse communicates her concern while for instance bathing an unconscious patient, is obviously important. The stimulus of a constant familiar voice or repetition of a familiar tune — and nowadays these may be utilised in the form of tape-recordings — may eventually produce a response and help to re-establish the patient's AL of communicating.

Of course, a number of patients who are admitted to hospital may have been blind or deaf or dumb or partially paralysed for a period of time. It is particularly important that the nurse discovers what the individuals' usual coping mechanisms have been so that as far as possible, they can continue these practices and use their limited capacities for communicating to the optimum level.

Obviously communicating is not easy. Patients need and enjoy the human interest of social conversation and this is usually an effective way of establishing the basis of a relationship. But planned purposeful communication is also required. Observing and listening, as well as asking appropriate questions, can help the nurse to assess the timing of planned communication and the level at which the information is given. Although effective communicating is not easy, it is possible for the student nurse to learn the skills.

EXPERIENCE OF PAIN

Of all the features of illness, pain is probably the most common. It is a peculiarly individual phenomenon. Because of its subjective nature, it is difficult to measure and only people afflicted can communicate their perception of its presence and intensity. Hence the reason for allocating the main discussion of pain to the AL of communicating. The relevance of the link with communicating is corroborated by McCaffery (1983) who considers that 'pain is what the patient says it is, existing when he says it does'.

Most people who know what it feels like to be in pain regard it as an unpleasant sensation and something to be avoided if at all possible. In fact, in some circumstances it can be a protective mechanism, a warning signal; it is the body's response to any number of stressors ranging from the invasion of pathogens to physical injury to mental trauma.

People bereft of the ability to feel pain are therefore constantly in danger of accidentally being burned, bruised or cut, and of failing to recognise the onset of disease. At the opposite pole are people who experience pain even in the absence of any apparently painful stimulus. These two extremes are part of the phenomenon of pain.

Physical aspects of pain

Pain is manifested by the nervous system, one of the physical systems aligned with the AL of communicating in our model, and research carried out over the past 20 years has greatly increased our understanding of the phenomenon. At the site of pain certain chemicals are released; they sensitise the nerve endings and help transmit the impulse to the spinal cord, from where it is relayed to the thalamus resulting in consciousness of the pain, then on to the cerebral cortex where the type, intensity and location of the pain are recognised. However, the painful stimulus can be so intense that the impulse is not transmitted to the brain and an immediate response is initiated by a reflex action, which is processed in the spinal cord. The classic example of this is the reflex withdrawal of the hand on touching something very hot.

For a long time it was thought that painful stimuli were received by special pain receptors in the tissue and transmitted along special pain pathways to a pain centre in the brain. However, this theory, called the *specificity theory*, does not account for the complexities of pain perception. A more acceptable explanation was provided by *pattern theory* which assumes that the pathways in the central nervous system are not narrowly specific but deal with patterns of impulses, pain therefore being transmitted along pathways which convey other sensations too.

One of the widely accepted theories of pain is the *gate theory* put forward by Melzack & Wall in 1965 and clearly discussed in their 1982 publication, *The Challenge of Pain*. As the name suggests, gate theory proposes the idea that there is a mechanism at spinal cord level which acts as a gate. It can decrease or increase the number and intensity of pain signals which reach the brain from the peripheral sensory receptors. Also, impulses from the higher centres of the brain (for example, anxiety or suggestion) can descend and modulate the ascending pain impulses. The gate-control theory helps to explain some of the strange features of the pain experienced, such as why the amount of pain perceived does not necessarily correlate with the intensity of the painful stimulus and why the emotional status of the person appears to influence the process of pain perception.

In fact the role of the brain itself in suppressing pain sensations is now accepted as an area of knowledge crucial to understand. In 1975, Hughes & Kosterlitz (Medicine, 1984) discovered a powerful pain-blocking chemical which they called endorphin, present naturally in the human brain and spinal cord. Since then several such substances (endorphins) have been identified, as well as some non-opiates (enkephalins) which are produced in the body and they all have a complicated part in closing the gate to pain. These discoveries add a new and important dimension to understanding the physiology of pain.

Perception of pain

This aspect of the pain experience is one of the most fascinating. It concerns the individual's interpretation of the meaning of the signals received in the brain — his perception of the pain.

Individuals vary in their perception of pain. Two people can be given an injection and one may find it excruciating while the other may hardly feel it. Pain perception also varies in the same individual under different circumstances.

The influence of suggestion on the intensity of pain is increasingly being recognised. For example the 'placebo effect' is well-known: placebo drugs (often, innocuous confections of sugar) can relieve a person's pain simply because of the implicit suggestion that 'drugs make pain better' (Alagaratnam, 1981).

Past experience of pain is another important factor and children are influenced by the attitudes of their parents to pain. Some mothers make a great fuss about even a fairly minor injury whereas others reserve attention for more severe pain; as a result the children concerned will adopt different ways of responding to pain.

Cultural factors, too, are recognised as influencing the way people grow up to perceive and react to pain. In Western societies childbirth is generally considered to be a painful experience, whereas in some other parts of the world women appear to experience little pain in labour. Members of some tribes in India and Africa engage in ritualistic ceremonies involving piercing of the lips and cheeks with needles and stakes: they do not appear to experience pain and the resulting wounds heal quickly.

It is often said that these variations in the perception of pain are the result of people's different 'pain thresholds' — some people having a low threshold and feeling only slightly painful stimuli, and others having a high threshold and being immune to everything except the most intensely painful stimuli. In fact, all people have the same 'sensation threshold' (that is, the point at which sensation of any kind is experienced): it is the '*pain perception threshold*' — the point at which the sensation of pain is experienced — which varies between individuals.

Of course, the ability to perceive pain requires a fully functioning nervous system and any damage to the sensory nerve endings, sensory tracts in the spinal cord or the involved areas of the cerebral cortex of the brain will interfere with pain perception. For example, there may be no perception of pain affecting the lower limbs in a person paralysed from the waist down. Sometimes, on the other hand, there is an increased sensitivity to pain and this often occurs in neuritis, an inflammatory condition affecting nerve tissue. Level of consciousness is also relevant; as the level lowers, the pain perception threshold is correspondingly depressed.

Reaction to pain

Like the perception of pain, the reaction to pain is highly individual. Despite these individual differences, however, there are physiological manifestations of acute pain which can be observed in all people: the pulse becomes more rapid, blood pressure rises; breathing quickens, skeletal muscle tenses and the skin may become pale and sweaty. Anorexia, nausea, restlessness, irritability and insomnia may also occur.

Again, like the perception of pain, the way an individual reacts to pain is largely determined by upbringing, personality and sociocultural factors. Cultural differences are very distinct; 'keeping a stiff upper lip' is the British reaction, whereas people of Latin origin characteristically express their feelings by crying and groaning aloud.

The reaction to chronic pain is different. Acute pain is characterised by a well-defined pattern of onset, with associated subjective symptoms and objective physical signs. In contrast, chronic pain has an insidious onset, lacking the objective signs commonly noted with acute pain (Foley, 1985); indeed, chronic pain sufferers may be less able to describe their perception of pain. Chronic pain is sometimes extremely complex, causing personality changes and psychological disturbance. Over time, pain makes people anxious and depressed or irritable and aggressive. The tiredness caused by pain lessens the person's ability to control and tolerate the continuous pain. Often when the chronic pain is associated with a malignant disease the person's reaction is to concentrate his whole attention on his pain and everything else is ignored, but Trevelyan (1988) gives an account of the successful control of chronic pain which included equal parts of physiotherapy, relaxation training and psychological management. The consultant who runs the Pain Clinic says 'We don't assess decrease in pain, we aren't actually changing the pathology; measuring activity levels is more valuable'.

Types of pain

Pain manifests itself in different ways according to the location, cause, intensity and duration. There is no one definition, but it is possible to categorise pain into various types. For example *superficial* pain is felt in the skin and subcutaneous tissue often with an obvious cause such as heat, pressure or mechanical trauma; *deep pain* usually involving muscles and joints may be described as 'aching' or 'gnawing'; *visceral pain* often is associated with a specific organ, for example the 'tight' pain of angina when there is a reduction in oxygenated blood reaching the myocardium; *neuralgic pain* arises from damage to peripheral nerves and is often caused by infection, inflammation or poor circulation; *referred pain*, for example angina, may be accompanied by shoulder pain; *phantom limb pain*, a tingling pins-and-needles pain experienced in an amputated limb, may continue for months although eventually it does disappear.

A different kind of pain occurs in the absence of apparent physical stimuli — *psychogenic pain*. Increasingly it is being recognised that psychological factors can cause pain and it is not imaginary; to the person experiencing the pain, it is real (Sofaer, 1984).

Assessment of pain

Because pain is a subjective experience and such a complex phenomenon it is not easy to assess. Obtaining the person's own description of the pain, obtaining a history and observing the individual's reaction to pain are the main methods of assessment.

The location of the pain is one of the first facts to ascertain. The person may be able to point to or describe the gross area involved, such as in the arm or may need help to locate it more specifically.

The temporal pattern of the pain may be important in diagnosis, for example, whether stomach pain occurs before, during or after a meal. The time of the onset of the pain, the duration and the time at which it gets worse or less or better can be established from questioning.

The intensity of pain must be assessed as the patient's own perception and is not necessarily reflected by the pain reac-

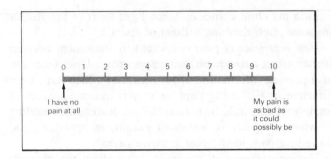

Fig. 7.4 A 'painometer'

tion. An effective way of finding out how intense the patient's pain is, and how the intensity varies, is to use a 'painometer'. This is not a scientific instrument but simply a continuum drawn on a card (Fig. 7.4) which the person is shown and asked to point to the appropriate rating. This method is more informative than spontaneous verbal statements such as 'I can't bear it' or 'It's terrible' and patients can use their own assessments as the yardstick of whether or not it is improving. Seers (1987) used a painometer and a pain relief scale in her research to study postoperative pain.

The reaction to pain, if observed carefully, may provide important information particularly when the person has difficulty in communicating verbally or has a depressed level of consciousness. Pallor, rapid breathing, a raised blood pressure and excessive sweating may accompany intense pain. Nonverbal cues may assist with assessment. Facial gestures such as screwing up the face or gritting the teeth are common reactions to pain. Body posture may also be relevant; for instance with stomach pain people often curl up whereas with chest pain they may want to lean forward or lie on the affected side. Crying and groaning may occur and if the pain is intermittent yet intense, the person may shout aloud or shriek.

The character of the pain is the way it is described. Some of the ways in which pain can be described have already been mentioned; 'aching', 'gnawing', 'tightness', 'tingling' are a few of the words commonly used. Some others are 'stabbing', 'burning', 'twisting' and 'shooting'. Sometimes the description is a comprehensive statement of the pain being experienced; for example, the patient may say 'I have a sharp pain in my chest when I breathe in' or 'I have a burning pain when I pass water' or 'I get cramp-like stomach pains with my periods'.

Factors precipitating the pain are important elements for identification in assessment. Pain is often related to everyday activities of living such as eating and drinking, eliminating, breathing, working and playing, to name a few. Whether pain is associated with mobility or whether it occurs even at rest is of crucial importance. Environmental factors such as noise, and psychological factors such as anxiety or fear may also precipitate pain. The person may describe without difficulty what precipitates the pain: 'The pain in my chest comes on when I get short of breath, for instance after climbing a flight of stairs'.

Past experience of pain is relevant in assessment because it may affect subsequent pain experiences. Discussion can also provide information about measures which have been effective in alleviating pain, or it may indicate sources of anxiety which could be reduced by adequate understanding of what to expect, for instance regarding an operation, and so reduce pain in the postoperative period.

Having gathered all the information about the person's experience of pain, the assessment must be documented so that continuity of care can be provided by the health care team, and to provide guidelines for documentation, Mc-Caffery (1983) discusses the use of selected assessment tools including the London Hospital Pain Observation Chart and the McGill Home Recording Card.

Of all health care staff, nurses are probably the most involved with ongoing assessment of pain. Writing about pain assessment, Camp & O'Sullivan (1987) quote several research findings which indicate the inadequacy of pain documentation — and by inference, the inadequacy of pain assessment. One study showed how features of acute and chronic pain influence nurses' estimates of pain experience, pain relief action, and attitudes towards pain. Another project noted lack of correspondence between observer inferences and patient self-reported pain; and another showed that nursing inferences were made by observing appearance and behaviour rather than asking the patient to describe the pain. Camp & O'Sullivan therefore decided to ascertain the degree of congruence between pain as described by medical, surgical and oncology patients and the related documentation of pain assessment. Their findings showed that documentation was conspicuously lacking, and nurses documented less than 50% of what the patient reported, in fact primarily only location, medication and the fact that the patient complained of pain. They concluded that because the nurse's role is vital to effective pain management, more education on the role of pain management is required.

Their project was conducted in the USA but Sofaer (1983) in the UK also suspected from a review of literature that nurses do not always recognise when a patient has pain; and their knowledge of pain relief and of analgesics may be inadequate. In her project, she studied the practicality and effectiveness of a clinically-based educational programme on pain management for nurses of all levels in four surgical wards.

Control of pain

The relief of pain and suffering is one of the most important objectives in health care and in many instances, some form of medication is used — by the oral, sublingual, rectal, intramuscular, spinal or parenteral routes. Nurses do not prescribe medications, but they do have a considerable role in relation to their administration and even when the medical practitioner physically administers the drug, for example a local anaesthetic block, nurses still have responsibilities in preparing and supporting the patient before, during and after the treatment. Patients primarily look to the nurse for pain relief and the nurse, along with the individual concerned, assesses the individual's current experience of pain before administering the prescribed drug and evaluating the effect. It is important therefore that nurses understand how analgesics work. Sofaer (1984) describes some commonly used narcotic (acting on the central nervous system) and non-narcotic (acting on the nerves at the site of the pain) drugs; their efficacy in pain control and their side-effects. Included in her discussion is the use of patient-controlled analgesic therapy (PACAT) which is suitable for adults who are rational and not in circulatory shock. It requires purpose-built equipment in which a previously programmed drug injection is connected to a venous cannula in the patient's arm or hand. A preset dose can be delivered over a predetermined time by the patient activating a press-button switch. This is done when the patient feels the need for pain relief but there is a built-in mechanism to prevent overdosage, and Sofaer quotes studies which indicate that patients are enthusiastic about the method, and side-effects are minimal.

Sofaer's research study was related to pain relief for patients in surgical wards which in general terms was acute pain and relatively transient. On the other hand, Regnard & Davies (1986) discuss the use of analgesia and methods of administration especially in relation to relief of chronic pain in patients who have advanced cancer. But pain control is possible not only in hospital. Harris (1988) talks about the new generation of drug delivery systems which offer the patient a large measure of personal control, and the possibility of staying at home, or even at work, because efficacious pain control techniques are now available.

Quite apart from pharmacological remedies prescribed by the medical practitioner, there are other pain therapies, some of which lie directly within the province of the nurse. Any sensory distraction or diversion such as change of position, application of heat or cold and relaxation techniques (Sims, 1987) may provide competition to stimuli which prevent them getting through the 'gate' and therefore reduce the pain signals. Also rubbing or lightly slapping an injured part can reduce the pain. Transcutaneous electrical nerve stimulation (TENS) is another 'competitive' measure; electrodes are attached to the skin over a painful area and a mild current is generated to compete with the pain stimuli (Latham, 1987). Acupuncture and biofeedback (Broome & Khorshidian, 1982) also come into this category. Many of these techniques, both pharmacological and non-pharmacological, are described as they relate to nursing by McCaffery (1983), and Melzack & Wall (1982) make the point that:

. . . as a result of hundreds of experiments there is a limit to the effectiveness of any given therapy; but happily the effects of two or more therapies given in combination are cumulative.

Some particular skills for helping to relieve pain when the patient is a child are described by Williams (1987) and Fradd (1988) and mentioned on page 345.

In several countries, special multidisciplinary pain control clinics have been established as a focus of specialised knowledge and in the UK there are over 200 pain clinics (Holmes, 1987). Patients come with a variety of problems including pain associated with arthritis, cancer, orthopaedic disabilities and back pain. Different treatments are offered including local analgesic injections, transcutaneous nerve stimulation, manipulation, acupuncture and psychiatric assessment, and those who need inpatient treatment are admitted. In instances of malignant pain, cordotomy may be performed where the anterolateral tract is cut between the cervical one and two vertebrae (C1 & C2) under local anaesthetic, or intrathecal catheters may be inserted through which analgesia is administered, but these patients can be discharged home after a few days into the care of the district nurse.

The search for new and more effective techniques of pain control goes on year by year. Anything which seems promising is investigated with hope and, at various times, different methods seem to be in vogue. These clinics offer diverse methods of pain control which can be summarised under three headings — physical, psychological and pharmacological:

physical methods of pain control	change of position
	applications of heat/cold
	massage and vibration
	electrical stimulation techniques
	neurosurgical techniques
	acupuncture
psychological methods of pain control	communicating
	sensory distraction and diversion
	music therapy
	relaxation techniques
	desensitisation
	hypnosis
	biofeedback
pharmacological methods of pain control	analgesics (local and general)
	drugs to treat the cause of the pain
	tranquillisers to reduce anxiety
	anaesthetic blocking agents (for example, epidural anaesthesia)
	inhalations

Pain control remains a major challenge and at the Pain Research Foundation, a registered charity, doctors and nurses are investigating causes of pain as well as the efficacy of various treatments (Holmes, 1987). However, the availability of drugs is not universal and politicoeconomic factors influence methods of pain relief. The World Health Organization (in 1988) estimates that there are 3.5 million people with severe or moderate pain as the result of cancer. As over half of them live in developing countries where it is difficult to procure or to afford oral narcotics, pain relief by other than pharmacological means assumes enormous importance. Any discussion of pain illustrates yet again the relatedness of physical, psychological, sociocultural, environmental and politicoeconomic factors.

Patients may complain of pain in any part of the body and in many instances it is not possible to see the cause, so for our model for nursing, McCaffery's (1983) definition is used 'Pain is what the patients says it is existing when he says it does'. As already stated, the problem of pain is therefore associated in our model with the AL of communicating. In the proforma for documentation of the Nursing Plan suggested in this textbook, the nurse would normally assess and chart the incidence of pain under the AL of communicating unless it were AL-specific; for example if someone had a respiratory infection and had a related pain in the chest, when pain would be recorded under the AL of breathing. Examples of pain related to specific ALs are mentioned in the appropriate AL chapter in Section 3.

Individualising nursing

The first part of this chapter reflects the Roper, Logan and Tierney model — the nature of the AL of communicating; the relationship of the lifespan to the AL; the effect of an individual's dependence/independence status; and the influence of physical, psychological, sociocultural, environmental and politicoeconomic factors on the AL. Mainly, the first part provides examples of potential problems occurring in everyday living, and what might be done to prevent them from becoming actual problems. In the second part of the chapter, a selection of actual problems and discomforts which can be experienced by people in relation to the AL have been described. This provides a background of general knowledge about the AL as such.

While describing the Roper, Logan and Tierney model for nursing, general information was provided about individualising nursing (p. 51) which, in fact, is synonymous with the concept of the process of nursing.

Out of this background of general knowledge about the AL of communicating, and about individualising nursing, it should then be possible to extract the issues which are relevant to one individual's current circumstances (whether in a health or an illness setting), i.e. make an assessment of relevant issues according to the individual's stage on the lifespan; according to current level of dependence/independence; and take into account the relevant physical, psychological, sociocultural, environmental and politicoeconomic factors. Collectively, this information would provide a profile of the person's individuality in living for this AL, and therefore guides the nurse in devising a plan for individualising nursing.

As indicated earlier in the text, this assessment would be achieved by various means such as observing the person; acquiring information about the person's usual habits in relation to this AL partly by asking appropriate questions, partly by listening to the patient and/or relatives; and using relevant information from available records, including medical records. The collected information could then be examined to identify any actual problems being experienced with the AL and these could be arranged in some order of priority. The nurse might also recognise some potential problems — not all possible potential problems but those which are relevant. Realistic goals, mutually agreed with the patient when this is possible, could then be set to prevent potential problems from becoming actual ones; to alleviate or solve the actual problems; or to help the person cope with those which cannot be alleviated or solved. Of course, some of the patient's problems with this AL, although identified from the nursing assessment, may well be out with the scope of nursing intervention. In such instances, after discussion with the patient when appropriate, these problems may be referred to other members of the health care team such as medical staff, dieticians, physiotherapists or social workers.

Keeping in mind what the person can and cannot do unaided, the nursing interventions to achieve the mutually set goals could then be selected according to local circumstances and available resources.

Following implementation of the interventions, their effects could be evaluated in relation to the goals set, and if goals were not reached, they could be revised or rescheduled, or even discarded.

It is worth repeating here that although discussed in four phases — assessing, planning, implementing and evaluating — individualising nursing is not a linear progression; it assumes a built-in responsiveness to feedback at any of the phases, giving ample allowance for change within the overall framework. Also, during an illness episode, an important consideration is rehabilitation of the individual, and planning for this could commence as soon as the person enters the health care system. Another important feature is the professional judgement needed to discontinue the nurse/patient relationship when it is no longer relevant.

This chapter has been concerned with the AL of communicating. However, as stated previously, it is only for

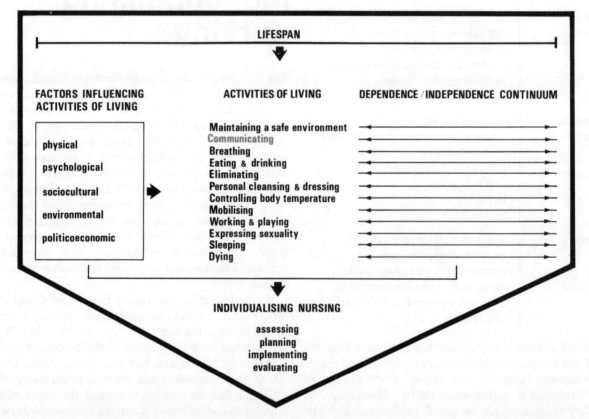

Fig. 7.5 The AL of communicating within the model for nursing

the purposes of discussion that any AL can be considered on its own; in reality, the various activities are closely related and do not have distinct boundaries. Figure 7.5 is a reminder that the AL of communicating is related to the other ALs and also to the other components of the model for nursing.

REFERENCES

Action for the Dysphasic Adult Group (ADA) 1987 How to help the dysphasic patient with speech and communication. ADA, London

Alagaratnam W 1981 Pain and the nature of the placebo effect. Nursing Times 77 (43) October 28: 1883–1884

Alderman C 1988 Conveying calming care. Nursing Standard 32 (2) May 14: 28–29

Ashworth P 1985 Don't forget to talk to him. Nursing Mirror 160 (18) May 1: 50–51

Ball M, Hannah K, Gerdin-Jelger U, Peterson H 1988 Nursing informatics: where caring and technology meet. Springer-Verlag, New York

Bax M 1986 Baby can you hear me? Community Outlook in Nursing Times 82 (37) September 82 (37): 41–45

Bond M 1988 Understanding assertiveness. Nursing Times 84 (9) March 2: 61–64

Bond S 1982 Relatively speaking 2: communicating with families of cancer patients. Nursing Times 78 (24) June 16: 1027–1029

Boore J 1979 Prescription for recovery. Royal College of Nursing, London, p 76

Broome A, Khorshidian C 1982 Psychological treatments of chronic pain. Nursing Times 78 (31) August 4: 1305–1306

Burnard P 1987a Sharing a viewpoint. Senior Nurse 7 (3) September: 38–39

Burnard P 1987b Counselling — basic principles in nursing. The Professional Nurse 2 (9) June: 278–280

Burnard P 1988 Empathy: the key to understanding. The Professional Nurse 3 (10) July: 388–391

Camp L, O'Sullivan P 1987 Comparison of medical, surgical and oncology patients' descriptions of pain and nurses' documentation of pain assessments. Journal of Advanced Nursing September 12: 593–598

Cartwright A 1964 Human relations and hospital care. Routledge and Kegan Paul, London

Chalmers C 1985 Talking to stroke patients. Nursing Times 81 (32) August 7: 41–42

Chisnell J 1988 District nurses' work with postoperative patients. Nursing Times 84(3) January 20: 54

Cowan V 1987 Documentation. Add-on Journal of Clinical Nursing 3 (14) February: 527–529

Darbyshire P 1987 Relatives — sour grapes. Nursing Times 83 (37) September 16: 23–25

Donnelly D 1987 Focus on disability: registered hopeless? Nursing Times 83 (24) June 17: 49–51

Ernsberger R 1988 Scanning fingers. Newsweek CX11 (14) September 26: 3

Ernsberger R, Robinson C 1987 Bringing the blind 'on-line'. Newsweek CX (7) August 17: 3

European Economic Community 1983 European Charter on the rights of patients. EEC, Brussels

Faulkner A 1985 Getting it right — counselling. Nursing 2 (38) June: 1132–1134

Fessey C 1988 Communication difficulties and assertivenss/negotiation skills. The Add-on Journal of Clinical Nursing 3 (27) March/April: 1002–1005

Foden R, Beauchamp T 1986 A history and theory of informed consent. Oxford University Press, Oxford

Foley K 1985 The treatment of cancer pain. New England Journal of Medicine 313: 84–95

Ford M, Fox J, Fitch S, Donovan A 1986 Light in the darkness. Nursing Times 83 (1) January 7: 26–29

Fradd E 1988 Tug of love. Nursing Times 84 (41) October 12: 32–35

Glasper A, Gow M, Yerrell P 1989 A family friend. Nursing Times 85 (4) January 25: 63–65

Haddon C 1987 Dogs that can take care of disabled people. Sunday Telegraph August 16: 3

Hardcastle M 1988 First impressions. Nursing Times 84 (21) May 25: 69–70

Harris L 1988 Something to live for. Nursing Times 84 (32) August 10: 25–28

Hayward J 1975 Information — a prescription against pain. Royal College of Nursing, London

Helman C 1984 Culture, health and illness. Wright, Bristol

Holmes P 1987 Breaking the pain barrier. Nursing Times 83 (5) February 11: 51–52

Hunter L 1987 Keyboard rehabilitation. Nursing Times 83 (32) August 12: 45–47

Keighley T 1987 Data protection. Add-on Journal of Clinical Nursing 3 (14) February: 524–525

Kiernan C, Reid B, Jones L 1983 Signs and symbols. Heinemann Educational, London

Koch B, Rankin S 1987 Computers and their applications in nursing. Harper and Row, London

Labun E 1988 Spiritual care: an element in nursing planning. Journal of Advanced Nursing 13: 314–320

Latham J 1987 Transcutaneous nerve stimulation. The Professional Nurse 2 (5) February: 133–135

Lelean S 1973 Ready for report, nurse? Royal College of Nursing, London, p 14

Lindsay M 1983 The roaring deafness. Nursing Times 79 (5) February 2: 61–63

McCaffery M 1983 Nursing the patient in pain. (Adapted for the UK by B. Sofaer). Harper and Row, London

McEvoy P 1988 Introduction to the counselling process. The Professional Nurse August: 456–460

Macleod Clark J 1988 Communication: the continuing challenge. Nursing Times 84 (23) June 8: 24–27

Macmillan M 1987 Informed consent. Senior Nurse 7 (3) September: 12

Maguire P 1985 Consequences of poor communication between nurses and patients. Nursing 2 (38) June: 1115–1118

Medicine 1984 Unlocking pain's secret. Time 24, June 11: 40–47

Melia K 1986 Dangerous territory. Nursing Times 82 (21) May 21: 27

Melia K 1988 To tell or not to tell. Nursing Times 84 (30) July 27: 37–39

Melzack R, Wall P 1982 The challenge of pain. Penguin, Harmondsworth

Milne C 1988 Laryngectomy. Nursing Standard 2 (29) April 23: 36–37

Moore D 1988 Confidentiality: all sewn up? Senior Nurse 8 (6) June: 6–7

Nursing and Computers 1988 Proceedings from the 3rd International Symposium on 'Nursing Use of Computers and Information Science' (Dublin). C V Mosby, St Louis

Parnell J 1982 Continuity and communication. Nursing Times Occasional Paper 78 (9) March 31: 33–40

Pearce J 1988 The power of touch. Nursing Times 84 (24) June 15: 26–29

Pearson A 1985 Getting it right — interprofessional communication. Nursing 2 (38) June: 1129–1131

Raphael W 1969 Patients and their hospitals. King Edward's Hospital Fund, London

Ratcliffe J 1988 Worth a try. Nursing Times 84 (6) February 10: 29–30

Regnard C, Davies A 1986 A guide to symptom relief in advanced cancer. Haigh and Hockland, Manchester

Roper N, Logan W, Tierney A 1983 Using a model for nursing. Churchill Livingstone, Edinburgh

Rowden R, Jones L 1983 A diversional programme for patients with cancer. Nursing Times 79 (11) March 16: 25–27

Royal College of Nursing, Association of Nursing Practice 1985 Guidelines for nurses who work with the hearing-impaired. RCN, London

Royal National Institute for the Blind 1987 Helping visually handicapped people in hospital. RNIB, London

Sawyer J 1986 Speech impairment after a stroke. Nursing Times 82 (3) January 15: 39–41

Seaton A 1989 Control of substances hazardous to health. British Medical Journal 298(6677) April 1: 846–847

Seers K 1987 Perceptions of pain. Nursing Times 83 (48) December 2: 37–39

Sims S 1987 Relaxation training as a technique for helping patients cope with the experience of cancer; a selective review of literature. Journal of Advanced Nursing September 12: 583–589

Sofaer B 1983 The effect of focused nursing education on postoperative pain relief; a pilot study. In: Proceedings of the First Open Conference of the Workgroup for European Nurse Researchers. Swedish Nurses Association, Stockholm

Sofaer B 1984 Pain: a handbook for nurses. Harper and Row, London

Tompkins J 1988 A good sign (Makaton). Nursing Standard 32 (2) May 14: 31

Trevelyan T 1988 Prevailing over pain. Nursing Times 84 (33) August 17: 45–47

Turton P 1989 Touch me, feel me, heal me. Nursing Times 85 (19) May: 42–44

United Kingdom Central Council 1984 Code of Professional Conduct for the Nurse, Midwife and Health Visitor, 2nd edn. UKCC, London

United Kingdom Central Council 1987 Confidentiality — an elaboration of Clause 9 of the 2nd edition of the UKCC Code of Professional Conduct. UKCC, London

United Kingdom Central Council 1989 Exercising accountability: a framework to assist nurses, midwives and health visitors to consider ethical aspects of professional practice. UKCC, London

Vousden M 1987 Do you really need to know? Nursing Times 83 (49) December 9: 28–30

Watson P 1986 Towers of Babel. Nursing Times 82 (49) December 3: 40–41

Wells R 1986 The great conspiracy. Nursing Times 82 (21) May 21: 22–25

Williams J 1987 Managing paediatric pain. Nursing Times 83 (36) September 9: 36–39

Wilson-Barnett J 1978 Factors influencing patients' emotional reaction to hospitalisation. Journal of Advanced Nursing 3 (May): 221–229

Wilson-Barnett J 1988 Patient teaching or patient counselling? Journal of Advanced Nursing 13 (March): 215–222

Yule W 1988 Dyslexia. British Medical Journal 297 (6647) August 20–27: 501–502

ADDITIONAL READING

Carr E 1989 Waking up to post-operative pain. Nursing Times 85 (3) January 18: 38–39

Coles J 1987 The child in the intensive care unit. The Add-on Journal of Clinical Nursing 3 (16) April: 608–611

Devlin R 1989 Helping disabled mothers. Community Outlook in Nursing Times 85 (15) April 12: 4–12

French S 1989 Mind your language (people with disabilities). Nursing Times 85 (2) January 11: 29–31

Moore D 1988 Confidentiality: all sewn up? Senior Nurse 8 (6) June: 6–7

Office of Health Economics 1988 Stroke. OHE, London

Salter M 1988 Altered body image. Wiley, London

Vaughan B 1989 Autonomy and accountability. Nursing TImes 85 (3) January 18: 54–55

Wells R 1988 Ethics and information. Senior Nurse 8 (6) June: 8–10

8

Breathing

The activity of breathing

'Taking the first breath' is of crucial importance at the birth of every baby and determines whether or not the infant will have a viable existence as a human being. From then on breathing seems effortless and people are not usually consciously aware of the activity of breathing until some abnormal circumstance forces it to their attention.

THE NATURE OF BREATHING

Physiologically speaking, breathing in is called inspiration, breathing out is expiration and the whole process is referred to as respiration. Inspiration is concerned mainly with the intake of oxygen from the atmosphere, and expiration with the expulsion of carbon dioxide and because of the site at which this occurs, it is called 'external respiration'. The whole point of breathing is to convey oxygen (O_2) from the atmosphere to each cell in the body so that it can create the energy to engage in its various activities. The cell is the basic unit of all life and respiration is the most fundamental of its processes; respiration is needed for all cellular activities and in the process carbon dioxide (CO_2) is formed as a waste product of metabolism. Because of the site at which this occurs, it is referred to as 'internal respiration'. The CO_2 is absorbed into the blood, in which it is transported along the cardiovascular system and arrives in the lungs to be breathed out as expired air. In very broad functional terms the requisites to achieve both external and internal respiration are:

- adequate oxygen in the atmosphere
- a functioning respiratory system
- a large moist surface in the lungs where the oxygen

129

and blood are in close proximity to allow exchange of O_2 and CO_2

- a physical 'bellows' arrangement (the thoracic cage) with muscles to operate it and nerves to control the muscles
- a 'transport' system, the blood
- a 'carrier' in the transport system, the haemoglobin
- thin-walled capillaries in close proximity to the cells where O_2 and CO_2 can be exchanged
- healthy cells which are capable of using the O_2 and releasing CO_2

This complex integrated activity is in constant use to collect O_2 from the atmosphere; transport it in the blood to the cells; collect the cells' CO_2; and transport it to the lungs where it is released to the atmosphere. It is evident that the action of the heart and blood vessels are complementary to breathing. It is therefore logical to expect that impairment at any point in this complex sequence of the cardiopulmonary system is going to affect the exchange of gases and the individual's ability to 'breathe'. It is not the intention in this book to describe these complex biological processes in detail, but further comment is made in 'Physical factors' on page 130 about the need to integrate knowledge from other disciplines, into nursing.

In the model of living and the model for nursing the 12 ALs are the main component and each is the subject of a chapter (Chs 6–17). In the remainder of the first part of this chapter, the other four components will be focused on the AL of breathing.

LIFESPAN: EFFECT ON BREATHING

At birth it may be necessary to suction the baby's upper respiratory tract to remove any debris collected during the birth process, but for most people, the AL of breathing is an independent activity throughout the lifespan. However, the fact that there is a direct relationship between age and the rate of breathing (and also pulse rate and blood pressure) is relevant knowledge in the present context.

Rate of breathing is measured by counting the number of times the chest wall rises and falls over a given period. An infant's rate of breathing may be up to 44 per minute but in children it is about 20 per minute and the range of normal for adults is 12 to 18 breaths per minute. In the older person, however, the breathing rate increases and respirations are shallower. These changes are due to the decreasing elasticity of the lungs and less efficient gaseous exchange between the alveoli and the pulmonary capillaries.

The pulse rate also varies in relation to age, the average of 140 beats per minute in the small baby decreasing gradually to around 70 beats per minute in adulthood. Males tend to have a slightly lower rate than females. The pulse rate tends to remain stable at the adult level for the rest of a person's life, unless altered by disease processes.

Blood pressure increases with age. In infancy the blood pressure is around 90/60 whereas in adulthood the average is 120/80, with little change in the later years unless due to the effects of disease. Adults with pressures above 140 mmHg systolic and/or 100 mmHg diastolic are referred to as hypertensive; adults with pressures below 100 systolic are considered to be hypotensive.

DEPENDENCE/INDEPENDENCE IN BREATHING

For most of the ALs, the dependence/independence continuum is closely related to the lifespan, during which a state of dependence in the early years is the norm. Breathing is the exception; it is the only AL which the majority of people perform independently right from birth throughout the entire lifespan, until the moment of death. In health, changes in dependence/independence status for breathing do not occur and therefore further discussion of this component in the context of the model of living is not required. However, certain illnesses do cause loss of independence for breathing and some of the reasons for dependence (on nursing care, oxygen and mechanical aids) are outlined in the second part of this chapter (p. 136) in the context of the model for nursing.

FACTORS INFLUENCING BREATHING

Commonly occurring activities such as speaking, laughing and eating cause minor alterations in the breathing pattern, though rarely is the individual really aware of these adjustments. Even in the healthy person, however, a number of factors can in a more obvious way influence the rate, depth and regularity of breathing, pulse rate and blood pressure. These are: the degree of physical activity, and the body's physiological response to stressors (physical factors); changes in mood and emotion (psychological factors); and, of course, the composition of inhaled air and the presence of abnormal constituents in the atmosphere (environmental factors). The fourth group of factors included in this component of the model — sociocultural factors — is only tangentially relevant in the West, but deserves mention under its own heading. Under the fifth heading, politicoeconomic factors, control of pollution is mentioned, and the problem of smoking is discussed from this particular point of view.

Physical factors
The physical factors most directly influencing the AL of breathing are of course the body structures and functions required for this AL. In biological terms these are the organs which collectively form the respiratory system, the function of which is to provide every cell in the body with

oxygen. To accomplish this, the blood, together with the vessels and organs comprising the circulatory and lymphatic systems are also relevant physical factors which influence the AL of breathing. In human biology terms, therefore, in the model for nursing the AL of breathing is not only juxtaposed with the respiratory system but also with the cardiopulmonary system. The purpose of this juxtaposition is to provide guidance when devising a nursing plan which takes account not only of nurse-initiated interventions, but also the nursing interventions which result from medical prescription and the suggested documents on page 54 accommodate this.

During vigorous exercise in the healthy adult there is a normal physiological increase in respiratory rate, because the muscles require more oxygen. To transport the oxygen more quickly, the heart beats faster so the pulse rate is simultaneously increased; in fact, respiration and pulse rates are related in a ratio of 1:4, and an alteration in one is usually accompanied by an alteration in the other. Conversely when the body is resting, particularly when sleeping, the respiratory rate and pulse rate are usually decreased.

Not only rate but the rhythm of breathing can be affected during such physical activities as talking, laughing, eating, singing, yet seldom are these variations given conscious thought. Even sneezing and coughing, if transient, are rarely pondered over as a deviation in the normal pattern of breathing.

Many people are now aware that cigarette smoking is a physical factor which can influence the respiratory system, but fewer people know that it can also affect the cardiovascular system. Disturbance in one or other, or both of these systems can affect the AL of breathing. Other systems can also be influenced by the inhalation of tobacco smoke and more ALs may be affected. For example, eating and drinking can be influenced by cancer of the mouth, throat, oesophagus and pancreas. Expressing sexuality is the AL associated with fetal damage from tobacco smoke causing low birth weight and even stillbirth. The AL of eliminating is affected when there is cancer of the bladder and kidney and smoking predisposes to these conditions. (Health Education Authority, 1987).

Tobacco smoke contains carbon monoxide (CO) which binds with haemoglobin in the red blood cells to form carboxyhaemoglobin which does not easily exchange oxygen. Consequently there is a reduction in the blood's oxygen-carrying capacity of between 10 and 15%, so it is understandable that there can be such widespread effects throughout the body. CO increases the permeability of arterial walls to cholesterol and this predisposes to atherosclerosis which increases blood pressure. The nicotine increases the heart rate and is another factor which raises blood pressure. The combination of nicotine and CO also seems to have the effect of increasing the viscosity of blood by making the platelets more sticky, predisposing to thrombosis. The condensate from tobacco smoke is deposited in the smoker's lungs and causes local tissue damage including cancer.

'Smokers' cough' is an explanation given frequently for a cough with expectoration of phlegm. Increasingly frequent incidents of bronchitis may occur and there is usually difficulty in breathing caused by narrowing of the small bronchial tubes. There are changes in the minute air sacs in the lungs which decrease the area of membrane available for gaseous exchange; the condition is called chronic obstructive pulmonary disease. In 1984 it caused more than 27 000 deaths in England and Wales (Health Education Authority, 1987). The impaired microcirculation in the lungs causes backlog problems in the pulmonary arteries and veins which is the beginning of chronic heart failure. Also in England and Wales in 1984 the death rate from lung cancer in men was 107.4 per 100 000 deaths, and in women it was 38 per 100 000, however the gap is narrowing. Data from Scotland shows that lung cancer in women has doubled in the last 10 years.

Coronary heart disease is the leading cause of death in the UK which has one of the highest mortality rates in the world from this disease (Health Education Authority, 1987). Men are more likely victims than women, and in general the risk increases with age, and in association with smoking, high blood pressure, lack of exercise, high blood cholesterol and diabetes. There is an increasing risk of coronary heart disease in the presence of more than one of these factors, together with a predisposing family history. The risk is also related to the number of cigarettes smoked daily, and the number of years of smoking. Those who smoke 20 cigarettes daily are estimated to double their risk of dying from coronary heart disease before the age of 65, and the risk is trebled for those who smoke 40 cigarettes daily.

Not only smokers are exposed to these risks. There is increasing evidence that there are other hazards of tobacco smoke, and these are 'mainstream smoke' which is in contact with a smoker's respiratory tract from its entry to its exit; and the 'sidestream smoke' which, as well as being exhaled into the atmosphere, includes the smoke curling from the end of the cigarette. The 'involuntary' smoker inhales 'sidestream smoke' from both these sources. Pownall goes on to say:

Levels of nicotine and carbon monoxide have been found at double the levels of mainstream smoke. Benzoa-pyrene has been found at three times, toluene at six times, and the carcinogenic dimethylnitrosamine at 50 times mainstream levels.

It is difficult to determine the scale of ill health caused by passive smoking, but Pownall (1987) quotes an estimate of 1000 deaths per annum in Britain. People who are chronically exposed to sidestream smoke may have a decreased lung function and may have an increased risk of lung cancer. There may be added danger for people who suffer from lung or heart disease. Children are also affected by sidestream smoke and in smoking households are more prone to chest problems and upper respiratory tract infections. Particularly disturbing is information from Cancer Research Campaign's education and child studies research group. Children were 1.5 times more likely to have frequent absences from school if their parents smoked, particularly the mother. In primary school they do not do so well in exams and there is an increased risk of their becoming smokers (Nursing Times, 1989). There is no doubt about the fact that cigarette smoke causes widespread damage to people's well-being, not only to those who smoke, but also to those who are subjected to a smoke-laden atmosphere.

Yet in 1986 there were still 35% of men and 31% of women in the UK who smoked (OPCS Monitor, 1988). Although these figures show that smokers have become a minority group in the population, the size of the figures leaves no room for complacency. This is apparent from data released by the Central Statistical Office in January 1989 which showed a 2.2% increase in smoking when the period from January to September 1988 was compared with the same 9 months in 1987.

It is not only adults who risk physical pathology by smoking. The Office of Population Census and Surveys (OPCS) conducted a survey in 1986 among secondary school children in England and Wales and found that 10% smoked regularly; 12% of these were girls and 7% were boys. Stewart & Orme (1988) wrote, 'The aim must ultimately be to try and ensure that children neither "drift" into smoking, nor are coerced into it: at best it should be an informed choice.' The role of nurses in helping to prevent children from smoking will be discussed in the second part of this chapter.

It is pertinent here to re-state that in the model for nursing, the component — 'Physical factors influencing the ALs' — is interpreted in a mainly biological context and that the respiratory, circulatory and lymphatic systems were juxtaposed to the AL of breathing. Consequently another physical factor influencing both internal and external respiration is the condition of shock which is basically a manifestation of circulatory failure. With decreased venous blood reaching the respiratory surface membrane, there is decreased exchange of O_2 and CO_2 so that there is a concomitant respiratory failure with a change in the body's electrolyte balance. First-aiders are taught to recognise 'collapse' and render help by using the mnemonic ABC:

Airway   — ensure that it is clear
Breathing   — mouth to mouth
Circulation   — external cardiac compression

The objective is to keep the collapsed person alive until more sophisticated equipment to maintain these bodily functions is available in a hospital setting. The nurse's role

in cardiopulmonary resuscitation will be discussed in the second part of this chapter.

As well as the biological processes related to smoking and the phenomenon of shock, there are others which become active in response to perceived danger — sometimes called environmental stressors. The response increases the rate and depth of respiration, as well as the heart rate, blood pressure and flow of blood to the muscles. In extreme form, these increases are part of the 'fight or flight' syndrome facilitating man's survival. However for most of the time most people's reaction to fear is much less intense. Physiologically the body reats to anxiety in a similar way, but frequently the reaction is of much longer duration. Anxiety can be troublesome and most poeple can be helped to overcome its effects by learning simple relaxation techniques, many of which involve controlled breathing as practised in chanting, transcendental meditation and yoga. Currently there is great interest in helping tense people to relax and lower their blood pressure and pulse rate by constant visual technological monitoring of these functions called biofeedback.

As the feeling of anxiety is so unpleasant, everyone, sometimes consciously but mostly subconsciously, attempts to avoid it. To do so, everyone indulges in an enormous diversity of coping mechanisms in an attempt to reduce stressful anxiety to a tolerable level. For those who are employed it may involve going home to family, and learning to leave work worries behind; for others, who perhaps live alone, it may mean the discipline of organising non-work time in a recreational way, and many local authorities are offering those who are unemployed the means to minimise stress by reduction of entrance fees to sports facilities and so on. In all these examples, the goal is to achieve relaxation and thereby prevent increased blood pressure which can predispose to conditions such as coronary heart disease and stroke.

Psychological factors
In very general terms the AL of breathing can be seen to be influenced by a variety of psychological factors. Certain emotional events in life can affect the individual's breathing. Sadness and grieving, for example, may affect the rate and depth of respirations resulting in audible and visible activities such as sighing and sobbing.

And at some time or another, everyone has had the experience of being suddenly startled; fright is often accompanied by an indrawn, gasping respiration followed by an increase in breathing and pulse rates. The two quite different emotions of anxiety and pleasurable excitement may also cause an increase in breathing and pulse rates and even minor, fairly transient pain can have a similar effect. Emotions, such as anxiety and fear, and circumstances which produce stress, can also increase the blood pressure. Hypertension (high blood pressure) is sometimes thought to be caused by stress and anxiety; but the part played by temperament and emotional factors is difficult to assess. However there is no doubt that worry about high blood pressure is only likely to exacerbate the problem.

Smoking was discussed as one of the physical factors influencing breathing but there is also a psychological dimension. One of the problems about smoking is that it produces a state of dependence.

Dependence on tobacco is a form of addiction. In an attempt to help people to recognise the complex set of circumstances which precede the state of absolute dependence on any chemical substance be it tobacco, alcohol or drugs, the World Health Organization (1975) has defined three types of dependence:

- *social dependence:* the person depends on a chemical in order to conform to the behaviour patterns of his particular community
- *psychological dependence:* the person depends on a chemical to provide enjoyment and/or suppress or come to terms with mental or emotional conflicts
- *physical dependence:* the person becomes dependent on a chemical for normal functioning

It seems that dependence on tobacco grows insidiously over the years. In many instances it starts as social dependence perhaps even at an early age while at school. It may be that there is oral gratification in having a cigarette between the lips; or the act of inhaling gives a special pleasure; or the feeling of relaxation may be associated with exhaling; or perhaps the greatest attraction lies in having something to do with the hands which would otherwise fidget. Sooner or later there is physical dependence, and some people in spite of determined effort to give up smoking find it impossible.

Those who do manage to give up smoking may suffer from unpleasant psychological symptoms for several weeks: for example, depression, irritability, anxiety, restlessness and lack of concentration. These are symptoms which result from the withdrawal of nicotine.

Sociocultural factors
Smoking as a physical factor influencing the AL of breathing has already been discussed, but there is also a sociocultural dimension to smoking. Formal adherence to some religions does not permit smoking. There are also other social groups of people who work together to promote anti-smoking activities, and others who equally fervently extol the rights of smokers.

Quite apart from the spitting associated with 'smokers' cough, there is a normal secretion of phlegm from the upper respiratory tract, most of which is swallowed, and in many cultures children are socialised into disposing of any excess phlegm by using a tissue. However, when people are outdoors, they sometimes spit this secretion onto the street, which can be offensive to onlookers. And when there is secretion from the lower respiratory tract, usually caused by chronic infection, coughing expels it into the upper respiratory tract. If it is expelled onto the street it can be dangerous, because, for instance, any microorganisms dry, are wafted in the dust and can be inhaled by other people, thereby influencing the AL of breathing by causing chest infection. During the process of dessication the microorganisms have acquired an 'environmental dimension' and this is an example of the relatedness of the factors influencing breathing.

It is interesting that currently in some Third World countries, there are notices on public transport and in public places exhorting people to refrain from spitting, along with reminders that spitting spreads disease — notices which were common, certainly in the UK, about four decades ago but now no longer in use. It is also relevant to note that policemen in the UK report spitting as one of the assaults perpetrated against them and were recently concerned that it might transmit AIDS although this fear is unsupported by currently available knowledge.

Environmental factors
Some environmental factors were discussed in general in the model of living (p. 30) and in the model for nursing (p. 48); here they are focused to the AL of breathing. The aspect of the environment which is obviously most relevant to consider in relation to this AL is the atmosphere. It is logical to expect that the composition of inspired air will affect the rate, depth and rhythm of breathing. Atmospheric air is a mixture of gases; it has a variable humidity; it contains microorganisms and it has a temperature characteristic of an area's geographical location and altitude. But how do these factors affect breathing?

Oxygen. Every cell in the human body requires oxygen and each time a person breathes, 4% of the oxygen content of inspired air is retained for cell metabolism.

At high altitudes, the air has a lower oxygen content than at sea level and even at moderate heights, the human respiration rate will increase in an attempt to compensate. On the other hand, too high a concentration of oxygen would support combustion too readily and be incompatible with life.

Nitrogen. Although present in atmospheric air, it cannot be used by the human body; it is in the form of an inert gas and acts as a diluent to the oxygen.

Carbon dioxide. Exhaled air contains 4% more carbon dioxide than inhaled air. In the process of preserving the ecological balance, plants and other vegetation, during photosynthesis, utilise carbon dioxide by retaining the carbon as a form of food and releasing the oxygen into the atmosphere and so the cycle of gas exchange between humans/animals and the plant world goes on.

Water vapour. The air breathed by humans is moistened by the water vapour in the atmosphere, thus preventing irritation of the respiratory mucous membrane. On the other hand, expired air has picked up some of the body's water so has a higher water content than inspired air, and saturation is reached when the water vapour begins to condense, visible on the breath when atmospheric temperature is low.

If the atmospheric humidity is very high, perspiration lies on the skin and the body cannot cool itself by the process of evaporation. For this reason, living in a very hot climate where there is high humidity can cause discomfort and in extreme cases heat exhaustion, one of the features being respiratory distress.

Environmental temperature. In a temperate climate, at sea level, the environmental temperature is usually lower than body temperature and consequently, some heat is lost from the body with each breath. Most people find this a reasonably comfortable environment for living, working and playing. When the environmental temperature is considerably higher, it is more difficult to maintain a comfortable balance between the human body and the atmosphere and, in extreme cases, heat exhaustion will result. Conversely, when the environmental temperature is low, the loss of body heat may cause chilling of the whole body and hypothermia (see Ch. 12) will result.

Microorganism content. Dispersed throughout the atmosphere are many millions of microorganisms; most are non-pathogenic but some, when inhaled, can cause infection in the respiratory tract, for example the common cold. Microorganisms fall to the floor or settle on objects in a room by force of gravity, and convection currents can recirculate them in the atmosphere and perpetuate the possibility of inhalation by man.

Pollutants. While out-of-doors in and around an *urban area*, man is frequently exposed to possible abrasion of the tissue in the respiratory tract by inhalation of smoke containing minute particles which are the products of combustion in domestic heating systems, industrial furnaces and transport vehicles. Condensation around the solid particles produces fog, often referred to as smog, a reminder that the smoke is the real hazard.

In many large cities, attempts have been made to reduce this health hazard by encouraging the use of smokeless fuels for household purposes. Some governments have passed legislation making it obligatory that grit is extracted before furnace smoke is released into the atmosphere; that street-cleaning machines spray water on the dust before sweeping; that garbage collection vehicles have mechanisms to prevent dust from dispersing into the atmosphere. At an international level, the World Health Organization is studying and monitoring the problem of atmospheric pollution and assisting with the exchange of information about prevention on a worldwide scale so that the air, so necessary to human life, will be less of a health hazard.

In the *work situation*, there may be exposure to respiratory abrasion from industrial waste particles, organic and inorganic, for example from linen, hemp, wool, metal, stone and coal. The coal-mining industry has a long history of protective practices to prevent the onset of the dreaded disease, pneumoconiosis, which develops when coal-dust particles become embedded in the lung tissue and eventually cause gross impairment in the capacity to breathe. Inhalation of minute particles of asbestos can cause cancer of the lung and a detailed Code of Practice has been designed in the UK to help workers protect themselves from the hazard. In this instance, even more widespread education is necessary because articles such as ironing boards and cooking pot stands have asbestos insets, and householders sometimes use asbestos for lagging pipes and insulating roofs.

Workers who are at risk in these types of industries are encouraged to use the appropriate preventive measures provided and to have regular chest X-rays so that any adverse effects will be promptly detected and treated. At international level, the International Labour Organization (ILO) has taken measures to encourage governments to provide employees with protection from several types of respiratory health hazards.

Another hazardous environmental factor has been identified in the last two decades. Water droplets from infected humidifier cooling towers, and stagnant water in cisterns and shower heads, are now known to transmit Legionnaires' disease. It is primarily a type of pneumonia and undoubtedly influences the AL of breathing.

At *home*, householders can pollute the air by failing to provide good ventilation, thus increasing the concentration of products from expired air. The oxygen and carbon dioxide content does not reach dangerous levels but the increased temperature and humidity is conducive to rapid multiplication of microorganisms. If poorly ventilated, the household atmosphere may also be permeated with unpleasant odours from the kitchen or toilet accommodation. Inhalation of leaking gases from appliances and from paraffin stoves can cause headaches, drowsiness or indeed, in large quantity, may render the occupants unconscious.

One of the most recent and interesting areas of research into ways of combating the ill effects of pollution concerns the use of ionisers (Lim, 1982). In the atmosphere there are positive ions (molecules which contain an electrical charge and which adversely affect human beings, for example causing headaches) and negative ions (which have a stabilising effect on both body and mind). It has been shown that negatively ionised air, for example in the office or classroom, results in improved performance and a feeling of well-being. Lim cites examples, and goes on to discuss some of the various medical settings in which ionisers have been tried out: for example, in burns units; in efforts to combat infection in hospital; and for patients suffering from anxiety and associated stress symptoms. Work on the effects of ionised air is still in its very early stages but there appears to be possible application in combating pollution in urban areas, in the work situation, at home — and in health care settings too.

Politicoeconomic factors

Many of the topics discussed in the preceding section have an obvious politicoeconomic dimension: for example, the problem of atmospheric pollution. That problem is primarily a responsibility of government and in many industrialised countries legislation exists to control and reduce the hazards associated with atmospheric pollution for city dwellers and workers at risk. However, individuals have responsibilities too; for example, to comply with the requirement to burn smokeless fuel or to wear a protective breathing mask when engaged in certain types of work. In such ways individuals minimise risks to others and avoid hazards which might affect their own breathing.

There are many other ways in which politicoeconomic factors can influence the implementation of preventive activities to reduce, for example, the risk of coronary heart disease and stroke in those people who have a symptomless raised blood pressure. Before setting up 'well persons' clinics' or in some areas imaginatively called 'MOT clinics' (an abbreviation for the Ministry of Transport's road-worthiness certificate required annually for vehicles which are 3 years old or more), extensive advertising (which is expensive) is necessary to inform members of the local community of the desirability of using this facility. Setting up the clinic costs money; it has to be available at times convenient to members of the local community, which may involve overtime payment of staff. It will involve the cost of medication for those found to be 'at risk'. Some health authorities, when allocating their financial budget, do not give priority to these preventive activities. This introduces an ethical dimension to the debate, namely, should the decision of a health authority deprive members of the local community who have a 'silent' raised blood pressure, of the facilities to prevent it causing coronary heart disease or stroke?

And with regard to cigarette smoking, the debate continues about the politicoeconomic factors related to it. Mention has already been made of this problem in terms of its physical effects on the body, and in relation to the development of dependence, a psychological state. Consideration of smoking as a politicoeconomic issue is yet another perspective. Most governments are concerned that smoking is a recognised and serious threat to health and are aware of the fact that treatment of smoking-related disease is a drain on the finances available for health care. However, at the same time, the government obtains revenue from the tax on cigarettes and so there are two sides to the economics of the problem.

Many other groups with health interests engage in education and mount vigorous campaigns against smoking: for example, ASH (Action on Smoking and Health) which was set up by the Royal College of Physicians, and the National Society of Non-smokers which was founded in 1926 and may be best known for its instigation of an annual National 'No Smoking' Day.

However, the money spent on prevention by the government and all the various organisations is infinitesimal compared to the millions of pounds spent on sales promotion by the cigarette companies. Anti-smoking advertising campaigns play a part in bringing about changes in smoking behaviour but a variety of approaches is needed, aimed at both the individual and at society as a whole. Programmes in schools have a crucial role in attempting to stop people ever starting to smoke; advice and information by doctors and other health professionals remain important, for healthy people as well as those suffering from smoking-related disease; improved methods to help people to give up smoking are being developed, for example the use of nicotine gum and behavioural techniques; and, for the protection of non-smokers from sidestream smoke, there has been a gradual increase in restriction on smoking. Over the past few years such protection has been most noticeable on public transport, particularly on planes and trains, where a majority of seats are designated 'No smoking', indeed on some short flights smoking is prohibited. Many restaurants have followed suit. Some work places have always had a 'No smoking' rule, necessary because of the work undertaken, and employees are aware of this before being employed there. However, at other work places, there is governmental encouragement to separate smokers from non-smokers, Another method is to have a 'No smoking' rule while working, but to provide a smoking room which can be visited in the rest periods.

So far in this chapter, the AL of breathing has been discussed in relation to the other three components of the model — lifespan, the dependence/independence continuum and the five factors influencing the ALs: physical, psychological, sociocultural, environmental and politicoeconomic factors. From the interaction of all these components, individuality in breathing develops.

INDIVIDUALITY IN BREATHING

The purpose of the model of living is to describe how a particular person develops individuality in the Activities of Living. The following is a résumé of topics which have mainly been concerned with the components of the model of living. These topics are relevant when considering a person's individuality in relation to the AL of breathing.

Lifespan: effect on breathing
- Age vis à vis rate of breathing
  pulse rate
  blood pressure

Dependence/independence in breathing
- Independence normal in health
- Dependence associated with ill-health

Factors influencing breathing
- Physical — characteristics of breathing (rate, depth, rhythm, sound)
  - level of activity
  - cough (if any)
  - smoking (habits if smoker; exposure to sidestream smoke if non-smoker)

- Psychological — dependence on tobacco
  - motivation to stop smoking } smokers
  - knowledge of and attitudes to smoking
  - effects of emotional status on breathing

- Sociocultural — safe expectoration

- Environmental — exposure to air pollution; at home at work
  - knowledge of and attitudes to air pollution

- Politicoeconomic — knowledge of and attitudes to air pollution prevention of smoking-related disease

Breathing: patients' problems and related nursing

Knowledge of a person's individual habits in the Activities of Living is the basis on which individualised nursing can be developed. Whereas some of the ALs are characterised by tremendous variation in individual habit, this is not so with breathing because it is primarily a physiological function which requires minimal conscious activity on the part of the person.

At the initial nursing assessment, people, if they are given the opportunity, can tell how they perceive any problem they have with this AL, and nurses can bear in mind the various topics noted in the preceding part of this chapter. If coughing is mentioned, the nurse can enquire when it occurs; whether or not it is productive of sputum; charac-

teristics of the sputum (p. 145); whether or not there is breathlessness; the relationship of breathlessness to exercise and so on. Certainly in all instances the person's age has an important bearing on the characteristics of breathing. For example mouth breathing in children can be indicative of enlarged adenoids which should alert the admitting nurse to the possibility of impaired hearing when assessing the AL of communicating, thus again demonstrating the relatedness of the ALs. If the patient is a smoker, then detailed information about smoking habits should be collected. This may be relevant in the context of understanding the patient's disease; and would be utilised in the context of health education concerning smoking; more will be said about this later in the chapter.

While assessing the AL of breathing the nurse would have some other questions in mind:

- does the individual breathe normally?
- what factors influence the individual's breathing?
- what knowledge does the individual have about breathing?
- has the individual experienced any difficulties with breathing in the past (or a longstanding breathing problem) and, if so, how have these been coped with?
- does the individual appear to have any problems (actual and/or potential) with breathing at present and are any likely to develop?

Other questions may be pertinent because in the model for nursing the AL of breathing is concerned not only with the respiratory system, but also with the cardiovascular system.

- has the individual ever been unduly conscious of the heart beating, probably faster, without an obvious cause such as circumstances causing fear or excitement?
- has the individual ever experienced more than transient cold in the extremities?
- has the individual experienced pain in the chest or legs on walking?

The objective in collecting this information is to discover the patient's usual habits in relation to the AL of breathing; whether there is any impediment to independence in breathing, remembering that cardiovascular problems can impede breathing; previous coping mechanisms in relation to breathing difficulties; and any current or incipient problems with breathing.

Of course, for patients admitted specifically for investigation or treatment (medical or surgical) of an actual breathing problem, in other words, when there is dysfunction of either of the body systems required for breathing (respiratory system and circulatory system), nursing assessment would require to be much more detailed as discussed by Boylan & Brown (1985) and Walker (1984). While observing, listening to what patients say and asking questions, nurses should bear in mind the patient's medical diagnosis and any information already obtained from the medical records or medical staff. However, it is not within the scope of this text to deal in any detail with specific disease processes or their medical treatment. That is not to imply that such knowledge is not necessary — for it is — and many nursing interventions for patients with breathing problems are the result of medical prescription; thinking about the proforma on page 57 should help students to differentiate between these and nurse-initiated interventions. Rather here, the intention is to provide only a general introduction to patients' problems with the AL of breathing and the related nursing, mainly for the benefit of the beginning student.

The healthy individual gives very little conscious thought to the vital, life-long activity of breathing. But when for whatever reason there is some interference with respiratory function, there is need for competent treatment of the cause. The cause may lie in the respiratory system itself, or in the circulatory system; or it could be excessive loss of blood (haemorrhage), resulting in 'air hunger'. Whatever it is, the interference may be sudden and dramatic calling for rapid emergency action and if the difficulty is more than transient, there is a need to provide support for a very anxious, distressed person. The feeling of suffocation and the inability to control such a vital function as breathing can be frightening. The person with less sensational respiratory difficulty must have equally competent, supportive care because a reduced capacity to breathe can disrupt the function of many other activities of everyday living; and if the incapacity is prolonged, may necessitate a considerable change in lifestyle.

A good nurse can help someone to 'breathe freely' or 'get his breath' in more senses than one, not least by caring for him in such a way that it restores or reinforces the way he sees himself as a worthwhile individual who is respected and valued by others.

Ashworth, 1979.

CHANGE OF ENVIRONMENT AND ROUTINE

When patients who have problems with the AL of breathing are to be nursed at home, there may have to be changes in the environment, for example, if possible it is better for all concerned if a single bed is used which is easily accessible from both sides. There may also have to be modification of the daily routine to accommodate for instance learning about the inhaling from nebulisers. This is a subject clearly described by Barnes (1988), and cleaning them efficiently is described by Barnes (1987).

However, the patient may have to be admitted to hospital. Irrespective of the individual's diagnosis, merely coming into hospital can alter the patient's normal breathing activity. The ward temperature may be so warm that the patient feels he is 'suffocating'; or the central heating may reduce the atmospheric water content causing irritation to the nose and mouth; or the odours peculiar to hospital may be unpleasant; or the strangeness of the surroundings may be so overwhelming as to produce the rapid, shallow breathing which often accompanies anxiety. And of course, the accompanying emotional upset can increase the pulse rate (Nursing Standard: Wall Chart, 1988).

Unless occupying a single room, patients may also have problems about smoking. If a heavy smoker, they may feel restricted and irritated by rules about limitations on indulging in this activity. If a non-smoker, they may abhor the enforced stay in an atmosphere of stale smoke or may be apprehensive about the fire hazards when fellow patients seem careless about extinguishing cigarettes.

Nurses must be alert to these circumstances and within the constraints of communal living attempt to accommodate the requirements of both smokers and non-smokers, as far as it is possible. The risk of fire in hospitals on account of smoking was mentioned in the context of maintaining a safe environment (p. 92), and nurses should be ever vigilant on this account.

Change of environment and routine which results in reduced exercise can contribute to the potential problems of deep vein thrombosis with possible consequent pulmonary embolism. It is relevant to mention them here, because these conditions pertain to the cardiopulmonary system, but there is further discussion on page 252 in the context of decreased mobilising related to possible nursing interventions.

CHANGE IN BREATHING HABIT

Many people erroneously believe that problems associated with breathing indicate only disorders of the lungs or upper airways. As mentioned earlier in the chapter, it can be deduced that any alteration to the cardiopulmonary sequence of events associated with respiration will have an effect on the individual's capacity to breathe and the patient may experience problems related to change in rate, rhythm and character of breathing.

Rate

Apart from atmospheric changes, the *rate* of respiration may be increased if there is:

- obstruction in any part of the respiratory tract such as a fragment or a swelling which narrows the lumen of respiratory passages
- loss of functioning tissue in the respiratory tract because of injury or disease
- defect in the intercostal muscles or diaphragm perhaps because of injury, or disease of the nerves serving those muscles as in poliomyelitis

- defect in the circulatory system such as impaired cardiac action which impedes circulation, or reduction in the size of the blood vessel lumen because of the deposit of fatty plaques as in atherosclerosis
- decrease in the number of red blood corpuscles as in haemorrhage, or reduced haemoglobin in the red blood corpuscles which occurs in iron deficiency anaemia

Usually these defects cause an increase in respiration rate as the body tries to make up for the O_2 deficit by breathing faster but in some instances such as head injury, brain tumours, or meningitis when the respiratory centre is depressed, the respiration rate is slower. A decrease is also associated with toxic conditions or with the intake of certain drugs (such as morphine) which depress the respiratory centre; indeed overdosage of morphine will cause respiratory arrest.

Rhythm
The *rhythm* involves the time interval between each respiration (which should be equal) and the depth of respiration. Usually deep slow breathing occurs when a patient is in coma, and shallow restrained breathing occurs in for example pleurisy when the patient is attempting to diminish the sharp stabbing pain caused by inflammation of the pleura. In a type of breathing known as Cheyne-Stokes breathing there is a marked and somewhat eerie change of rhythm found in a variety of conditions where the patient is critically ill. It begins slow, shallow and quiet, becomes deeper and noisier then dies away; and may be followed by a short period of apnoea (cessation of breathing), then the cycle recommences.

Character
The *character* of the patient's breathing may also be altered. Loud snoring or stertorous breathing is associated with brain injuries and alcoholism; a harsh grating sound called stridor occurs when there is obstruction of the larynx; a grunting note on expiration may occur in pneumonia; and wheezing is associated with asthma.

These are all subjective assessments and can be detected by the ear unaided, but by using a stethoscope various sounds can be identified which are indicative of the state of the lung tissue: constrictions, consolidation and the presence of excess mucus and fluid.

Moderate change in habit
There are various self-care remedies for mild forms of respiratory distress. Even a common cold causes discomfort when breathing because of congestion in the upper respiratory tract. Mortimer & Froud (1984) discuss the general nursing care of people who have this condition, together with the several other respiratory infections causing a moderate change in breathing. In addition the article puts these changes into a practical control of infection context.

Distress may be more marked in those who have asthma, and knowledge about its aetiology, treatment and control has increased in the last few years. There are 2.5 million sufferers in the UK (Barnes, 1988). The patient's problems are principally dyspnoea, wheezing and coughing. The article goes on to explain how asthmatic people can learn to manage their condition and describes the work of a nurse-run asthma clinic. Hek & Carswell (1986) report a small study conducted in three general practices in England; of the 86 children about whom data were gathered by questionnaire, 13 were newly diagnosed as having asthma. One recommendation was the appointment of a nurse to visit families at home and advise on individual management. Another article by Agius & Gregg (1984) discusses the role of the practice nurse in the management of asthma. There are illustrations of two different flow meters and a Nebuhaler, just one of the inhalers available, which can deliver drugs by inhalation so that they act more quickly, and can therefore be given in lower dose.

The writers describe how children need to learn how to use inhalers efficiently; and the nurse's role in assessment and treatment. In response to a report from the Royal College of Physicians (1981) — Disabling chest disease: prevention and care — Bagnall & Heslop (1987) describe the educational work which developed (after their appointment as Respiratory Health Workers) and its effects on the patients whom they visited at home. The Royal College of Physicians report (1981) estimated that 300 000 men of working age in the UK are potentials for invalidity pension because of dyspnoea from one cause or another, posing a considerable social and politicoeconomic burden.

A remedy which can be used at home to relieve upper respiratory infection is the steam inhalation to which menthol crystals may be added; it helps to loosen abnormal secretions in the respiratory tract and thereby eases breathing. A Nelson's inhaler may be used but an ordinary spouted domestic jug and towel serves the same purpose. Whether in home or hospital, care must be taken to ensure that steam inhalation equipment is handled carefully to prevent spillage and scalding, and to prevent irritation to the eyes. When use of steam is dangerous, specially designed apparatus such as a croupette (with canopy) or a croupaire (without canopy) may be used to humidify the atmosphere; they can be used continuously without the exertion of holding equipment and without the anxiety of scalding so are particularly useful for children who have respiratory problems, or for confused patients.

Marked change in habit
For the patient, severe difficulty with breathing (dyspnoea) is a distressing symptom which requires immediate attention. Though distressing it does in fact indicate that a

compensatory body mechanism is attempting to convey more O_2 to the cells. Every movement of the body uses up O_2 and produces CO_2 so it is obvious that everything should be done to spare the patient unnecessary activity. Lying flat, normally the most restful position, is however contraindicated as it further embarrasses breathing; when flat the abdominal organs slide against the inferior aspect of the diaphragm and inhibit its movement, and the rib cage also has limited expansion.

The patient must therefore sit up in a well-ventilated room and indeed often requests to be near an open window. In hospital, special beds may be available which help to maintain the sitting position and are often more comfortable for the patient and easier for the staff, but if these are not available, the nurse should be skilful in helping the patient to find a comfortable sitting position well supported by pillows. A bedtable with a pillow on which the patient may lean forward supported on the arms sometimes gives considerable relief and is restful. Many patients find it more comfortable however to sit well supported in an armchair and, at home, a person with chronic breathlessness usually prefers to do so. The inability to breathe except when in the sitting position is called orthopnoea.

Breathing is such a vital activity of daily living and marked difficulty causes patients great anxiety and distress so the nurse must adopt a quiet, calm manner when carrying out procedures and should anticipate their needs as much as possible.

There are occasions when the breathless patient cannot be lifted out of bed for bed-making, and changing a bottom sheet with the patient in the sitting position is more difficult than when lying flat so every move in the procedure should be planned beforehand so that the patient is spared unnecessary, oxygen-consuming exertion.

Because they are gasping for air, they are breathing through the mouth as well as the nose, and the mouth can become very dry so a drink in a covered container should be at hand, and should a reduced fluid intake be prescribed, a pleasantly flavoured mouthwash can be comforting. Milky drinks may have to be followed by oral hygiene if the mouth is to be kept clean and comfortable and cracked lips require an application of vaseline (p. 218).

Apart from the change in rate, rhythm and character of breathing associated with respiratory distress, other effects on total body functioning may cause the patient distress. Nervous tissue is particularly sensitive to oxygen deficit and the patient with respiratory problems may show signs of impaired brain function: headache, dizziness, drowsiness, restlessness, faulty judgement and disorientation. Nurses must therefore be on the alert for indications of abnormal behaviour and remember that such symptoms are often reversible if the O_2 supply is improved.

The patient's colour may also be altered. Cyanosis, a bluish tinge in the skin, the lips, the nail beds and in mucous membrane is indicative of respiratory distress. The muscular system too reacts to oxygen deficit and the person tires easily and feels exhausted on very slight exertion. People who are breathless require skilful nursing. Activities and relatively minor anxieties with which they would normally cope unaided assume abnormal importance when they are fighting for breath, and nurses must not be irritated by their frequent attempts to seek attention, and to seek reassurance of the presence of a nurse.

In an attempt to hasten the transport of available O_2 to O_2-deprived cells the heart beats faster to keep up with demand, so the pulse rate as well as the respiratory rate may be greatly increased during respiratory distress. If distress proceeds to imminent respiratory failure, it is a medical emergency and after ensuring that the airway is clear, mechanical ventilation must be instituted as described on page 144.

Another marked change in breathing habit is hyperventilation; it is characterised by rapid shallow breathing, chest pain, anxiety and a tingling sensation in the fingers and toes. It is associated with high anxiety and arousal states and the faulty breathing can change the blood pH to a level of alkalinity which can produce tetany. Early recognition and treatment is necessary to prevent this happening. Once diagnosed, a paper bag into which the patient breathes and re-breathes expired air usually relieves the symptoms. This simple method works because the inhaled air has a higher than normal level of carbon dioxide, and thus corrects the low level in the blood (Glover, 1986).

Change in pulse

The origin of the pulse beat arises in the heart and it is responsible for supplying an adequate amount of venous blood to the diffusing surface of the pulmonary alveoli. As has already been described, inhaled air exchanges 4% of its oxygen to this circulating blood, while at the same time 4% of the blood's carbonic acid which changes to carbon dioxide is diffused into it, to be exhaled. This is essential for maintenance of the blood pH within the normal range of 7.45 to 7.55 (Boylan & Brown, 1985). Some heart diseases can lessen the amount of blood reaching the pulmonary alveoli and can therefore interfere with this aspect of the blood pH regulating mechanism. Also the disadvantageous change in blood pH can occur at the 'internal breathing' sites in the body which involves the metabolic activity of each cell. It is not the objective of this text to deal with these complex phenomena, but the foregoing facts are merely mentioned to help the beginning student who is learning about the Roper, Logan and Tierney model for nursing to appreciate that the AL of breathing includes 'internal' as well as 'external' respiration involving the close functional relationship between the respiratory and cardiovascular systems.

Everyone's heart beats at a characteristic rate and this is transmitted via the arteries as the pulse. The pulse rate can be counted by gentle compression of an artery as it passes over a bone, the most usual site being the radial artery. Various medical conditions can lower the pulse rate to less than 60 beats per minute (bradycardia), although it has to be remembered that healthy athletes can achieve this lower rate after a period of intensive training. A decreasing pulse rate can be indicative of an increasing intracranial pressure and it is for this reason that patients suffering from cerebral conditions, including head injuries, require to have the pulse counted hourly or even half hourly. Drugs, however, may be prescribed to deliberately reduce the heart rate; digitalis preparations are taken to slow and strengthen the heart beat, but in order to prevent the drug reducing the rate too drastically, the pulse is checked regularly to ensure that it does not drop below 60 beats per minute in an adult.

Various medical conditions can raise the pulse rate and if it is over 100 beats per minute, the term tachycardia is used. It characterises such diverse conditions as cardiac failure, fever, haemorrhage, shock and thyrotoxicosis, when accurate pulse counting is essential to monitor the patients' response to treatment.

Change in blood pressure

The blood exerts pressure on the walls of the vessels in which it flows. In the living body, arteries are full of blood which causes a continuous stretch in their elastic walls. When the left ventricle contracts and discharges blood into an already full aorta, the increased pressure produced is known as systole. In the adult the systolic blood pressure is around 120 millimetres (mm) of mercury (Hg) that is, it supports a column of mercury in a sphygmomanometer 120 mm high.

When the heart is resting with no discharge of blood from the aorta the pressure within the blood vessels is termed diastolic pressure and is around 80 mmHg. Blood pressure is expressed therefore as $\frac{120}{80}$ mmHg.

A sphygmomanometer and stethoscope are required to assess the blood pressure, if the procedure is performed manually. The sphygmomanometer's inflatable cuff, acting as a tourniquet is used to compress the brachial artery until no pulse is discernible. As the inflated cuff gradually deflates, a stethoscope is placed over the bend of the elbow to detect the returning pulse.

The sounds were first described by Korotkoff and take his name. They consist of:

- phase 1 a clear tapping recorded as the systolic pressure
- phase 2 a softening of the sound
- phase 3 return of sharper sound
- phase 4 abrupt muffling — diastolic 4
- phase 5 disappearance of sound — diastolic 5

Traditionally in the UK, the muffling sound of diastolic 4 is recorded as the diastolic pressure. In the USA it is customary to record diastolic 5 as the diastolic pressure.

There is ample evidence (Thompson, 1981) of inaccurate measuring of blood pressure. Bell & Siklos (1984) report a small study of preoperative patients and recommend that baseline blood pressure measuring, and pulse counting should be carried out at the end of the initial assessment, rather than at the beginning of the admission procedure, when patients are likely to be more anxious.

Change in pulse and blood pressure in shock

Changes in both pulse and blood pressure are manifested in the condition of shock.

Basically shock is a state of circulatory failure. The average adult body contains about 6 litres of blood and if all the innumerable blood vessels were widely open simultaneously, there would be insufficient blood to fill them. The body functions with this relatively small volume of blood by controlling the muscle tissue in the walls of the small arteries (arterioles), thereby narrowing (vasoconstricting) or widening (vasodilating) the lumen. The control is very exact and normally it is a state of vasoconstriction. However, when the control is disturbed and the lumen of many arterioles are simultaneously vasodilated, the volume of blood is insufficient to maintain effective circulation and there is some degree of shock.

The most common causes of shock are the inhibition of vasoconstriction due to:

- loss of blood, as in haemorrhage
- loss of plasma, as in severe burns
- loss of electrolytes, as in continued vomiting and/or diarrhoea, and heat exhaustion
- alteration in permeability of blood vessel walls, as in injured tissue
- severe pain
- severe fright

When there is, for example, loss of blood or plasma, (sometimes called hypovolaemic shock) the reason for circulatory failure is more readily understood and expected because there is actual loss of circulatory volume and the treatment is intravenous infusion to replace the lost fluid (Herbert, 1984). But in instances of severe pain or severe fright there is no loss of fluid; shock (sometimes called neurogenic shock) is due to reduced vasoconstriction. It is just as important to expect and recognise the body's warning signals of neurogenic shock so that it can be effectively treated.

In shock, the body defences immediately try to compensate by permitting the vessels supplying blood to vital organs such as the brain, heart and kidneys to continue to do so, while the supply to muscles, skin and intestines is severely restricted. In a severe form of shock, the body temperature falls; the blood pressure falls; the pulse increases; the person complains of feeling cold; the skin is grey, cold and moist; and there is generalised prostration. If the cause of shock is treated satisfactorily, these adverse changes will be reversed but if not, the blood pressure falls further and death will ensue.

There is another type of shock produced by cardiopulmonary failure, sometimes called cardiogenic shock or cardiac arrest which requires special mention. Immediate treatment is essential as the brain is damaged when deprived of oxygen for as short a time as 3–5 minutes. It is estimated that every year in Britain 60 000, i.e., 60% of deaths from myocardial infarction (one cause of cardiogenic shock) occur before the patients reach hospital (Goodwin, 1988a). Goodwin lists various parts of the world where teaching about cardiopulmonary resuscitation was offered to citizens, together with the opportunity to acquire the necessary practical skills, after which there was a decrease in these preventable deaths.

A report from the Royal College of Physicians in 1987 states that an average of three patients in the UK die daily from cardiac arrest occurring in hospital, most of them in general wards where there is a need for nurses to provide Basic Life Support until the 'crash team' arrives, usually within 3–5 minutes (Wynne & Marteau, 1987). They report a study in London to assess the Basic Life Support skills which include clearing the airway, applying external cardiac compression, and mouth-to-mouth breathing. The project included 53 registered nurses who qualified at 43 different hospitals in the UK. None of them performed adequately, and 30 were assessed as completely ineffective. Other references testify to doctors' and nurses' inadequate skills for carrying out Basic Life Support.

Resuscitation techniques are continually undergoing re-evaluation as more research knowledge becomes available. The ABC sequence is now accepted as the best method. The mnemonic stands for Airway, Breathing and Compression. A flaccid tongue obstructing the airway is illustrated in Figure 8.1 and it is prevented by using the jaw lift or jaw thrust illustrated in Figure 8.2. For breathing, it is recommended that two ventilations (usually mouth-to-mouth) of 1–1½ seconds allowing for deflation between them, should be carried out initially, and then repeated after 15 external chest compressions, there being at least 80 compressions per minute (Newbold, 1987a). The Royal College of Nursing AIDS Working Party (1986) recommends that devices for cardiopulmonary resuscitation should be readily available to enable this procedure to be carried out without direct mouth-to-mouth contact. Advanced Life Support is usually carried out by a medical member of the 'crash team' and consists of tracheal intubation and attempts to restart the arrested heart (Newbold, 1987b).

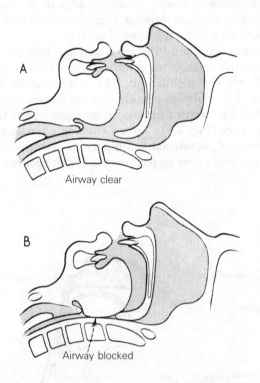

Fig. 8.1 Flaccid tongue and jaw muscles interfering with breathing

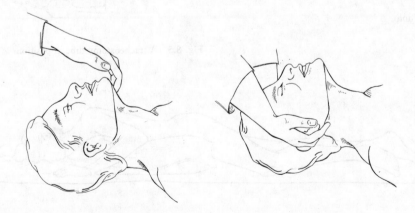

Fig. 8.2 Jaw lift, jaw thrust: the recommended method for preventing a flaccid tongue obstructing the airway

To finish this section about 'Change in breathing habit' it is important to raise some of the ethical issues which may need to be considered in relation to resuscitation. When, for example, the person is terminally ill, or in the older age group, or for some reason is suffering from irreversible brain damage, the case for resuscitation is sometimes raised; also, if it is unlikely that the person will survive without the aid of sophisticated life-support techniques such as prolonged mechanical ventilation. These instances can only be judged on individual criteria. The decision to commence resuscitation techniques and to discontinue them is usually made by a team of health professional staff, and often close relatives of the patient are involved in the decision.

CHANGE OF DEPENDENCE/INDEPENDENCE STATUS FOR BREATHING

Obstructed air passages

To maintain independence in the crucial activity of breathing, the most obvious need is the maintenance of a clear airway in the upper respiratory tract. To achieve this goal in some newborn babies, mucus, blood and amniotic fluid are removed from the respiratory tract. Conscious patients will cough to remove obstructions but those in an altered state of consciousness (p. 328) must be carefully observed as the cough reflex is depressed and it may be necessary to clear their air passages mechanically. In emergency situations nurses may have to do this with a finger, suitably protected against clenching of the teeth by for instance, wrapping with a wad of tissues. In a hospital setting, clearance may be achieved by using a catheter and suction to the mouth or nose, or by inserting an artificial airway into the throat in order to keep the tongue forward and the airway patent (Fig. 8.3). Patients in an altered state of consciousness (coma) should be kept in the semiprone position to facilitate drainage from the mouth and prevent accumulation in the pharynx (Fig. 8.4).

Obstruction due to excessive secretion may however be beyond the reach of an artificial airway or a catheter inserted via the mouth/nose, and a *tracheostomy* may be required. An incision is made into the trachea, and a tube inserted and secured in position by tapes tied at the back of the neck (Fig. 8.5). The air entering a tracheostomy is not warmed, moistened and filtered as normally occurs in the nose and upper respiratory tract so the patient is more

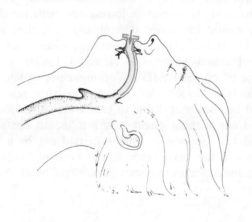

Fig. 8.3   An airway in position

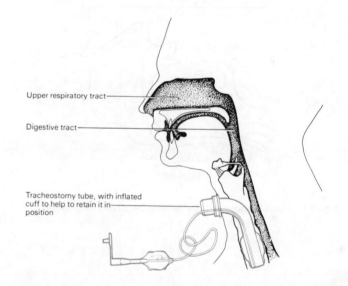

Upper respiratory tract

Digestive tract

Tracheostomy tube, with inflated cuff to help to retain it in position

Fig. 8.5   A tracheostomy tube in position

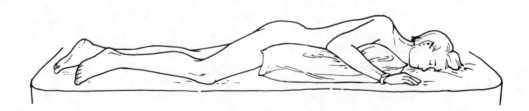

Fig. 8.4   Patient in semiprone position

liable to infection . The removal of secretions by suction is therefore performed using a sterile catheter and gloved hands and the inner cannula of the tube can be removed for cleansing and replaced by a sterile substitute cannula (de Carle, 1985; Allan, 1987; Allan, 1988). There is always a risk of mucosa damage; to minimise this the suction catheter should be less than half the diameter of the tracheostomy tube. The suction apparatus pressure gauge should be between 100 and 120 mmHg. Instillation of normal saline to moisten mucus has little or no value, but the administration of water vapour has been proven to be effective (Regan, 1988).

To conscious patients, tracheostomy suctioning can be a most alarming procedure and must be carefully explained, although when the use of a tracheostomy is a long-term measure, patients may eventually learn to carry out the suction themselvs. When they are in control of the situation they usually feel less dependent.

In the initial stages the patient may develop an irritation of the skin around the tracheostomy but a soothing keyhole dressing under the flange of the tube usually brings relief. The tapes holding the tube in position may cause distress and should be checked to ensure that they are sufficiently tightly tied to hold the tube securely without causing skin irritation. When soiled, the tapes should be changed not only for comfort but for prevention of infection, and the patient may be concerned about the appearance. It is not common but there are occasions when air gets into the tissues around the tube and it causes a rapidly spreading puffiness in the surrounding tissue which crackles when touched. The surgeon must be informed so that he can relieve the obstruction and ease the patient's discomfort and distress.

Usually the patient who has a tracheostomy will want to sit in an upright position and this is desirable because it lessens the danger of chest complications.

Reflecting the relatedness of the ALs, communicating is a problem when patients have a tracheostomy because they are unable to talk, so a pad and pencil should be provided to lessen the frustration which comes with this type of dependence and a handbell must be within hand reach so that they can summon help. Sometimes a light gauze dressing is placed over the opening of the tube and when patients are shown how to place a finger over the dressing, it is possible though difficult to speak.

Initially there may be difficulty with feeding and sometimes thickened fluids are easier to manage than thin liquids. Mouthwashes and mouth care are comforting and also help to prevent infection.

With the aid of a tracheostomy, excessive secretions which are reachable by insertion of a catheter can be removed but there may be secretions at a lower level in the respiratory tract, impeding the passage of O_2 from the alveoli to the capillaries. *Postural drainage* may be needed for this problem.

It is important in the first instance to teach deep breathing exercises. The patient is then helped into a position, depending on the site from which secretions must be drained, which will encourage the excess mucus and pus to move by gravity into contact with healthy tissue and initiate coughing. Postural drainage usually involves leaning over the side of the bed then coughing and spitting into a large receptacle placed on the floor which is suitably protected by a disposable paper sheet so the nurse must ensure privacy as this is a somewhat undignified position to adopt, and most people dislike coughing and spitting in public. The physiotherapist in these circumstances can be an important member of the health team and may assist with vibration and percussion movements over the affected lung area (Thompson, 1984), but the nurse usually has to assist the patient. The appearance and odour from the sputum may cause the patient distress and the receptacle should be removed as soon as possible.

The exertion involved in this technique of postural drainage usually leaves patients exhausted and the nurse must help them into a comfortable position in bed to recover, then provide facilities for sponging the face and hands and for rinsing the mouth. Despite the unpleasantness to the patient, postural drainage can bring quite dramatic relief especially in the morning after wakening: secretions gather during sleeping hours when there is relatively little change in body position.

Oxygen insufficiency
Oxygen insufficiency renders patients dependent, not only on the apparatus via which oxygen will be administred, but also on the medical staff for safe prescription and the laboratory staff for monitoring the blood gases and acid/base status. Patients depend on nurses having adequate knowledge and skills to us the apparatus so that maximum benefit is achieved without risk. They depend on nurses' sensitivity to their anxiety and nurses should offer patients every opportunity to retain as much independence and decision making as possible.

The apparatus via which oxygen can be administered is usually selected from a variety of facemasks, nasal cannulae, T-pieces which are used in conjunction with an endotracheal tube or a tracheostomy, and oxygen tents. Oxygen tents are now rarely used for adults, but in modified form such as incubators and head tents they are useful for babies and young children. Some of these types of apparatus are illustrated by McMillan (1984) and Jamieson et al (1988). The doctor's prescription will include the type of apparatus, the rate of flow and the duration of therapy. An introduction to the types of apparatus follows.

Facemasks. Modern facemasks are usually transparent and are made of plastic. Many of them are disposable which is a considerable contribution to prevention of infection. They fit over the nose and under the jaw and are anchored in this position by a strap attached to either side, passing along the cheeks and round the back of the head, so all these areas should be inspected for signs of any response to friction and/or pressure. Some air is breathed in (entrained) around these masks but with well fitting masks and a high flow of oxygen, an inspiratory concentration of 60% or more can be achieved (Boore et al, 1987). Masks are prescribed when oxygen is needed for a relatively short time and the lungs are not diseased. They are not suitable for people with chronic chest conditions because the respiratory centre has become less sensitive to carbon dioxide, but there are masks which have a small adjustable valve facilitating a more reliable percentage, and some masks can have several different valves fitted so that percentages of inspired oxygen from 24 to 60 can be achieved.

If it is a patient's first experience, the placing of a mask on the face of a person who is already breathless can be frightening and the nurse should remain until anxiety is at least diminished if not completely allayed. Patients need to be encouraged to control the rate and depth of respiration because, as noted in the previous paragraph, this contributes to the decreasing or increasing of the percentage of oxygen reaching the lungs for diffusion into the blood.

While the mask is in position, it is not possible for the patient to talk and this barrier to communication increases anxiety, so a bell or buzzer within reach with which to summon assistance is a physical nursing intervention allied to the goal of decreasing anxiety. Understandably, the mask must be removed for eating and drinking; however, in some instances oxygen has to be given via nasal cannulae during the meal. The mask should be dried and the patient provided with facilities to sponge the face before it is replaced. Because of the drying effects of increased oxygen intake, oral hygiene is necessary and nursing interventions for the prevention and treatment of cracked lips.

Nasal cannulae are less restricting than a face mask as, while in situ, they permit speech, eating and drinking. Also there is less facial perspiration but this type of apparatus can be just as frightening to the patient. The central part has two light plastic tubes which are inserted into each nostril. A tube on each side passes along the cheek and is supported on the top of each ear lobe and descends to form a Y-junction with the tube leading to the oxygen supply. They deliver 30–50% oxygen at a flow rate of 2–6 litres per minute (McMillan, 1984). Nasal toilet is essential because of the drying effect of oxygen in such close proximity to the mucosa. The potential problem of sore and painful nares is discussed in the next paragraph.

T-piece. In the presence of facial injury and/or surgery it is obvious that masks cannot be used, so a nasopharyngeal airway or endotracheal tube is left in situ and oxygen administered by attaching a T-piece. Use of the nasopharyngeal airway has the potential problem of sore and painful nares. Applying Vaseline, or putting Vaseline gauze around the tube may help; however it may be neces-

sary to spray the area with a local anaesthetic. When using an endotracheal tube, it is obvious that the natural humidifying function of the nasal mucosa is not available to the oxygen, so the use of a humidifier is essential, especially when oxygen at a greater than 40% concentration is given. There are three hazards — infection, overheating and condensation — all of which involve nursing responsibilities and particular observations. This applies when patients are receiving oxygen regardless of the apparatus (McMillan, 1984).

The oxygen supply may be piped to the ward or it may be stored in cylinders which stand at the bedside and cylinder changes should be effected outside the ward as the noise involved in changing a cylinder head can be acutely distressing to an already anxious patient.

Emergency O_2 equipment in the ward should be checked daily to be ready for use, and empty cylinders must be clearly marked and removed from the ward precinct as quickly as possible.

Any supply of oxygen presents a fire hazard. It is the nurse's responsibility to ensure that when oxygen is in use, a warning notice is placed on the cylinder and the dangers explained to the patient, to visitors and to fellow patients. Smoking is forbidden; mechanical toys, electric bells and heating pads are removed; bedmaking and hair combing should be done with care to avoid creating static electricity; and every member of staff should know how to use the nearest fire extinguisher and raise the fire alarm.

Some nurses, especially those unfamiliar with the equipment used for administering oxygen, humidifying it, or for managing assisted ventilation (which is the topic of the next section) express anxiety about the equipment. Most of it is in fact relatively straightforward to use if manufacturer's instructions are followed carefully, and opportunity for supervised practice following demonstration is provided. It is essential for nurses to know how to check that the equipment is functioning properly, how to clean it after use and, most importantly, how to minimise the patient's discomfort while it is in use. After all, the nurse's primary responsibility and concern are for the patient and not the machine, but that priority is only possible if the nurse feels familiar and confident with the equipment concerned.

Mechanical defects

Anything which interferes with the mechanics of breathing is going to cause problems for the patient. A defect in the respiratory muscles or the nerves supplying them means that the patient cannot breathe without mechanical assistance. Artificial ventilators can be divided into two groups; firstly, those operating on the principle of negative pressure on the outside of the chest (the traditional 'iron lung') which was used in the polio epidemic in the 1950s. Some of these original 'iron lungs' have been restored and are being used to patients' advantage in the respiratory unit in the UK (Campbell, 1984). A cuirass is an updated version working on the same principles. It encloses the chest, and an accompanying pump produces the negative pressure for inspiration, and elastic recoil causes expiration. Secondly there are ventilators which operate on the principle of positive pressure which forces air from a power-driven source into the lungs by means of a tracheostomy tube causing the chest and lungs to expand. The technical aspects of artificial ventilation are often bewildering, and caring for patients can appear daunting. But the nursing of ventilated people follows the same principles as care of the totally dependent person. Prevention of sensory monotony, orientation to time and place, maintenance of nutritional status, and prevention of pressure sores assume a high priority. Even if such patients cannot talk, nurses should continue to explain procedures, and to inform them of what is going on around them. After a period on the ventilator, full return to spontaneous breathing may take several days or weeks. Weaning from the respirator is usually determined by the patient, but for a few patients this is not possible. All such people need psychological help to come to terms with the many changes involving self-image and self-esteem (Milne, 1988).

Some of the people who require to be ventilated for life may be able to live at home, but many wide-ranging issues need consideration to make this possible (Corrigan, 1984). There are also some ventilation-dependent children; they suffer not only from lack of exercise, but they also experience frustration and boredom stemming from their total dependence on a machine. With some ingenuity, swimming and sunbathing have been used as effective therapies (Carter, 1988).

Patients who require artificial ventilation are highly dependent for the AL of breathing and they and their families require considerable emotional support.

As long ago as 1979, Ashworth's research indicated that of all types of, respiratory problems, the greatest difficulties were experienced by the patient whose breathing was being maintained artificially via a tracheal tube and who was also paralysed by drugs or the pathological condition which caused the respiratory failure. She wrote:

Speech and other forms of communication may be impossible except perhaps blinking of the eyelids and other small movements. It can be very frightening to be unable to indicate needs or feelings, and also very frustrating. To add to the problem, even experienced nurses may find it very difficult to go on talking to someone who appears unresponsive, who cannot talk, move, smile or perhaps open their eyes.

In a small study in five intensive care units it was found that there was a correlation between the amount of communication by the patient and by the nurse: the less the patient communicated, the less intentional communication there was by the nurse. An awareness of this should encourage nurses to seek to maintain communication (and to encourage relatives to do so too) even with apparently unresponsive patients, for the reason Ashworth gave:

To someone who is aware yet totally helpless and unable to control even his own breathing, it is essential to have people to talk to him by name about things which interest and concern him, if he is not to lose his sense of identity and to feel like 'just another body in a bed'.

SOME SPECIFIC PROBLEMS ASSOCIATED WITH BREATHING

Cough

Coughing can cause considerable distress to the patient, may interfere with many daily activities and may even prevent sleeping. If sputum is produced the patient should be helped to cough in order to remove the excess secretions and reduce the possibility of superimposed infection. Postoperatively, especially after thoracic and abdominal surgery, patients are encouraged to do deep breathing exercises and to cough for this very reason. They usually find it reassuring, if nurses 'splint' the surgical incision with their hands as patients often fear that the sutures will give way because of the muscular effort involved.

Coughing is a frequently encountered respiratory problem and is really a reflex protective mechanism used by the body to expel foreign material from the respiratory tract. There are various observations which nurses should make:

Character. A 'dry' cough has little expectoration; a 'loose' cough is associated with the production of sputum; a short restrained, suppressed cough accompanies pleurisy and pneumonia; there is a short, frequent, dry cough in early tuberculosis; a breathless, distressing cough is associated with cardiac conditions.

Duration and frequency. A cough is described as continuous in untreated pneumonia for example, and as spasmodic in asthma.

Time. With many disease conditions coughing is worse in the morning when the patient awakens and changes body position.

Effect on the patient. A cough can be irritating but shallow, or it may involve strenuous effort and leave the patient exhausted.

Expectorant drugs may be prescribed when a cough is productive of sputum, but when it is unproductive, irritating and preventing sleep, soothing cough syrup can be given to reduce discomfort and permit longer periods of rest.

Sputum

Sputum is usually the outcome of coughing. It is a secretion poured out from the irritated lining of the respiratory tract and consists mainly of mucus but if associated with an infection, pathogens will also be present.

Patients can be very distressed by the appearance of sputum and by having to spit in front of other people. If the amount is small, they may prefer to spit into a tissue which is folded and placed immediately into a disposal bag at the bedside. Otherwise they may use a disposable sputum mug which has the lid replaced when not in use.

There are several observations of the sputum which the nurse should make:

Quantity. The daily amount may have to be measured.

Consistency. In acute conditions sputum is sticky and tenacious; in long-term conditions it is often more fluid; if associated with infection it is purulent.

Colour. Sputum is usually greenish-yellow in the presence of pus; blood stained in mild tuberculosis and pneumonia.

Odour. Malodorous sputum is usually associated with infectious conditions such as abscess of the lung, bronchiectasis or pulmonary gangrene and large quantities of foul-smelling sputum are expectorated (it is this type of condition which often requires postural drainage). It is sometimes necessary to send a specimen of sputum to the laboratory for bacteriological investigation. It is therefore necessary for nurses to realise that sputum can contain pathogenic bacteria, and meticulous handwashing is essential to remove any transient flora which can include the opportunistic *Pneumocystis carinii*. Pneumonia caused by this organism is the main presenting disease seen in AIDS, and is by far the most frequent cause of death in persons with AIDS (Atkinson, 1989).

Haemoptysis

Coughing up blood is called haemoptysis and may vary in severity from mere streaking of the sputum, a common symptom in bronchitis, to a massive haemorrhage. Coughing up frank blood is alarming to the patient and to those in the vicinity, so the bed should be screened. The nurse should remain with patients and they should be helped into a comfortable position, which usually by choice will be sitting up supported by pillows. Unless massive and resulting in sudden death, the bleeding will stop provided the patient can rest quietly. Usually a sedative is ordered immediately, and the calming effect of the drug enables the patient to control the cough and to use it effectively instead of dissipating energies in useless coughing bouts which merely aggravate the bleeding. When nursing patients who are HIV seropositive or who have AIDS, linen soiled with blood must be placed in a water soluble plastic bag labelled with a hazard warning and then double bagged in accordance with local practice for the processing of infected linen. Blood may spill onto the floor or furniture and should be dealt with immediately using an appropriate chemical disinfectant for example, sodium hypochlorite (10 000 parts per million available chlorine) and disposable towels. Nurses should wear disposable plastic aprons and gloves during these procedures (Royal College of Nursing AIDS Working Party, 1986).

The patient's face and hands should be sponged and a mouthwash offered. Careful observation is subsequently required and restlessness may be an indication that a further episode will occur.

However small in amount, haemoptysis should be considered as potentially serious and should be reported to the nurse in charge or the doctor. Carcinoma of the lung and pulmonary tuberculosis are common causes of haemoptysis.

Allergy

Allergy can cause discomfort in breathing. Substances in the atmosphere which have no obvious adverse effect on most people can cause acute discomfort to those who are allergic. Attacks of sneezing with profuse watery nasal discharge, nasal obstruction and watering of the eyes are associated for example with the condition known as hayfever, which is probably an antigen-antibody reaction. The usual antigen is pollen from grasses, flowers, weeds and trees and as grass pollen is the most common cause in the UK, the disorder is at its peak during May to July. de Mont (1985) states that 8 million people in Britain seek treatment for seasonal allergic rhinitis (hay fever) each year. Alderman (1988) describes its causes, effects and treatments. Allergies may however also be due to odours or fumes or sudden changes in temperature. The episode usually lasts for a few hours and can be controlled by drugs such as decongestants and antihistamines although often a complete cure cannot be found. Allergies are an inconvenience rather than a disease but can be disrupting to social life and to domestic/work activities.

Palpitation

While collecting information about the AL of breathing, the patient may report being conscious of a rapid, forceful beating of the heart. Listening carefully to the patient, the nurse may discover that it only occurs after exercise, or when lying down. If it occurs in other conditions, ascertainment of whether or not it is regular or irregular has relevance to the medical diagnosis and the information should be shared with the doctor. In the first two instances mentioned, though it is disconcerting, it is not usually indicative of disease.

Choking

It is very discomforting when food 'goes the wrong way'. Most people experience this phenomenon at some time in their lifespan. It usually results in a bout of coughing accompanied by excessive watering of the eyes. Should the face become livid, immediate action is necessary to dislodge the foreign body. The choking person will probably be standing to maximise contraction of the abdominal muscles in order to produce effective coughing. The helper stands behind the person; puts one hand as a clenched fist on the person's abdomen so that the midline of its lower border is just above the umbilicus; covers the 'fist' with the other hand; applies pressure with both these positioned

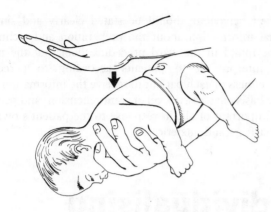

Fig. 8.6 Back blows for removal of foreign body in small children

hands and directs it upwards to dislodge the obstruction. It is a frightening experience and the person may be best comforted by touch such as holding the hand until the breath has been regained and the person can talk comfortably.

In the case of choking in small children, a finger sweep of the mouth may cause sufficient retching to dislodge the 'foreign object'. If this fails, the adult should sit on a chair, put the knees lower then the hips, place the child face down on the downward sloping thighs. The child's upper chest and lower neck should be supported by one hand while the other hand should apply back blows (Fig. 8.6).

Pain
The main discussion about pain is in the chapter on communicating (p. 121). In this chapter it will be discussed as a manifestation in the cardiopulmonary system required for the AL of breathing. Given that pain in any part of the body may cause alterations in the normal breathing pattern, pain in relation to the respiratory tract itself is of two main types:

a. pain made worse by coughing and experienced behind the sternum — the type of pain associated with inflammation of the trachea
b. sharp, stabbing pain made worse by deep breathing and coughing and caused by inflammation of the pleura

Note should be made of the site, onset, duration, and intensity and any precipitating factors. As with pain of any kind every attempt should be made to remove the cause or minimise the effect and if these measures are unsuccessful, to help the patient to cope with pain. In many instances, assisting the person into a comfortable position will help and someone with pleuritic pain will usually lie on the affected side. If an unproductive cough is the cause, soothing cough syrup may alleviate the discomfort and if antibiotics are prescribed for an inflammatory condition they will counteract the infection and therefore relieve the pain-producing inflammation.

There are instances when chest pain which affects the activity of breathing is really cardiac pain sometimes referred to as angina; the site is characteristically behind the sternum or across the chest. It is usually described as being crushing in character and there may be radiation down one or both arms or even into the neck and shoulders or through to the back. The patient can become profoundly shocked and cardiac arrest may occur and it requires immediate treatment (p. 141). This type of pain is also a feature of myocardial infarction (p. 141) and it must be relieved so that the shocked state may be reversed. A number of patients with this condition are admitted to intensive coronary care units which have highly specialised health teams skilled in emergency treatment.

Rehabilitation of patients with heart disease, particularly myocardial infarction and cardiac surgery, is crucial if patients are to regain their confidence and return to optimal functioning in the community. It is now well recognised that the physical effects of heart disease are influenced by both psychological and social well-being. Consequently education and emotional support for both patient and family increase the chance of a full recovery. They need information about, and sometimes practice at, such activities as exercise, relaxation, stress management, safe drug taking, a healthy diet, alcohol intake and of course help with stopping smoking and losing weight if appropriate.

Prevention of coronary heart disease is indeed better than cure. There is a 'heart chart' to assess a person's risk of developing coronary heart disease. For each of the following criteria — family history, blood pressure, lung expansion, smoking, fat in diet, weight, alcohol, stress, exercise, aerobic fitness (step test) — there is a numerical allocation of 0 to 4. The higher the score the greater the risk (Deans & Hoskins, 1987). Permission is given for photocopying the chart and it is suggested that health visitors, occupational health nurses and practice nurses are particularly well placed to use the charts. However, all nurses should bear it in mind when assessinng patients.

Deep vein thrombosis usually produces pain in the calf muscles, although it can also be a painless condition. It is a potential problem which can become an actual one in women who take oral contraceptives for a prolonged period. Deep vein thrombosis is also a potential problem postoperatively; almost all postoperative thromboses begin during, or within 72 hours of operation. Different preventive routines are used such as compression stockings worn for 5 days, calf compression during operation, and injections of low-dose heparin for 5 days (Smith, 1985). As a routine preventive measure, all patients who are having less exercise than usual should be encouraged to breathe deeply and exercise the feet several times daily. It is customary in some hospitals for the physiotherapist to initiate this preventive activity, but it is necessary for nurses to encourage its continuance at intervals during the day.

The calf muscles can also be the site of ischaemic pain because atheromatous plaques in the arteries supplying the lower limbs are preventing the flow of an adequate blood supply. However, if the person is mobilising and experiences such pain, pausing for a minute or so permits the person to walk a little further. Smoking should be discouraged because the chemicals in smoke are considered to reduce the efficiency of blood supply to the calf muscles. After examination of the blood there may be a prescription for medication to lower the blood cholesterol; and there may also be dietary modification to assist in lowering the blood cholesterol. Encouragement is usually necessary to help these people to persevere with walking as it helps in the development of collateral circulation. Obese people will be advised to reduce their intake of calories (Kilojoules).

Local pain arising in the medial aspect of the lower legs can also be caused by superficial ulcers which are a manifestation of impairment in the cardiovascular system. Severe pain is more frequent in arterial ulcers — those secondary to arterial insufficiency — but they are only responsible for 8–10% of all leg ulcers (Smith, 1988): they have a less favourable prognosis than venous ulcers which are estimated to comprise 75% of leg ulcers. The new types of wound dressings have improved the healing of all types of leg ulcer (Morgan, 1987).

Intravenous infusions and blood transfusions are frequent forms of treatment and they may cause problems which manifest in pain. The most common problems are extravasation of fluid into the tissues and phlebitis (Jamieson et al, 1988). When phlebitis develops there is a potential problem of thrombus formation; the thrombus can become an embolus which commonly lodges in the lungs when the condition is called pulmonary embolism (Speechley & Toovey, 1987). The pain from pulmonary embolism is of the pleuritic type (p. 147).

Anxiety about investigations
Sometimes investigations which are carried out to assess dysfunction in the respiratory system cause discomfort or pain. Probably the most commonly used investigative technique is X-ray which is not in itself painful, although it may cause discomfort if performed in conjunction with the introduction of an opaque dye to outline the bronchi and bronchioles, a bronchogram. Respiratory function tests are sometimes prescribed and they may cause discomfort. A bronchoscopy on the other hand, may be painful and can be alarming; a tube is passed into the upper respiratory tract and the tissue lining can be viewed by means of a lens in the eyepiece (Twohig, 1984; Allan, 1987). In all these procedures, the patient will have some anxiety about what he will be expected to do, how he will react and what the result will be.

The nurse must take time to explain any preparation involved prior to the procedure, and what to expect during and after. Any relevant instructions about the patient's expected behaviour should be stated clearly and simply. Factual information about the preparation and technique will be found in the ward procedure book but the nurse must interpret it to patients according to perceived preparedness of each patient to receive the information; and on the basis of assessed level of comprehension; and perhaps most important of all, in response to the patient's own expressed fears and anxieties.

Individualising nursing

To individualise nursing, nurses need to know about the person's individuality in living which is discussed in the first half of this chapter. While describing the model for nursing, general information was given about individualising nursing (p. 51) which in fact is synonymous with the concept of the process of nursing. The assessment would be achieved by various means such as observing the person, acquiring information about usual habits, partly by asking appropriate questions; partly by listening to the person and/or relatives; and partly by using relevant information from available records, including medical ones. The collected information could then be examined to identify any actual problems being experienced with regard to breathing and these could be arranged in an order of priority. The nurse might also recognise some potential problems — not all possible potential but those which are relevant. Mutually agreed realistic goals could then be set to prevent potential problems from becoming actual ones; to alleviate or solve the actual problems; or to help the person cope with those which cannot be alleviated or solved.

Keeping in mind what the person can and cannot do unaided, the nursing interventions to achieve the mutually set goals could then be selected according to local circumstances and available resources.

Following implementation of the interventions, their effect could be evaluated in relation to the set goals, and if goals were not reached, they would then be revised or rescheduled, or even discarded. It is worth repeating that although discussed in four phases — assessing. planning, implementing and evaluating — individualising nursing is not a linear progression; it assumes a build-in responsiveness to feedback at any of the phases, with ample allowance for change within the overall framework.

During an illness episode, an important consideration is rehabilitation of the individual, and planning for this could commence almost as soon as the person enters the health system. Another important feature is the professional judgement needed to discontinue the nurse/patient relationship when it is no longer relevant.

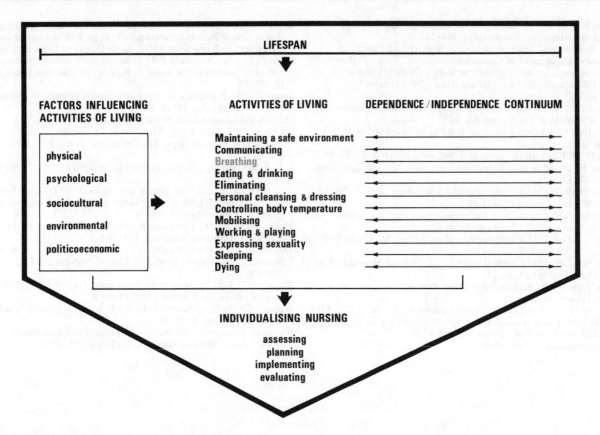

LIFESPAN

FACTORS INFLUENCING ACTIVITIES OF LIVING

physical

psychological

sociocultural

environmental

politicoeconomic

ACTIVITIES OF LIVING

Maintaining a safe environment
Communicating
Breathing
Eating & drinking
Eliminating
Personal cleansing & dressing
Controlling body temperature
Mobilising
Working & playing
Expressing sexuality
Sleeping
Dying

DEPENDENCE/INDEPENDENCE CONTINUUM

INDIVIDUALISING NURSING

assessing
planning
implementing
evaluating

Fig. 8.7 The AL of breathing within the model for nursing

This chapter has been concerned with the AL of breathing. However, as stated previously it is only for the purpose of discussion that any AL can be considered on its own; in reality the various activities are so closely related and do not have distinct boundaries. Figure 8.7 is a reminder that the AL of breathing is related to the other ALs and also to the various components of the model for nursing.

REFERENCES

Agius L, Gregg I 1984 The role of the practice nurse in the management of asthma. Nursing: The Add-On Journal of Clinical Nursing 2 (28) August: 815–819

Alderman C 1988 Not to be sneezed at. Nursing Standard 2 (30) April 30: 37

Alimo A, Hannah D 1987 Rehabilitating heart patients. Nursing Times 83 (14) April 8: 40–42

Allan D 1987 Tracheostomy. Nursing Times 83 (45) November 11: 36–38

Allan D 1988 Suctioning. Nursing Times 84 (10) March 9: 46–47

ASH (Action on smoking and health) 1986 Women and smoking. Scottish Health Education Group, Health Education Centre, Woodburn House, Canaan Lane, Edinburgh EH10 6SG

Ashworth P 1979 Psychological and social aspects of respiratory care. Nursing 1st Series (7) November: 295–299

Bagnall P, Heslop A 1987 Chronic respiratory disease: educating patients at home. The Professional Nurse 2 (9) June: 293–296

Barnes K, Clifford R, Holgate S T 1987 Bacterial contamination of home nebulisers. British Medical Journal 295: 812

Barnes G 1988 Asthma: latest developments in care. The Professional Nurse 3 (9) June: 364–366, 368

Bell M, Siklos P 1984 Recording blood pressure: accuracy of staff and equipment. Nursing Times 80 (26) July 4: 32–34

Boore et al (eds) 1987 Nursing the physically ill adult. Churchill Livingstone, Edinburgh, p 782

Boylan A, Brown P 1985 Respiration: observations. Nursing Times 81 (11) March 13: 35–38

Campbell D 1984 An inspired tale of the old iron lung. Nursing Mirror 159 (15) October 24: 32–36

Carter B 1988 Simple (Chronically ventilated children). Nursing Times 84 (13) March 30: 38

Corrigan A 1984 Home ventilation. The Add-On Journal of Clinical Nursing 2 (28) August: 840

Deans W, Hoskins R 1987 Preventing coronary heart disease. The Professional Nurse 2 (10): July 328–329

De Carle B 1985 Tracheostomy care. Nursing Times 81 (40) October 2: 50–54 Occasional Paper 81 (6)

de Mont A 1985 Summer fever. Nursing Times 81 (24) June 12: Community Outlook: 20–30

Draper P 1987 Taking blood pressure. Nursing Times 83 (10) March 11: 58–59, 62

Durie M 1984 Respiratory problems and nursing intervention. Nursing: The Add-On Journal of Clinical Nursing 2 (28) August: 826–828

Glover A 1986 Hyperventilation. Nursing Times 82 (49) December 3: 54–55

Goodwin R 1988a Cardiopulmonary resuscitation. Nursing Times 84 (34) August 24: 63, 65–68

Goodwin R 1988b Cardiopulmonary resuscitation in children. Nursing Times 84 (35) August 31: 48–51

Hek G, Carswell F 1986 Asthma: anxiety attacks. Nursing Times 82 (29) July 16: Community Outlook: 23–24

Herbert R 1984 Maintaining the circulating volume. Nursing: The Add-On Journal of Clinical Nursing 2 (26) June: 766–768

Jamieson E M et al 1988 Guidelines for clinical nursing practices. Churchill Livingstone, Edinburgh, p 104–117

Jenkins M et al 1987 Smoking policies at work (Heath Education Authority) Department of Community Medicine, King's College School of Medicine and Dentistry of King's College, London

Lim D 1982 Clearing the air. Nursing Times 78(6) February 10: 256–257

McMillan E 1984 Oxygen therapy. Nursing: The Add-On Journal of Clinical Nursing 2 (28) August: 822–825

Milne C 1988 Care of the patient on ventilation. Nursing Standard 2 (17) January 3-0: 26–27

Morgan D 1987 Leg ulcers. Nursing Times 83 (12) March 25: 53–54

Mortimer B, Froud A 1984 Respiratory infections. Nursing 2nd Series 28: 831–835

Newbold D 1987a Critical care: external chest compression — the new skills. Nursing Times 83 (26) July 1: 41–43

Newbold S 1987b Critical care: the physiology of cardiac massage. Nursing Times 83 (25) June 24: 59–60, 62

Nursing Standard 1988 Finger on the pulse. Nursing Standard (Wall chart) 2 (47) August 27: 22–23

Nursing Standard 1987 Common arrhythmias. Nursing Standard (Wall chart) 4 (2) October 24: 24–25

Nursing Times 1989 Child smoking: nurses must act. Nursing Times 85 (3) January 18: 8

Pownall M 1987 A killer cloud. Nursing Times 83 (16) April 22: 18–19

Regan M 1988 Tracheal mucosal injury — the nurse's role. Nursing: The Add-On Journal of Clinical Nursing 3 (29) August/September: 1064–1066

Royal College of Nursing 1986 Second report of the RCN Working Party. Nursing guidelines on the management of patients in hospital and the community suffering from AIDS. Royal College of Nursing, London

Royal College of Physicians 1981 Disabling chest disease: prevention and care. Journal of the Royal College of Physicians of London 15 (2): 69–87

Smith K 1985 Preventing postoperative venous thrombosis. Nursing Mirror 160 (20) May 15: 29–30

Smith S 1988 Doing the legwork. Community Outlook: 17–18

Speechley C, Toovey J 1987 Problems in IV therapy.
1. The flow slows or stops. The Professional Nurse 2 (8) May: 240–241.
2. Inflammation, pyrexia, tachycardia and rigors. 2 (12) September: 413
3. Oedema, tachycardia, itching and faintness. 3 (3) December: 90–91

Stewart A, Orme J 1988 Why do adolescents smoke? The Professional Nurse 4(2) November: 81, 84–86

Thompson D R 1981 Recording patients' blood pressure: a review. Journal of Advanced Nursing 6: 283–290

Thompson M C 1984 Physiotherapy — essentials of chest care. Nursing: The Add-On Journal of Clinical Nursing 2 (27) July: 796, 798–800

Twohig R G 1984 Respiratory function tests. Nursing: The Add-On Journal of Clinical Nursing 2 (927) July: 807–810

Walker M 1984 Observation in the newly admitted patient. Nursing Times 80 (26) July 4: 29–32

Wynne G, Marteau T 1987 Race against time (Cardiopulmonary resuscitation). Nursing Times 83 (30) July 29: 16–17

9

Eating and drinking

The activities of eating and drinking
The nature of eating and drinking
Lifespan: effect on eating and drinking
Dependence/independence in eating and drinking
Factors influencing eating and drinking
Individuality in eating and drinking

Eating and drinking: patients' problems and related nursing
Change of environment and routine
   Timing of meals
   Serving of meals
   Alteration in appetite
   Hospital meals
   Pre- and post-meal activities
   Children in hospital
Change in eating and drinking habit
   Modification of habitual food intake
   Modification of habitual fluid intake
Change in mode of eating and drinking
   Nasogastric feeding
   Gastrostomy feeding
   Intravenous feeding
Change of dependence/independence status
   Problems associated with physical dependence
   Problems associated with emotional/psychological dependence
Some specific problems associated with eating and drinking

Individualising nursing

References

The activities of eating and drinking

Human life cannot exist without eating and drinking, such is the essential nature of this activity. It takes up a considerable part of each day since apart from the time involved in eating of meal, food has to be procured and prepared; indeed in some instances it has to be grown by the individual family. In most cultures it is the women who select, buy and cook the family's food. However in many industrialised societies, with the movement towards a greater sharing of parental and domestic activities, this is beginning to change and men are playing a much more active part in matters related to food and feeding.

THE NATURE OF EATING AND DRINKING

The human body is a highly complex collection of millions of cells. The cycle of each cells's growth and development as well as the constant cell activity requires an energy source, and the source of all energy used by the body is obtained from eating and drinking. At subsistence level, human beings will eat almost any available food, often in its raw state, in order to meet the basic need for sustenance. In more affluent societies however, it is possible to make a choice about what will be eaten; there probably will be a mix of cooked dishes and food in its natural state; and quite elaborate rituals may be associated with the setting, the utensils used, the presentation of the meal, and the choice of accompanying drinks.

Nearly all solid food has a high water content but as most of the body consists of water, an additional intake of fluid is essential to continued human existence. Actually the newborn baby's diet is entirely fluid, mainly in the form of milk or water but as children get older, they quickly learn that fluid intake can consist of a wide variety of beverages.

Human milk of course is the natural food for infants, and the sucking reflex is present at birth. As the baby grows, milk on its own does not supply enough nutrients to satisfy appetite so semi-solid and solid foods are introduced to the diet; and the child becomes proficient in chewing as the teeth appear. The sense of taste is developed too: milk is somewhat bland in flavour and as solids are added, the child learns to experiment with a variety of tastes. Nevertheless even in the same family, there are individual differences related to food and drink; there may be large appetites and some small, some may be quick eaters, some may be slow. Even at a young age, each individual is consciously aware of this essential AL of eating and drinking; indeed throughout life, the waking day is punctuated by meals — breakfast, lunch, supper or some variation of these words — and many other Activities of Living are arranged around them.

Fluids and nutrients are necessary to facilitate multiplication of body cells until adult stature is reached. Thereafter, throughout all stages of the lifespan, the intake of fluids and nutrients replenishes the substances needed in all the cells to maintain an adequately functioning body, as well as to provide the energy for all the day to day activities. The study of food and the associated biological processes of growth, maintenance and repair is known as the science of nutrition and an outline of this subject is given on page 155.

Providing nutrients is the biological reason but eating and drinking also serve several other purposes in everyday living. During family mealtimes, for example, eating plays an important part in learning about the culture. The meal provides an opportunity for the young child to learn about the rituals of serving food, about the vessels from which different foods are eaten, and about the utensils used for certain items in the diet.

As children explore relationships with people both within and outside the family circle, they began to appreciate that food can have considerable social significance concerned with interpersonal relationships. In almost all cultures, eating and drinking are considered social occasions and offering a meal to visitors is one overt way of expressing friendship and hospitality. Eating and drinking in most societies are also an integral part of such diverse family ceremonies as birth, marriage and death; and of some national holiday festivities and religious festivals.

It is not surprising therefore that deep-rooted beliefs and attitudes are associated with the AL of eating and drinking.

LIFESPAN: EFFECT ON EATING AND DRINKING

It is not difficult to appreciate that the activity of eating and drinking will vary according to the individual's stage on the lifespan. The close relationship of the lifespan and the dependence/independence component is integral to the model, and this is certainly so for the AL of eating and drinking particularly for the very young, and in some instances at the other end of the age spectrum for the elderly.

The AL commences in utero. The physical growth and development of the fetus are dependent on nutrition received from the mother via the umbilical cord, so the quality and quantity of the maternal diet is important throughout pregnancy and features highly in health education during the prenatal period. The goal of health education is to enable pregnant women to make the best choices under the circumstances, particularly if they are adverse, and these may be as varied as inadequate food supply to the geographical area, or an inadequate financial income to buy the recommended diet.

Currently, if the mother has decided to breast-feed, it is customary to put the newborn infant to the breast almost immediately after delivery, or within 24 h (Fisher & Minns, 1986). In the infant stage of the lifespan, breast milk provides protection against infection and allergy, as well as nutrition for the baby in the form most suited to human infants. Provided the mother is taking a reasonable diet, the constituents of breast milk are present in the correct ratio for the human infant's digestive system; and the milk is sterile, at the correct temperature, available without elaborate preparation and is cheaper than formula milk (Francis, 1984). The intimacy of breast feeding is known to induce a special relationship between mother and baby, called 'bonding'.

Despite the acknowledged superiority of breast milk, the practice of breastfeeding is declining in the UK. In 1980, 74% of first-time mothers started breastfeeding their babies, but this had fallen to 69% in 1985, and of these, only 51% continued for 2 weeks, and only 26% for 4 months or more (Smith, 1988). Martin & White (1988), also using data collected in 1985, show another worrying reduction in breastfeeding among a specific group of mothers (often teenagers) who do not have partners. Only 44% of this group attempted to breast-feed compared to 52% in 1980. DHSS guidelines on infant feeding recommend that women should be encouraged to breast-feed for up to 1 year.

Regarding breastfeeding and women who are HIV seropositive, the DHSS's guidelines have been criticised for their 'dangerously excessive caution' (Feinmann, 1988). There are only four known cases of transmission of HIV infection via breast milk and Feinmann's article states that 'Two took place in Zaire, and in all cases the mother was infected by a postnatal blood transfusion'. Epidemiologists consider that the risk is small and that in the present state of uncertainty, breastfeeding should be actively encouraged.

The decreasing number of breastfeeding women already mentioned is not confined to the UK; it is prevalent in many countries throughout the world, and is accompanied by an increase in the number of babies who are bottle fed. Intensive marketing and advertising of 'breast milk substitutes' are known to be a contributing factor to the undesirable changes. In 1981 the World Health Organization issued an International Code of Practice on the marketing of 'breast milk substitutes' mainly for commercial firms, but it also recommended that health professionals should refrain from offering samples of these formulae (provided by sales representatives) to new mothers, or advertising them in any way, for example in maternity hospitals and clinics (Renn, 1987).

For a variety of reasons, however, bottle feeding may be the method of choice. In these circumstances, dried milk preparations are frequently used. It is most important that the amount is carefully calculated using the measuring spoon provided in the packet, and the prescribed measure of liquid (Jeff, 1989). Otherwise the baby may develop an electrolyte imbalance which can lead to a dramatic disruption of physiological processes. To prevent infection the bottle and teat are scrupulously cleaned and then sterilised between feeds, usually by immersion in a hypochlorite solution, which is discarded and replaced daily (Devlin, 1984). Close bodily contact between mother and baby during feeding enhances the 'togetherness' part of bonding.

As the infant grows, milk is no longer adequate for nutritional requirements and the process of weaning from breast or bottle-feeding begins. Semisolid foodstuffs, usually cereals, possibly fortified with minerals and vitamins, are offered on a spoon. Babies therefore have to develop a different eating skill; instead of sucking they have to cope with food on a spoon and manipulate the semisolid in the mouth before swallowing. Not surprisingly there is initial awkwardness and time must be given for experimentation.

Eventually infants begin to handle the spoon themselves and lift the food to the mouth. They experiment with gripping and controlling the spoon and tracing the spatial pathway from plate to mouth. The resultant 'messiness' is inevitable but patience and the presence of a warm supporting mother or mother substitute permit acquisition of the necessary dexterity. Gradually, solid foods are introduced into the diet and eventually the majority of children become independent in the necessary skills for eating and drinking. However, a minority of people have physical disabilities which prevent them from acquiring independence as they progress along the lifespan. More will be said about this later.

But what should children be eating? In the last 20 years, several research reports have associated a high fat intake, particularly saturated (animal) fats, with coronary heart disease. Consequently some nutritionists recommended that from an early age, children should be given a diet low in animal (saturated) fat; others believed that this is inappropriate as milk fat makes an important contribution to a child's available energy as well as supplying vitamins and trace elements (Holmes, 1987). The DHSS report (1988) should allay confusion; it recommends that skimmed milk should not be given to children under 2 years, but 2-year-olds can be given semi-skimmed milk, and 5-year-olds may be given skimmed milk.

Other general recommendations were for decreased salt and sugar, and increased fibre in the diet (of adults). There was concern that this dietary advice could be inappropriately applied to the under-5-year-olds. The British Dietetic Association reviewed the relevant literature and made recommendations, an important one being — energy requirements are dependent on age, gender and physical activity and must be met for each individual child to promote optimal growth (Holmes, 1987).

In the early 1980s a government-sponsored survey investigated the diets of British school children. A representative sample of 3285 children in two age groups — 10–11 and 14–15 years old — kept a diary of all food and fluid taken over a period of 7 days. Analysis of the data revealed a preponderance of biscuits, cakes, crisps, chips, soft drinks, sweets, sugar and white bread which were not indicative of a healthy diet (Walker, 1986). Cereal and toast were the most common breakfast foods, although some children went to school without having eaten any breakfast. In many families the characteristic family meal has tended to disappear and has been replaced by a 'grazing type of eating pattern' with a heavy dependence on convenience, processed and 'fast' foods (Dickerson, 1988). Although much is said and written about a healthy diet, there is no room for complacency, and nurses, as health educators, can help children to make wise food choices.

Throughout adolescence many people are physically active, expending a great deal of energy. Consequently the appetites of adolescents tend to be large and in the Western world seem to be satiated by high energy snacks rather than traditional meals. Many young people live away from home for the first time, and they become independent for providing their own diet. Some experiment with changing to, for example, a vegetarian diet. But in the interests of health, all should try to follow the main recommendations from the National Advisory Committee on Nutritional Education (NACNE, 1983) and the Committee on Medical Aspect of Food Policy (COMA, 1984). These are to eat sufficient food to maintain optimal weight for height, and to take adequate exercise. A decrease in salt and sugar intake is recommended. Dietary fat should provide a maximum of one-third of the total daily energy intake; and only one-third of this should be saturated (animal) fat and the rest should be made up of polyunsaturated fat. Alcohol should comprise no more than 4% of daily energy intake. And, of course, dietary fibre should be increased by eating wholegrain cereals, pulses, fruit and vegetables (Holmes, 1988a).

The variation in food and drink preferred by adults is legion and the variety becomes more obvious when there is a multiracial society. The two reports previously mentioned in the context of adolescents, were originally recommended to promote healthier eating practices in the adult population, and they should be continued throughout life. The prime objective of the reports was to prevent coronary heart disease (p. 153) but there are other diet-related diseases — diverticulosis, obesity, dental caries and periodontal disease. It is important in adult years to take sufficient exercise, because the increased metabolism is beneficial to the cardiovascular system in particular.

Going to the end of the lifespan the elderly person often has less appetite for food; there is usually less physical activity so there is not the same requirement for the energy-giving foodstuffs. There may also be less interest in cooking and preparing a meal for one, if the person is living alone, and hastily prepared snacks often do not provide the necessary vitamins, minerals. Deficiency of vitamins D and C, thiamine and folic acid are common in elderly persons admitted to hospital (Dickerson, 1986a). The most frequently occurring manifestations of malnutrition are severe weight loss and cachexia, iron deficiency anaemia, folate deficiency, scurvy, and osteomalacia. A less severe form of malnutrition called 'subclinical' is likely to be present in about 7% of the elderly population (Debenham, 1988). Being housebound may be due to apathy or dementia but a physical disability can also make it difficult or impossible to go out for shopping. There is usually an increasing dependence on others as the old person moves to the end of the lifespan and this will probably influence the choice of food and drink, and perhaps reduce the pleasure usually associated with this Activity of Living.

DEPENDENCE/INDEPENDENCE IN EATING AND DRINKING

Independence in eating and drinking obviously is associated with the individual's stage on the lifespan. There is the obvious dependence of the young and the potential dependence of the elderly. At any stage of the lifespan, persons previously independent for this AL can become dependent, temporarily or permanently, from either physical or psychological disability. Behaviourally disturbed people may not be able to leave home and go shopping for food; or decision-making may be difficult and so on. There are others who may have a hand or arm defect or who have diminished sight yet can still be independent for eating and drinking, provided they have the use of mechanical aids. These aids may be in the kitchen for preparing food, or

used when cooking and eating food and allow the individual to retain the maximum self-esteem and dignity despite a physical handicap. For a quite different reason mentally handicapped people too will often have eating and drinking problems and the importance of good positioning with a suitable size of chair and table, in a relaxed atmosphere, are basic to progressive independence.

There is now a range of feeding aids, not necessarily expensive, and a considerable literature (Yates & Whitehead, 1986) with collective ideas which have proved useful to physiotherapists, occupational therapists and speech therapists who have studied the problems of handicapped people so that they can achieve optimal independence in eating and drinking.

FACTORS INFLUENCING EATING AND DRINKING

Eating and drinking play a significant part in the everyday living pattern of all age groups and for most people they are pleasurable activities. However, there are many factors which can influence this AL and affect the individual's reaction to food and drink. The various factors are described, using the categories which appear in the model under the headings of physical, psychological, sociocultural, environmental and politicoeconomic factors.

Physical factors

In the model, physical factors are mainly of a biological dimension, and those related to the AL of eating and drinking are the ones required for three functions — ingestion, digestion and absorption; namely the mouth, oropharynx, oesophagus, stomach and small intestine, together with the salivary glands, pancreas, liver and gallbladder which provide juices and enzymes to facilitate these three functions. For the purpose of the model, in human biology terms, the upper alimentary tract and the accessory organs of digestion are juxtaposed with the upper alimentary tract. The purpose of this juxtaposition is to provide guidance when devising a nursing plan which takes account, not only of nurse-initiated interventions, but also the nursing interventions which result from medical prescription, and the suggested documents on pages 56 and 57 take account of this.

To provide understanding of the problems faced by people who have feeding difficulties (discussed in the second half of this chapter), the body structure and function required for swallowing will be described. It is now customary to think of a 'preparatory stage' which includes appreciation of what, for that person, is a 'manageable mouthful' on a fork or spoon; then tracing the visuospatial pathway without spillage from vessel to mouth, so that food is brought to the mouth at an appropriately sequenced time interval. As the food arrives, the lips part, the mouth opens and food is deposited on the tongue, the lips close around the cutlery helping to remove the food from it; the fork or spoon is then withdrawn and the lip seal completed. The concept of physical factors has therefore to widen to include at least one functioning upper limb, or some other way of conveying food from a plate to the mouth, and this may mean the assistance of another person.

The next stage is variously called the voluntary, pre-swallow or oral stage (Cockcroft & Ray, 1985). It starts when the lip seal is formed around the food. Although the tongue is the sensory organ for taste, texture and temperature; it is also the motor organ for moving food in the mouth, to enable biting, chewing and grinding by the teeth on the preferred side. Correct apposition of teeth in the upper and lower jaws is necessary to accomplish this and the service of an orthodontist may be necessary to facilitate this. Correct apposition is equally important when fitting dentures. Saliva and mucus both help to soften the food and bind it into a bolus, which is rolled to the back of the tongue which is the lowest part of the ring of swallow receptors, the ring being completed by the pillars of the fauces at the sides, and the soft palate at the top.

The final stage of swallowing is involuntary; called the swallow or pharyngeal stage. Stimulation of the sensory ring is the beginning of a complicated reflex action; the soft palate moves upwards and backwards to prevent food rising into the nasopharynx with possible nasal regurgitation. The tongue rises to occlude food returning to the mouth which may cause dribbling or drooling. The glottis closes and the epiglottal folds close over the entrance to the larynx to prevent aspiration of food into the respiratory tract. Further assistance in this is provided by momentary cessation of breathing as the oropharyngeal constrictor muscles push the food into the oesophagus, along which it travels by peristalsis to the stomach and small intestine for subsequent digestion and absorption.

Body size is a visible physical dimension resulting from eating and drinking, and height and weight are measurable physical aspects. Also included in the concept of physical factors influencing this AL are the basic constituents of food. The study of food and the associated biological processes of growth, maintenance and repair are known as the science of nutrition and a brief outline of this subject follows.

Nutrition

From every country in the world comes an enormous variety of foodstuffs but when analysed, they can be classified into a few essential constituents:

- carbohydrates
- proteins
- fats
- vitamins

- trace elements (mineral salts)
- dietary fibre
- water

To function effectively each cell in the body requires these substances, and to maintain health and efficiency the individual must have a balanced daily intake of all these constituents. Carbohydrates, proteins and fats are oxidised in the body to provide it with energy and the amount of energy produced by these different nutrients can be measured (Dickerson, 1986b). In many countries, it is assessed in heat units called Calories — weight-watchers frequently maintain that they are 'watching' their Calories'. Since 1975 however, the United Kingdom has adopted the kilojoule (kJ), and SI (System International) unit for dietetic calculations. The kilojoule requirement for an individual varies with height, weight, age, sex, climate and occupation but roughly speaking, the daily intake for an adult female with a sedentary job might be around 8000 kJ (2000 C), for a pregnant woman around 12 000 kJ and for a man doing heavy physical work 16 000 kJ. To provide a balanced diet, a person on a diet of 8000 kJ (2000 C) might have:

about 4400 kJ (1100 C) carbohydrates	= 55% of the total
about 1200 kJ (300 C) proteins	= 15% of the total
about 2400 kJ (600 C) fats	= 30% of the total

Vitamins, mineral salts, dietary fibre and water are essential to health but do not provide kilojoules of energy.

Carbohydrates. The starches and sugars are composed of carbon, hydrogen and oxygen and are found in foods such as sugar, potatoes, cereals, fruit and vegetables, Before they can be used by the body they must be reduced to glucose.

1 gram of carbohydrate yields 16 kJ (roughly 4 C)

Carbohydrates provide heat and energy and can be stored in the liver as glucogen but when eaten in excess are deposited in the fat depots of the body as adipose tissue.

Proteins. The body relies on proteins for its supply of nitrogen, but they also contain carbon, hydrogen, oxygen, sulphur and phosphorous; they are broken down to amino acids prior to absorption. Protein foods are, for example, meat, fish, eggs, milk products, soya beans, peas, beans and lentils.

1 gram of protein yields 17 kJ (roughly 4 C)

These foods supply the essential amino acids for building and repairing body tissue. For this reason, children require a higher proportion of protein foods than adults, and people who have been ill may be prescribed a high-protein diet to replace damaged tissue and to replace weight loss.

Fats. Carbon, hydrogen and oxygen are present in fats but in different proportions to carbohydrates and before they can be absorbed they must be broken down to fatty acids and glycerol. The terms 'animal fats' and 'vegetable fats' have been superseded by 'saturated fats' and 'polyunsaturated fats' respectively. The latter terms not only designate content but they are less restrictive regarding source; for example, some saturated fats are of vegetable origin — coconut and palm oil; and some polyunsaturated fats found in fowl and fish are obviously of animal origin. A decreased fat intake was recommended by a report published in 1983 and one published in 1984 (p. 153). Since then the debate has continued, and it is now less certain that a low fat intake prevents coronary heart disease. A high blood cholesterol is certainly a causative risk factor in heart disease, and it is influenced by the amount and type of fat in the diet. But reducing fat consumption in those with a normal blood cholesterol does not influence the subsequent risk of coronary heart disease (Holmes, 1988b).

1 gram of fat yields 37 kJ (roughly 9 C)

In the body, fatty deposits are found around delicate organs like the eye or kidney to protect and maintain their position, and fats also have an important function in transporting fat-soluble vitamins but the general functions of fatty foods, as with carbohydrates, is to provide heat and energy.

Vitamins. Good health is dependent on vitamins and most cannot be manufactured in the body so they must be obtained from food. Vitamins are chemical compounds which are classified into two main groups:

fat-soluble vitamins: A D E K
water-soluble vitamins: B C P

Vitamins are required in only small amounts. In many instances their function is catalytic, as components of enzyme systems involved in essential metabolic reactions. Although not supplying energy to the body, some are needed for the regulation of energy; and some are needed for the regulation of tissue synthesis. They are required therefore for the general health of tissues and gross deficiency can lead to specific disease conditions for example rickets (lack of vitamin D); scurvy (lack of vitamin C); beri-beri and pellagra (lack of vitamin B). Vitamins are found in many foods; the fat-soluble are mostly in dairy products, fat meat and fish oils; and the water-soluble in fresh fruit and vegetables, nuts and the germ of cereals (Pownall, 1986).

Trace elements. Although required only in small quantities, these inorganic elements have many essential roles. They are components of body tissues and fluids, and of many specialised substances such as hormones, transport molecules and enzymes. For example, calcium and phosphorus are required for teeth and bone production; iron is required for red blood corpuscles; iodine is needed for the hormone secreted by the thyroid gland, an endocrine gland; sodium is important in the maintenance of the fluid volume in the body.

Sodium is an example of an electrolyte and the balance of the various electrolytes in the body is of critical importance. An electrolyte is formed when an inorganic compound such as salt (sodium chloride) is dissolved in water and dissociates into two or more electrically charged particles. For example, in the body, sodium chloride (Na Cl is the chemical symbol) is present in solution as sodium (Na^+) and chlorine (Cl^-). The desired range of the different electrolytes in the cell fluid and in the extracellular fluid is known. When, because of disease or loss of fluid from the body this electrolyte balance is upset, the function of body cells may be grossly impaired. Mineral salts are widely dispersed in foods, including meat, fish, dairy products, and vegetables.

Dietary fibre. The cellulose part of food which passes through the digestive tract and is excreted as part of the faeces is called dietary fibre. It does not at any time become part of the body structure but its bulk helps to stimulate muscular movement in the large intestine and promotes defaecation thus preventing constipation (Bennett, 1988). There is also evidence that the breaking down of fibre by colonic bacteria makes the stool more acid and this is one of the reasons why fibre is believed to reduce the amount of possible carcinogens (Burkitt, 1983).

Water. The chemical symbol H_2O represents water and signifies that each molecule is composed of two parts hydrogen to one part oxygen. Water is essential to life and makes up about two-thirds of the body weight. Death will follow if there is water deprivation for more than a few days as many body processes are dependent on its presence: water is the main constituent of all body fluids; many physiochemical changes take place in the environment of the body fluids; most nutrients and cellular waste products are soluble in water.

In a 24-hour period the adult human requires about 2500 ml of water and if the intake is inadequate or if the loss of water is excessive (urinary output does not usually exceed 1500 ml per day) the person will experience the sensation of thirst.

Normally, provided that an adequate well balanced diet is available, food and fluid intake is controlled by complex biochemical processes. There are centres in the brain which are sensitive to changes in the levels of nutrients and trace elements in the blood thereby controlling appetite and thirst (Holmes, 1986a).

Psychological factors

A minimal level of intelligence is necessary to master the skills used in the process of eating and drinking. This is apparent when observing a young child as he experiments intellectually as well as physically with the development of mealtime skills, and likewise it is apparent when observing mentally handicapped children whose intellectual development is impaired; they often have great difficulty in acquiring eating and drinking skills (Anderson, 1983).

A certain intellectual level is also required for the acquisition and application of the knowledge needed to select and prepare a diet which will maintain health, and a great deal of time and effort are expended by the government, the health professions and the media in health education to interest the general public in desirable eating practices. The acquisition of knowledge is required also to apply appropriate food hygiene practices when handling food; and to dispose of food waste in such a manner that it will not attract vermin and flies which have the potential to harbour and spread pathogenic microorganisms to humans.

The individual's emotional state may sometimes affect food intake. The child's excitement prior to a holiday, the anxiety associated with examinations, the stress of a change of job may well reduce the accustomed intake for that individual. These however are usually transient. Loss of appetite or lack of desire for food over a prolonged period can be indicative of a more serious disturbance in emotional states and is referred to as anorexia nervosa. It has a peak incidence in adolescence especially among young women, although the number of men is increasing. Despite evidence to the contrary, the individual views herself as fat (distorted body image) and will refuse to eat or will deliberately vomit following food intake. Anorexia nervosa is usually considered to be a disturbance in personality development, often in the relationship with one parent. However, research has shown that when people with a 'normal' appetite are starved, the higher mental functions are impaired. There is selfishness, withdrawal from social activities and a decreased interest in sex, together with increasing self-centredness and rigid thinking, so that compromise cannot be considered. All these manifestations have been seen in people with anorexia nervosa (Wright S J, 1986).

In contradistinction some people use food as a source of comfort and security. Overeating in the majority of people leads to obesity (p. 164), and those who are comfortable with their body image will not be motivated to lose weight. However the doctor may advise a reduction in weight, for example, if surgery becomes necessary, or if arthritis develops in the joints of the lower limbs.

Compulsive overeating means that the person no longer has control over what is eaten although aware of the enormous quantity being eaten. There is usually a morbid fear of becoming fat, but this is avoided by self-induced vomiting or laxative abuse or both. 'Binge eating' has long been recognised as a feature in some people with anorexia nervosa and obesity. It is only in more recent years that it has been identified in people who are not suffering from either of these psychological problems influencing eating, and it is called bulimia nervosa (Savage, 1984).

Currently alcohol dependence/abuse is a major problem in many countries of the world. Usually the onset of de-

pendence on alcohol is insidious, starting with social drinking but when out of control, the habit can lead to irresponsible behaviour, petty crime or even assault, and bring distress not only to the individual but to family and friends. It is discussed in more detail on page 169.

Sociocultural factors

In certain cultures it is customary to take meals in the home in a special room set aside for the purpose but there are many variations, and it may be accepted practice to eat under a tree, round a camp fire or in a tent. Not only the setting but the style of eating may vary considerably. Some societies make use of fingers, others use chopsticks, and yet others use knives, forks and spoons; some eat food from a communal bowl, others from individual plates or bowls; some sit cross-legged on the floor, others customarily use a chair. In a few cultures there may even be segregation of the sexes at mealtimes with adult males eating together but separately from adult females eating together. More commonly, however, the meal is an occasion when all members of the family are sharing news about the day's activities although in some industrialised countries, the increasing use of 'fast' foods and the consuming dominance of TV-viewing are altering the pattern of mealtime socialising.

Certain religious groups have definite rules about the choice and preparation of specific items on the menu. For example orthodox Jews must prepare and serve dairy products and meat dishes separately, while the Koran forbids Muslims to touch pork and alcohol, and the devout Hindu will not eat animal products. There are however other groups who, not for religious reasons, are vegetarians and will not eat animal products.

With the interaction of these many variables, and remembering the interaction of the five groups of factors influencing the AL of eating and drinking, it is not surprising that each person develops an individual pattern related to this AL.

Environmental factors

Physical environmental factors can affect the choice of food. Obviously geographical position, soil fertility, climate and rainfall will determine the type of food which can be grown locally, and will also influence the meat, fish and poultry content of the diet. Nowadays, for industrial nations with their extensive import/export networks, reliance on local food is not such a dominant feature of everyday living but it is crucial for about two-thirds of the world who are dependent on local produce.

Availability of fuel is also a consideration. Although certain groups such as Eskimos eat raw fish and seal, it is customary in most countries to improve the palatability of food by cooking many of the vegetables and fruit fibres, and the flesh of fish, fowl and animals. Also some form of fuel is needed for preservation of food for example in bottling, canning or deep freezing, and making storage possible.

However, careful planning for storage of new food, whether scarce or abundant, may be negated if the environment is plagued by vectors such as cockroaches, flies, mice and rats. Not only can they deplete the supply; they may 'spoil' food by contamination with excreta and make it unfit for human consumption, or they may even transfer pathogens which can lead to food poisoning (p. 159).

Food is imperative for human existence but an adequate supply of water is even more important. Three-quarters of the world's surface is water but getting an adequate supply of fresh, clean water which is safe to use for drinking and cooking is one of the world's pressing problems. Most of the world's water is salt and in the oceans; only 3% is fresh and only a small amount of that is accessible as a public water supply. Many of the world's women and children have to walk miles to draw water from a stream or well which may be inadequate for all the Activities of Living; when a safe supply is available on tap, water is so much taken for granted. Accessibility and distribution of food and water in the local environment certainly contributes to the ease of eating and drinking.

In a slightly different sense, the environment is obviously taken into account by restaurateurs who consider that the ambience of the environment can contribute to food and drink enjoyment. Noise, hustle and bustle are not thought to be good for digestion and many hoteliers give considerable thought to the provision of carpeting, lowered lights and soft background music as an environmental aid to both the physiological and psychological enjoyment of eating and drinking.

Politicoeconomic factors

Any consideration of eating and drinking presupposes that food and drink are available. This is not always the case, indeed, about half of the world's population is hungry. In certain areas even now, hundreds of people die every day due to starvation, and many thousands of others are undernourished because they have insufficient food to eat. There are many complex reasons for this maldistribution of food throughout the world, such as infertile soil, inferior seed, inadequate crop rotation, overgrazing, soil erosion, lack of irrigation, lack of knowledge and lack of finance, all of which contribute to a poor yield. Some parts of the world, too, are more liable to suffer from natural disasters such as drought, floods or pestilence which result in crop failure or even large-scale famine. When this occurs, scarcity creates an increase in the price of food which often takes it beyond the financial reach of lower income groups so the people are undernourished or may in fact 'starve to death'. Considerable attempts have been made at national and international levels to redress these gross inequalities but still the problem remains, much of it due to economic

and political constraints highlighted in the Brandt Report as long ago as 1980.

Protein is the most expensive food nutrient to process and protein-calorie malnutrition is a widespread and serious problem especially in the first years of life. Very young children are highly susceptible to lack of adequate nutrients, and in developing countries babies who have initially been breast-fed may suffer severe nutritional deficiencies, especially of protein, when they are weaned. One of the gross manifestations of protein deficiency in young children is kwashiorkor.

The WHO (World Health Organization) collaborates with the FAO (Food and Agricultural Organization) and UNICEF (United Nations Children's Fund) in the Protein-Calorie Advisory Group set up by the UN and it is paying particular attention to the development of low-cost, protein-rich weaning foods suitable for local production in developing countries. Enhancing self-help is a much more enduring policy than encouraging import of foreign-produced foodstuffs to an undernourished or malnourished nation.

To help to prevent malnutrition in the older person, some countries have instituted a 'meals-on-wheels' service. At a small cost or free of charge in cases of financial hardship, a cooked meal is delivered in the middle of the day to the home of those who, because of physical disability or frailty, are unable to go shopping for food or are disinclined to cook for themselves. For those elderly people who are still ambulant, voluntarily organised local luncheon clubs are becoming popular. They provide a cooked nutritious meal and have the advantage of being a social event (Holmes, 1989).

Of course malnutrition can exist in the midst of plenty, and indeed is associated with obesity (p. 164). Insurance companies are becoming hesitant about issuing policies to grossly overweight people because statistics show that compared with their slim contemporaries they are more susceptible to, for example, coronary disease, bronchitis and diabetes mellitus.

Because of the link with disease and dysfunction, a number of industrialised countries are greatly exercised about the need to change their national dietary habits and are attempting to adopt a standard approach to recommendations for the whole population. By and large they include proposals to reduce fat intake to around 30% of total energy intake, of which only 10% should be saturated fatty acids; to reduce average salt and sucrose intakes and to increase dietary fibre. In the UK, probably the best known reports advocating these changes are from the National Advisory Committee on Nutritional Education (NACNE, 1983) and from the Committee on Medical Aspects of Food Policy (COMA, 1984). They are discussed briefly on page 153. They were discussed at length on the radio and television and were written about in the national press, suggestions being made that political manoeuvring had delayed publication of both reports because of the implications for agricultural policy, food manufacturing techniques and EEC regulations (Janes, 1986).

There is no point in exhorting the nation to eat a healthy diet if the food and water provided are not free from the potential of causing illness in the consumers. Most countries have government Food Laws about the standard of hygiene to be maintained in, for example food retail outlets and restaurants, and the food additives and colourings that may be used (Holmes, 1986a), and the pesticides to be used for spraying crops. Because of the tremendous advances in food technology in the last few decades, many of these laws are now inadequate, and the UK government is having to respond to public pressure about the increasing incidence of illness arising from microbial contamination of food. From one decade to another, the pathogens present in food are not necessarily the same ones, and this applies to the foods transmitting the pathogens.

In 1988 eggs and chickens were incriminated as transmitters of Salmonella infection. The public became alarmed and the sale of these foods dropped dramatically. Since they are perishable goods, large numbers had to be destroyed, for which the producers received compensation from the government, but not the victims of Salmonella poisoning. Further response from the government included advice to consumers about such activities as storing, preparation for cooking and details of cooking these possibly infected foods to render them safe to eat. But in a paper read at a National Environmental Health Seminar, reported by Reid (1989), it was argued that the producer and not the consumer should be the principal guardian of clean food. A plea was made for effective legal control over the wholesomeness of food offered by the producers, as it was evident that without such control, consumers can die. One piece of evidence is that in 1984, an outbreak of Salmonella poisoning in a hospital resulted in 19 deaths of elderly people (Alderman, 1988).

Listeriosis is a disease with flu-like symptoms, yet it kills one in three victims. UK government figures show that the number of cases is rising, but of the 705 reported since 1986, only four have been associated with food, and it is alleged that 1 in 15 cooked chicken products were infected with listeria (O'Byrne, 1989). The causative microorganism is *Listeria monocytogenes*; its presence is widespread and it can withstand a wide range of temperature from 2 to 15°C. It is recommended that domestic refrigeration of precooked foods should be at 2°C and that such foods should be heated to 70°C before eating; any food left over should not be reheated. After purchase, these foods should be put in the fridge or freezer as soon as possible. However, these guidelines may well change, as listeria have been found to reproduce at temperatures as low as freezing and have survived at more than 90°C (Turner, 1989).

Yet another example of a ubiquitous microorganism is *Campylobacter jejuni/coli* which only in the last decade has been identified as a cause of disease in humans. In the late 1970s it was found in faeces from people suffering from diarrhoea and by the late 1980s it had become the most common bacterium associated with diarrhoea in humans in the UK. It has been found in chickens, and handling raw chicken has caused the disease, as well as eating inadequately cooked chicken (Alderman, 1988).

There are other pathogens which gain entry to food and drink, and can cause disease in humans. It is claimed that irradiation of food would remove *all* pathogens thereby rendering food safe to eat and drink. An opinion poll of a representative sample of 1500 people in 1987 found that 84% thought that the irradiation ban should remain. However, if further research answers many of the queries which surround this technology, and the public gain confidence in it, it may well be that the government in the future will change the Food Laws in order to provide the safest possible food and drink. These are examples of the necessity for nurses to continually update their knowledge.

The drinking of alcohol can be influenced by several politicoeconomic factors. For example there are usually laws about where and under what circumstances alcohol can be sold. In some countries it can only be sold from government controlled premises, and from licensed social institutions such as public bars, restaurants and hotels. In others, it is more readily available, for instance in superstores, along with groceries and other household commodities. This means that drinking alcohol is not confined to the hours set by some governments for drinking in licensed premises. There may be a minimum age at which people can buy alcohol, or drink it in a licensed place, and there is usually imposition of a fine for selling alcohol to under-age drinkers. Also there is usually a maximum permitted level of alcohol in the blood when driving a vehicle. Yet, among the young in the UK, 39% of drivers aged 20–24 who are killed in road accidents have blood alcohol levels over the legal limit (British Medical Journal, 1988). Alcohol dependence/abuse and the problems which it can cause related to other ALs are discussed in the appropriate chapters of this section.

INDIVIDUALITY IN EATING AND DRINKING

Individuality is the final component of the model to be introduced. From the preceding discussion it is evident that there are many dimensions of the other components of the model which contribute to the development of individuality in the AL of eating and drinking. Below is a résumé of the main points in the discussion.

Lifespan: effect on eating and drinking
- Nutrition in utero
- Breast/bottle-feeding and weaning in infancy
- Increasing skills in eating and drinking during childhood

- Prudent diet during adolescence and adulthood
- Reduced appetite/potential nutritional deficiency in old age

Dependence/independence in eating and drinking
- Special utensils
- Mechanical aids
- Kitchen gadgets
- Special transport for shopping

Factors influencing eating and drinking
- Physical
  — state of mouth and teeth
  — swallowing
  — intact digestive system
  — nutrition
  — physical proficiency in shopping for/preparing food
  — physical proficiency in taking food and drink
  — appetite/thirst regulation
- Psychological
  — intellectual capacity to procure and prepare food and drink
  — knowledge about diet and health
  — weight control
  — distorted body image
  — alcohol dependence/abuse
  — food hygiene
  — disposal of food waste
  — attitude to eating and drinking
  — emotional status
  — likes and dislikes
- Sociocultural
  — family traditions
  — cultural idiosyncrasies
  — religious commendations/restrictions
- Environmental
  — climate and geographical position
  — facilities for procuring/growing food
  — distance from home to shopping area
  — availability of transport
  — means of cooking
  — means of storage
  — vectors and food spoilage
- Politicoeconomic
  — malnutrition/finance
  — choice of food and drink
  — quantity and quality of food and drink
  — published national reports about healthy diet
  — safe food

Eating and drinking: patients' problems and related nursing

Unless they are detrimental to health, it is desirable that during an episode of illness, the patient's individual habits of living are changed as little as possible. It is therefore important that the nurse should know about these habits, and use the knowledge to devise an individualised nursing plan (p. 56)

In order to individualise nursing for this AL, it is necessary to assess the activities of eating and drinking. Assessing involves observing the patient; acquiring information about eating and drinking habits by asking appropriate questions, and by listening to the comments and questions raised by the patient and family; and using relevant material from available records such as medical records. The nurse would be seeking answers to the following questions:

- how often does the individual usually eat and drink?
- what does the individual usually eat and drink?
- when does the individual eat and drink?
- where does the individual eat and drink?
- what factors influence the way the individual carries out the AL of eating and drinking?
- has the individual any long-standing difficulties with eating and drinking and how have these been coped with?
- what problems, if any, does the individual have at present with eating and drinking and are any likely to develop?

Of course the nurse does not necessarily ask these actual questions because much of the information can be acquired in the course of conversation with the patient and by observation. For example, if there has been recent weight loss, the clothes may hang loosely, or if the change has been weight gain the clothes will probably be tight.

The information can then be examined to identify, in collaboration with the patient when possible, any problems being experienced with the AL and these can be arranged if necessary in priority. The nurse may recognise potential problems and these can be discussed with the patient. Mutual realistic goals can then be set to prevent potential problems from becoming actual ones; to alleviate or solve the actual problems; or to help the patient cope with those which cannot be alleviated or solved. Keeping in mind what the patient can and cannot do, the nursing interventions (and any action the patient has agreed to undertake) to achieve the set goals can then be selected according to local circumstances and available resources. These interventions should be written on the nursing plan along with the date on which evaluation will be carried out, in order to discern whether or not they are achieving the stated goals.

Other members of the multidisciplinary health team are usually involved in the care programme, such as occupational and speech therapists, dietitians and doctors; and it is important that the individualised nursing plan is congruent with the team's mutually agreed objectives for the patient. On the Nursing Plan proforma suggested by Roper/Logan/Tierney (p. 57) there is a section for appropriate entries of this type in order to indicate the relationship between nursing interventions derived from medical/other prescription and nurse-initiated interventions.

However before nurses can begin to think in terms of individualised nursing, they require a general idea of the conditions which can be responsible for, or can change, the dependence/independence status for the AL of eating and drinking and which can be experienced by the person as a problem in carrying out the AL. The remainder of this section is a general discussion of the types of patients' problems related to eating and drinking and the relevant nursing.

They are grouped under headings which indicate how the problems can arise:

- Change of environment and routine
- Change in eating and drinking habit
- Change in mode of eating and drinking
- Change of dependence/independence status
- Some specific problems associated with eating and drinking

Many factors can influence the highly individualised activity of eating and drinking. Disease or injury to the digestive system itself may interfere with the activity, or with the individual's capacity to benefit nutritionally from the activity. In addition, disease and pain affecting other body systems can cause disturbance of the appetite and may well alter the individual's intake of food and drink. Admission to hospital however, irrespective of cause, almost always produces some degree of stress and anxiety and can create problems related to this important activity of eating and drinking.

CHANGE OF ENVIRONMENT AND ROUTINE

Not all people experiencing a problem related to eating and drinking change their environment; many of them remain at home, and may visit the local health clinic or surgery for advice and support from the doctor or practice nurse. Should the problem be persistent vomiting, perhaps associated with food poisoning, then the routine related to eating and drinking will be changed as they follow the prescription. This may be to have frequent mouthwashes to relieve oral discomfort; take sips of fluid as soon as the nausea and vomiting stops; and if the sips are tolerated, increase the volume; then gradually take semisolid food; increase the amount and introduce 'solid' food until the normal dietary intake is resumed.

Most people are well accustomed to changes of diet while on holiday or during business trips but in these instances, they are usually in control of their decisions about eating and drinking. In hospital however this is not usually so, and mealtimes and their associated activities often come to have increased significance. Individuals may be hypersensitive to alterations in the timing of meals and the methods of serving them; they may be apprehensive about the availability of facilities related to hygiene activities; they may be easily irritated by distracting influences; they may be much more apprehensive about fluctuations in appetite. For young children in particular, the change in environment and routine in hospital will be bewildering and their developing mealtime habits therefore may be considerably disrupted.

Timing of meals
Patients newly admitted to hospital often have no idea of the mealtime programme: whether to expect a cooked or a continental breakfast; whether the main meal is served in the middle of the day or in the evening; whether they will be allowed to have snacks between meals. Some patients may have heard of the need to fast prior to surgery and certains tests, and be concerned about the discomfort of feeling hungry or thirsty.

Nurses can allay some of the anxiety by offering information and also by providing opportunities for patients to ask questions so that they can feel reassured about what they are expected to do in continuing this important AL. Most patients understand that in an establishment as complex as a hospital, it is usually necessary to have set mealtimes; indeed, some find that meals give a certain degree of order to the day, providing stable time-points in an otherwise bewildering situation.

However, in the interests of financial economy, meal preparation for several hospitals is increasingly being centralised, leaving nursing staff in the wards with little control over the timing of meals. Appetite is often fickle during illness, and a patient may be ready to eat an hour after the routine meal has been served. Or a patient may be away from the ward, perhaps in another department, at the mealtime and may be hungry on return. Some hospitals are solving these problems by installing a microwave oven in the ward kitchen, so that meals pre-cooked in the central kitchen can be re-heated. When the cook-chill process was introduced into some hospitals in the early 1980s, there were high hopes that it would provide cheaper, hot, nutritional meals, at the times patients required them (Turner, 1989). The food is cooked and then fast-chilled and stored for up to 5 days in controlled low temperatures, and re-heated immediately before eating. The method gives flexibility to kitchen staff regarding time of cooking, types of food served, and individual ward mealtimes. However, there is debate about the possibility of this method transmitting pathogenic microorganisms such as Salmonella, *Listeria monocytogenes* and Campylobacter (p. 159). And the debate continues providing an example of the necessity for nurses to continually update their knowledge.

Serving of meals

In hospital, patients may find that the way of serving meals is a problem because it is so different from their usual routine. Even though most people are accustomed to 'tray' meals in self-service restaurants, few are used to having all meals served in this manner.

People do not usually choose to be in bed while taking a meal, so for the minority of patients who are bedfast, eating and drinking may become a formidable task especially if they must remain in a recumbent position, or attached to various pieces of equipment associated with their treatment.

If bedfast patients can sit up at mealtimes, the nurse should help them into a comfortable position and ensure that they are adequately supported with pillows before placing the bedtable in an appropriate position ready for the meal-tray. Many people like to drink with a meal and, unless it is contraindicated, most patients have a water-jug and glass on the bedside locker so the nurse should check that it is within easy reach.

Functionally-designed hospital furniture has improved over the last few decades. Chairfast patients can have a bedtable lowered to receive the mealtray so that they are in the usual position for eating and drinking. They can then eat and drink in their usual style, which might be using modified cutlery and crockery, or even being fed by another person. Ambulant patients will enjoy meals more if sitting at a table; in fact, in new and upgraded wards, a dining area is frequently included in the design of the ward unit.

Meals should be served in a calm, unhurried manner if patients are to enjoy what is really a social event in their day. The nurse should appreciate the symbolism attached to food, indicative of hospitality and caring. Associated with this symbolism, the very acts of serving and accepting food provide an opportunity for establishing and maintaining the important relationship between nurse and patient.

Particularly in a psychiatric hospital, group dining may be a deliberate therapeutic measure to give patients an opportunity to solve some of their problems by practising the social behaviour associated with mealtimes.

Alteration in appetite

Most people have personal idiosyncrasies about food choice and even when an appropriate, attractive meal is served, patients may not feel inclined to eat. If they are feeling unwell, or homesick, or unused to the type of food served, they may not eat adequately and the nurse must be interested in the 'used' tray. Over a century ago (1859) Florence Nightingale observed:

A nurse will often have patients loathing all food and incapable of any will to get well who just tumble over the contents of the plate or dip the spoon into the cup to deceive the nurse and she will take it away without ever seeing that there is just the same quantity of food as when she brought it, and she will tell the doctor too that the patient has eaten all his diets as usual when all she ought to have meant is that she has taken away his diets as usual.

The stress and anxiety associated with admission to hospital may result in lack of appetite, albeit temporarily. Early establishment of rapport with newly admitted patients may help to minimise it. Unpleasant sights and odours may diminish appetite and nursing activities need to be planned so that the ward atmosphere is free from malodour at mealtimes. Pain, particularly of a chronic nature, can interfere with appetite and if it is possible, pain-control regimes could take mealtimes into consideration so that patients are relaxed, free from pain and can anticipate the meal with pleasure. Loss of appetite occurs when there is nausea and/or vomiting and these are discussed on page 171.

Anorexia (loss of appetite) is a symptom of several diseases, and when the disease is treated, normal appetite is usually re-established. Reduction in appetite can affect the body's response to medication therapy. Conversely, both the side- and therapeutic effects of drugs can interfere with food intake by either increasing or decreasing appetite (Holmes, 1986b).

Anorexia is a common and serious symptom in patients with cancer. They experience such unpleasant changes in taste sensation, that they can reject food which relatives have carefully prepared especially for them, and this can cause family tension. Warning relatives that this might happen, and assuring them that the rejection is not personal, usually helps them to cope with the problem. In one study (Stubbs, 1989), items causing the greatest taste changes (in descending order) were meat, bacon and ham, fried eggs, tea, coffee, alcohol, sweets and chocolates. A nursing contribution is to encourage patients to regard food as an essential medicine to be taken at regular intervals throughout the day until treatment is successful. A high-protein breakfast may help with the problem of meat aversion which has been found to increase as the day progresses. Helping people who are experiencing changed taste sensation demands individualised nursing.

Anorexia nervosa, over-eating, obesity, compulsive over-eating, binge-eating and bulimia nervosa are all related to alteration in appetite. As they have a psychological dimension, they are discussed in the section 'Psychological factors influencing eating and drinking' (p. 156).

As nutrients are essential for the repair of body tissue, it is imperative that nurses know about the therapeutic value of food, and either report verbally on patients' appetites and food intake at the 'end of shift' handover, or record the information on the patients' nursing notes.

Hospital meals

In recent years hospital meals have been influenced by various reports about healthy eating. Information about healthy eating was contained in a report published in 1983 and another one published in 1984 (both are discussed on p. 153). The information was available to the public, indeed the title of the 1983 report was 'Proposals for nutritional guidelines for health education in Britain'. Both reports were discussed on the radio and television and they were written about in the national press and in non-professional journals. Consequently many people currently admitted to hospital have a higher expectation of hospital meals, to which most hospital catering departments are responding. The *Nursing Times* was concerned about these reports and mounted a 'Care about food' campaign in 1985. It advocated that in each hospital a multiprofessional Food Policy Committee should be convened. It invited nurses to supply information about current practices in the hospitals in which they worked. This information was published on a 'Feedback' page from time to time. Approximately 1 year after the initiation of the 'Care about food' campaign, Wright (1986) evaluated the results on a nationwide basis and concluded that there was a move towards healthier and more varied menus available for patients, and for staff in hospital canteens.

In those hospitals in which a menu provides an assortment of food, it is customary for the desired items for meals on the following day to be ticked on a menu card in the evening. Some provide for the selection of a large, average or small portion. Helping patients to choose meals from the next day's menu can offer nurses an opportunity to talk about the important links between nutrition and health (Nursing Times, 1985). But it means having a sufficient number of nurses on the evening shift. Some hospitals cope with the anticipated lack of evening staff by helping the patients fill in the menu cards in the afternoon. If there are visitors present, they too could benefit from the discussion about choice of diet. But, there are instances of patients who, having forgotten what they ordered the day before, refuse to eat the food (Sanford, 1987). A clinical nurse specialist in a nutrition team states her reservations about the designation of 'non-nursing duties' to mealtime activities, and says that in some cases the ward clerk or maid fills in the menu cards, and removes the uneaten food (Carlisle, 1988).

Not all hospitals provide a mealtray service; some serve food from a mobile heated trolley and those patients who are able, make their decision when they are told what is available. This avoids the problem of removal of heavy covers and cling film inherent in a mealtray service; it provides for size of helping to be adjusted to current appetite, and patients may well be reassured to see nursing staff serving food, and taking an interest in the meals.

Yet, despite the publicity given to 'healthy eating' in the media as a result of the two national reports in 1983 and 1984, and the *Nursing Times* 'Care about food' campaign in 1985, Taylor, in 1988 wrote '. . . the sad fact remains that a high percentage of hospital patients continue to suffer from malnutrition'. She goes on to say that nurses are frequently blamed for this, possibly because they are constantly with patients and are, therefore, potentially able to influence what they eat. She addressed openly the frequent interprofessional conflict between dietitians and nurses and wrote about 'the former not allowing sufficient flexibility and understanding of the practical difficulties involved in getting food into patients'. She says that nurses should be 'encouraged to value the humanistic skills which result in patients getting fed'.

However, even when hospital meals are adequate, some patients will complain about them. There may be cause for dissatisfaction but grumbling about food may be a manifestation of some more covert need, for example lack of information about the treatment programme, upset of usual routine, lack of attention; the discerning nurse will investigate the significance of dietary complaints.

Pre- and post-meal activities

The majority of patients who are not bedfast will be able to continue their habitual pre- and post-meal routines such as handwashing, visiting the toilet and cleaning the teeth. Bedfast patients may experience considerable concern because they are no longer independent for these activities but nurses can reduce anxiety by ensuring that these facilities are made available.

Patients will be reassured if they actually see members of the nursing staff wash their hands in preparation for serving meals and/or helping with feeding activities. This is important for general hygiene reasons but it is also important in order that food will be free from contamination by pathogenic microorganisms. Prior to meal-serving, the nurse may have been dressing wounds, or helping a patient who is vomiting or she may have been handling a bedpan. In an establishment such as a hospital, it is crucial that all food-handlers should be scrupulously careful about hand cleanliness because potentially they can infect the food of many people, and people who are more susceptible to infection because they are already suffering from some disorder which has precipitated entry to hospital.

As a pre-meal activity, it is important for nurses to plan their work so that unpleasant sights, sounds and smells will not ruin the patient's appetite for food and drink. As far as possible, treatment appointments in other departments of the hospital should be scheduled for other times of the day, and doctors' rounds should avoid mealtimes.

Children in hospital

Admission to hospital can adversely affect the eating and drinking pattern of people in any age group but for young children, the trauma of separation from mother is compounded by the bewilderment engendered by a change of environment. They are unhappy and confused. In addition, the food will probably be different and will almost certainly be differently served, so recently cultivated home routines for eating and drinking will be broken and their social learning in this AL may be interrupted. It is not surprising if their eating and drinking habits are affected and this may manifest itself as loss of appetite, or refusal to eat, or regressive behaviour with loss of independence in feeding. Nurses can often help to prevent this by asking the parents about the child's likes and dislikes, and previous eating and drinking routines. It is often helpful to children if a parent remains with them during mealtimes.

Moore (1985) says that hospitals have a duty to encourage good eating habits in children. The NACNE report did not put forward a reason why children should not be weaned onto a diet with less fat and less refined and processed foods. The COMA report excluded the under-5s regarding less saturated fats, and suggested that they continue to drink whole milk. However Moore (1985) discusses the subject further, concluding that children do not need the saturated fat from milk if they are taking a healthy mixed diet. Smallman (1987), in the context of malnutrition among children in hospital, describes how to assess those 'at risk' by using a range of assessment tools, including measurement of the mid-upper-arm circumference and grasping the skin at the same site in a calibrated caliper.

CHANGE IN EATING AND DRINKING HABIT

Dietary habits often change during illness. Usually the change is transient but sometimes patients may have to be helped to re-educate themselves about eating and drinking habits on a life-long basis.

Modification of habitual food intake

During illness appetite may range from extreme hunger as is found in uncontrolled diabetes mellitus to utter lack of interest in food when, for example, a patient has a high fever. When in hospital, the range of need is catered for by providing meals which vary in texture and quantity. The variations can be described broadly as normal diet; light diet which contains no fatty, highly-seasoned foods; soft and fluid diets which are 'light' but are in semi-solid or liquid form and used for ill patients or those who have ingestion, digestion and absorption problems.

Some patients, however, whether at home or in hospital, are advised to accept modifications in diet as part of the treatment for a specific disease condition and some may rebel against this suggested restriction of food choice. When patients are grossly overweight for example, it should be ascertained whether or not they are willing to accept a diet which is reduced in its daily kilojoule value, perhaps as low as 4000 kJ, and although this entails an overall reduction in dietary intake it usually involves a gross reduction in foodstuffs which have a high carbohydrate content. Patients often find great difficulty in altering life-long eating habits which involve shunning foods they enjoy, and also they feel hungry. They need much encouragement to resist unsuitable food and drink, and need help to learn about a balanced food intake even after a successful loss of weight. The amount of self-discipline required by patients to maintain a *low carbohydrate/low kilojoule* diet should not be underestimated and their efforts require frequent reinforcement. Before making a plan, it is helpful if overweight people keep a diary of everything eaten and the fluids taken; whether or not they were hungry at the time, as well as their mood. This usually highlights the snacks taken without noticing and when they felt vulnerable. Naturally height will be measured and a weight chart is a visible reminder of any change. Overweight people are then encouraged to make a diet plan; some cope better if they take a small meal at a 3- or 4- hourly interval. Foods containing fibre provide bulk and usually diminish the feeling of hunger. Some people manage best if they join a slimming club, all of which aim at permanent behavioural change related to eating and drinking habits (Ibbotson, 1988). In recent years, proprietary preparations of Very Low Calorie Diets (VLCDs) have gained in popularity. They are particularly tempting to morbidly obese people who can buy these products without going to the doctor. Of course they do not help people to change their eating and drinking habits and this is essential for maintenance of the reduced weight (Fine, 1987).

Young people who are diagnosed as having diabetes mellitus, however, need to develop slightly modified eating and drinking habits on a lifetime basis. A diet with very restricted carbohydrate was recommended up to 1982. Since then, the British Diabetic Association's recommendations allow greater carbohydrate intake, while restricting fat, and continuing to restrict sucrose and other simple sugars. There is more emphasis on controlling total energy intake, which means controlling all food intake, instead of the previous restriction of only carbohydrate foods (Ibbotson, 1986). Indeed the modern diabetic diet is similar to the advocated healthy diet, which means that family cooking need not be so complicated.

Initially these patients may be brought into hospital for tests but once diagnosed and on a regime where they understand the need to balance diet/insulin/exercise, the injections of insulin will deal with the defective carbohydrate metabolism provided the carbohydrate intake is controlled. These people can lead a normal life once they are educated to cope with the diabetic state — and it is a lifelong state. Those who develop diabetes when in the older age bracket are usually obese and the diabetic state can often be contained with a *low carbohydrate/low kilojoule* diet.

Obesity and diabetes mellitus are examples of conditions which necessitate modification in carbohydrate/kilojoule intake but sometimes the fat intake presents a problem. Patients who have infective hepatitis (a form of jaundice) have this type of problem so a *low fat* diet is indicated until the liver recovers from the infection. The problem may be with a specific aspect of fat metabolism, however. People with coronary artery disease may be advised to omit a particular form of fat from the diet, namely saturated fat which is found in lard, butter and other animals fats. It has been found that when dietary intake of saturated fats is greatly reduced the level of blood cholesterol is reduced. High blood cholesterol seems to be associated with the deposition of fatty plaques in the arterial wall and this is conducive to coronary artery disease and myocardial infarction. Those who have had 'heart attacks' are therefore advised to take unsaturated rather than saturated fats in the diet and as with diabetics, this diet is usually advocated for the remainder of the patient's life.

There are occasions when *food and fluid intake is prohibited*; before an anaesthetic and before certain investigations, the patient may be asked to fast for several hours. An explanation with clear instructions about timing is usually all that is required for most adult patients though in *Nil by Mouth?*, Hamilton-Smith as long ago as 1972, deplored the great variations in practice many of which have no scientific basis. 15 years later, in 1987, Thomas reported a small replication of this study and found that no substantial changes had occurred. However, in the same year, Hunt (1987) reported an ongoing operational research project highlighting the complexity of a multidiciplinary approach that was necessary to overcome many of the 'planning' problems which require to be solved before nurses at clinical level can use research findings related to a research-based period of preoperative fasting.

An unnecessary length of preoperative fasting means that patients arrive in the operating theatre in an (albeit temporary) malnourished state, but in the ensuing postoperative days, they may not be able to take adequate nourishment, thereby continuing the malnourishment which is not conducive to wound healing. Hunt's project was based on the physiological necessity for fasting from food for 6 hours, and from fluid for 4 hours prior to an anaesthetic.

In a paediatric ward as well as explaining the reason, any food or drinks on the bedside locker should be temporarily removed. It is important to check whether or not a patient may have a snack on return from an investigation: it may be some time before the next meal is scheduled. If the nurse does not make and serve the snack herself she should ensure that the dietary staff have been requested to do so and that the patient receives it.

Prior to surgery, a patient is often given by injection a drug called atropine which reduces secretion in the mouth and respiratory tract and therefore reduces the danger of inhalation of fluid during anaesthesia. Patients should be told to expect that they will feel thirsty and experience a feeling of dryness in the mouth.

Modification of habitual fluid intake

Problems with fluid intake are often more urgent than those associated with food intake. Fluid deprivation can only be tolerated for a few days and in a 24-hour period the adult human requires about 2500 ml of fluid.

There are obvious reductions in fluid intake when it is impossible to procure drinking water — in dramatic shipwreck and desert rescues for example — but excessive fluid output from the body is the usual cause of *dehydration*. It may be found in any condition featuring high fever, vomiting or diarrhoea and also occurs when there is severe haemorrhage, severe burns, untreated diabetes mellitus and untreated diabetes insipidus. It may occur in milder form. Some elderly people with weak bladder control may deliberately reduce their intake in the hope that it will reduce the need to ask for a bedpan; or the patient who is mentally handicapped may be unable to make decisions about the adequacy of intake; or intake may be depleted during prolonged unconsciousness.

In the early stages of dehydration fluid is withdrawn from the skin and tissues in order to maintain the blood volume while simultaneously the kidneys excrete less urine in order to conserve body fluid. If the cause of dehydration is not treated effectively however, more serious effects ensue. Such patients are thirsty and the tongue looks dry and leathery. There is lethargy, and the eyes (and fontanelle in a baby) appear sunken. The skin loses its natural elasticity and has a wrinkled appearance. Urinary output is not only reduced, but the urine is highly concentrated (Turner & Turner, 1988). In extreme cases, blood volume is reduced causing deficient circulation, and in turn the kidneys fail to excrete waste products. Renal failure and death may ensue.

Where there is mild dehydration, the nurse should encourage the patient to drink and ensure that freshly procured drinks of a desired flavour, perhaps with ice, are available. When there is gross dehydration, intravenous fluids will be required usually in the form of a saline infusion as salt will have been lost along with body fluid.

Any gross loss of fluid is accompanied by a dramatic loss in body weight and records must be maintained of weight, fluid intake, all forms of output — urine, faeces, vomitus — and note made of excessive perspiration. The usual treatment is oral rehydration and it is discussed on page 186.

In contradistinction to dehydration the patient's body may retain an excess amount of fluid and the condition is called *oedema*. Oedema is most commonly seen when the heart, as a pump, is not functioning normally. The resulting swelling — it is recognisable by the way the skin in affected areas 'pits' on pressure — is most obvious in the dependent parts of the body such as the feet, ankles, legs and if the patient is sitting in bed or a chair, in the sacral area. The patient may be distressed by the ugly appearance of swollen ankles, the discomfort, the reduced mobility. If pressure sores are to be prevented, the stretched 'devitalised' skin in affected areas requires special care. When there is gross imbalance fluid will also collect in the pleural and peritoneal cavities causing respiratory difficulty and the patient will then be breathless and uncomfortable, so a procedure to aspirate the fluid may be medically prescribed to alleviate the distress: this will necessitate specific nursing interventions.

It is logical to expect that a patient who has oedema should take a *low fluid/low salt* diet. Again, individual likes and dislikes regarding time and content of fluid intake should be discussed with the patient and a suitable regime adopted. These patients often appreciate a pleasant tasting mouthwash at hand even during the night. Regarding salt intake, condiments are removed from the food tray but salt substitutes may be used for flavouring.

Only a few examples have been cited which involve changes in eating and drinking habits, but in all instances it must be remembered that merely imparting information to the patient does not guarantee advice will be followed. Explaining the reason for a special diet is essential and should take into account the patient's socioeconomic, cultural, religious, moral and ethical values. Wherever possible advice should be related to the usual dietary habits of the individual and modifications rather than drastic change should be attempted.

If the patient must continue a special diet for some time, advice may be required in relation to purchase of certain foods, perhaps unaccustomed foods, and home budgeting may need to be adjusted. When a dietitian is not available to provide such a service, the nurse must inform and assist the patient thereby providing an excellent opportunity to offer health education related to nutrition and food handling should this be necessary. It is important to remember too that a long-term dietary alteration may affect not only the individual but the family, and the nurse should be able to make helpful suggestions about food preparation so that patients do not feel ostracised at meal times or that they are creating extra work because of changes in their daily activity of eating and drinking.

CHANGE IN MODE OF EATING AND DRINKING

Some people, either temporarily for a short or long period, or permanently, are deprived of their usual mode of eating and drinking. If, for any reason, food cannot be ingested, nutrients can be introduced into the gastrointestinal tract and the generic term 'enteral feeding' describes this change of mode in eating and drinking. It includes tube feeding by the nasogastric route, as well as by gastrostomy, duodenostomy and jejunostomy. If a tube can be placed in the upper gastrointestinal tract, nasogastric feeding is usually implemented. If this is not the case, one of the 'ostomy' routes is selected. In the 1970s tube feeding was not so widely used, but with the introduction of various fine bore tubes and recognition of the problem of malnutrition in hospital patients, enteral tube feeding is gaining favour. A fine bore tube can be passed via the skin into one of the 'ostomy' sites, and of the three already mentioned, jejunostomy has become the preferred route as it reduces the risk of reflux into the oesophagus (Wood, 1986). When for any reason there is malabsorption from the small intestine, nutrients are introduced into the venous system and this is called 'parenteral feeding'. These changed modes of eating and drinking will now be discussed.

Nasogastric feeding

When nasogastric feeding is required, the problem for conscious patients is that they are deprived of the sensual pleasure of smell, taste, temperature and texture of food which normally stimulates the flow of saliva and starts the first stage of digestion as well as maintaining moistness of the mouth for comfort and for speaking. Mouth care is therefore very important and a little Vaseline applied to the nostril is usually comforting. Proprietary feeds are available for nasogastric feeding through a fine bore tube and feed contamination has to be avoided (Taylor, 1988a and 1988b). Food and drink can be swallowed in the presence of a nasogastric tube and some nutritionists suggest this 'weaning' process before final removal of the tube. Frank, sensitive discussion with these patients is necessary about how they are going to cope with the social and cultural dimensions of this AL if the treatment has to be prolonged (Bladen, 1986). This cannot be the case for unconscious patients, but the goal is the same; it is to help to preserve life by introducing an adequate supply of nutrients and fluid.

Gastrostomy feeding

After the surgical formation of a fistula between, for example the stomach or jejunum and the skin, nutrients are introduced via a catheter which stays in the fistula. One distinct advantage of 'ostomy' over nasogastric feeding is that patients can usually learn to feed themselves and quickly become independent for feeding and mouth care, although they are dependent on the apparatus and the commercial feeds.

Intravenous (parenteral) feeding

The foregoing methods, although not using the usual oral route for the ingestion of food and fluid, do involve direct entry of nourishment to some part of the digestive tract. In some instances when it is not possible to provide nutrition via the tract itself, food nutrients dissolved in fluid to prevent malnutrition and dehydration, may have to be administered straight into the bloodstream by means of an intravenous infusion — parenteral feeding. The choice to be made by the nutrition team is whether to infuse into a peripheral vein (Fig. 9.1) or a central vein. A disadvantage when using a peripheral vein is that the solutions used are often hypertonic and can damage the lining of the vein causing phlebitis and thrombosis. The past tense might be more appropriate now because in the last decade knowledge about the elements in food and fluids has increased and some isotonic solutions are available, but they are expensive. Peripheral venous feeding continues to be used; combinations of fat with either amino acids and/or glucose in solution are infused and these substances are less hypertonic than previously (Pascoe 1986, pp 287, 289).

Central venous feeding is now more common than previously and the subclavian vein is the most frequently used route. In Pascoe's article (1986) there is a photograph of a central line in situ, having been inserted through the right subclavian vein. The final part of the article discusses weaning patients from total parenteral nutrition. But a small number of patients have to rely on central venous

feeding permanently and when they become independent in using this process are discharged into the community with close liaison between the hospital nutrition team and the community services. Pascoe (1986) likens these programmes to those of home dialysis for people with chronic kidney failure. It has to be remembered that these people are deprived, not only of the sensual pleasure of eating and drinking, but also of the social and psychological pleasures associated with family meals, as well as dining out. Some of them benefit from chewing food and discreetly disposing of it into a tissue (Dewar, 1986).

Oral and dental hygiene was mentioned in the context of nasogastric feeding; they are no less important in people who are being fed intravenously, either peripherally or centrally; temporarily or permanently. Care of the mouth is discussed on page 218.

CHANGE OF DEPENDENCE/INDEPENDENCE STATUS

For a variety of reasons patients may require assistance with the actual activity of eating and drinking, and this should be given graciously and with dexterity so that they will be protected from needless embarrassment resulting from their lack of independence in this AL. The ability to help oneself to food and drink is usually taken so much for granted until circumstances occur which interfere with this activity of living and result in problems of dependence, either temporarily or permanently.

Problems associated with physical dependence

Posture
Even something apparently simple such as a change of physical posture may create ingestion and swallowing problems, for example when patients are forced to lie flat when eating. The distress, difficulty and even indignity suffered by patients in such circumstances should be appreciated by nurses and dealt with sensitively.

Such patients may have to be fed by a nurse, and it is almost impossible for them to feel relaxed if the nurse is standing over them. Nurses should therefore be seated when feeding patients. Obviously food on the plate will have been prepared so that it can be lifted to the mouth by one piece of cutlery, a fork or spoon, whichever the patient prefers. The question arises, should the nurse sit at one side, facing the same way as the patient, so that the nurse's hand can mimic the movement of the patient's preferred hand when lifting food from plate to mouth? Or should the nurse sit facing the patient? Perhaps patients can be asked about their preference which should be written on the nursing plan, so that nurses on each shift offer the same sort of help. Liquids may be interspersed throughout the meal or offered at the end according to the

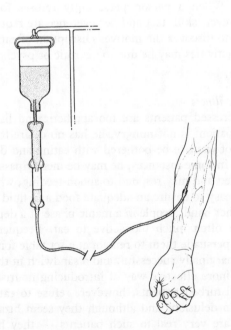

Fig. 9.1 Intravenous feeding

patient's wishes. Liquids can be given from a spouted feeding cup but a drinking straw usually allows better control of the flow and nowadays, angled straws made from materials which can withstand warm fluids make mealtimes less difficult for people who require help with feeding.

Oral hygiene is often required before and after the meal and it is a cardinal rule that, unless contraindicated (for example when a patient is unconscious, or is on restricted fluids) anyone who needs special oral hygiene, needs also to be helped to take oral fluids in order to keep the mouth tissues in a healthy, comfortable state.

Physical handicap

The majority of people who become physically handicapped live at home. When assessing their dependence/independence status for eating and drinking one has to start with the early preparations. Can they go shopping for food? Can they prepare food in the kitchen? Can they cook it? If they cannot be helped to go shopping themselves, usually the social services can make arrangements for their shopping to be done by another person. In the UK there are many centres where gadgets which can help with preparing and cooking food are displayed. There are several devices available for 'stabilising' food or containers which is the key problem for a one-handed person, for example vegetables can be mobilised on a spiked board to accomplish peeling and chopping. There are 'tip-up' stands to enable pouring from teapots and kettles, as well as non-spill cups, plate guards, unbreakable crockery and several types of modified cutlery. The occupational therapist can often make useful suggestions which will help the patient to retain independence and dignity at mealtimes. Spilling of food and soiling of clothes are distasteful to most people, especially when eating in the company of others who are not at a physical disadvantage.

However, there are some people whose physical handicap precludes them from achieving independence and they remain dependent for feeding throughout the lifespan. Non-progressive brain damage (usually at birth) can result in spasticity of muscles, and/or inability to control muscular movement so that the limbs, and perhaps the head and neck, are never still; there is continuous purposeless movement. Speech therapists have highlighted the complexities of feeding such people, and Anderson (1983) wrote a book, *Feeding — a guide to assessment and intervention with handicapped children*, to help parents and professionals working with children who have profound learning difficulties, including learning to eat and drink. Though described in clear language there is no doubt about the complexity of eating and drinking. Such handicapped people may be admitted to a general hospital for a reason other than the handicap. If the usual 'feeder' cannot attend all mealtimes, nurses should observe the technique so that they can provide 'continuity of feeding' when necessary.

Respiratory distress

Understandably, breathless patients will appreciate soft foods which do not require unnecessary effort in chewing. Foods such as steaks and vegetables are obviously contraindicated and dry foods such as biscuits can be dangerous if inhaled during a breathless episode so should either be avoided or accompanied with fluid to moisten them. Breathless patients need extra time to eat and should be spared the effort of speaking during a meal though not ignored; any verbal communication can be done mainly by the nurse. It may be necessary to give smaller amounts of food more frequently and every attempt should be made to provide interesting meals which are easy to digest but nutritious.

Impaired vision

Occasionally blind patients are admitted to hospital, or as a result of an accident or operation (for example, removal of a cataract) a patient may temporarily have the eyes bandaged. In these circumstances the food should be cut into mouth-size pieces and the type of food described when served. In most instances, the patient should be helped to retain independence in eating but where necessary the nurse should give assistance.

Problems associated with emotional/psychological dependence

Stress

At some time or other in their lives, most people have experienced emotional stress and one of the manifestations of anxiety can be loss of appetite. The stress and the accompanying upset of the AL of eating and drinking are usually transient. When a person persistently refuses food and fluid, however, skill, tact and perseverence are required by the nurse to discover the motive. Disruption of eating and drinking activities may be due to neurotic or psychotic disorders.

Psychiatric illness

Many depressed patients are too apathetic and listless to eat. The patient is not hungry, he has no desire for food, he does not want to be bothered with eating and drinking activities. In some instances, he may be merely passive and uninterested and may respond to spoon-feeding, when it is relatively easy to ensure an adequate food and fluid intake. On the other hand, people in a manic phase of a depressive illness are often much too active to eat. Frequently attempts to persuade them to remain at a set table for a meal are only marginally successful, and a sandwich in the hand may be a more effective way of introducing nourishment.

Some disturbed patients, however, refuse to eat. They suffer from delusions and although they seem bizarre the delusions are very real to such patients — they have no money to pay for food; they are unworthy; their 'bowels are blocked'; the food has been poisoned; a voice is telling them not to eat. At every mealtime, therefore, they require persuasion to eat and having done so, may vomit in order to avert the awful consequences they think will ensue if they retain the food in their body.

Other problems with eating which have an emotional connotation may be exacerbated by advertisements in the media in Western countries which propagate the message that to be slim is to be attractive. Indeed, health professionals in the health promotion aspect of their work reinforce this image. Most people make dietary choices which (together with the exercise they take) enable them to feel reasonably comfortable with their psychological body image regarding its physical shape and size. However for a minority of people, mainly young women (usually adolescents), their eating programme gets beyond their control, and they experience feelings such as shame, and guilt at their behaviour which can include undereating, over-eating, self-induced vomiting achieved by drinking large amounts of water; over-use of laxatives, diuretics, and even self-administered enemas (Biley & Savage, 1984). Three names are given to the conditions which may include one or more of these behaviours — compulsive eating, anorexia nervosa and bulimia nervosa. They are not mutually exclusive and people can have periods when any one of the three predominates (p. 157).

Anorexic people appear to lack insight into the disorder, making it difficult for them to accept the necessity for treatment. The goal is restoration of body weight and adequate eating habits, together with psychological adjustment involving reduction of weight phobia, and the development of methods of coping with emotional conflict.

Mental handicap

More and more attention is being paid to helping mentally handicapped people to acquire the functional skills required in everyday living. A clinical psychologist, Scott (1986), gives an account of how a student nurse helped a 27-year-old severely mentally handicapped and totally blind man who had been in hospital since childhood to achieve independence for feeding. The ambitious behavioural programme required great commitment and perseverance, but the article states that 4 years later the man was still feeding himself. Such a long-lasting achievement is surely worth the necessary commitment and perseverance.

Alcohol abuse

It is relevant to consider 'alcoholism' here, as not only is it associated with the AL of drinking, but it inevitably changes individuals' dependence/independence status. Factual information about the volume and frequency of alcohol intake required to produce the state of dependence is difficult to obtain, because only individual drinkers know this, and both volume and frequency may be minimised or maximised when giving information for a 'drinking history'.

It is estimated that 20% of general hospital beds in the UK are occupied by those who drink at levels harmful to health, and it is increased to approximately one-third of patients in psychiatric wards. However early identification and intervention have been effective. Doctors and nurses are increasingly being encouraged to identify those patients 'at risk' before severe health problems develop, or alcohol dependence is established. In a research project Maynard & Rowland (1988) developed a brief alcohol screening questionnaire which took 1–2 minutes to complete; the objective was to identify patients 'at risk' from alcohol-related problems. For the purpose of their study 'excessive drinking' was defined as 36+ units of alcohol per week for men, and 24+ for women. A unit of alcohol is a half pint of beer or lager; a glass of wine; a glass of fortified wine (port or sherry); or one 'standard' measure of spirits. Watts (1987) gives further advice about 'defining alcohol abuse'; as does the booklet *That's the limit* (1986) published by the Health Education Council, London.

The development of alcohol dependence is usually insidious. In some countries, wine drinking may be a normal part of mealtimes and in many societies, people can enjoy a drink socially without experiencing any compulsion to take more. Some people, however, come to be dependent on alcohol and this may manifest itself in behaviour which is atypical for that person such as disregard for personal appearance, unpunctuality, irritability or absence from work. Excessive drinking may also lead to irresponsible behaviour, petty crime, casual sexual activity which can be sexual abuse, and even disorderly behaviour amounting to assault, perhaps involving police custody. All these deviations bring attendant distress to family and friends.

Sometimes the problem is less easy to detect because the person appears to function adequately in everyday activities yet needs to imbibe at increasingly frequent intervals during the day in order to cope with commitments. As might be expected, the affected individual begins to suffer from malnutrition because the appetite for food decreases; weight is then lost and health deteriorates. Eventually there are economic overtones as more and more money is spent on procuring alcohol to the detriment of the family budget, and work capacity may become impaired, often to the point of loss of employment.

In the UK, various voluntary associations work in conjunction with the National Council for Alcoholism. One is for ex-alcoholics and is called Alcoholics Anonymous (AA), a world-wide association. Members of local branches meet frequently to give each other moral support in the long and continuous process of refraining from drinking alcohol. Another is called the A1-Anon Family Group which is for the spouse, friends and relatives of the alcoholic, and they help one another to cope with the many problems of alcoholism which impinge on family life and cause untold upset.

Despite efforts to provide treatment for alcohol abuse, the problem seems to be growing. There is evidence to suggest that alcohol intake is increasing among all groups in our society but particularly among women and particularly among women in the 18–25 age group (Dunbar & Morgan, 1987). These findings have considerable significance not only because drinking is starting in a younger age group but because excessive drinking during pregnancy can have adverse effects on fetal development resulting in a range of abnormalities termed Fetal Alcohol Syndrome (Sulaiman et al, 1988). Although most studies about FAS come from the USA, it occurs in many parts of the world and in many races. Even in the postnatal period, the effects of alcohol abuse during pregnancy can be exhibited in the newborn. Symptoms of alcohol withdrawal have been observed within 6–12 hours of birth. McKnight & Merrett (1987) recognise alcohol consumption in pregnancy as an area for antenatal education.

Symptoms of 'withdrawal' are perhaps more easily identified when an alcohol abuser is suddenly deprived of alcohol as may occur after an accident requiring immediate surgery and a stay in hospital. Withdrawal symptoms featuring restlessness, agitation, hallucinations, delirium and disorientation may occur, together with tremor and shaking; the term used for the condition is delirium tremens. The patient may decide to use the incident to seek treatment and if so requires sensitive handling and a great deal of encouragement to proceed. Help may be obtained in one of the special centres which have been created for those who are highly motivated to overcome the uncontrollable craving for liquor. However there is a movement away from intensive therapeutic intervention and prolonged inpatient stay. It is often considered preferable to help the alcoholic and the family within their own environment, mobilising community resources (Kennedy & Wright, 1988). In this context, inpatient care is seen as a phase within an overall treatment plan, and not sufficient in itself.

Currently in the UK there are vigorous campaigns to educate the public about the dangers of alcohol abuse in an attempt to prevent the distress associated with dependence on alcohol and all its sequelae.

Health professionals in the community are educating patients to cope with their drink problem (Ryder & Hart, 1986). So that health professionals can help people to use alcohol with social and personal responsibility, an education and training programme has been developed.

SOME SPECIFIC PROBLEMS ASSOCIATED WITH EATING AND DRINKING

Sore mouth

A sore mouth can be an actual problem of which patients are all too aware. When one considers the many structures forming the mouth — the tongue, teeth, gums, inner cheeks, upper palate, tonsils and the salivary glands which pour their secretion into the mouth — one realises that there has to be location of the 'soreness' before appropriate nurse-initiated intervention can be planned.

A sore tongue for example can be due to something as straightforward as the sharp edge of a damaged natural tooth, or friction from dentures. The nurse-initiated intervention will be vigilant oral hygiene described on page 218. Application of a local anaesthetic gel will produce temporary relief to facilitate eating and drinking, but an appointment with a dental member of the health team will be necessary. On the other hand, a sore tongue can result from insufficient intake or poor absorption of vitamins B and C and dietary iron, contributing to different types of anaemia. If investigations confirm these causes, there will be a medical prescription to remedy them and it will include the consequent nursing interventions such as drug administration, as well as those which are nurse-initiated.

'Toothache' is applied to several phenomena — the constant dull ache from dental caries, and the throbbing ache from a root abscess, as well as the jagging pain when an exposed nerve is in contact with hot or cold fluid or food. Obviously dental treatment is required for these conditions and a dental appointment has to be made for long stay patients. In an emergency, to provide relief, the usual household remedies can be used, for example the application of oil of cloves and use of a local anaesthetic gel to facilitate toothbrushing so that the healthy teeth are not compromised. Soft food can be offered when chewing triggers toothache, and food and fluids at body temperature will be appreciated when there is an exposed nerve.

Inflammation of the gums (gingivitis), the tongue (glossitis) and the whole mouth (stomatitis) can occur when the natural oral flora (non-pathogenic commensals) are compromised, that is the state of colonisation ends and infection begins (p. 75). The subject is important because the change can be caused by treatments such as antibiotics, chemotherapy and radiotherapy: it can also be changed by a specific infection such as AIDS. For example, the fungus Candida albicans, a normal commensal in the mouth, can become pathogenic causing thrush. Some patients have found Redoxon mouth washes refreshing, and half a Redoxon tablet left on the tongue effervesces and cleans, and helps the person to feel more comfortable. Gentian violet mouthwashes three times a day, for 4 days, may also be recommended. Or antifungal tablets may be medically prescribed to be retained in the mouth for as long as possible four times daily for at least 4 days. Part of the resultant nursing intervention is helping patients to understand the prescription and to resist resorting to chewing the tablets, as well as continuing the full course even if they think that the condition has been 'cured' after only 2 or 3 days.

A sore mouth is always a potential problem in

dehydrated patients and those with insufficient flow of saliva; febrile and·ill patients are also at risk of developing an actual problem, and information about ways of preventing this happening is on page 218.

A sore mouth can be due to complicated pathology such as cancer when the nursing interventions ensuing from the medical prescription will be additional to the already suggested nurse-initiated interventions.

Problems with swallowing

Knowledge about the complex activities related to swallowing (p. 155) is essential to facilitate understanding of the problems which can be experienced with this part of the AL of eating and drinking. Much of the recent knowledge about feeding patients has been contributed by speech therapists who realised that treatment for the motor and sensory neuromuscular dysfunctions involved in speech impediments, whether congenital or acquired as a result of disease, were in fact related in many instances to swallowing.

With the increased multidisciplinary interest in patients who have feeding and swallowing problems, 'Feeding aids resource centres' are being developed in various parts of the UK. In some areas a specialist 'feeding team' has been established comprising occupational therapist, physiotherapist, speech therapist and sometimes a technical aids officer (Caunter & Penrose, 1983). The team carries out a full assessment and, in conjunction with nurses, plans suitable individual programmes so that people with these problems can achieve their optimal independence, according to their circumstances, to achieve the goal of optimal nourishment without loss of social or psychological dignity. It is important that nurses record the amount of food and fluid taken, as well as the rate of progress towards optimal independence.

After a stroke, many people have feeding and swallowing difficulties. Re-educating the feeding mechanism is a necessary nursing contribution which requires guidance from the dietitian and speech therapist. Frequent practice at biting a Bikkipeg strengthens the relevant muscles. A syringe may be used to place a small quantity of liquid in inner lip, followed by a facilitated swallow. It is accomplished by placing a hand under the person's lower jaw, and raising it, thereby moving the tongue up and back in readiness for swallowing (Cockcroft & Ray, 1985).

Re-learning to swallow has been further helped by the development of a sensory stimulating loop which can be fitted to an upper denture if one is worn. If the patient has natural teeth, the loop is fitted to a dental plate (Knowles & Selley, 1988). Nurses can also contribute more to the rehabilitation of people's post-stroke lip dysfunction by attending to 'food catches' on the lips during feeding, and the escape of food from the mouth. As each of these dysfunctions has social and psychological implications for the patient, it is important for nurses to help with re-learning of eating and drinking independently and with dignity

(Carr & Hawthorne, 1988). A training programme which was originally developed by Heimlich was used to re-train swallowing in a 78-year-old man who in the previous 3 years had been fed by nasogastric tube (Axelsson et al, 1986).

Handicapped people, whether it is a mental and/or physical handicap, often have eating problems; these can be associated with hyposensitivity, hypersensitivity, sucking, biting, chewing, swallowing and drooling. They are rarely present singularly; for example, the presence of a speech problem may accompany disability in sucking, chewing and swallowing; drooling is usually due to lack of sensation and swallowing less frequently than normal (Cauriter & Penrose, 1983). Anderson's book (1983), mentioned on page 168 in the context of 'Problems associated with physical dependence', is equally applicable here in the context of 'Feeding and swallowing problems related to eating and drinking'.

Nausea

This condition is easily recognised by the person experiencing it but difficult to describe. It occurs in waves, may be accompanied by excess salivation, pallor and sweating, and is often a precursor of vomiting. Almost always there is loss of appetite. Nausea may merely be a manifestation of over-indulgence in food and drink but can also occur associated with anxiety states, post-anaesthesia, jaundice, dysfunction in the digestive tract, or the ingestion of drugs which irritate the lining of the digestive tract, or pain anywhere in the body. It may also be a symptom in the early months of pregnancy probably due to hormonal changes in the mother's body. It may also occur as an undesirable side-effect after administration of, for example, morphine or digoxin, in which case the drug may be stopped, or given in a reduced dose. Nausea can also be a reaction to cytotoxic drugs. Patients with cancer may be debilitated and the additional problem of nausea is very distressing. To relieve it, acupuncture is increasingly being used. In one project, 105 patients, all of whom had experienced severe sickness during a first course of cytotoxic chemotherapy, were prescribed acupuncture. Most achieved a 'very good' result which was no sickness during the subsequent 8 hours. The technique can be repeated. Other parts of the trial included patients experiencing postoperative and morning sickness and they produced similar results (Dundee, 1988).

Nausea is distressing to the sufferer and the nurse should be comforting and supportive. Some people find it helpful to suck ice when feeling nauseated, others prefer a peppermint flavour, still others find it helpful to lie down in a quiet, well ventilated room. For some a modification of diet, avoiding the nausea-producing food or drink is all that is required. For others an anti-emetic drug may be medically prescribed to be given subcutaneously to relieve the discomfort until the cause is isolated and treated.

Vomiting

Nausea may be followed by expulsion of the stomach contents. In instances where vomiting is persistent it can lead to dehydration because of the excessive loss of body fluids. It is important for the nurse to observe:

time of occurrence
— early morning: related to pregnancy, renal disease
— soon after a meal and giving relief from pain: related to gastric ulceration

character and appearance
— containing undigested food: related to indiscretion of food and drink
— containing red blood: related to rupture of a blood vessel in the upper digestive tract
— containing dark red digested blood ('coffee grounds'): related to gastric ulceration
— containing brown foul-smelling material ('faecal vomit'): related to intestinal obstruction

manner of ejection
— effortless and in small quantities: related to intestinal obstruction
— with much pain and retching: related to gastritis and gastric ulceration
— projectile and without warning: related to head injuries, pyloric stenosis (obstruction due to narrowing of the pyloric orifice)

any accompanying diarrhoea/constipation

Whatever the form, the nurse should procure, and help the patient to hold the vomit bowl, and assist by wiping his mouth with a tissue. The bed should be screened. Usually patients find it comforting if a hand is placed on their forehead and nurses' behaviour conveys assurance and sympathy without disgust at such episodes which are undoubtedly unpleasant for both patient and nurse. Most people find it easier if in a sitting position with the head over a basin but if it is necessary to lie flat, the head should be turned to one side and supported, and the patient should be helped into a side-lying position.

It is important to remove vomitus and any soiled linen from the vicinity of patients as quickly as possible. Should the vomit contain frank blood, or the linen be soiled with blood, and the patient has serum hepatitis, or is a carrier of the hepatitis B virus, or is HIV seropositive, or has AIDS, then the nurse must carry out the procedure recommended by the health authority when removing the vomit bowl and soiled linen. Facilities should be provided for them to sponge the face and hands and have a refreshing mouth-wash. A specimen of vomitus should be retained for inspection, as it may be helpful in diagnosis of the cause.

Observation of patients who are in an impaired level of consciousness (p. 328) which includes recovering from an anaesthetic is of critical importance. Death can readily result because of respiratory obstruction caused by vomit being sucked into the airway; during such states, patients should be turned on to one side in the semi-prone position with all pillows removed until consciousness is regained and with it, the protective cough reflex.

Heartburn

A burning sensation behind the sternum, often accompanied by regurgitation of an acid-like fluid into the mouth is called heartburn. Other terms used for the condition are pyrosis and waterbrash. Usually it occurs following meals and is frequently associated with a gastric ulcer or a hiatus hernia (herniation of abdominal contents into the thorax) but clears up when the ulcer heals or the hernia is repaired. It may be alleviated however by maintaining a sitting position following meals and sometimes, taking an oral alkaline mixture effectively prevents its occurrence. If these measures are unsuccessful a mouthwash helps to counteract the discomfort.

Flatulence

Some patients complain of 'wind' or flatulence. Two types are recognised. Inevitably some air is swallowed when eating and sometimes when the stomach contracts, the air can be expelled up the oesophagus and produces what is termed belching. In some cultures it is a mark of appreciation following an enjoyable meal; in Western culture belching is usually considered to be an embarrassment. As a single feature, gastric flatulence is not generally considered to be pathological but can cause a great deal of discomfort or even pain and may be relieved by taking a peppermint sweet, or a drink of peppermint water which is usually more effective when given in hot water. Intestinal flatulence is discussed on page 197.

Halitosis

Halitosis literally means a foul-smelling breath and although the sufferer may not be aware of the condition, it is apparent to those in the vicinity. The condition is being discussed in this section of problems related to the AL of eating and drinking because it can be caused by infected gums or decayed teeth and dental attention may be indicated. It also occurs in very ill patients or those who are not taking sufficient fluid and food to keep the mouth clean and healthy. In such instances, the mouth and tongue become coated with a film consisting of bacteria, dead cells and decaying food and it is a nursing responsibility to provide frequent mouth care which will prevent or reduce halitosis and help the patient to feel more comfortable. Unless contraindicated, the patient should be helped to drink as much fluid as possible.

Exhaustion, emaciation, cachexia

The word cachexia, in the last 2 decades has been associated with cancer and more recently with AIDS. Gross loss of weight can be the patient's problem which motivates a visit to the doctor. On the other hand, the loss of weight may occur after the first course of treatment whether it is radiotherapy alone or combined with cytotoxic chemotherapy. Cancer involves a proliferation of cells which require increased metabolism, and there is some evidence that it is abnormal metabolism (Woods, 1989). She says that in the current state of knowledge there can be a place for aggressive use of parenteral nutrition (p. 167) in these patients to allow better tolerance of chemotherapy and radiotherapy.

Food allergy

Many authors of scientific papers prefer to retain the term 'allergy' for reference to immunological mechanisms only, and suggest the use of 'idiosyncrasy' or 'food intolerance' to describe an adverse reaction to food (Hall, 1987). For the people who suffer, the terms will seem irrelevant. They may experience swelling in different parts of the body; heavy perspiration unrelated to exercise: fatigue not helped by rest; bouts of tachycardia; fluctuations in weight; and the symptoms come and go. Although some patients will have strong suspicions as to which foods provoke the symptoms, history alone should not be relied on and is no substitute for controlled clinical observation, 'elimination dieting' and challenge with suspected food allergens.

The problems of food allergy can be more dramatic in a baby and may involve for example vomiting, diarrhoea, abdominal colic, rash, respiratory distress, irritability and general failure to thrive (David, 1985). Diagnosis is difficult but identification of the cause and treatment may be life-saving.

Pain

Pain in the digestive tract may occur because of an inflammatory condition, an obstruction, a hiatus hernia, an unusual growth, and may be accompanied by vomiting.

Varying degrees of pain occur in most diseases of the upper gastrointestinal tract, often related to the intake of food and often at a specific time interval after meals. Foods which are difficult to digest — fried foods, rich carbohydrates and highly spiced foods — are particularly liable to cause pain and most frequently it is experienced in the epigastric region. The degree or duration of pain from gastric ulceration can often be reduced by taking an oral dose of an alkaline mixture, but in principle, pain should be dealt with by treating the cause.

Pain in a hollow muscular tube like the digestive tract can be experienced as *colic*, a severe sharp shooting pain. Colic is a discomfort not uncommonly experienced by babies and it may accompany many types of disorder affecting the digestive tract.

Referred pain (p. 123) can be a feature of gallbladder disease, and the patient feels the pain in the region of his scapula (shoulder blade).

Anxiety about investigations

To assess deviations in the capacity to eat and drink, and any pain/discomfort in the digestive tract, various investigations are carried out, some of them very elaborate and requiring sophisticated equipment. The most commonly used in relation to this AL of eating and drinking are probably X-ray, which may or may not be combined with a barium swallow or barium meal; gastric secretion tests, and gastroscopy, with or without a biopsy. The actual technique of X-ray is not painful; the barium swallow and barium meal are distasteful; the gastric secretion test causes discomfort but the gastroscopy can be alarming and may even be painful. Nevertheless in all circumstances, the patient will have some anxiety about what he will be expected to do, how he will react and what the result will be.

The nurse must therefore take time to explain any preparation involved prior to the procedure and what to expect during and after. Any relevant instructions about the patient's expected behaviour should be stated clearly and simply. Factual information about the preparation and technique will be found in the ward's procedure book but the nurse must interpret it to the patient according to her perception of his preparedness to receive the information.

Feedback about the result of tests are usually of crucial importance to the patient and are given by the doctor or the nurse in charge of the ward/clinic/health centre.

Whatever the nature of the illness, all patients require a healthful diet delivered in the manner most suitable to the circumstances. The nutrition of patients must be seen as part of the total care and may well determine the success or failure of other treatments. Maintaining or regaining appropriate nutritional status is a crucial aim of treatment, and although it is the responsibility of a health care team, nurses are important members. Nurses are with the patient when meals are served and have the opportunity to note if they take the food and fluid, enjoy eating and drinking or if, as quoted earlier, the patients 'just tumble over the contents of the plate or dip the spoon into the cup to deceive the nurse'.

Individualising nursing

The first part of this chapter reflects the model — the nature of the AL of eating and drinking; the relationship of the lifespan to the AL; the effect of the individual's dependence/independence status; the influence of physical, psychological, sociocultural, environmental and politicoeconomic factors on the AL. In the second part of the chapter, a selection of actual and potential problems which are experienced by people in relation to the AL have been described. With this background of general knowledge about the AL, it should be possible to incorporate such information (when it is relevant to the person's current circumstances) in an individual nursing plan.

While describing the model for nursing, only general information was given about individualising nursing (p. 51) which in fact is synonymous with the concept of the nursing process.

Out of this background of general knowledge about the AL of eating and drinking, and about individualising nursing, it should then be possible to extend the issues which are relevant to an individual's current circumstances (whether in a health or illness setting), that is, to make an assessment of relevant issues according to the individual's stage on the lifespan, according to current level of dependence/independence; and take into account the relevant physical, psychological, sociocultural, environmental and politicoeconomic factors. Collectively, this information would provide a profile of the person's individuality in relation to this AL.

As indicated earlier in the text, this assessment would be achieved by various means such as observing the person, acquiring information about the individual's usual habits in relation to eating and drinking, partly by listening to the patient and/or relatives; and partly by using relevant information from available records. The collected information could then be examined to identify any actual problems being experienced with the AL and these would be arranged in an order of priority. The nurse might also recognise some potential problems — not all possible potential problems, but those which are relevant. Mutually agreed realistic goals could then be set to prevent potential problems from becoming actual ones; to alleviate or solve the actual problems; or to help the person cope with those which cannot be alleviated or solved.

Keeping in mind, what the person can and cannot do unaided, the nursing interventions to achieve the mutually set goals could then be selected according to local circumstances and available resources.

Following implementation of the interventions, their effects could be evaluated in relation to the goals set, and if goals were not reached, they would then be revised or rescheduled, or even discarded. It is worth repeating here that although discussed in four phases — assessing, planning, implementing and evaluating — individualising nursing is not a linear progression, it assumes a built-in responsiveness to feedback at any of the phases, with ample allowance for change within the overall framework.

During an illness episode, an important consideration is the rehabilitation of the individual, and planning for this should commence almost as soon as the person enters the

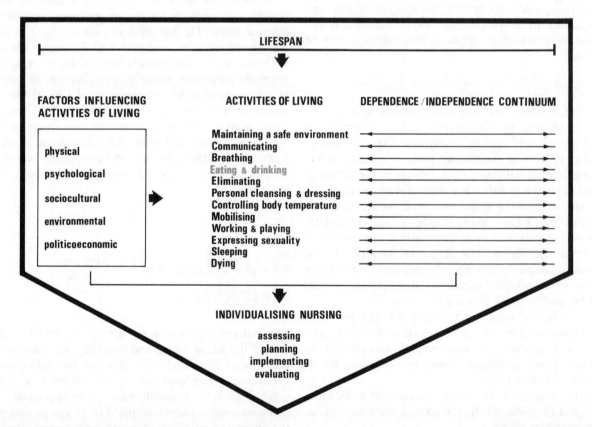

Fig. 9.2 The AL of eating and drinking within the model for nursing

health system. Another important feature is the professional judgement required to discontinue the nurse/patient relationship when it is no longer relevant.

This chapter has been concerned with the AL of eating and drinking. However, as stated previously it is only for the purpose of discussion that any AL can be considered on its own; in reality the various activities are so closely related and do not have distinct boundaries. Figure 9.2 is a reminder that the AL of eating and drinking is related to the other ALs and also to the various components of the model for nursing.

REFERENCES

Alderman C 1988 Bad taste (Food-borne disease) Nursing Standard 2 (40) July 9: 28–29

Anderson C A 1983 Feeding — a guide to assessment and intervention with handicapped children. Jordanhill College of Education, Glasgow, Scotland

Axelsson K, Norberg A, Asplund K 1986 Relearning to eat late after a stroke by systematic nursing intervention: a case report. Journal of Advanced Nursing 11 (5) September: 553–559

Bennett M 1988 The fibre squad. Nursing Times 84 (4) January 27: 160–161

Biley F, Savage S 1984 Anorexia nervosa. Nursing Times 80 (31) August 1: 28–32

Bladen L M 1986 Enteral nutrition. Nursing: The Add On Journal of Clinical Nursing 3 (8) August: 281–285

Brandt W 1980 North-South: a programme for survival. Pan Books, London

British Medical Journal 1988 Alcohol services: exhortations rather than commitment. British Medical Journal 297 July 23: 241–242

Burkitt D 1983 Don't forget fibre in your diet. Dunitz, London, p 66–68

Carlisle D 1988 Food for thought (hospital food does not have a sparkling reputation). Nursing Standard 2 (15) January 16: 28

Carr E K, Hawthorne P 1988 Lip function and eating after a stroke: a nursing perspective. Journal of Advanced Nursing 13: 447–451

Caunter M, Penrose J 1983 Solving feeding problems (mentally handicapped people). Nursing Times 79 (51) December 21: 24–26

Cockcroft G, Ray M 1985 Feeding problems in stroke patients. Nursing Mirror 160 (9) February 27: 26–29

COMA (Committee on Medical Aspects of Food Policy) 1984 Diet and cardiovascular disease: Report on health and social subjects, no. 28. DHSS, HMSO, London

David T 1985 Intolerant babies. Community Outlook March: 22, 27–28

Debenham K 1988 Meeting nutritional needs. Nursing Times 84 (13) March 30: 32–34

Devlin R 1984 The great sterilising debate. Nursing Times (Community Outlook) 80 (27) July 11: 246

Dewar B J 1986 Total parenteral nutrition at home. Nursing Times 82 (28) July 9: 35, 37–38

DHSS 1988 Present day practice in infant feeding: third report. Report of a working party of the panel on Child Nutrition, Committee on Medical Aspects of Food Policy. HMSO, London

Dickerson J 1988 The food chain. Nursing Times (Community Outlook) 84 (6) February: 15–16, 18

Dickerson J W T 1986a Hospital induced malnutrition: a cause for concern. The Professional Nurse 1 (11) August: 293–296

Dickerson J W T 1986b Nutrition in health and illness. Nursing: The Add-On Journal of Clinical Nursing 3 (8) August: 303–307

Dunbar G C, Morgan D D V 1987 The changing pattern of alcohol consumption in England and Wales, 1978–1985. British Medical Journal 295 October 3: 807–810

Dundee J W 1988 Acupressure as an antimetic. Acupuncture in Medicine. V (1) August: 22–24

Feinmann J 1988 Breast is still best (HIV infection). Nursing Times 84 (28) July 13: 21

Fine G 1987 International conferences on obesity. Nursing: The Add-On Journal of Clinical Nursing 3 (16) April: 616–618

Fisher C, Minns H 1986 Successful breastfeeding. The Professional Nurse 1 (12) September: 329–331

Francis D E M 1984 The infant feeding controversy. Nursing: The Add-On Journal of Clinical Nursing 2 (22) February: 635–638

Hall D E 1987 Adverse food reaction. The Professional Nurse 2 (6) March: 183–184

Hamilton-Smith S 1972 Nil by mouth? Royal College of Nursing, London

Health Education Council 1986 That's the limit. Health Education Council, London

Holmes A 1986 Food additives. Nursing: The Add-On Journal of Clinical Nursing 3 (8) August: 293–295

Holmes S 1986a Nutritional needs of medical patients (interaction of drugs). Nursing Times 82 (17) April 23: 34–36

Holmes S 1986b Determinants of food intake. Nursing: The Add-On Journal of Clinical Nursing 3 (7) July: 260–264

Holmes S 1987 Sweet nothings (Report on children's diet). Nursing Times 83 (27) September 23: 32–34

Holmes S 1988a Current dietary recommendations. Nursing Standard (Special supplement) October 1: 5–6

Holmes S 1988b Does a high fat diet cause heart disease? Nursing Times 84 (13) March 30: 34–35

Holmes S 1989 Nutrition and the elderly. Nursing 3 (37) May: 18–21

Hunt M 1987 The process of translating research findings into nursing practice. Journal of Advanced Nursing 12 January: 101–110

Ibbotson M 1986 Living with a diabetic diet. The Professional Nurse 2 (3) December: 69–71

Ibbotson M 1988 Not another diet? The Professional Nurse 3 (8) May: 299–301

Janes E 1986 Changing our eating habits. Nursing: The Add-On Journal of Clinical Nursing 3 (7) July: 268–272

Jeff S 1989 Inaccurate measurement of baby milk powder. Journal of the Royal College of General Practitioners 39: 113

Kennedy J, Wright S 1988 Sobering thoughts. Nursing Standard 2 (26) April 2: 22–23

Knowles C, Selley W 1988 Relearning to swallow after a stroke. Nursing Times 84 (36) September 7: 46–47

Martin J, White A 1988 Infant feeding 1985. HMSO, London

Maynard A, Rowland 1988 The battle of the booze. Nursing Standard 2 (42) July 23: 32

McKnight A, Merrett D 1987 Alcohol consumption in pregnancy — a health education problem. Journal of the Royal College of General Practitioners 37 February: 73–76

Moore J 1985 Feeding sick children. Nursing Times 81 (51) December 18/25: 29–30

NACNE (National Advisory Committee on Nutritional Education) 1983 A discussion paper on proposals for nutritional guidelines for health education in Britain. Health Education Council, London

Nursing Times 1985 Pick a plateful. Nursing Times 81 (12) March 20: 40

O'Byrne J 1989 Food poisoning alert. Nursing Standard 18 (3) January 28: 8–9

Pascoe D A 1986 Total parenteral nutrition. Nursing: The Add-On Journal of Clinical Nursing 3 (8) August: 286–289, 291–292

Pownall M 1986 Vitamins, glorious vitamins. Nursing Times 82 (30) July 30: 49–50

Pownall M 1987 Ray treatment for food. Nursing Times 83 (22) June 3: 43–44

Reid L 1989 Food for thought: on food laws. Evening News April 7: 9

Renn M 1987 Is breast second best? Nursing Times 83 (6) February 11: 19–20

Ryder D, Mark P 1986 A context for drinking. Community Outlook September: 27–28, 30

Sanford J 1987 Making meals a pleasure. Nursing Times 83 (7) February 18: 31–32

Savage S, Biley F 1984 Bulimia nervosa. Nursing Times 80 (32) August 8: 42–45

Scott D 1986 Time and patience. Nursing Times 82 (32) August 6: 36–37

Smallman S 1987 Nutritional assessment of children in hospital. Nursing Times 83 (5) February 4: 55–57

Smith S 1988 Battle of the breast. Nursing Times 84 (34) August 24: 21

Stubbs L 1989 Taste changes in cancer patients. Nursing Times 85 (3) January 18: 49–50

Sulaiman et al 1988 Alcohol consumption in Dundee primigravidas and its effects on outcome of pregnancy (study). British Medical Journal 296: 1500–1503

Taylor M 1988 Food, glorious food. Nursing Times 84 (13) March 30: 28–30

Taylor S J 1988a A guide to NG feeding equipment. The Professional Nurse 4 (2) November: 91–93

Taylor S J 1988b A guide to nasogastric feeding. The Professional Nurse 3 (11) August: 439–442

Thomas E A 1987 Preoperative fasting — a question of routine? Nursing Times 83 (49) December 9: 46–47 (Occasional paper 83 (7))

Turner T 1988 Milk of human kindness? Nursing Times 84 (8) February 24: 19

Turner T 1989 A chilling business? Nursing Times 85 (5) February 1: 19

Turner J, Turner A 1988 Helping the dehydrated patient. Nursing Times 84 (18) May 4: 40–41

Walker C 1986 The fats of life. Nursing Times 82 (19) May 7: 20–21

Watts M 1987 Defining alcohol abuse. Nursing: The Add-On Journal of Clinical Nursing 3 (20) August (Psychiatric nursing supplement 1–4)

Wood S 1986 Nutritional support: an overview of general principles. Nursing: The Add-On Journal of Clinical Nursing 3 (8) August: 301–302

Woods M 1989 Tumour takes all. Nursing Times 85 (3) January 18: 46–47

Wright M 1986 We're getting there. Nursing Times 82 (9) February 26: 16–19

Wright S J 1986 Altered body image in anorexia nervosa. The Professional Nurse 1 (10) July: 260–262

Yates J E, Whitehead G 1986 Aids to feeding. Nursing: The Add-On Journal of Clinical Nursing 3 (7) July: 244–248

10

Eliminating

The activity of eliminating

Eliminating is an activity of living which all individuals perform with unfailing regularity throughout life. Whatever people are doing, wherever they are, and regardless of the time of day, they respond to the need to eliminate and this response is an integral activity of everyday life. One of the most interesting characteristics of this AL is that, by custom, it is performed in private. In public buildings, and even in the family home, the provision of a place affording privacy to the individual for eliminating is considered to be essential. Even in societies which emphasise the communal nature of activities of living, eliminating is normally a private activity and the products of elimination are concealed from the public eye.

For the excretion of these waste products quite separate systems of the body are involved. However, they are being discussed together as one activity of living because, as far as the individual is concerned, they are virtually inseparable. The AL of eliminating comprises *urinary elimination* and *faecal elimination*.

THE NATURE OF ELIMINATING

So essential is the nature of eliminating that even a unicellular organism must eliminate the waste products of the metabolic processes which are constantly going on within it. In many multicellular organisms however, separate systems deal with the elimination of urine and faeces. In human beings the urinary system produces and excretes urine; whereas the large bowel or colon produces and excretes faeces — the colon has customarily been described as part of the 'digestive system' but in this text is called the defaecatory system. Eliminating is so necessary that the newborn baby excretes waste matter (meconium) from the bowel, and urine from the urinary bladder shortly after birth by reflex (involuntary) response to a stretch stimulus from fullness in the bowel and bladder. Eventually voluntary control over reflex evacuation of the bladder and bowel is achieved. When necessary though, the desire to eliminate can be suppressed for a considerable time until there is a suitable time and place.

Whereas the AL of eating and drinking is for the sole biological purpose of providing the essential nutrients for living, the AL of eliminating is for dealing with the waste products from utilisation of food and drink. The main purpose of eliminating urine is to dispose of unrequired fluid intake and dissolved chemicals which the body cells are not immediately requiring (and which cannot be stored) so that the body is correctly hydrated, in electrolyte balance and thereby in overall acid/base balance. The main purpose of excreting faeces is to rid the body of indigestible cellulose and unabsorbed food but faeces also contains shed endothelial cells, intestinal secretions, water and bacteria. The nature of the products of eliminating — urine and faeces — will now be discussed.

Urine

Urine is secreted throughout the 24 hours but production slows during sleep, so that voiding is unnecessary during that period. The first urine voided on waking is usually darker in colour due to its concentration. Otherwise the colour ranges from amber to straw-coloured.

Urine has a specific gravity of between 1.015 and 1.025 and is normally acidic with a pH (a hydrogen ion concentration) of about 6. It is composed of about 96% water, 2% salts (especially sodium and potassium) and 2% nitrogenous waste (urea). When recently voided it has only a slight smell but after exposure to air, it decomposes and begins to smell of ammonia.

A high fluid intake results in a high urine output and vice versa. However, the normal urine output is around 1 to $1\frac{1}{2}$ litres in 24 hours; the usual frequency of micturition is from 5 to 10 times in that period.

Faeces

The first stool of the infant is a sticky, greenish-black substance called meconium which has accumulated in the bowel from about the fifth month of prenatal development. This consists of mucus, endothelial cells, amniotic fluid, bile pigments and fats. Meconium is passed several times in the first days of life. Then a brownish-green stool is passed and, a few days later, the baby's excreta become yellow in colour. A breast-fed baby has softer, brighter yellow stools than a bottle-fed baby whose stools are paler, more formed and with a slightly offensive smell. Once the infant is weaned and beginning to have a balanced diet of normal foodstuffs, the faeces begin to take on their familiar composition.

Faecal matter in the adult is normally brown in colour, soft in consistency and cylindrical in form. There is an odour from faeces due to the action of bacterial flora in the intestine and the smell varies according to the bacteria present and the type of food ingested. Faeces are normally composed of water (75%) and solid matter (25%) made up of quantities of dead bacteria, some fatty acids, inorganic matter, proteins and undigested dietary fibre. With regard to number and size of stools, the collection of epidemiological information shows that people in rural third world countries excrete two stools a day with a total weight of between 300 and 500 g, whereas the average for people in Western society is one stool daily weighing between 80 and 120 g (Burkitt, 1983).

In Burkitt's reference it is also stated that the time taken from ingestion of food to its output as faeces is termed 'intestinal transit time'. Again there is difference in this time between people in rural third world countries and Western societies — approximately $1-1\frac{1}{2}$ days in the former; and about 3 days in young healthy adults in the latter, the time increasing in the elderly to 2 weeks. If carcinogens are formed in the bowel, their contact with the lining membrane will be minimised by rapid transit time.

An acid stool is produced by bacteria breaking down the unabsorbed dietary fibre, and faecal acidity is thought to be one of the factors which reduce the amount of potential carcinogens in the bowel.

It is likely that in the next few years more information will be available about the function of faeces in preventing not only bowel disease but also disease in other parts of the body. This shows very clearly the importance of constant updating of knowledge.

LIFESPAN: EFFECT ON ELIMINATING

The lifespan clearly has relevance to eliminating and as a component of the model of living will now be focused to this AL.

It has already been pointed out that even the newborn infant voids both bladder and bowel involuntarily. An important milestone in childhood is the acquisition of voluntary control over elimination. Although toilet training helps the child to learn to recognise the signals of the need to eliminate, it cannot really hasten the development of voluntary control because this is dependent on maturation of the required components of the nervous and musculoskeletal systems.

The time to start toilet training a child depends partly on age, and partly on each individual child's 'readiness' to begin. One of the first indicators of 'readiness' for toilet training is awareness of having a full bladder. Soon the child begins to warn the mother that the potty is needed and at this stage can begin to do without nappies during the day. Control over defaecation is gained before control over urinary elimination.

By 3 years of age many children can go to the toilet on their own and are beginning to be able to do without toileting during the night. Children of 4 are usually competent in the social skills associated with elimination and, by school age, have developed independence and also a feeling of desire for privacy while eliminating.

Gradually when children have gained control of both activities they can make decisions for themselves about where and when they will eliminate. Sometimes children may misuse these newly acquired skills to manipulate the parents, for example by 'wetting' to attract attention, or by referring to eliminating activities in company to cause embarrassment. Attitudes develop not only to the activities, but also to the products of the activities. Whereas society's attitude to ingestion of food is that it is pleasant, desirable and in the main carried out in the company of others; its attitude to elimination of the waste from food — faeces — is that it is unpleasant, sometimes offensive, intensely personal and carried out in privacy.

At the other end of the lifespan, eliminating habits established in childhood may undergo change. Often in the process of ageing the bladder loses its tone, and the kidneys become less efficient, so that older people sometimes need to eliminate smaller amounts of urine at a more frequent time interval than when younger. The process of ageing can also manifest in the bowel as sluggishness of muscular action and there can be decrease in the volume of faeces as many older people eat less; these conditions can predispose to chronic constipation.

DEPENDENCE/INDEPENDENCE IN ELIMINATING

The lifespan component of the model of living which was discussed previously is clearly relevant to the concept of dependence/independence for eliminating. For everyone there is a *natural dependence* in the early years and for some there is a return to a varying level of dependence in the later years. There are others who are not capable of achieving independence as they progress through the stages of the lifespan because of congenital conditions as diverse as abnormality of the bowel or bladder, of the nerves supplying them, or physical abnormality of the limbs, or mental handicap. Anywhere along the lifespan people's dependence/independence status can change because of trauma to, or disease of, the bowel or urinary system, or indeed the cause may be in the nervous system. Because the AL of mobilising is a necessary part of eliminating, trauma or disease affecting the musculoskeletal system can also change a person's status on the dependence/independence continuum for the AL of eliminating.

The concept of 'aided independence' is applicable to eliminating. People who for example experience physical decline in advancing years can be helped to retain their 'independence' by provision of a grab rail near the toilet to help them regain the standing position. Should there be stiffness of the hips which makes sitting difficult, a removable raised toilet seat can be used.

FACTORS INFLUENCING ELIMINATING

So far two components of the model of living — the lifespan and the dependence/independence continuum — have been described in their relationship to the AL of eliminating. Here, the third component, 'Factors influencing the ALs', will be focused to eliminating; the factors are physical, psychological, socioeconomic, environmental and politicoeconomic and they will be described in that order.

Physical factors

To be able to eliminate in the normal way a person has to have fully functioning urinary and defaecatory systems. This not only means intactness of the organs comprising these systems but also of the sensory and motor nerves supplying them. Beginning students will acquire detailed knowledge of these body structures and functions in the biological components of the curriculum; it is important to integrate and synthesise the acquired knowledge into the 'Nursing Component'. Such knowledge of biology is necessary not only for understanding the pathological conditions which can occur in these systems, and the effect which they can have on the AL of eliminating; but also for understanding the nursing interventions ensuing from medical prescription for investigation and treatment of the pathology.

Gender influences this AL since usually men stand while passing urine and women sit; this is taken into consideration when providing facilities, particularly in public buildings.

Currently everyone is being exhorted to eat more dietary fibre. It increases the bulk of faeces which in turn increases the motility of the bowel resulting in a soft stool that is easy to excrete regularly. By definition a low-residue diet is non-bulk forming and has the opposite effect. Changes in diet can therefore alter an individual's established defaecation pattern (p. 156).

However, the AL of eliminating involves much more than simply the physical acts of micturition and defaecation. The person must be able to reach the toilet (which often is situated upstairs in homes and public buildings), to adjust clothing, to sit on a toilet and rise from it. Post-elimination hygiene too, including the use of toilet paper and handwashing, has to be carried out. It is apparent that eliminating is closely related to the equally complex AL of mobilising.

Psychological factors

A minimum level of intellectual ability is required to learn the many skills involved in eliminating. If the learning is started too early or is very strict some people think that it can contribute to a rigid personality. The development of concepts of modesty and privacy are also important to enable a person to appreciate and conform to the prevailing social customs.

If people are to achieve and maintain a healthy state of eliminating they require knowledge about the relationship of this AL to the amount of fluid taken into and lost from the body; the amount of fibre in the diet, and the type of exercise to keep the abdominal and pelvic floor muscles effective in the act of eliminating.

A person's attitudes and beliefs about this AL may well influence the way it is carried out. For example in a public toilet some people never sit on the 'communal' seat, as they believe that it can carry infection; others flush the cistern to drown the noise of their own eliminating.

Certain emotions may affect the AL of eliminating. Most people have experienced the urgent need to empty the bladder when facing a stressful situation such as an examination. Depression often causes apathy and sluggishness and this can influence eliminating, usually resulting in constipation.

Sociocultural factors

The fact that different words are used in different cultures for the process and products of eliminating is interesting. Alternatives such as nappy or diaper tend to be perpetuated from one generation to the next. Likewise the names used for the products of elimination are important, and those used by one cultural group might be considered vulgar by another. Indeed even within a culture, different words may be used by those in different social classes; and in many instances it is family convention which influences the words used. When children first start school they may well be exposed to those from a mix of social classes and as they discover some of these differences they may need help in continuing to use the words selected as family convention.

The child is eventually able to go to the particular place provided for eliminating and gradually there is socialisation according to the concept of privacy and modesty for this AL. There can be difference in the name given to this place, and while the word 'toilet' has a wide acceptance, others such as lavatory and bathroom are used. In most cultures there are 'public toilets' or 'conveniences' for use by people who are away from home and they are usually labelled separately for males and females.

Some strict post-elimination activities are specified by several religions and are transmitted to each succeeding generation. Of course it is desirable that everyone is socialised into acquiring adequate and safe hygiene activities related to eliminating in the interest of preventing infection, particularly the diarrhoeal diseases.

Environmental factors

It is all too easy for those who are used to flush toilets which are attached to a water carriage system of sewage disposal to think that these are the norm. But in some parts of the world people are fortunate if they have chemical toilets, or indeed latrines (earth toilets) which will be discussed in the politicoeconomic section. All three types are designed so that the person can sit on them, but in some countries it is customary to provide a toilet which is a hole in the ground filled with water, on either side of which are foot plates, and elimination is achieved in the squatting position which is functionally an efficient position. In some parts of the world there is no amenity and people 'go into the bush' to defaecate where the surrounding earth may be too hard and dry to be scooped to cover the faeces; it is therefore an attraction for flies which can transmit infection to food causing one of the diarrhoeal diseases.

Whether or not an inside toilet is available in a home will obviously influence several aspects of this AL. Most homes have only one toilet and it may be within the bathroom or separate from it. If separate, unless the room has handwashing facilities within it, it may be less easy to uphold standards of hygiene. This applies equally if members of several households have to share a toilet which is not within the home. If to reach the toilet one has to go right outside, then in bad weather the feeling of the need to defaecate may go unheeded which could predispose to constipation.

Politicoeconomic factors

It is difficult for us to realise that only a little more than 100 years ago cholera was rife in the UK and still is in some parts of the world. Mortality and morbidity from the diarrhoeal diseases of typhoid, paratyphoid, the dysenteries and enteritis was, and in some countries still is, high. The realisation in the first half of the century that there is a faecal-oral route for spread of such infection led to the increasing introduction of water carriage systems of sewage disposal resulting in a gradual reduction in the incidence of diseases spread by this route. Of course such schemes cost money, and they are dependent on decisions made by a country's government.

In developing countries where the financial budget is not considered sufficient to warrant the implementation of an extensive water carriage system of sewage disposal (the water may not be available), local people in the villages are being encouraged to construct earth toilets. Some countries are using their economic aid from other countries to accelerate this programme in an attempt to achieve the World Health Organization's goal 'Health for all by the year 2000'.

In many countries there is legislation about for example the sanitary requirements for campsites, public toilets, and toilets in public buildings. Minimally, cold water has to be provided for post-elimination handwashing in an attempt to prevent outbreaks of the diarrhoeal diseases.

INDIVIDUALITY IN ELIMINATING

There are many different factors responsible for shaping each individual's personal eliminating habits. Childhood training and the customs of the person's family and society are important among these.

The actual times of voiding urine vary according to the individual's personal daily routine. Most people void on waking, before going to sleep, and before or after meals. Children and elderly people often make sure they go to the toilet regularly at 2- or 3-hourly intervals in view of their lesser bladder capacity and control.

For most people, defaecation is performed at a set time of the day when time and privacy are available. Various research reports in the 1950s and 60s showed that the frequency of defaecation varied within as wide a range as three bowel actions per day and three per week and that only habits outside this range should be regarded as unusual.

The many people who firmly believed that daily evacuation of the bowel was essential for health, were reassured that this was not so, and there was a general lessening of tension. However, epidemiological information was being collected from developing third world countries and those in which economic development had led to adoption of a Western way of life, particularly related to diet (Burkitt, 1983). Based on this epidemiological evidence there is a return to the belief that daily evacuation of at least 150 g, and preferably 250 g of faeces is desirable. It can only be achieved by increasing the dietary intake of fibre, but it will take time to convince members of the public that a somewhat drastic change in eating habits is necessary in the interest of health.

The purpose of the model of living is to highlight a person's individuality in living. It can be seen from the discussion so far that there are several dimensions to each of the components of the model of living which can influence the acquisition of individuality in eliminating: and a résumé of the variables described at each component of the model follows:

Lifespan: effect on eliminating
- Involuntary voiding in infancy
- Childhood training for continence
- Loss of muscle tone in old age

Dependence/independence in eliminating
- Relevant to lifespan
- Congenital conditions
- Disease/trauma
- Dependence on aids/on people

- Total dependence

Factors influencing eliminating
- Physical — fully functioning urinary and defaecatory systems
  — ability to reach the toilet, manipulate clothing, carry out post-eliminating toilet, wash hands

- Psychological — intellectual ability
  — concept of modesty, privacy
  — response to toilet training
  — attitude to eliminating

- Sociocultural — knowledge about diet/eliminating
  — word for products of elimination
  — cultural group/social class/family convention
  — word for place of eliminating
  — post-elimination hygiene/religion

- Environmental — type of toilet
  — handwashing facilities

- Politicoeconomic — money available for prevention of diarrhoeal diseases

Eliminating: patients' problems and related nursing

It is important that during an episode of illness the patient's individual habits of eliminating are changed as little as possible, unless they are detrimental to health. It is therefore imperative that nurses know about these individual habits and use this knowledge to implement an individualised nursing plan. The information can be gleaned by nurses bearing in mind the topics noted in the preceding résumé while discussing the AL of eliminating with the patient. It is useful, particularly during the initial assessment phase of the process of nursing if the nurse has in mind the following questions:

- how often and when does the individual eliminate urine/faeces?
- what factors influence the way the individual carries out the AL of eliminating?

- what does the individual know about eliminating urine/faeces and post-eliminating hygiene?
- what is the individual's attitude to eliminating?
- has the individual any longstanding problems with eliminating urine and faeces, and if so, how have these been coped with?
- what problems if any does the individual have at present with eliminating urine/faeces and are any likely to develop?

The emphasis during assessment is on the discovery of the patient's usual routines, what can and cannot be done independently, and any coping mechanisms that have been used previously for problems or discomforts which might well be of a chronic or recurring nature. Relevant information from medical records will be noted. In collaboration with the patient whenever possible, any actual problems with the AL of eliminating will be identified.

The nurse may well recognise potential problems which may or may not be recognised by the patient and these will of course be discussed with the patient. Mutual realistic goals will be set, to prevent potential problems from becoming actual ones; to alleviate or solve the actual problems; or help the patient cope with those which cannot be alleviated or solved. The nursing interventions and when relevant any activities which the patient agrees to do to achieve the set goals will be selected according to local circumstances and available resources. These will be written on the nursing plan together with the date on which evaluation will be carried out to discern whether or not they are achieving or have achieved the stated goals. As the interventions are implemented, it will be written in the patient's nursing notes. All these activities are necessary in order to carry out individualised nursing related to the AL of eliminating.

However, before nurses can begin to think in terms of individualised nursing they need to have a generalised idea of the kind of problems which patients can experience related to the AL of eliminating. These will be discussed together with relevant nursing activities which are encountered early in a nursing career. They are grouped together under five headings:

- change of environment and routine
- change in eliminating habit
- change in mode of eliminating
- change of dependence/independence status for eliminating
- some specific problems associated with eliminating.

CHANGE OF ENVIRONMENT AND ROUTINE

From time to time most people experience some disruption to their individualised eliminating habits as a result of a change in environment and routine. Going on holiday inevitably means adapting to a different timetable, doing different things, and making do with whatever toilet facilities are available, even if sometimes these are unfamiliar and unsavoury! If the holiday is a lazy one, it is possible that the less active routine will cause constipation; on the other hand, diarrhoea may be the result of sampling unfamiliar foods. The same sort of problems can be experienced by people who are admitted to hospital.

Admission to hospital

Disruption to established eliminating habits seems to be a common consequence of admission to hospital.

When patients are admitted because of problems associated with urinary elimination or faecal elimination, doctors and nurses ask all sorts of questions about these activities; specimens of urine or faeces are collected and tested and sometimes special procedures such as catheterisation are a necessary part of treatment. Certain communications between patients and staff centre round eliminating. These body functions are no longer private and personal; they seem to the patients to have become everybody's business and not unnaturally they may feel anxious and embarrassed.

Even those patients whose reason for admission is not specifically related to eliminating problems may at assessment be found to be experiencing a problem with this AL. Other patients may encounter difficulties with this AL because of the hospital environment. In particular many patients become bothered by the lack of privacy.

Lack of privacy

Previously in the patient's adult life no-one has asked daily whether or not he has had a bowel movement. This is a routine in many hospitals and some patients who have not been admitted because of a bowel complaint may well consider this an invasion of their privacy.

Curtains round beds may provide visual privacy but they do not provide aural privacy for those patients experiencing urinary or defaecatory problems when giving related information to doctors and nurses. Nurses can help by modulating their voices; choosing to talk with the patient when the beds on either side are empty; or inviting the patient into a room in which nurse and patient can talk without interruption.

For ambulant patients, in many hospital wards which were built in the days when the majority of patients were nursed in bed, toilet facilities are inadequate for the needs of today. Often there are too few toilets or those available are too far away to be readily reached; many are too small for wheelchairs or walking aids; and some are too cold for comfort, or so public that they deny any real privacy.

Nurses may not be able to do much about the inadequacy of facilities in the ward, but they can make the most of what exists. For example, toilets should be kept clean and free from the clutter of sluice equipment, and air fresheners can be used to minimise malodour. (Aerosols are not recommended as some contribute to destruction of the ozone layer which is currently a cause of international concern.) Patients using the toilet should be afforded as much privacy as possible. How often do nurses thoughtlessly 'pop in' to ask if patients are ready to be helped back to bed when a call system could be provided which would avoid this situation?

Unfamiliar routine

If the imposed ward routine for the patients' AL of eliminating is not the same as their individual habit then they are more than likely to have a problem. For example, individuals who usually have a bowel movement immediately after breakfast may find this is not possible because they are expected to stay in bed awaiting the doctor's round. Some people, accustomed to getting up during the night to pass urine, may feel apprehensive about continuing this routine for fear of disturbing other patients.

When showing the newly admitted patient where the toilet facilities are, and discussing things such as when it may be necessary to use a bedpan or provide a specimen of urine, the nurse can take the opportunity to find out as much as possible about the patient's eliminating habits and later to record any relevant information. It is only when an assessment has been carried out that potential problems can be identified and the necessary nursing planned.

As far as possible, patients should be enabled to maintain any deeply ingrained individual habits of eliminating. Bedpan or urinal 'rounds' impose a routine on all patients and it is much better to accommodate each individual's accustomed routine whenever possible.

CHANGE IN ELIMINATING HABIT

Even if conscious, deliberate attention were not paid, for example to how frequently the bladder was emptied, a person probably would notice a marked increase or decrease in the frequency of passing urine and faeces. Should there be a marked change in the colour, odour or consistency of either urine or faeces a person would be likely to notice it too.

As changes in eliminating habit are often indicators of some dysfunction of the urinary or defaecatory systems (or even other body systems) nurses have a responsibility to be able to recognise any change in a patient's urine or its elimination, and faeces and their elimination. Recognition of changes is only possible if the nurse understands what constitutes 'normal' and has data from assessment on the individual patient's norm.

Changes in urine and its elimination

Change in colour. Several factors can cause a change in colour, sometimes transient and not necessarily pathological.

Pale urine may be due to temporary diuresis as a result of excessive fluid intake, or it can result from taking a diuretic drug, or it may be of a continuous nature as in the condition of diabetes mellitus.

Dark urine may mean that it is concentrated as a result of dehydration (p. 165) when less urine is excreted; the colour will lighten as the patient increases fluid intake. Or it may be caused by the presence of bile pigments (urobilin or bilirubin) due to disease of the liver or gallbladder. The urine will become pigment-free as the disease responds to treatment.

Coloured urine can result from the intake of some foods. Carotene contained in carrots as well as other vegetables and fruits can make urine a bright yellow; beetroot and blackberries can make the urine red.

Medications can also change the colour of urine; an antibiotic called rifamycin makes it an orange-red colour. Naturally, patients should be warned about this.

A smoky colour is indicative of 'occult' (hidden) blood from high in the urinary tract; it is so mixed with the urine that it has lost its identity as blood. On the other hand, urine which is red from frank blood usually means that the bleeding is lower in the urinary tract.

Change in odour. The characteristic odour of urine may change to sweet-smelling, a manifestation of diabetes mellitus. Part of the treatment of diabetic patients is teaching them to test their urine to make sure that it does not contain excess glucose. Decomposing urine smells like ammonia. An infected urine has an offensive fishy smell, and there may be frank pus (pyuria) in the case of severe urinary infection. The patient may need to increase perineal hygiene (p. 203), and be meticulous about changing underwear to prevent odour. In the case of dependent patients this of course would be a nursing activity.

Change in frequency. A change in the number of times a patient passes urine may or may not be accompanied by an alteration in the total amount of urine voided in 24 hours and accurate data are required to establish this.

Increased frequency can vary from that due to the anxiety associated with admission to hospital, and special procedures, tests and so on, to a totally demanding 'urgency' that dominates the patient's life, even disturbing sleep. This type is a very disabling condition. It is often a manifestation of urinary infection (cystitis), a common problem of women and older people.

The frequent voiding of small amounts of urine, although an inconvenience to the person, is actually helpful in combating the infection. The pathogenic microorganisms are not allowed to remain for long in the urinary tract and so excessive multiplication is prevented. When increased frequency of micturition in an older person is not due to urinary infection, it may be attributed to loss of muscle elasticity reducing sphincter control or deterioration in cerebral function.

Decreased frequency is closely associated with decreased

output and it can result from obstruction, water retention (oedema), kidney disease and dehydration. It is particularly important for nurses to recognise decreased frequency in older patients, since impairment of their thirst mechanism can put them at risk of dehydration. If suspected, the nurse can examine the lips and mouth for dryness, another clue to dehydration (p. 165).

Change in quantity. Marked deviation from the patient's norm is dangerous because it can result in fluid imbalance. As soon as the change is recognised the patient's fluid intake and output will probably need to be measured and this is a nursing responsibility but depending on patients' competence, they may be able to help with the measuring and recording on a fluid balance chart.

A decreased output (oliguria) or total absence of urine (anuria) indicates that either urine is not being produced normally by the kidneys as in renal failure, or that its excretion from the bladder is being blocked. In the case of blockage which can be caused by prostatic enlargement, there is retention of urine in the bladder causing a midline abdominal swelling over which there is a dull sound on percussion. It is potentially dangerous and most uncomfortable; indeed, it can be very painful. Sometimes the pressure in the overfull bladder forces urine through the urethral sphincters when the condition is referred to as 'retention with overflow'. Because of the mechanical nature of the blockage, the bladder has to be drained by a catheter (p. 191). The condition can arise postoperatively when some patients experience difficulty in re-establishing micturition and the nurse should report whether or not the patient has passed urine early in the postoperative period.

An increased output can be expected when patients are taking diuretic drugs, their purpose being to increase urinary output in people with oedema. Several of the hypotensive drugs are combined with a diuretic, and nurses need to be aware of this when nursing patients with high blood pressure. Over 2 litres in 24 hours constitutes a pathologically increased output of urine (polyuria). This condition is often associated with excessive thirst (polydipsia) and increased fluid intake, characteristic of the diabetic condition.

Collecting urine specimens. Collecting urine specimens is a common nursing activity but the nurse should remember that it is probably a new experience for the patient. Careful instruction is therefore necessary and ascertainment of whether or not it has been understood. Explanation of the reason for the procedure will help the patient to accept it, and of course privacy and dignity should be maintained throughout.

A specimen of urine can be collected in a clean container at any time — in the toilet at home, in a health clinic, outpatients' department or a hospital ward. It is not usually necessary for this to be mainstream urine (Wallis, 1984). 'Mainstream' means that the first flow is passed into the

toilet, the mainstream of approximately 30 ml is collected in the clean container, and the remainder passed into the toilet. A urine specimen is observed for colour, tested for specific gravity and pH, and for biochemical tests for glucose, ketones, protein, bile and blood. It is necessary for the nurse to know whether or not a woman is menstruating, as, if so it may give a false-positive reading for blood in the urine.

A midstream specimen of urine is collected when bacteriological examination in the laboratory is necessary to confirm or deny the presence of pathogenic microorganisms, and to identify their sensitivity to different microbial agents. Obviously the goal is to collect urine which is uncontaminated by microorganisms from the lower end of the urethra and the perineum. To accomplish this, the first flow is passed into the toilet (or other vessel), the midstream of approximately 30 ml is passed into a sterile jar and the remainder into the toilet. A research report states that vulval cleaning with swabs and soapy water prior to taking midstream urine specimens in general practice, for laboratory culture, provided no more reliable results than specimens obtained without preparation (Bradbury, 1988). However, health authorities vary as to instruction about this procedure. Should an antiseptic be advocated for pre-specimen swabbing, then the area must be thoroughly rinsed to prevent any of it contaminating the specimen, there to continue its bactericidal action and resulting in a false report.

Procuring urine specimens from babies is notoriously difficult. A leakproof nappy is available, which on trial resulted in satisfactory specimens from babies in hospital and at home, in the first 6 weeks after birth (Goodinson, 1986). It can be used for a random specimen, or for a 24-hour specimen, explained below.

Early morning specimen of urine. The name implies that it is the first urine excreted in the morning: it is more concentrated than daytime urine and is particularly useful for pregnancy tests and tuberculosis tests.

24-hour collection of urine is necessary when the test involves detection of a substance which is not secreted at an even rate throughout the 24 hours. The first urine passed at, for example 08.00 hours, is discarded. All urine is collected in a vessel, from which it is poured into a large container. At 08.00 hours the next day, the bladder is emptied and the urine added to the collection. For some tests, the contents of the container are stirred and a specimen poured into a glass jar for transfer to the laboratory. In other instances the container and its contents are sent to the laboratory.

Strict cleanliness is essential when collecting any of these specimens. When urine is being collected for bacteriological culture, there is a danger of the hands becoming contaminated with transient flora; and the environment and nurse's uniform can be contaminated from urine splash

(p. 193).

Catheter specimen of urine. A specimen of urine can be collected by introducing a catheter into the bladder using an aseptic technique. The vessel into which the urine flows must also be sterile and capped immediately. As soon as the flow ceases, the catheter should either be withdrawn or clamped, otherwise microorganisms can have access to the catheter lumen and travel to the bladder.

Urine specimens from an indwelling catheter. A discussion of collecting urine specimens would not be complete without considering that in many instances, specimens need to be collected from the apparatus attached to an indwelling catheter (p. 192). It may be a single specimen which is required or a 24-hour specimen.

Finally it is pertinent to point out that urine is included in the list of 'body fluids' which can transmit the AIDS group of viruses (Royal College of Nursing, 1986). These nursing guidelines state that disposable plastic aprons and gloves should be worn when exposure to 'body fluids' is anticipated, and those related to this section are: collection of specimens for ward or laboratory analysis; invasive nursing procedures such as catheterisation: attending to patients' sanitary needs, and for the disposal of excreta; and when dealing with spillages of 'body fluids'. The Infection Control Committee in each local area issues recommendations which it requires its personnel to implement, with the objective of preventing the spread of infection, and students should be familiar with them.

Changes in faeces and their elimination

Changes in appearance. A disorder of the digestive system may be indicated by a change in the appearance of faeces. Absence of bile, as in biliary obstruction, produces putty-coloured stools. Some obstructive, infective, inflammatory or malignant diseases can cause the faeces to contain blood, which if not visible to the naked eye but detectable by chemical testing is called 'occult blood'. If blood is mixed with the faeces, causing it to look black and shiny, it is known as melaena and comes from a distal site such as the stomach or small intestine. Or it may be evident as frank red blood which, if on the surface of the stools, comes from a local site, and most commonly from bleeding haemorrhoids. Steatorrhoeaic stools, those mixed with mucus and fats, occur in some metabolic disorders. Bulky stools containing undigested food material indicate faulty absorption. Drugs may affect the colour of faecal matter; iron products stain the stool black. Malformed stools, often pencil-like, are indicative of obstruction in the bowel.

Changes in frequency. A healthy person normally has a fairly regular pattern of defaecation. A deviation from this to a decreased frequency is called constipation; change to an increased frequency is diarrhoea.

Constipation. Lack of unabsorbable fibre in the large bowel results in constipation. Research evidence has confirmed the high correlation between low fibre intake and constipation in hospital patients (Mallillin, 1985). Other studies report a reduction in the use of aperients and enemata after increasing the fibre content of hospital diets (Beveridge, 1986; Thomas, 1987). Dietary fibre is important because it adds bulk to the faeces, making defaecation easy and more frequent. It appears that the diet of Western societies contains much less fibre than is common in societies in rural Africa; consequently the faeces of Western adults have much less bulk and constipation occurs frequently as a result (p. 178).

This observation of distinct cultural differences leads to the conclusion that increasing the amount of dietary fibre is likely to prevent constipation. Cereal fibre is more effective than fruit or green vegetable fibre and the easiest way to improve the diet is to take a bran cereal or add small amounts of millers' bran to fruit or cereal.

In a published interview (Swaffield, 1979), which is still relevant, Denis Burkitt a well known gastroenterologist was asked 'How does the average person tell if he's constipated?' and the reply was 'Simply by weighing the stools. All you have to do is have some letter scales in the bathroom, and some bits of newspaper or old margarine tubs or whatever and weigh the stools for about four days. . . . We should excrete *at least 150 grams daily*, preferably 250 grams.' In the article it states that the average daily stool in Western society is about 120 grams, and as low as 50 grams in some old people.

Whether constipation is an actual or a potential problem, the goal on the nursing plan will be to re-establish the patient's usual frequency of defaecation (unless it was unsatisfactory), and promote ease of defaecation. The nursing intervention would be to ensure that the patient understands the following preventive activities:

- eat a balanced diet which includes fibre-containing foodstuffs (e.g. wholemeal bread, bran cereals, green vegetables, salad and fruits)
- maintain an adequate fluid intake
- take as much exercise as possible
- maintain usual habits of defaecation or establish satisfactory habits
- respond to the sensation of a full bowel
- avoid undue worry about bowel habit
- promote ease of defaecation by using abdominal and pelvic floor muscles

Nurses can do a great deal to prevent constipation by educating all patients to follow this routine.

For the treatment of constipation most people think of taking medicine — aperients or laxatives — and unfortunately this is a widespread practice in the Western world. For some people it becomes a frequent, even a daily habit;

this is dangerous because the bowel muscle loses its natural tone. But of course aperients are useful when constipation is a temporary problem, for example in response to a change of environment and routine. They should never be taken when there is accompanying abdominal pain, nausea or vomiting. Aperients are estimated to cost the UK National Health Service £8 million a year (Booth & Booth, 1986), so prevention of constipation is a worthy goal of a nurse-initiated preventive intervention. Although aperients can be bought without a medical prescription, it is still the custom in most hospitals for them to be prescribed by the doctor but they are administered, evaluated and documented by the nurse. Booth & Booth (1986) after consulting the British National Formulary compiled a useful list of the most commonly used aperients, suppositories and microenemas, using the column headings — 'name, starts working in, how it works, side-effects, cautions, dose, price'.

When constipation is a chronic problem particularly in elderly people, Shreeve (1985) advises that aperients should not be given as a first treatment, but Micralax (one of the available microenemas), volume 5 ml, can soften and mobilise a large mass of impacted faeces in 5 to 15 minutes due to its 'peptising' action. Shreeve says that by avoiding the introduction of large quantities of fluid into the colon this preparation does not produce water intoxication and electrolyte imbalance. It can therefore be used even for children, very ill adults and frail elderly people; the exception is those suffering from inflammatory bowel disease (Booth & Booth, 1986).

Constipation postoperatively is common, particularly after surgery affecting the gastrointestinal tract. This occurs because there is temporary loss of peristalsis. If this loss persists longer than the initial postoperative period, it develops into a serious condition called paralytic ileus.

However, a much more common complication of constipation is faecal impaction.

Faecal impaction. This condition has already been mentioned; faeces hardens and accumulates in the colon and rectum, making defaecation difficult or impossible. It is a distressing condition for patients because, although they may feel the need to defaecate, they are unable to, and abdominal distension and rectal pain cause severe discomfort. Sometimes small amounts of liquid faecal matter bypass the hardened faeces and leak from the anus and this may be wrongly diagnosed as faecal incontinence. Faecal impaction is probably the commonest cause of incontinence in the elderly, particularly those in institutions (Alderman, 1989). In some instances, if the chemical action of one or more evacuant microenemas does not break up the faecal mass, an olive oil microenema may be introduced into the rectum and retained for as long as possible in order to soften the faeces thereby facilitating manual removal using a gloved hand. Gentle hand movement is essential to avoid damaging the mucous membrane. It is an unpleasant procedure for both patient and nurse, and great sensitivity is necessary to preserve the patient's privacy and dignity.

Diarrhoea. This is yet another change in eliminating habit; it is the condition in which faeces contain excess water and the frequency of defaecation is markedly increased. Diarrhoea is a common symptom and may be the result of something as benign and self-limiting as pre-examination nerves or something as serious as carcinoma of the colon.

Acute diarrhoea has a sudden onset and usually ends rapidly. It is often the result of an infection such as food poisoning, or it may occur from an infectious disease such as typhoid which affects the digestive tract. Chronic diarrhoea exists when the symptoms persist. Ulcerative colitis is an inflammatory condition of the bowel which causes chronic diarrhoea. People who suffer from this often become very debilitated and their lifestyle may be completely dominated and disrupted by this unpleasant disease.

Over time, diarrhoea poses a danger to health because of the excessive loss of fluids and salts, incomplete absorption of nutrients from food, and incomplete synthesis of vitamins. If untreated, patients will suffer from a multitude of problems. They will become dehydrated and suffer from fluid and electrolyte imbalance, and will lose weight and strength. Medical management may include intravenous administration of fluids and dietary supplements.

Children require special mention — as diarrhoeal diseases are still a major cause of morbidity and mortality, more so in the developing countries, but still so in the Western world. It is estimated that in the UK, 5% of children under 1 year of age will develop gastroenteritis, but only 10% of these require hospital admission (Khatib, 1986). When diarrhoea is accompanied by excessive vomiting, intravenous rehydration and appropriate drugs are common medical prescriptions, together with 'therapeutic' starvation followed by cautious reintroduction of diet. Studies conducted by health workers in the developing countries have challenged these dogma by demonstrating the success of oral rehydration programmes as advocated by the World Health Organization and United Nations Childrens Fund (UNICEF). There are now several centres in the UK which employ oral rehydration and minimal modification of diet as an outpatient treatment, and early results show less discomfort and weight loss for the child, less parental anxiety and a financial saving (Candy, 1987).

Nursing activities, based on assessment of the individual, vary according to the severity and duration of the diarrhoea. Feeling the need to defaecate urgently can be distressing for older children and adults, so, to alleviate fear of soiling, availability of a toilet or commode is essential. The patient should be encouraged to drink more than usual in order to replace fluid lost and to take a nourishing diet which is reduced in fibre-containing foods. Washing of the perianal area and the application of cream can help to alleviate skin soreness around the anus which is caused by the liquid faeces.

Because diarrhoea is often caused by infection, great care must be taken in the disposal of the patient's faeces. Regular handwashing (p. 93) is necessary by both patient and nurse to prevent spreading the infection. Of course, handwashing is necessary whenever faeces are dealt with, such as when collecting a specimen of this excrement.

Collecting a specimen of faeces. A specimen for bacteriological laboratory examination is obtained by asking the patient to defaecate (without also passing urine) into a clean bedpan and, using a spatula or disposable spoon, a small portion of faeces is put into a special sterile container. Stool collections for several days may sometimes be required, for example in cases of steatorrhoea when estimations of amounts of fat in the faeces are made while fat intake in food is controlled. Whenever nurses are involved in the collection of specimens of faeces they must take care to avoid contamination of themselves and their clothes, and adopt a meticulous handwashing technique.

Incontinence of urine

By custom the word incontinence refers to the involuntary excretion of urine. Incontinence of faeces will be discussed later. When there is both urinary and faecal incontinence, the term 'double incontinence' is used.

When considering the subject of incontinence, few people give any thought to the very complicated phenomenon whereby throughout the day and night most children achieve continence by the age of 3. Norton (1988) gives an account of the complexities which all continent adults have mastered, yet about which the majority of both lay and professional people know very little. However there are some children who do not achieve continence and 1–2% of adults continue to be bed wetters.

If healthy children continue to wet themselves after the age of 5, or regress to this behaviour after a period of dryness, they can be described as being incontinent of urine. The size of the problem of nocturnal enuresis is estimated as affecting 55% of girls at 2–3 years; 3% at 7 years and 0.05% at 17 years: whereas it is 66% of boys at 2–3 years; 7% at 7 years, and 1% at 17 years (Sillitoe & Reed 1986). The most effective treatment for bedwetting is based on conditioning principles. A urine-sensitive pad is connected to a battery-operated alarm by the bedside; urine in the pad completes the electrical circuit, activates the alarm and wakes the child who then goes to the toilet. It has been used successfully with mentally and physically handicapped children (Sillitoe & Reed, 1986), as well as with 'normal' children.

Over the last decade the plight of many incontinent adults has received some publicity and there is a helpful leaflet published by the Disabled Living Foundation.

'Adult bed-wetting: causes, sources of help, remedies'. Manley (1984) reviews two reports — *The problem of promoting continence* published by the Royal College of Nursing and *Action on incontinence* a report of a working group (King's Fund project paper, no. 43). These two reports published in 1983 contain information which is still 'up-to-date' and they make it clear that incontinence is a condition which all nurses will have to deal with at some time in their career, since such patients are to be found in geriatric, gynaecology, medical, mental handicap, paediatric, psychogeriatric, surgical and urology wards as well as in their own homes and whenever disabled and handicapped people might be.

A comparison of the number of incontinent people in different age ranges and institutional or community settings is provided by Egan et al (1988). An extensive 4-year survey revealed that of those in the 5–14 age range, 15.3% were in an institution while 84.7% were cared for at home; of those in the 15–64 age range, 44.4% were in institutions while 55.6% were at home; and in the 65+ range, 54.3% were in institutions and 45.7% were at home.

The total number of incontinent people is difficult to estimate as so many of them are not in the care of the health or social services, but the experts working in this field give the figure of 3 million in the UK (Manley, 1984). Part of the problem is in defining 'incontinence'. The International Continence Society defines urinary incontinence as 'a condition where involuntary loss of urine is a social or hygienic problem'. Millard (1979) compares incontinence with a definition of continence 'that state of continence which involves the ability of the individual to identify an acceptable place for elimination; to be able to get to that place; and be able to hold excreta until that place is reached'. Another part of the problem is in defining different types of incontinence arising from, for instance, a neurogenic bladder.

Neurogenic bladder

To begin to understand the complexities of incontinence one can examine the term 'neurogenic bladder'. It is used when there is interference with the nerve supply to the bladder, and it can result in various types of incontinence. In one type the desire to pass urine may be appreciated but there is no cerebral inhibition so the bladder contracts resulting in urge incontinence, and evacuation of the full bladder. In another type the full bladder empties reflexly with no sensation. Yet another variation is the atonic bladder which fills so full that the pressure stretches the sphincters and urine dribbles out continuously (overflow incontinence or retention with overflow). Such dribbling incontinence can also occur when the sphincters are incompetent and the bladder no longer acts as a reservoir. The medical diagnosis for people with these different types of incontinence can be as diverse as a stroke (cerebrovascular accident), spina bifida, paraplegia, peripheral neuropathy in diabetes mellitus, multiple sclerosis, a brain tumour, dementia or a head injury. This list shows clearly that incontinence is a symptom and not a disease; it presents the patient with a problem related to the AL of eliminating and the patient requires nursing help to cope with it (p. 193) since the damage to the nervous system cannot be cured. Norton (1983) discusses various ways to assist voiding; she says that clean intermittent self-catheterisation is probably the single most significant advance in the management of patients with a neurogenic bladder. And as tribute to this advance, an article written by a young woman who had tried to cope with incontinence for $2\frac{1}{2}$ years is included (Sibley, 1988). She was visited by a continence adviser, who taught her the technique of clean intermittent self-catheterisation which facilitated being continent once more, and she explains what it has meant to her.

Dribbling incontinence

Dribbling incontinence can come from the non-neurogenic bladder if there is obstruction in or pressure on the urethra from such conditions as an enlarged prostate gland, a full rectum, or a cystocele. There is therefore a mechanical reason for the ensuing retention of urine and when there is sufficient pressure in the bladder it stretches the sphincters and produces dribbling incontinence. The treatment of the cause will theoretically cure the incontinence but in a few instances it is followed by a different type of incontinence.

Urge incontinence

Urge incontinence can also occur in the non-neurogenic bladder. Awareness of the desire to pass urine is immediately followed by passage of urine; this can be a small or large amount while the person is on the way to the toilet. Naturally people are very distressed about this problem and the more anxious they become the worse the condition gets. They perceive bladder fullness at a smaller and smaller volume of urine until they can be voiding every 10 or 15 minutes: the bladder musculature (detrusor) is unstable, and current thinking favours a plan for bladder training. It starts at the person's frequency, and aims to increase the time interval between passage of urine, after evaluation reveals that each short-term goal has been achieved, until eventually the long-term goal of voiding at a 3- or even 4-hourly interval is achieved. Obviously this demands committed patient participation and meticulous recording of constantly changing short-term goals, and their achievements. It may be that some people with urge incontinence could manage such a programme at home; others may need hospital admission for such a detailed and quickly changing plan.

Stress incontinence

Stress incontinence occurs because of insufficiency of the urethral sphincter mechanism; it is known to be the commonest form of incontinence in women of all ages (Norton, 1986). Should coughing or sneezing or running for a bus — indeed anything which increases intraabdominal pressure occur, the compromised sphincters permit escape of urine. Return of competence to the sphincters can be accomplished by perseverence with pelvic floor exercises (Montgomery, 1986). Thomas (1988) maintains that midstream interruption of the flow of urine contributes to strengthening of pelvic floor muscles.

Heap (1987) discusses stress incontinence in the context of midwifery, and states that assessment of women should include a full obstetric history, the circumstances in which urine escapes, urinalysis to exclude urinary tract infection, and a urodynamic assessment to measure bladder pressure and function.

Although the foregoing is a short account of different types of incontinence for the sole purpose of understanding the subject, in reality there can be mixed causes of a person's incontinence. This can be the case for a large group of people who are physically and/or mentally handicapped. Children and adults with physical handicaps which impair their appreciation of the sensation of bladder distension, or render them unable to cope independently with the AL of eliminating, often suffer permanently from incontinence. These people need to be helped to cope with this problem so that they can lead as normal a life as possible. Often the best approach is to utilise special appliances available (p. 190) but sometimes long-term catherisation is necessary.

Incontinence and mental handicap

There is a high incidence of incontinence among those who are severely mentally handicapped because there is often damage to the nervous system and this may impair the individual's ability to exercise voluntary control over elimination. Even if there is no physical defect, mentally handicapped people usually have difficulty in coping independently with the AL of eliminating. However, if they are helped to learn the skills of independent toileting, incontinence often can be overcome. An effective method of toilet training is by the use of behaviour modification procedures.

This approach to teaching involves very careful and gradual shaping of new behaviour using reinforcement techniques. Detailed behavioural assessment is carried out first and, from evaluation, changes in behaviour are monitored. The effectiveness of behaviour modification toilet training with severely handicapped patients in a ward environment was evaluated as part of a research project carried out by Tierney (1973). She found that nurses once trained in the techniques involved had considerable success in toilet training patients by this method. Others have continued the use of behavioural techniques to achieve urinary and faecal incontinence in mentally handicapped people

(Turner, 1988); the article presents a chart of the sequence of actions used, a reward being given as each is achieved.

Promoting continence
As well as the size of the incontinence problem in people of all ages, both at home and in institutions, there is the financial cost of the nursing service and the equipment required, the major part of the money being spent on pads and pants to contain incontinence (Royal College of Nursing, 1983). Promoting continence also has a financial cost, but with its successful implementation, it may well be that it can be financed by the money saved on containing incontinence. Added to this there is the personal psychological and sociological cost to incontinent people and their carers, and nurses cannot ignore the words used in the literature to explain their plight — degrading, demoralising, distasteful, distressing, embarrassing and humiliating are just some examples. These psychological reactions are a response to loss of control over the acts of micturition and defaecation which, for the majority of adults, have been a private and personal responsibility ever since continence was achieved in early childhood (Faugier, 1988). A consequent loss of self-esteem is understandable. There can also be a devastating effect on people's social life and it is therefore essential that nurses learn to use sensitivity and empathy when communicating with them (Faulkner, 1988). There is now considerable literature about this subject and if the available knowledge were translated into practice using a positive attitude, many incontinent people would regain continence. An individualised approach is absolutely essential if success is to be achieved and the framework of the nursing process — assessing, planning, implementing and evaluating — can accomplish this.

Detailed information about the characteristics of the person's incontinence is essential before a plan can be devised for promoting continence. 'Toilet charting' defines the pattern of the problem and provides baseline data about, for example, time of passing urine into a receptacle and time of incontinence episodes. A simple measurement of the degree of incontinence might be useful: one of the published ones includes pants damp, clothes damp, clothes wet, and surroundings wet (Rooney, 1987). In the discussion about stress incontinence on page 188, the quickly changing short-term goals were mentioned; toilet charts can be used for recording the achievement of each short-term goal; the setting of the next goal and so on.

Information about fluid intake is relevant because some incontinent people think that by restricting intake the problem will improve, whereas it may be exacerbated by the resultant concentrated urine which is a bladder irritant. Impaired mobilising, manual dexterity, eyesight and hearing may all be contributing factors and should be borne in mind at the initial, and during ongoing, assessment (Bayliss, 1988). It is also important to know about the toilet facilities in the home environment in order to set realistic goals.

As pressure in the bladder or rectum is raised, the pelvic floor muscles normally constrict and close the urethra and anus until a sufficient quantity of urine or faeces is ready for voiding. Inefficient pelvic floor muscles cause stress incontinence and there are various exercises for strengthening these muscles (Mongomery, 1986). As mentioned previously, midstream interruption of urine flow also helps to strengthen the pelvic floor muscles. Muscle strengthening from exercise demands time and perseverance to achieve the long-term goal of continence. However, each day in which there has been a decreased number of times of involuntary escape of urine could have something positive, may be a gold star, added to the chart to reinforce morale and perseverance.

Swaffield (1988) says ' The problem for continence advisers is why — when they have educated, when they have taught communication skills and assessment — do nurses then find it so difficult to promote continence among patients in long-term wards?' The positive and negative variables pertaining to the patients and staff in these wards were identified and analysed: two themes were revealed — motivation of patients and staff, and institutionalisation (p. 283). The article ends with discussion of intrinsic and extrinsic motivation, knowledge of which can help nurses to develop a positive attitude to promoting continence.

Incontinence of faeces (encopresis)
Despite the increasing publicity now given to urinary incontinence, faecal incontinence still carries a high degree of social stigma. A young man describes the shame, misery and sense of isolation he felt, when, in his mid-20s he became incontinent of faeces as a result of inflammatory bowel disease (Thomas, 1987). Turner (1987) in a detailed article describes how continence of faeces is normally achieved, and points out how unfortunate psychological associations can be made in the early period of life which can later in childhood result in constipation. Lack of dietary fibre and fluid can further predispose to constipation in children. As faeces collects in the rectum and descending colon, it is 'dried' by absorption of fluid. Bacterial action in the colon and secretion of mucus can liquify the external surface of the mass of faeces and this fluid is expelled involuntarily as episodes of 'faecal incontinence'. Treatment for constipation and prevention of its recurrence was mentioned on page 185.

In adults the problem of faecal incontinence is probably under-reported because, not only is it a taboo subject, but the afflicted person can only interpret it as regression to a status associated with the early years of life, and feel bewildered and demoralised. Norton (1986), estimates that about one adult in 200 living in the community suffers regular faecal incontinence. Alderman (1988) describes the many different causes but states that faecal impaction is probably the commonest cause: patient assessment is discussed followed by possible nursing interventions. In a later article, Alderman (1989) discusses the social consequences of faecal incontinence and suggests that nurses can do much to prevent some of the problems which can lead to incontinence. Alderman makes it clear that the majority of sufferers can be cured, but for those people with intractable faecal incontinence advice is required about 'protective pads and garments to ensure the best quality of life possible' . . . .

Nursing the incontinent patient

For both ambulant and bedfast patients there are body-worn and bed drainage fabrics so that the skin is no longer in constant contact with urine. There are several different 'pad and pant' systems on the market, none of which is universally suitable for all incontinent people. In an ideal world, all types would be available to nurses helping these people, so that the one best suited to, and most acceptable by the wearer would be an individualised decision after trying several of them. In the real world nurses need to discover which pads and pants are available locally to help achieve the patient's goal of containing incontinence. This also applies to the bed drainage fabrics. However, some male incontinence can be coped with by penile sheath drainage. Blannin (1987) lists some causes of male incontinence and gives practical advice on how to cope with the condition. Gonsalkovale & Lawless (1987) tested two types of penile sheath in geriatric wards; the comparison was made in relation to comfort, changing times and cost-effectiveness.

When there is incontinence of faeces the patient does need to be changed immediately. In many ways it is easier for the nurse to manage an episode of faecal incontinence in a bedfast patient. Coping with such an episode in an ambulant patient is a more problematic task: this was highlighted some time ago, in the research done by Reid (1976). Her observations of the nursing management of incontinence revealed how ill-equipped are many hospital wards for enabling nurses to adequately wash patients and change their day clothes. Either the patient needs to be taken to his bed if this is to be managed properly, or the toilet facilities require to be adapted to provide the nurse with appropriate facilities. Some modern hospitals are equipped with bidets and these permit thorough washing of the perineum and indeed enable many patients to carry out this personal cleansing procedure themselves.

In hospital the use of a drawsheet over a plastic sheet is still common practice as it allows easy replacement of one item of linen with minimum disturbance to the patient in bed. However, drawsheets tend to allow urine to pool under the patient; they also slip and crease readily which is particularly undesirable if pressure sores are to be avoided. The use of incontinence pads is not an ideal solution either because they are seldom effective in containing the urine in one area and frequently cause irritation to the skin and therefore they too may contribute to pressure sore development. Sudocrem is better for treating incontinence-related dermatitis than conventionally used zinc cream; it also has bactericidal properties (Anthony et al, 1987).

At home, however, protection of the bed is very necessary because most families are without a large resource of linen, and laundering wet and soiled linen becomes a major task for relatives, one which may be impossible if they are elderly or infirm. In the UK some areas have a laundry service through which bed linen is loaned and laundered and this is a tremendous help for a family when coping with an ill member at home.

Supporting the patient. The importance of the nurse showing discretion, tact and kindness when helping patients who have problems with the AL of eliminating cannot be overemphasised. It is especially important when nursing incontinent patients. Some nurses do not find it a pleasant activity and it is sometimes difficult for them not to feel annoyed or disgusted at having to deal with another person's excreta. However, such a feeling must not be conveyed to the patient who should never be scolded or made to feel like a child. Realising that it is probably equally distasteful to patients, communicating and understanding of their feelings by sympathetic and tactful nursing can turn what might otherwise be an unpleasant nursing activity into a satisfying and important aspect of nursing.

Because incontinence may make people feel ashamed and cause them to lose dignity it may cause loss of interest in personal appearance which can mean being less attractive to other people including those of the opposite sex. For those who are sexually active there is an even bigger problem. Nurses are becoming less reticent than previously to discuss with incontinent people how to continue expressing their sexuality, including being sexually active if they so desire.

In this section the term 'continence adviser' has been mentioned several times, and merits some amplification. The Association of Continence Advisers in the UK started in 1981 as a multidiciplinary group of professionals. Each member of the multidisciplinary group has a role in assisting the incontinent person. In alphabetical order the team consists of chiropodists, doctors, nurses, occupational therapists, physiotherapist, radiologists, supplies officers and technicians. At the Association's instigation the subject of incontinence has been discussed in parliament, and there have been television and radio programmes on the subject. From April 1987 in the UK there has been television advertisement about available products and Swaffield (1987) and White (1988) report on these promotions. The role of the nurse continence adviser is described by Turner (1988), but there is variation in interpretation of the role to suit local circumstances. The Association of Continence Advisers in the UK started its first biannual journal as a

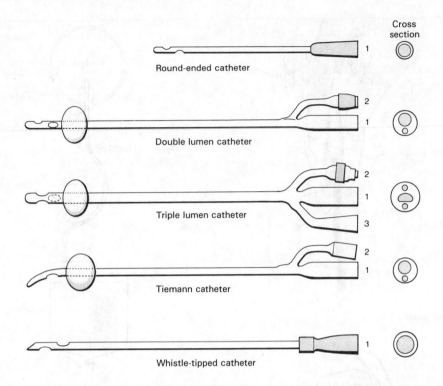

Fig. 10.1 Selection of catheters in common use. Key: 1 = channel for urine flow; 2 = channel for balloon inflation; 3 = channel for irrigating fluid flow

supplement in the *Nursing Times* in 1987. The journal will contain up-to-date information about the latest research-based knowledge related to promoting continence of urine and faeces.

CHANGE IN MODE OF ELIMINATING

For various reasons it sometimes becomes necessary for urine or faeces to be removed from the body by an alternative or artificial route. For the patient, this causes problems arising from the imposed change in mode of eliminating.

Urinary catheterisation

Urine can be drained to the exterior through a tube — a catheter — inserted into the bladder via the urethra. This may be required once only, for example to ensure an empty bladder pre-operatively, or to relieve a distended bladder post-operatively. Catheterisation may be required intermittently, perhaps to measure the amount of urine remaining in the bladder after normal emptying. In all these instances, a simple straight catheter is used (the one for females is shorter than the one for males) and the urine is collected in a sterile measuring vessel, the whole procedure being carried out using aseptic technique. Clean (not aseptic) intermittent self-catheterisation was mentioned on page

188 in the context of coping with neurogenic bladder. Seth (1987) provides a brief historical survey of the activity followed by details of the types of people for whom it is a satisfactory solution to the problem of incontinence, and the article includes instruction necessary for female and male self-catheterisation. In a later article, Seth (1988) illustrates how available catheters over the last 40 years have improved with the objective of increasing patient comfort. Alderman (1988) also discusses and illustrates the types of catheter available for self-catheterisation.

An indwelling catheter attached to a drainage system is required by some of the people who have no control over passing urine. It is recommended that it is used for as short a time as possible, but there are people for whom it solves the problem of incontinence on a long-term basis.

The procedure of catheterisation. An aseptic technique must be used in order to prevent the introduction of pathogenic microorganisms into the urinary bladder. A selection of catheters in common use is shown in Figure 10.1, and insertion of a catheter into the female urethra is shown in Figure 10.2; Figure 10.3 illustrates the insertion of a catheter into the male urethra. Infection is a common and potentially dangerous complication of catheterisation and Johnson (1986) says that urinary tract infection is the commonest hospital-acquired infection. It accounts for approximately 30% of all such infections (Fig. 6.7, p. 94) and at least 500 deaths per year in the UK. By using a

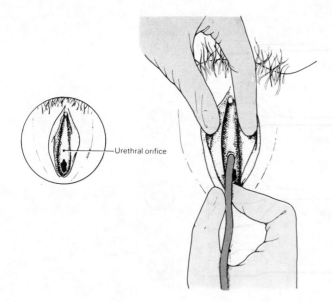

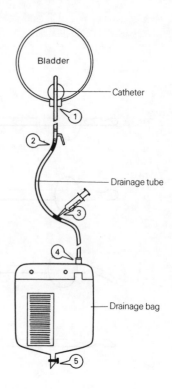

Fig. 10.2   Female catheterisation

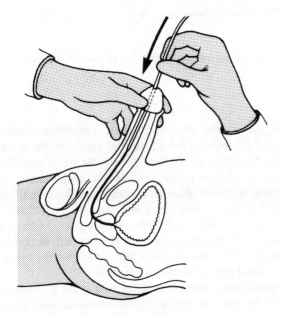

Fig. 10.3   Insertion of catheter into male urethra (Reprinted with permission from Jamieson et al 1988 Guidelines for clinical nursing practices, Churchill Livingstone, Edinburgh.)

Fig. 10.4   Points at which bacteria can enter a urinary drainage system 1- the urethral orifice; 2- connection of catheter and drainage tube; 3- where sample of urine taken; 4- connection of drainage tube and collecting bag; 5- drainage bag outlet.

system of urinary drainage the likelihood of urinary infection is significantly lessened. However, recent research (Mulhall et al, 1988a) has cast doubts on the efficacy of some nursing practices which were observed. They were mainly concerned with the five points at which bacteria can enter what was previously and often still is, called a closed urinary drainage system. They are illustrated in Figure 10.4 and will now be mentioned briefly.

1. *The urethral orifice*, also called the meatal space and the pericatheter space. Microorganisms entering via the urethral orifice travel along the potential space between the outer catheter surface and the urethral mucosa. It has to be remembered that the urethra has a natural bacterial flora of commensals, that is, it is colonised (p. 74); some commensals are potentially pathogenic, and any injury by catheter to the urethral mucosa will encourage the change of state from colonisation to auto-infection. Mulhall et al (1988b) state that 'Cleansing of the meatal region is desirable on social grounds. However, there is no firm existing evidence to support the use of antiseptics.' It is obvious that further research is required to guide acceptable intervention on 'social grounds', or on validated grounds for 'prevention of urinary tract infection'. Application of knowledge from microbiology suggests that 4-hourly washing of the perineum would keep the natural flora within the limits with which the body's defence system can cope.

2. *Connection of catheter and drainage tube.* The logical reasons for breaking this seal are when a substance has to be injected into the bladder, or when a bladder washout becomes necessary. Both these interventions would be carried out using aseptic technique. Inadvertent breaking of this seal is not specifically reported in the literature.

3. *Where sample of urine taken.* A specimen of urine can be withdrawn by steadying the part and piercing the tube

with a sterile widebored needle attached to a large sterile syringe. The nurse's hands must have been washed to remove both resident and particularly transient flora (p. 75), some of which may be pathogenic organisms, particularly in a hospital setting. A plastic apron will protect the nurse's uniform from any splash while transferring urine into a specimen jar. Afterwards meticulous hand washing is obviously essential to prevent cross-infecting another patient. Urine as a 'body fluid' capable of transmitting the AIDS viruses was mentioned on page 185. *The drainage tube* requires mention. Its purpose is to provide an uninterrupted downhill flow of urine, so it should never be above bladder level. The downhill flow is necessary to prevent stasis of urine in the bladder, especially important if the urine is known to be infected (bacteriuria).

4. *Connection of drainage tube and collecting bag.* It is necessary to break this seal when changing the collecting bag, whether it is of the single use type, or of the reusable type in which there is an outlet at the base for emptying urine. Before separating the drainage tube and collecting bag, placement of a clamp on each, helps to minimise urine splash. As soon as they are separated, the end of the drainage tube is in contact with the atmosphere which may contain pathogenic microorganisms, so time-wise minimal exposure is desirable. The nurse's hands require to have been effectively washed both before and after replacement of a collecting bag.

5. *Drainage bag outlet.* These are only present on the reusable bags and there are several types available. The results of one study indicated that nurses can contaminate their hands with microorganisms during bag emptying (Glenister, 1987). Assessment of visible hand contamination on emptying seven different types of drainage bag was achieved by the addition of methylene blue to the urine bag, and measuring the area of splash. After bag emptying, a drop of blue dye remained on the end of the outlet tap; Glenister suggests that the outlet needs to be wiped with an absorbent/disinfection cloth at the end of the procedure, but Mulhall et al (1988) state that 'There is very little evidence in existing literature concerning the value of disinfecting taps on drainage bags.' They consider that a sensible precaution would be to dry the tap thoroughly to prevent multiplication of bacteria.

Ascending infection along the surface of the urethra to the bladder has been mentioned; it can also occur via a contaminated drainage system (Blenkharn, 1988). In an attempt to avoid it, prevention of backflow during bag emptying is accomplished by the bag remaining below the level of the bladder. There are now several devices fitted to drainage bags to prevent backflow but scientific and clinical evidence of their effectiveness is inadequate (Mulhall et al, 1988). Although the various drainage systems are visually 'closed', and the term 'closed urinary drainage system' is in common use, Lanara (1987) calls these 'open drainage systems' — they are open in a microbiological context because, on emptying they are open to the air. Closed systems have a second collection bag below the first and separated from it by a valve. The valve is opened to drain urine from the upper to the lower bag; it is then closed before the tap at the bottom of the lower bag is opened, thereby preventing access of air to the system. Evidence to support the microbiological 'openness' of the outlet tap in a single bag drainage system is provided by Blenkharn (1988).

The patient's problems. In this section so far, the emphasis has been on the equipment available and the technique of catheterisation, rather than on the patient, but consideration of the patient is all-important whichever type of catheterisation is used. Patients who are catheterised have a variety of problems to contend with. They are subjected to the embarrassment of the procedure and then have to put up with the inconvenience of having a tube and bag attached to the body. Patients have to get used to the difficulties this presents when carrying out such activities as bathing, walking or getting in and out of bed. They may also be embarrassed about explaining the appliance to visitors. Not least, such patients are at risk of developing a urinary infection. Helping patients to come to terms with such varied problems demands sympathetic and skilful nursing.

People with indwelling urethral drainage systems are being discharged home, and of course before they leave hospital they need information about their catheter system and practice in managing it to prevent urinary tract infection. Roe (1988) carried out a study to discover nurses' knowledge about catheters and the advice which they gave to patients and relatives about caring for the drainage system at home. After analysing the data Roe wrote, 'Teaching patients and carers about catheter care is not a recognised priority in nursing practice'. The study then investigated patients' understanding and knowledge of their catheters. 67% of patients stated that no one had given them an initial explanation of how to care for the apparatus. A commercial firm provides a free booklet to help to increase patients' understanding of, and knowledge about catheters (Roe, 1987).

Another experienced nurse developed a teaching programme for nurses to help them in their role as health educators (Wright, 1989). She also produced a written guide for catheterised patients who are being discharged with a catheter in situ: permission is given for it to be photocopied. McCullough (1989) carried out a small survey of 12 men to find out how they coped with their urinary drainage system at home. They were asked what advice they had been given about fluid intake; method of meatal cleansing; how often to renew the night bag; how to keep the night bag clean; how often to renew the day bag; handwashing; avoiding constipation and exercising. It is evident from the literature that patients require to have opportunity for practising self-care before discharge from hospital.

Urinary diversion

If urethral excretion of urine is not possible at all, as occurs in some diseases affecting the lower urinary tract, a permanent method of urinary diversion becomes necessary. For patients this involves a drastic change in their mode of eliminating. Urostomy is the overall name given to various surgical procedures which are used to bypass the bladder; urine is diverted from the two ureters into a stoma which opens onto the abdominal wall. Like the other output stomas (colostomy and ileostomy) the excretion flows involuntarily into a bag-like appliance which is fitted over the stoma and adheres to the surrounding skin. The urostomy bag has a tap at the base for emptying the urine, so what was said about teaching people to manage an indwelling catheter drainage system is pertinent here. The apparatus also has an anti-reflux valve to prevent back-flow of urine when the person lies down. Adults requiring this type of surgery may well have been ill for some time and may be depressed that the bladder condition is not improving. Communication with them needs to be especially sensitive and empathic as they try to come to terms with a change in body image related to the AL of eliminating, which in itself has such private and personal overtones. The principles of nursing are the same as for other 'ostomy' people and are discussed on page 195. There is a Urostomy Association in the UK where people can gain and give support by sharing for instance, a practical detail about care of the appliance which has been found useful.

Interest in and concern for people who have any kind of stoma has been demonstrated by nurses specialising in stoma care. The trend began in the USA in 1958 but the first stomatherapist was not a nurse but an 'ileostomist'; stoma care nursing was pioneered in the UK at St Bartholomew's Hospital in London in 1969, and it is estimated that there are now upwards of 200 stoma care nurses in the UK (Dyer, 1988).

Renal replacement therapy (renal dialysis)

Other changes in the mode of eliminating become necessary when conventional treatment for 'chronic renal failure' is not adequately removing waste products from the blood. The medical diagnosis changes to 'end-stage renal failure' and other means of removal become necessary for these people who have not enjoyed good health, probably for many years. The generic name for these treatments is 'renal replacement therapy' and it includes peritoneal dialysis, haemodialysis (renal dialysis), and renal transplantation, and these will be discussed albeit briefly.

Peritoneal dialysis is a relatively new treatment which started in the USA in 1978 (Stevens, 1988). For many patients it is now the first line of treatment and is the most rapidly expanding area in renal replacement therapy

(Milne, 1988). In the UK its increase has been matched by a decrease in the number of patients on home dialysis (Stevens, 1988). The peritoneum is used as the dialysing membrane and the dialysing fluid is introduced via a catheter passed through the abdominal wall and anchored there. Fluid from a plastic bag passes through the catheter and remains in the abdomen for 4–5 hours, after which it is drained back into the bag. The process is repeated four or five times daily and the continuous clearance of waste products maintains a more stable blood chemistry and avoids the peaks and troughs which can occur with haemodialysis. This lessens the feeling of exhaustion experienced by people in end-stage renal failure, and gives greater dietary freedom and often a free fluid intake (Milne, 1988). As with any invasive technique, there is a risk of infection and people on peritoneal dialysis need to know how to recognise it, and what to do when it occurs. Milne's article describes how one dialysis unit carries out individualised teaching plans. The full title of this technique — continuous ambulatory peritoneal dialysis — shows that it is compatible with people carrying out their normal daily routine, obviously modified to accommodate the periods of infusion and withdrawing of fluid. However, such people need a lot of support and encouragement as their life literally depends on their commitment to complying with the exacting routine.

Intermittent peritoneal dialysis is the least popular of the three dialyses. Treatment time is 9–10 hours, three or four times weekly and many people cannot fit this regime into their lifestyle. It has been found useful in acute renal failure and for some types of drug overdose (Boore et al, 1987).

Haemodialysis may be the treatment of choice for acute renal failure but as this is a reversible condition it is usually a short-term, life-saving treatment. It can also be used for short periods to rest the peritoneum when infection supervenes in that form of dialysis. Haemodialysis involves the continual removal of blood from an artery into a closed circuit containing a thin membrane which is bathed with dialysing fluid. This, just like the kidney nephrons, removes urea and other waste products from the blood before it returns to a vein and into the general circulation. The process is usually carried out overnight, several nights a week. All people requiring any form of dialysis are stabilised in a hospital dialysis unit where many learn to be independent. Some return to the unit to carry out their treatment independently; others return because they require supervision during treatment.

Approximately two-thirds become independent on home dialysis. Another person, usually a family member, learns to manage the technique and this can strain family relationships. Some people on haemodialysis experience almost immobilising exhaustion at times, others tire easily. As well as coming to terms with the essential demanding routine, there is usually restriction of diet and this may affect not only appetite but also put certain constraints on socialising and family relationships. But since the stark alternative is death, this unrelenting routine has to be continued for life or until a kidney transplant is available. A few special holiday centres provide dialysis machines and people on renal dialysis can go to these centres, dialyse at night and enjoy a holiday during the day.

Unfortunately, few countries can afford to provide dialysis treatment and kidney machines for all those who require them. Without them many people die each year. When economic resources for health care are limited, many moral dilemmas face those responsible for allocating finance, as in this case, deciding who should have the available machines.

Renal transplantation offers a new hope for people with end stage renal failure, but it is not a first treatment for many, because there are not enough donor kidneys available. The system in some countries is distribution of donor cards so that people can carry with them notification of their willingness to have their kidneys used in the event of sudden death. Some other countries have an 'opt-out' system whereby, unless a person carries an opt-out card, in the case of sudden death, the kidneys can be removed for donation. Currently a system of 'required request' is being discussed in many countries. In the case of an unconscious dying patient, the doctor would be required to ask the family whether or not the patient had expressed any objection to his/her organs being used for transplant. If the patient's wishes are not known, the doctors would be required to ask the family if they had any objection. The public are being encouraged to think about these possibilities, so that, should a family tragedy occur, the 'required request' from the doctor will not be perceived as meddlesome or offensive, but as a duty which has to be carried out.

Undoubtedly the quality of life is greatly improved for most people who have had a kidney transplant. They no longer need a kidney machine; there is usually a gradual reduction in dietary restriction and fluid intake, and their energy level rises.

Recently there has been concern about payment being made for donation of a kidney and some countries are in the process of legislating against this.

Ileostomy/colostomy

People at an early stage on the lifespan may need to have a stoma — urostomy, ileostomy or colostomy. They may be newborn babies, children and teenagers. If the stoma is permanent, children incorporate it into their body image, but the older child or adolescent has to go through the same sort of psychological grieving experiences as adults (p. 335). Health visitors, community nurses, school nurses and occupational health nurses all make an important contribution to the adjustment of this group to 'being different' yet still valued as an individual, and

having an important contribution to make in developing their potential talents. Parents and school nurses should ensure that the teaching staff are aware of the implications of stoma surgery (Johnson, 1988). Children express their sexuality in many different ways; however, after puberty, for most people who are confronted with needing a stoma, the AL of expressing sexuality assumes importance (p. 298). They experience fear and anxiety about matters such as: whether they will still look attractive; will the appliance show under their clothes; will they smell; will they be able to have sex; and will they be able to conceive? (Bell, 1989).

In the older age group bowel cancer can be the reason for creating a colostomy. Some surgeons regard stoma formation for cancer as lifesaving (Donaldson, 1989), but Devlin (1985) refers to ostomists as 'people who have traded death for disablement'. There is no doubt that new ostomists have to face many problems and anxieties before they feel able to return to their previous social activities. Elcoat (1988) writes:

It is therefore essential that the care planned for patients undergoing this type of mutilating surgery reflects realistic goals to enable them to achieve psychological wellbeing and become rehabilitated, resuming an undiminished role in society.

In 1978 it was estimated that there were 52 000 people with a stoma in the UK (Health Services Development, 1978). In that year, the UK government circulated to all health authorities; recommendations on the precision of stoma care, yet Dyer (1988) states that there were approximately 200 stoma care nurses in the UK.

From this information it is obvious that not all people with a stoma can have access to a specialist nurse. Surveys of patients and trained nurses about the teaching and counselling support for new stoma patients have confirmed that many wards do not have access to the services of a full-time specialist nurse. To help nurses in these wards, to help patients who are undergoing stoma surgery, the specialist stoma nurses share their up-to-date attitudes, knowledge and skills by publishing articles in appropriate journals.

With regard to ileostomy, the effluent is fluid, so the external appliance may have an outlet tap at its base via which the contents of the bag can be emptied into the toilet, thus reducing the frequency of application of a clean bag to the skin. The fluid is strongly alkaline and may contain proteolytic enzymes, so prevention of leakage from the appliance, and extra protection of the peristomal skin are essential.

Regarding a colostomy, its site will determine consistency of the effluent; from a transverse colostomy it will be a semisolid stool which collects involuntarily in a closed bag which is removed daily, followed by application of a clean bag. The faecal content of the used bag has to be flushed away before wrapping in a plastic bag or newspaper, sealing, and placing in the household refuse system. The effluent from a sigmoid colostomy resembles a normal stool, and cleansing of the bag before disposal requires cutting and eversion before flushing, wrapping, sealing and placing in the refuse bin. It is little wonder that many adults and elderly people find it aesthetically unacceptable. Harlow (1988) investigated the disposal of used stoma bags and states:

So we not only have physical and psychological problems with disposal of soiled stoma bags, but also social and ecological ones.

Stoma care nurses spend much of their time reassuring patients that they can lead a virtually normal life postoperatively, and yet we are still in the Dark Ages when it comes to disposal. We could make a start by insisting that every public lavatory has a bin for disposal of soiled appliances. . . . It should be mandatory for all toilets in public buildings, hotels, guest houses and restaurants to have adequate facilities.

It is hoped work will progress on the biodegradable bags and perhaps surgical techniques will also improve so that permanent stomas requiring bags will be things of the past.

Meantime, however, we need to promote a sense of social responsibility for those people who do have a stoma so that they can experience an acceptable quality of living.

Currently a vast selection of appliances is available to colostomists and most can be tailored to suit individual requirements (Airey et al, 1988). Some people with a colostomy eventually manage a daily evacuation at a particular time and are sufficiently confident to wear only a dressing over the stoma or a stoma cap. Others irrigate the bowel above the stoma each morning to minimise involuntary passing of faeces into the appliance during the day and between irrigations some only wear a stoma cap. These groups have less skin soreness, probably from minimisation of leakage. In spite of improvements in materials and design, patients' main problems continue to be skin soreness, leakage from the bag, and the odour and sound of the involuntary passage of flatus.

CHANGE OF DEPENDENCE/INDEPENDENCE STATUS FOR ELIMINATING

The concept of a dependence/independence continuum is useful when focused to the AL of eliminating because movement can be in either direction. Many patients are only temporarily dependent on the nurse for example for inserting a suppository or giving an enema and they quickly regain independence. On the other hand when a person succumbs to disease of the urinary or defaecatory system the dependence may be for information and advice about the condition; it may be about short-term changes, for example in diet and fluid intake and how abatement of the condition can be evaluated until the previous state of independence has been regained. For others, the change in dependence/independence status can be caused by limited mobility, confinement to bed or psychological disturbance and these will now be discussed.

Limited mobility

As mentioned earlier (p. 179) several physical skills are involved in the AL of eliminating. Any limitation on mobilising obviously reduces a person's potential for independence. A person who is unable to walk easily, or for any distance, will have difficulty in getting to and from the toilet, especially one which is situated upstairs. Those confined to a wheelchair may have problems when having to rely on public toilets unless there are facilities specially designed with an entrance ramp and the cubicle door wide enough to allow the wheelchair through. Someone with an arm in plaster or with hands badly affected by arthritis has a different problem. That person will be able to get to the toilet but may be unable to undress and dress or use toilet paper.

Any impairment of movement, be it of the arms and/or legs, may render a person incapable of managing to use the toilet without assistance.

Particular problems arise for the patient in hospital whose mobility is completely restricted on account of confinement to bed.

Confinement to bed

When for any reason confinement to bed is prolonged, there may be loss of tone in the gastrointestinal and trunk muscles which may predispose to constipation. Urinary stasis can occur especially if the patient is nursed in the supine position, since urinary flow from the kidneys to the bladder is assisted by the force of gravity. The attendant sluggish flow of urine is conducive to the formation of stones (calculi). In addition, when there is reduced muscular activity, there are fewer acid waste products in the urine so it tends to be alkaline — another condition which favours stone formation.

Nursing activities include supervising an adequate fluid and dietary fibre intake and encouraging the patient to use all muscles as much as possible. Some patients may require help from the physiotherapist in learning to exercise their abdominal and pelvic floor muscles.

Patients confined to bed or the bedside area are totally dependent on the nurse for help with the AL of eliminating. Unless a patient is too ill or incapacitated to move, a commode at the bedside is preferable to a bedpan. In a study, four groups of patients had their heart rate, oxygen consumption and blood pressure measured after using a bedpan, and after using a commode. Use of a commode produced no more cardiovascular stress than use of a bedpan (Nursing Times, 1986). This is not surprising as being perched on a bedpan is not very comfortable and it is almost impossible for a woman to use toilet paper to dry the perineum without her hand coming into contact with the urine in the pan. Handwashing facilities must be provided; it is the single most important method of infection control (p. 93).

However, there are patients for whom there is no alternative to a bedpan, such as those on traction, or attached to monitors. They need to be lifted on and off the bedpan and the nurse needs to carry out post-elimination hygiene in such a way as to minimise their embarrassment because they probably have not been helped in this way since they were small children.

Whether using a bedpan or a commode at the bedside, patients will probably experience embarrassment knowing that the bedcurtains do not mask either smell or noise when urine, faeces and flatus are being passed. Whenever possible it would seem to be desirable to transfer patients to the toilet in a wheelchair or a Sanichair.

Psychological disturbance

Various mental abilities are necessary for people to appreciate and conform to the various social customs associated with elimination. Knowledge is also needed to understand the importance of disposing of excreta hygienically, to recognise abnormalities of urine and faeces which may indicate the presence of disease, and to prevent the occurrence of problems such as constipation and urinary infection.

Psychological disturbance which results in confusion, depression or disorientation may mean that people do not remember when they last went to toilet, for example, so they may keep returning absent-mindedly or else forget to go again when necessary. Other patients become incontinent because they fail to recognise the signals of a full bladder or rectum, or recognising them, fail to respond to them. Sometimes patients who are disorientated, particularly at night, cannot find their way to the toilet and others may be so confused that they eliminate indiscriminately in their beds or on the ward floor.

People who are mentally handicapped are by definition slow learners. At one time their incontinence was accepted as inevitable. However, many of them are now helped to achieve both urinary and faecal continence by the use of behavioural modification techniques which were mentioned on page 188.

Loss of consciousness results in loss of the ability to respond to a full bladder or bowel and the unconscious patient becomes totally dependent on others for ensuring that urine and faeces are removed and disposed of. The nurse should carry this out in a manner that acknowledges the human dignity of the unconscious person.

It is impossible to capture on paper the large variety of patients' problems which necessitate assessing, planning, implementing and evaluating any change in either direction on the dependence/independence continuum related to the AL of eliminating.

SOME SPECIFIC PROBLEMS ASSOCIATED WITH ELIMINATING

Pain related to eliminating

The general discussion of pain is on page 121; here it will be focused to the AL of eliminating, and considered as pain which can be experienced in any part of the urinary or defaecatory systems. The pain from an overfull bladder, and pain experienced when trying to expel hard, dry faeces have already been mentioned.

Dysuria is the name given to painful micturition. The problem for the patient is a burning sensation as urine is passed and a constant feeling of an overfull bladder and a frequent urge to pass urine. There may be a constant dull ache in the groin. Some preventive and comforting activities for this condition are mentioned on page 203.

Ureteric colic is usually caused by a stone moving in one of the ureters and the muscular contractions on, and the irritation caused by the stone produces the patient's problems which are excruciating pain, restlessness and sweating. The condition usually constitutes an emergency admission to hospital where muscle relaxant and pain killing drugs will be prescribed by the doctor unless surgery is imminent when the prescription will be for preoperative drugs.

Tenesmus is the medical name for painful, ineffectual straining to empty the bowel. People with this problem should be advised to see the doctor because the cause can be as diverse as proctitis, prolapse of the rectum, rectal tumour or irritable bowel syndrome. Meantime, a warm bath may be comforting.

Flatulence is gaseous intestinal distension. The intestinal flora produce some gas which is normally expelled per rectum. Some people experience excessive gas production which can be embarrassing as it produces borborygmi — rumbling noises caused by the movement of gas in the intestines; it can also cause abdominal distension which can be painful. It can sometimes be moved towards the rectum by contraction of the abdominal muscles. Carminatives taken orally may be effective, the most usual one being peppermint in the form of sweets or peppermint water; others are cinnamon, cloves, ginger and nutmeg. Sometimes a warm bath can result in the passing of flatus. Alternatively a long hollow lubricated tube can be passed along the colon while the free end is immersed in water, through which the flatus can be seen to bubble. This is an intimate procedure and patients require not only an explanation of what to expect, but also an empathic approach by nursing staff.

Haemorrhoidal pain is increased on defaecation. Haemorrhoids ('piles') are dilations of the terminal parts of the veins which lie in the submucosa of the anal canal. The doctor can prescribe medication, which when applied locally reduces the inflammation and discomfort. Constipation predisposes to haemorrhoids: should a nursing assessment reveal this problem then teaching about prevention and ordering a high fibre diet are possible nursing interventions to achieve the goal of a soft bulky stool which is easy to pass.

Postoperative pain on defaecation is feared by many patients after abdominal or urogenital operations and this may predispose to the problem of constipation. Discomfort will be alleviated to some extent by ensuring that faeces are soft and as easy as possible to pass without straining. The patient can also be advised to lean forward while sitting on the toilet, folding the arms against the abdomen to give support to the wound and increase intra-abdominal pressure.

Anxiety about investigations/surgery
In the diagnosis of the cause of a problem related to eliminating, the doctor may require to carry out certain medical investigations many of which, being concerned with intimate parts of the body, are anxiety-producing and distressing for patients. The fact that patients do experience discomfort and anxiety related to investigations was highlighted several years ago by Wilson-Barnett (1980). She points out that the level of anxiety is not necessarily related to the seriousness or invasiveness of the particular test and urges nurses to pay attention to the feelings of individual patients. The research also attempted to assess whether information and explanations about scheduled investigations would reduce anxiety. Barium enema was one of the investigations studied and it was found that explanation of the preparation for, and procedure of, a barium enema did help to make the patient feel less anxious.

An evacuant enema is still, in some hospitals, part of the routine preoperative preparation for surgery not involving the urinary and defaecatory systems. However, with the emphasis on holistic medicine it is gradually becoming a more selective procedure. There are a number of disposable evacuant enemas available; the microenema contains 5 ml of fluid and the hypertonic saline enemas contain 128 ml. Either, or both of these may be medically prescribed and thereafter, planning, implementing, evaluating and documenting the intervention is a nursing responsibility.

When investigation or surgery involves the defaecatory system it is obviously necessary to remove faeces from the bowel, and the enemas just mentioned may suffice or they may be combined with rectal lavage. This involves passing a wide bore catheter into the rectum through which a funnel full of water runs and is then returned into a bucket on the floor by lowering and inverting the funnel over it. This process is repeated until the returned fluid is clear and free from faecal flakes or stain and it can take up to 1 hour to achieve this (Roper, 1988). Another bowel preparation introduced in the 1970s is whole gut irrigation. From a flask containing either saline or mannitol, fluid

drips through a nasogastric tube into the stomach while the patient sits on a commode for several hours. It is regarded as the most efficient remover of faeces from the gut (Ratcliffe, 1988). His review of the literature highlights some of the adverse physiological changes and lack of patient acceptability. One of the research groups (Downing et al, 1979) made some recommendations to improve patient acceptability, including sedation, a separate room with radio and television, and a padded commode.

Some of these various methods are used prior to a barium enema and a low residue diet is often prescribed for the previous few days. Patients need to understand that another enema containing barium will be administered in the X-ray department and that after the X-rays are taken they can go immediately to the toilet to get rid of most of the heavy white chalk-like substance. Any residual barium will be passed in the next stool and the nurse needs to know and document when and how often there is a bowel movement.

Sigmoidoscopy usually requires some bowel preparation and possibly dietary modificaton before passage of a tube-like instrument into the bowel via the anus, through which the rectum and sigmoid colon can be viewed. The actual procedure is uncomfortable rather than painful but understandably some patients find it difficult to relax the anus in the presence of other people. Sigmoidoscopy is gradually being replaced by colonoscopy for which whole gut irrigation is usually necessary. The new fibreoptic colonoscopes can be manoeuvred through the colon to the caecum; light is transmitted by means of very fine glass fibres; photography and biopsy can be carried out if necessary. Whole gut irrigation, mentioned previously, is being done increasingly prior to any form of colorectal surgery.

The administration of evacuant enema prior to labour has become a controversial subject and many women are becoming more voluble about their objections. However, studies reveal that some women are so anxious about soiling during labour that they prefer to have an enema. After carrying out a randomised controlled trial with one group having an enema and the other not having an enema, the results did not support the routine use of enemas. But Drayton & Rees (1984) conclude that the state of the bowel must be assessed for each woman in labour and a mutual decision made as to whether or not an enema will be given.

Bowel preparation may be necessary when investigating urinary problems, for example, because of the proximity of the colon. If the kidneys and ureters require to be X-rayed, an empty bowel gives a clearer X-ray; and an intravenous injection of a radiopaque fluid is also necessary for the same reason. Many patients will not connect these procedures with investigation of their urinary problem, so they need an explanation. However, the radiopaque liquid may be injected directly into the renal pelvis by way of a fine catheter introduced through a cystoscope, an instrument which is introduced into the bladder via the urethra,

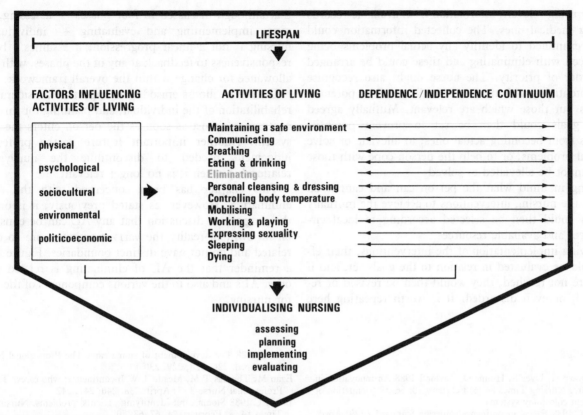

Fig. 10.5 The AL of eliminating within the model for nursing

and obviously patients require a different explanation in preparation for such an intimate procedure. It may be the bladder which has to be investigated after it has been filled with a radiopaque liquid introduced via a urethral catheter (see catheterisation p. 191). Or the examination may involve a micturating cystogram in which, after injection of a radiopaque liquid, sequential X-rays are taken during micturition. This can be part of an investigation into urinary incontinence, when an already demoralised patient requires extra psychological support. It may be provided by explanation of what to expect, and how the knowledge gained from breaking the social convention of privacy when passing urine, will enable realistic planning of interventions to relieve the distressing incontinence.

Individualising nursing

The first part of this chapter reflects the model of living — the nature of the AL of eliminating; the relationship of the lifespan to the AL; the effect of the individual's dependence/independence status; the influence of physical, psychological, sociocultural, environmental and politico-economic factors on the AL. In the second part of the chapter, a selection of actual and potential problems which are experienced by people in relation to eliminating have been described. With this background of general knowledge about the AL, it should be possible to incorporate such information (when it is relevant to the person's current circumstances) in an individualised nursing plan.

While describing the model for nursing, general information was given about individualising nursing (p. 51) which in fact is synonymous with the concept of the process of nursing.

Out of this background of general knowledge about the AL of eliminating, and about individualising nursing, it should then be possible to extract the issues which are relevant to an individual's current circumstances (whether in a health or illness setting) that is, to make an assessment of relevant issues according to the individual's stage on the lifespan; according to current level of dependence/independence; and take into account the relevant physical, psychological, sociocultural, environmental and politicoeconomic factors. Collectively, this information would provide a profile of the person's individuality in relation to eliminating.

As indicated earlier in the text, this assessment would be achieved by various means such as observing the person, acquiring information about the individual's usual habits in relation to this AL, partly by asking appropriate questions; partly by listening to the patient and/or relatives; and partly by using relevant information from available records including medical ones. The collected information could then be examined to identify any actual problems being experienced with eliminating and these could be arranged in an order of priority. The nurse might also recognise some potential problems — not all possible potential problems but those which are relevant. Mutually agreed realistic goals could then be set to prevent potential problems from becoming actual ones; to alleviate or solve the actual problems; or to help the person cope with those which cannot be alleviated or solved.

Keeping in mind what the person can and cannot do unaided, the nursing interventions to achieve the mutually set goals could then be selected according to local circumstances and available resources.

Following implementation of the interventions, their effects could be evaluated in relation to the goals set, and if goals were not reached, they would then be revised or rescheduled, or even discarded. It is worth repeating here that although discussed in four phases — assessing, planning, implementing and evaluating — individualising nursing is not a linear progression; it assumes a built-in responsiveness to feedback at any of the phases, with ample allowance for change within the overall framework.

During an illness episode, an important consideration is rehabilitation of the individual, and planning for this could commence almost as soon as the person enters the health system. Another important feature is the professional judgement needed to discontinue the nurse/patient relationship when it is no longer relevant.

This chapter has been concerned with the AL of eliminating. However, as stated previously, it is only for the purpose of discussion that any AL can be considered on its own; in reality the various activities are so closely related and do not have distinct boundaries. Figure 10.5 is a reminder that the AL of eliminating is related to the other ALs and also to the various components of the model for nursing.

REFERENCES

Airey S, Down G, Dyer S, Hulme O, Taylor I 1988 An innovation in stoma care. Nursing Times 84 (6) February 10: 56–59 (evaluation of a continent colostomy system)

Alderman C 1988 Faecal incontinence. Nursing Standard 2 (29) April 23: 32–34

Alderman C 1989 Faecal incontinence: social stigma. Nursing Standard 16 (3) January 14: 22–23

Anthony D, Barnes E, Malone–Lee J, Pluck R 1987 A clinical study of Sudocrem in the management of dermatitis due to the physical stress of incontinence in a geriatric population. Journal of Advanced Nursing 12 (5) September: 599–603

Bayliss V 1988 A private problem. Community Outlook November: 24, 26

Bell N 1989 Sexuality and the ostomist. Nursing Times 85 (5) February 1: 28–30

Beveridge C 1986 Catering for health can save money. The Health Service Journal 8: 1118

Blannin J 1987 Men's problems. Community Outlook February: 21, 29

Blenkharn I 1988 Urinary drainage systems: a new look. Nursing Times 84 (9) March 2: 72, 74, 76 The Journal of Infection Control Nursing

Boore et al 1987 Nursing the physically ill adult. Churchill Livingstone, Edinburgh, p 858

Booth B, Booth S 1986 Aperients can be deceptive. Nursing Times 82 (39) September 24: 38–39

Bradbury S M 1988 Collection of urine specimens in general practice: to clean or not to clean? The Journal of the Royal College of General Practitioners 38 (313): 363–365

Burkitt D 1983 Don't forget fibre in your diet. Positive health guide. Martin Dunitz, London

Candy C E 1987 Recent advances in the care if children with acute diarrhoea: giving responsibility to the nurse and parents. Journal of Advanced Nursing 12 (1) January: 95–99

Devlin B 1985 Second opinion. Health and Social Services Journal 95 (4931): 82

Disabled Living Foundation (undated) Adult bedwetting: causes, sources of help, remedies. Disabled Living Foundation, London

Donaldson I 1989 Communication can help ostomists accept their stoma. The Professional Nurse 4 (5) February: 242, 244, 245

Downing R et al 1979 Whole gut irrigation: a survey of patient opinion. British Journal of Surgery 66: 201–202

Drayton S, Rees C 1984 'They know what they're doing'. Nursing Mirror 159 (5) August 15: supplement iv–viii

Dyer S 1988 The development of stoma care. The Professional Nurse 3 (7) April: 226, 228, 229, 230

Egan M, Thomas T M, Meade T W Incontinence: who cares? The Professional Nurse 3 (7) April: 238, 240, 241, 242

Elcoat C 1988 Stoma care: identifying patients' problems. Nursing Times 84 (8) February 24: 67–68, 70

Faugier J 1988 Incontinence: hidden for whom? Senior Nurse 8 (3) March: 19–20

Faulkner A 1988 Too bad to mention? Nursing Times 84 (14) April 6: 70, 72

Glenister H 1987 The passage of infection. Nursing Times 83 (22) June 3: 68, 71, 73

Gonsalkovale M, Lawless J 1987 Looking for the perfect fit. Nursing Times 83 (40) October 7: 38–39

Goodinson S M 1986 The nurse as an innovator. The Professional Nurse 2 (3) December: 87–90

Harlow J 1988 Stoma care: waste disposal. Nursing Times 84 (8) February 24: 72, 75

Health Services Development 1978 The provision of stoma care. DHSS Publications HC 78, London

Heap J 1987 Too ashamed to tell. Community Outlook October: 14, 16, 18

Johnson A 1986 Urinary tract infection. Nursing: The Add-On Journal of Clinical Practice 3 (3) March: 102–105

Johnson H 1988 Growing up with a stoma. Community Outlook April: 15–16

Khatib H 1986 Acute gastroenteritis in infants. Nursing Times 82 (17) April 23: 31–32

Lanara V 1987 Catching infection from catheters. Conference report. Nursing Standard 1 (1) September 12: 6

Mallillin E 1985 Facts about fibre. Nursing Times 81 (47) November 20: 32

Manley R 1984 Winning the fight against apathy. Nursing Times (Community Outlook) April 11: 18

McCullough J 1989 Catheter care at home. Community Outlook March: 4, 6, 8

Millard P H 1979 The promotion of continence. Health Trends 11: 27–28

Milne C 1988 Continuous ambulatory peritoneal dialysis. Nursing Standard 2 (14) January 9: 29

Montgomery E 1986 Pelvic factor. Community Outlook September: 33–34

Mulhall A, Chapman R, Crow R 1988a Emptying urinary drainage bags. Nursing Times 84 (4) January 27: 64, 66

Mulhall A, Chapman R, Crow R 1988b Meatal cleansing. Nursing

Times 84 (4) January 27: 66, 69

Norton C 1983 Training for continence. In: Wilson–Barnett J (ed) Patient teaching. Churchill Livingstone, Edinburgh, p 153, 155–156

Norton C 1986 Nursing for continence. Beaconsfield Publishers, Beaconsfield

Norton C 1988 Incontinence can be prevented at all ages. The Professional Nurse 4 (1) October: 22, 24, 26

Ratcliffe P 1988 Whole gut irrigation: an acceptable risk? Nursing Times 84 (18) May 4: 33–34

Reid E A 1976 The problem of incontinence. Nursing Mirror 142 (14) April 1: 49–52

Roe B 1987 Catheter care: a guide for users and their carers. Available from H G Wallace Ltd, Unit A, Commerce Way, Colchester, Essex CO2 8HH

Rooney V M 1987 Toileting charts. Nursing: The Add–On Journal of Clinical Nursing 3 (22) October: 827–830

Roper N 1988 Principles of nursing in process context, 4th edn. Churchill Livingstone, Edinburgh, p 190

Royal College of Nursing 1983 The problem of promoting continence. Royal College of Nursing, London

Royal College of Nursing 1986 AIDS nursing guidelines. Royal College of Nursing, London, p 16, 20

Seth C 1987 Doing it yourself. Community Outlook October: 6, 11, 12

Shreeve C 1985 Bowel habits in the elderly. Nursing Mirror 160 (19) May 8: 20–21

Sibley L 1988 Confidence with incontinence. Nursing Times 84 (46) November 16: 42–43

Sillitoe R, Reed S 1986 Dry at night. Community Outlook March: 20, 21, 23

Stevens E 1988 End stage renal failure. Nursing (London) 3 (28) June–July: 1034–1036

Swaffield L 1979 Any questions? Nursing Times 75 (15) April 12: 94–95 Community Outlook

Swaffield J 1987 Find the right medium. Nursing Times 83 (15) April 15: 92

Swaffield J 1988 Motivating for continence. Nursing Times 84 (43) October 26: 56, 59

Thomas G B 1987 Is there anyone else out there? Nursing Times 83 (21) May 27: 32

Thomas L 1988 Eliminating incontinence. Nursing Standard 2 (17) January 30: 22

Thomas M 1987 More fibre makes sense. Nursing Times 83 (3) January 21: 39

Tierney A J 1973 Toilet training. Nursing Times 69 (51/52) December 20/27: 1740–1745

Turner A 1987 Childhood continence problems. The Professional Nurse 2 (4) January: 119–121

Turner A 1988 The role of the continence advisor. Senior Nurse 8 (3) March: 15

Turner A F 1988 Incontinence in people with mental handicap. The Professional Nurse 3 (9) June: 348–352

Turner A F 1988 Encopresis: family support must accompany treatment. The Professional Nurse 4 (3) December: 141–142, 144–146

Wallis M C 1984 The collection and testing of urine. Nursing: The Add–On Journal of Clinical Nursing 2 (29) 853–854

White H 1987 Setting up a service. Nursing Times 83 (46) November 18: 74–76

Wilson–Barnett J 1980 Prevention and alleviation of stress in patients. Nursing (Oxford) part 10 (February): 432–436

Wright E 1989 Teaching patients to cope with catheters at home. The Professional Nurse 4 (4) January: 191, 192, 194

Wright L 1974 Bowel function in hospital patients. The study of nursing care project reports. Series 1 Number 4. Royal College of Nursing, London, p 18

11

Personal cleansing and dressing

The activity of personal cleansing and dressing

Through the ages man has paid attention to his personal hygiene; there is archaeological evidence of the means whereby these activities were performed by members of previous civilisations. In each historical period there has been a gradual refinement of the articles used for cleansing the skin, hair, nails and teeth. Today, the ever increasing budgets of the cosmetic and hairdressing industries are indicative of an increased sophistication and interest in personal grooming.

The clothing and fashion industries have developed equally expansively. Clothes today are very different from past times; clothing worn by members of previous generations on formal occasions is evident from paintings. Also depicted are the clothes worn for leisure time activities and for different sorts of work. Progress in manufacturing processes has resulted today in a wide variety of 'easy-care' clothes for every conceivable occasion so that people can now enjoy this part of everyday living with less effort and greater variety.

THE NATURE OF PERSONAL CLEANSING AND DRESSING

The objective in most cultures is to socialise children into independent performance of personal cleansing and dressing activities, usually in privacy and in rooms set aside for these purposes. Even for those children who do not have their own bedroom, the bed and bedside area are symbols of privacy, and they usually dislike other members of the family 'interfering' with this area. For most people the attitude is inculcated from an early age that cleansing and clothing one's body is a personal concern, which if not carried out in privacy is accomplished in the presence of close family members only.

But the end result is observable by others, cleanliness and good grooming being commended in most cultures, while lack of these is deplored, particularly if accompanied by malodour and infestation. As there are several different activities concerned with personal cleansing, they will be discussed separately.

Washing and bathing. Most people clean the skin by washing with soap and water, rinsing and drying. It can be an 'all-over' wash using a basin of water, an immersion bath or a shower. The disadvantage of the immersion bath is that the bather is surrounded by the debris which is washed off the skin, and as the bath empties, some of this 'scum' adheres and has to be removed. The shower, in contrast, is said to be more hygienic and has the advantage that it saves space and water. Children are socialised by membership in the family into a frequency norm for their 'all-over' cleansing, such as daily or weekly, however it is accomplished.

Even the apparently simple activity of washing is implicated as important in the prevention of the spread of HIV infection and AIDS. Guidelines for theatre staff in particular,and health care workers in general recommend that, in the event of blood (or other body fluid) splashes to the skin, immediate washing with soap and water should be carried out (Sadler, 1987; Smith, 1988). This simple precaution applies equally to members of the general public, particularly those in contact with a person who is HIV seropositive.

Hand washing. Everyone is now encouraged to wash their hands before preparing or eating food and after going to the toilet. Notices to this effect are displayed in kitchens where food for large numbers of people is being prepared, and in toilets. This concern for more frequent hand washing resulted from the discovery that hands can act as a vehicle for the microorganisms that cause food poisoning and others that cause diseases of the bowel such as typhoid fever. If hand washing before meals is not feasible as on planes, finger wipes should be provided. Hand washing assumes a particular importance in the context of hospital care; yet, despite this, evidence suggests that patients' post-toilet hand washing is not routine (Pritchard & Hathaway, 1988) and nurses' hand washing is often inadequate and not carried out after all dirty activities (Gidley, 1987).

Frequent removal of the skin's natural oily secretion (sebum) may produce chafing, and broken skin is a route of entry for microorganisms which can lead to local infection. Dryness can be counteracted by using an emollient hand lotion after washing and adequate drying; when applied before sleeping it has maximum time to act.

Perineal toilet. The moist membranes in the female perineal area require special attention to maintain health and comfort and to avoid malodour. Females are encouraged to cleanse this area from front to back after elimination, especially of faeces. Microbiological data has confirmed that the majority of infections of the female bladder (cystitis) are caused by microorganisms that normally inhabit the bowel and are present in faeces and can therefore be in close proximity to the short urethra. Such organisms do no harm in their natural habitat but are pathogenic (disease-producing) in other organs.

Care of hair. A healthy condition is achieved by at least daily combing and/or brushing with a clean comb and brush; weekly hair washing is the norm for many people although daily washing is becoming more common in the younger age groups. Of all the personal cleansing activities, hair washing over the years has become the least 'private' (witness modern hairdressing salons). To cater for every kind of hair, there are numerous lotions and shampoos many of which help to keep the scalp free from dandruff. Spraying water over hair is thought to be the best way of completely removing shampoo, but many people still manage with a basin of clean water. Since hair grows daily, albeit slowly, most people have their hair cut at frequent intervals. Hair styles, which change with the fashion, are an important aspect of self-image and sexuality.

Care of nails. Cleanliness can be achieved by removing any obvious dirt with a blunt instrument before using a nail brush while hand washing. After drying, while the cuticle is still soft it can be gently pushed backward with the towel to prevent it growing down on to the nail. A ragged cuticle can provide an entry point for microorganisms and a whitlow can result. Cuticle cream helps prevent raggedness. For toe nails it is thought that if they are cut in a straight line, any pressure on the middle of the nail from the shoes will slightly raise the two sides and avoid an ingrowing toe nail. Finger nails are usually rounded to the shape of the finger end, although some people wear their nails long and pointed. A few occupations cannot be performed safely for the client by a person with long nails. For instance bakers, hairdressers and nurses are strongly encouraged to have short clean finger nails.

Care of teeth and mouth. Whereas many of the cells in the human body, if damaged, can be replaced the teeth cannot be. The best that can be done for decayed teeth is to remove the carous part by drilling and to fill the space with a metallic substance. To avoid dental caries, people must follow a rigorous routine of teeth and mouth care.

Fluoride protects the teeth; it is present naturally in some drinking water supplies throughout the world and is added artificially (in some countries) to others. Where it is not present or has not been added, fluoride-containing toothpaste should be used by all age groups.

Brushing the teeth with a slightly abrasive alkaline paste

or powder helps to remove plaque from the exposed tooth surfaces. Plaque is a sticky film of food and saliva deposits, cells shed from the mucous membrane and micro-organisms; it adheres to the surface of the teeth and is not easily removed. The presence of plaque still adhering to the teeth after cleaning can be revealed by using a dye disclosing agent. Plaque builds up quickly in the absence of cleaning and starts attacking the teeth shortly after the ingestion of sugars or refined carbohydrates. Therefore it is important that the teeth are cleaned immediately after eating sweet things. A good 3-minute brush at least once a day is recommended to remove plaque, best carried out before sleeping.

Vigorous up and down movement when brushing teeth is now discouraged and a rotary movement is recommended, not forgetting the backs of the teeth. The gums are also damaged by plaque and gum disease accounts for the loss of more teeth than any other cause in adulthood. Regular dental care, flossing between the teeth and adequate and proper brushing help to prevent gum disease. Recession of the gum, common in older age groups, encourages dental caries; desensitising toothpaste enables brushing to be accomplished without discomfort if the gums are painful.

Ideally food debris should be removed from the teeth after each meal. When tooth brushing is not feasible at these times, the abrasive action from chewing something fibrous like an apple or orange is helpful. A drink of water removes food particles from the mouth but is not so effective in removing them from between the teeth; dental floss or a tooth-pick can accomplish this.

In spite of improved knowledge about the causes and prevention of dental caries, many countries are experiencing an increased incidence of dental caries and a lowering of the average age at which people become edentulous and require dentures. The social changes whereby fizzy drinks and ice cream are readily available to children who eat and drink these simple sugar-containing confections between meals contributes to the problem. Sticky sugar adheres to the teeth; it breaks down into acid more readily than starch; acid in contact with tooth enamel for a sufficient time erodes it, and dental caries ensues.

Dressing. Changes in tradition and culture are reflected in clothes and each succeeding generation modifies dress to suit the changing environment and social conditions. Victorian crinolines would be difficult to manage as everyday clothes in today's fast-moving world and would certainly not fit in with the present-day attitude that clothes should be easy to launder and require minimal pressing and ironing.

Clothes are a medium of non-verbal communication. They can signify ethnic origin, level of income and social status, as well as personal preference of colour, style and fashion. They can convey mood: when well, people keep their clothes in good condition; when dejected, they frequently do not seem to notice stained clothes and down-at-heel shoes.

The manual skills required for independence in dressing are achieved by most people, but dressing includes much more than simply learning how to put clothes on. Children usually accept the type of clothing worn by members of the community in which they grow up. They learn that different clothes are worn for different occasions, such as for school and sport, and that a 'uniform' is worn by employees in many occupations.

Clothes which are next to the skin are in contact with sweat, sebum, epithelial scales and microorganisms. The latter have optimal conditions for rapid multiplication, consequently clothes worn during waking hours should not be worn for sleeping and ideally should be changed daily. Shedding of microorganisms attached to the scales from the skin into the atmosphere can be a means of spreading infection.

Sensible selection of clothing can reduce strain on the heat-regulating centre in the brain by the protection afforded against rain, wind, cold, heat and sun. Clothing can also protect from injury, an example being crash helmets. Most people dress for personal adornment and get great satisfaction from doing so. The activity of dressing offers the opportunity for making decisions which help to develop a feeling of self-direction, an important part of self-fulfilment. And last but by no means least clothes are a vehicle of communication.

LIFESPAN: EFFECT ON PERSONAL CLEANSING AND DRESSING

The AL of personal cleansing and dressing is performed throughout the lifespan but, in its various stages, there are some different concerns and preferences, and these are described in this section.

Infancy. During infancy, another person — usually a parent — attends daily to personal hygiene and dressing activities. For bathing the water is prepared at body temperature as an infant's skin is sensitive to heat. As well as a daily bath babies need to have any milk spillage removed immediately to prevent a sour odour. Because of their incontinent state the perineum and buttocks must be sponged and properly dried after elimination of urine and faeces, followed by application of a clean nappy or diaper which is non-irritant and absorbent. Excessive thickness between the legs should be avoided as the bones at this stage are still quite soft, being mainly organic matter. Loose-fitting and cross-over garments are chosen for the very young baby because even momentary confinement and darkening (as when clothes are drawn over the head) are frightening. Also the blinking reflex and tear glands do not work efficiently in early life.

At the crawling stage all-in-one suits are the most suitable daytime wear, for they will not impede the first attempts at standing unaided. As toddling is achieved, dungarees are useful as they afford some protection against the inevitable grazed knees. Gradually clothes characteristic of the culture are introduced. Night clothes should be made of non-inflammable material and pyjamas are safer than gowns which more easily catch fire.

The toddler can progress to the family bath where there is space to enjoy playing with toys so that bathing is associated with pleasure and relaxation. The cold water is run first to avoid overheating of the bath itself and scalding of the child. There are other dangers, too, for children at bathtime and so adult supervision is necessary throughout.

All clothes for children should fasten at the front and children should be able to dress themselves by the time they go to school. Children's clothes are now much better geared towards encouraging independence; for example, Velcro fasteners are provided instead of buttons and laces. Outdoor safety is also a concern of clothes' manufacturers these days. Road safety authorities are concerned about small children wearing coats with hoods, which can restrict hearing and vision as the wearer steps out on to the road. A fluorescent garment should be worn when children travel to and from school in inadequate daylight.

Care of the teeth is an extremely important aspect of this AL in the early years of the lifespan. There is considerable variation in the age at which a baby's first tooth appears but the usual teething period occurs when the baby is 6–9 months old, a time which as Steward (1988) describes can be somewhat trying for parents. While parents can help during this phase, they are vital in helping establish life-long teeth care habits.

The habit of regular and proper brushing of teeth can be established as soon as a young child is able to hold a toothbrush and, indeed, at that early stage, it is fun rather than a chore. Dental education is increasingly being brought to young children through playgroups and nursery schools, and to their parents through the mass media and child health clinics. The main recommendations are proper brushing; regular dental inspection; and minimum intake of sugar-containing foods (and drinks) and refined carbohydrates. Sweets are better given following a meal and should be avoided altogether for snacks between meals; preferable alternatives are savoury foods and fruit. Started at an early age, it is more likely that habits which avoid harm to the teeth can be established. Fluoride increases the resistance of teeth to decay, particularly when given during the developmental period, and it is recommended as a preventive measure by the British Dental Association and the World Health Organization. It can be administered systematically throughout childhood or topically by use of fluoride toothpaste (Cormack, 1983).

Childhood. Increasing development of the neuromuscular system allows children gradually to master the technique of attending to their own personal hygiene and dressing with supervision. Increasing psychological development permits practice in decision making about these activities resulting in eventual independence and individuality. During these stages children gradually develop a concept of modesty in relation to the AL of personal cleansing and dressing.

Adolescence. As adolescence is reached there are several changes in the skin activity which may require specific attention. There is usually increasing under-arm perspiration and most people need to use a deodorant and antiperspirant. Dandruff on the scalp can occur. Many adolescents, particularly males, have to contend with acne, sometimes sufficiently severe to warrant medical treatment. Obesity creates a risk of maceration in the skin folds, for example under the breasts and in the groins which can affect care of the skin and choice of garments. Also excessive tissue on the upper inner aspects of each leg can cause unpleasant chafing from the friction produced when walking.

Adolescence can be the period for experimenting with way-out fashions and new hairstyles and provided that they do not cause any harm, tolerance and good humour reap better rewards all round than continual derisory remarks. It can be seen as part of the young person's bid for independence and a means of communication, both with peers and other groups.

Adulthood. As adult years are reached the reasons for and time of personal cleansing activities, such as bathing, may vary according to work and recreation. The choice might be an invigorating cold bath on waking or a soothing hot bath before sleeping. A whole lifestyle is reflected in a person's clothes: those for work, for formal social occasions, for informal social occasions, for relaxation, for leisure time activities and for sleeping. Most adults have acquired the ability to dress according to the socially acceptable norm for their culture, whatever the occasion, and to derive pleasure from so doing. Hair styling, grooming and use of cosmetics are ways to express personality and sexuality.

Old age. In the declining years, elderly people may have increasing difficulty in managing some of the physical activities involved in cleansing and dressing, perhaps particularly getting into and out of the bath. Many gadgets are now available to enable older people to maintain their standards of personal cleanliness. Skin dryness may make moisturising lotions necessary to prevent excessive flaking. Failing eyesight and shaking hands may make it increasingly difficult for older people to retain their independence with conventional clothing. Back fastenings of garments are difficult to reach and front fastenings are therefore preferable; zips and Velcro tapes are easier to manipulate than small buttons or hooks and eyes. Many older people more readily feel the cold and may need to wear extra clothing to keep warm. Two layers of thin material (because of the entrapped air which is a bad conductor of heat) are warmer than one thick layer. Adequately warm clothing is a simple, but important, means of preventing hypothermia (p. 238) which is a particular threat to old people in severe winter weather.

Problems with the mouth and teeth are also common in old age. Geissler & McCord (1986) mention statistics which indicate that 74% of those over 65 and 87% of those over 75 are toothless and, of those who do retain their own teeth, the majority have gum disease and caries. They recommend that the elderly should be encouraged to receive regular dental care and to ensure that oral health is maintained by proper cleansing of dentures and regular brushing of natural teeth.

DEPENDENCE/INDEPENDENCE IN PERSONAL CLEANSING AND DRESSING

The close relationship within the model of the dependence/independence continuum and the lifespan is reflected in almost all of the Activities of Living, and the AL of personal cleansing and dressing is no exception. In infancy there is almost total dependence on others for cleansing and dressing activities; childhood is characterised by ever-increasing independence; and independence is expected in adolescence and throughout adulthood, except for those unable on account of physical or mental handicap, or during a period of illness. Declining physical and mental ability in the final stage of the lifespan may render an old person dependent on help, for example with bathing or cutting nails. A variety of aids are available on the market which can help people to cope independently with cleansing and dressing activities which they would otherwise be unable to manage. Some of the available aids are described later in this chapter within a more detailed discussion of dependence/independence for personal cleansing and dressing in the context of the model for nursing.

FACTORS INFLUENCING PERSONAL CLEANSING AND DRESSING

The way the AL of personal cleansing and dressing is performed varies among individuals and many different factors are responsible for this. In keeping with the model, this section is sub-divided into physical, psychological, sociocultural, environmental and politicoeconomic factors which influence the AL.

Physical factors

The physical body structures which relate directly to the AL of personal cleansing and dressing are the skin (the integumentary system) and its appendages (nails and hair), and the teeth. However, apart from these physical structures, the many activities associated with this AL require adequate functioning of the nervous, musculoskeletal and cardiopulmonary systems, among others.

Physical changes with ageing
Concerning the skin, nails, hair and teeth in particular, it is important to understand the physical changes which occur in the normal process of ageing. These changes have a direct as well as indirect influence on the ways in which personal cleansing and dressing activities are carried out. For example, because growth of teeth is a development of infancy and childhood, preventive dental care is especially important in these early stages of the lifespan. In adult years, care of the gums assumes as much importance as dental care because of the gradual shrinking of the gums with ageing. And, in later years of life, the loss of teeth and their replacement with dentures requires yet another form of attention.

Similarly, changes occur in the course of the lifespan in the physical properties of the skin, hair and nails. Again, these changes mean that personal cleansing and dressing requirements are different at different stages of the lifespan. In adolescence, for example, there are the problems of acne and greasy hair; whereas, in old age, it is dryness of the skin and hair — and brittleness of the nails — which pose different problems, requiring different solutions.

Individual physical differences
The changes in the skin, hair, nails and teeth which occur in the normal process of physical ageing give rise to differences in physical appearance at various stages in the lifespan. In turn, people alter personal cleansing and dressing activities; for example, by modifying make-up to suit skin changes and altering hair styles as hair changes in condition and thickness.

Even among people of the same age, there are individual physical differences in terms of appearance which, to a large extent, is portrayed in the colouring and characteristics of the skin and hair. Individuality is portrayed by such things as the propensity for blushing and the presence of freckles, moles or birthmarks. Pigmentation of the skin reflects an individual's ethnic origin but, even among Caucasians there are variations ranging from what we call 'fair-skinned' to 'dark-skinned'.

Physical hazards
Fair-skinned people are particularly at risk to one form of physical hazard, namely, the harmful elements of sunrays. They have less pigment in their skin and, therefore, less protection. While suntanning had become fashionable with the advent of summer holidays abroad, more recently attention has turned to its dangers. Skin cancer, particularly in the serious form of malignant melanoma, is on the increase in many countries, including the UK. The risk is higher in fair-skinned people and also in those with a

large number of moles. Since malignant melanoma is potentially curable if treated early, a major effort has been put into public education in recent years, both to encourage early detection as well as prevention (Nichols, 1988; Casey, 1988).

Sun is not the only form of physical hazard which can have an adverse, even dangerous, effect on the skin. Excessive heat, fire, cold, wind, pressure, friction and a whole range of chemical substances and diseases (e.g. infections and parasitic conditions) are other examples of physical hazards from which the skin requires to be protected.

Physical sex differences

The physical differences between females and males are relevant to discuss in relation to personal cleansing activities.

Female. Knowledge of the reason for effective perineal toilet (p. 203) will help to motivate girls to carry out this preventive technique. As the breasts develop, extra care is needed to avoid maceration in the lower skin fold; daily washing, powdering and support in a brassiere usually is sufficient preventive action. Girls require knowledge about the structure of their external genital organs so that they can remove excess secretion from the folds of skin and mucous membrane before it decomposes and causes an unpleasant odour. Psychological preparation for the onset of menstruation will help them to cope with its occurrence; during menstruation all glands are more active and a daily bath or all over wash is even more necessary. Girls acquire the behaviour of their cultural setting related to body hair; it can include removal of unwanted hair from the upper lip and legs, and from the female pubic area before the marriage ceremony.

Male. The bulbous end of the penis is the glans and the foreskin is the prepuce. Between the glans and foreskin at birth there are fine adhesions which prevent retraction of the foreskin and the necessity for cleansing under it. The adhesions dissolve in 6 months to 5 years when retraction of the foreskin is easily accomplished. If it is forcibly pulled back before this, the adhesions may be broken down and infection introduced. Boys are then taught to draw the foreskin daily over the glans and cleanse the circular skin fold. Like girls, boys must be taught that this cleansing is a necessary part of their personal hygiene to prevent unpleasant odour and infection. Before puberty boys need to be psychologically prepared for the possibility of 'wet dreams' (ejaculation of semen during sleep); they may wish to bath on waking to remove the characteristic odour of semen. At puberty they acquire the culturally determined behaviour of shaving or having a beard.

It is customary in some cultures for baby boys to have the foreskin removed (circumcision) shortly after birth. In other instances when parents wish to have a son circumcised they are usually advised to wait until he is toilet trained as this reduces the risk of infection. There is some evidence that there is less cervical cancer in women whose husbands have been circumcised.

Physical disability

Obviously, an individual's level of physical ability will determine the extent to which the various activities involved in personal cleansing and dressing can be carried out adequately; and people who are physically disabled may have difficulty in some aspects of this AL.

Psychological factors

Although modern society in general pays less attention to such things as dressing baby boys in blue and girls in pink, and adolescents nowadays tend to favour 'unisex' fashions, there are still basic differences in psychological outlook between the sexes with regard to the AL of personal cleansing and dressing.

Girls do tend to be more concerned with cleanliness and appearance, and boys may require greater encouragement to carry out personal cleansing activities with sufficient rigour. Adolescents of either sex may deliberately lower their standards of cleanliness as a form of protest against the authority of parents and teachers. On the other hand, their desire to be sexually attractive may result in a somewhat obsessional interest in appearance, make-up, hairstyle and clothes.

In later years, too, standards of cleanliness and dress often reflect personality and emotion; an extrovert is more likely to wear bright colours and the latest fashion than a shy person; and a person who is depressed is likely to lose interest in appearance, sometimes even to the point of neglecting essential, basic hygiene.

Attending properly to the AL of personal cleansing and dressing does require knowledge, for example about the importance of handwashing and the measures involved in preventive dental care. Therefore, lack of knowledge is likely to result in inadequate attention to cleansing and dressing activities which, in turn, may result in problems such as infection, infestation, skin disease and dental caries. People who are mentally handicapped and therefore, by definition slow to learn, require patient and repeated teaching in order to gain confidence and independence in personal cleansing and dressing activities.

Sociocultural factors

Not all cultures place the same value on cleanliness, and the personal cleansing pattern into which a person is socialised becomes deeply ingrained. Those used to a daily bath, shower or sauna may experience discomfort when facilities do not permit them to follow this pattern; conversely, people not accustomed to such patterns may find it strange to be in a country where this seems to be expected of everyone. Similarly, while some cultures place great value on cleanliness, others believe that the 'natural' smell of the body is normal and is part of sexual attractiveness.

There are ranges of norms for shampooing the hair (dryness or greasiness often being the deciding factor) and for cleaning the teeth, although many dentists would prefer that everyone accepted as their norm cleaning after meals and before going to bed at night. From a health point of view there is an essential norm for handwashing which is before touching food, and after elimination to prevent food poisoning and diseases spread by ingesting microorganisms from faeces.

There are still instances where culture dictates the type of clothing worn. In the West it has become acceptable for women as well as men to wear trousers; in some cultures it is customary for the men to wear robes and for the women to wear trousers. Religion still influences dress, for instance the clothing worn by monks and nuns. In most countries, not only culture and religion but also the law determine those parts of the body which must be clothed when in public. All of these sociocultural variations are more widely appreciated nowadays through the influence of the mass media and as a result of international travel.

Environmental factors

It is easy for those whose homes have a piped supply of hot water and a fixed bath or shower to presume that these facilities are available to all people. Again it is presumed that water will be available from a tap until the threat or reality of a water shortage reminds people that even such a basic amenity cannot be taken for granted. The AL of personal cleansing and dressing does require the availability of certain amenities in the home environment if the activities involved are to be adequately carried out.

This is true also of the work environment. Some industries expose the skin to risk from such things as coal dust, tar, soot, asbestos and other cancer-producing agents. Showers are considered to be more efficient than baths and the workers are encouraged to shower before going home. In some countries protective clothing may be obligatory if there is a known health risk to the workers.

The climate of the surrounding environment is another factor which influences the AL of personal cleansing and dressing. For example, in tropical climates there may be the need for more frequent bathing or showering to remove excessive perspiration. Many people in hot climates find that they are more comfortable in clothes made of cotton because it absorbs perspiration, and less comfortable in man-made fibres which are less absorbent. Garments made from man-made fibres and wool are useful for providing warmth in colder climates. White and light colours are chosen by people in sunny regions, since they reflect the sun's rays; in contrast dark colours, because they absorb the rays and are therefore warmer, are often the choice of people in cold climates.

Politicoeconomic factors

With the world shortage and consequent high cost of fuel, many people who have the facilities for a hot water supply are experiencing difficulty in affording it. This can apply especially to a nation's disadvantaged groups such as those on a fixed income, be it a pension or unemployment benefit. Some governments consider the amenity of a fixed bath sufficiently important to warrant a financial grant towards its installation in old property.

The importance of preventive dental care and treatment is recognised by those governments which provide a free (or subsidised) service for people unable to afford to pay for it themselves and/or who most need it: such as children, pregnant women, the elderly and the unemployed. The possible addition of fluoride to the water supply is something of a political issue.

There is certainly an economic dimension to the AL of personal cleansing and dressing at the individual level. Personal income determines the amount of money which can be spent on articles used for personal cleansing, such basic things as soap, shampoo, comb, hairbrush, tooth-brush, toothpaste and manicure tools. When income is limited, emphasis is less on appearance and more on basic health issues — the prevention of infection, skin irritation or disease, dental caries and infestation with lice.

Economics also enters into the number of clothes a person can buy: minimally a person needs to possess enough clothes to wash or dry clean them sufficiently often to prevent odour from dried perspiration or irritation to the skin from dirty fabric. For those who are impoverished, clothes become simply a matter of basic necessity and the person is denied the pleasure of attractive clothes and variety in dressing.

INDIVIDUALITY IN PERSONAL CLEANSING AND DRESSING

The purpose of the model of living is to highlight a person's individuality in the Activities of Living. Taking into account all the issues described in the foregoing discussion of the various components of the model (the list below provides a résumé), it should be easy to appreciate that people develop marked individuality in relation to the AL of personal cleansing and dressing.

Lifespan: effect on personal cleansing and dressing
- Infancy
  — skin care (incontinent state)
  — suitable clothing for mobility/safety
  — growth of teeth

- Childhood
  — developing independence and individuality
  — developing concept of modesty
  — importance of care of teeth

- Adolescence
  - increased underarm perspiration
  - problems of acne, greasy hair, dandruff
  - expression of feelings/individuality/sexuality through clothes, make-up, hairstyle
  - puberty (menstruation/ejaculation)

- Adulthood
  - routines related to working and playing
  - reflection of personality in appearance and clothes

- Old age
  - skin dryness
  - difficulties with bathing, care of nails and feet
  - difficulties with dressing
  - physical disability

Dependence/independence in personal cleansing and dressing

- Dependence in infancy/old age/illness
  - on people
  - on aids and equipment

Factors influencing personal cleansing and dressing

- Physical
  - stage of physical development
  - physical changes with ageing
  - individual physical differences
  - skin state
    colour
    bruising/scars/blemishes
    dry/moist
    turgid/wrinkled
    areas of discontinuity
    cleanliness
  - state of hands and nails
    cleanliness
    handwashing habits
    condition
  - state of mouth and teeth
    moist/dry mouth
    odour of breath
    teeth (number/condition, dentures)
    teeth cleaning routine
  - condition/style of hair
    type (dry/greasy)
    dandruff/lice
    hair washing routine
  - dress
    style/appropriateness
    standard of cleanliness/odour

  quality/suitability of footwear
  special clothing for work/play
  - physical hazards
  - physical sex differences
    female: perineal toilet
    breast care
    menstruation
    body hair
    male: cleansing foreskin
    shaving

- Psychological
  - sex differences/sexuality
  - standards related to personality/emotional state
  - knowledge (e.g. handwashing, dental care)
  - intelligence

- Sociocultural
  - values concerning cleanliness/appearance
  - social norms for cleansing/dressing routines
  - cultural influences/rules on dress
  - religious influences/rules on cleansing/dressing

- Environmental
  - bath/shower in the home
  - piped hot/cold water in the home
  - exposure at work to substances damaging to the skin
  - availability of bathing/handwashing facilities at work
  - climate

- Politicoeconomic
  - adequacy of necessary facilities for low income groups
  - personal income for articles for personal cleansing
  - personal income for essential clothing and footwear

Personal cleansing and dressing: patients' problems and related nursing

Detailed knowledge about a patient's individual habits related to personal cleansing and dressing activities is necessary if this important aspect of everyday living is to be given due emphasis in individualised nursing. In the past, when hospital nursing was highly routinised — with the emphasis on tasks more than on patients — little account was taken of the usual routines and established preferences of the individual. Patients had their faces washed and hair brushed on waking and, as soon as breakfast was over, nurses began on the 'bedbaths' and 'big baths' strictly according to bed position in the ward! ⟩

Such rigid routine completely ignored the fact that individual habits in everyday life are very varied. Some people bath in the morning, others at night; some never have a bath, always a shower (and vice versa); and while some people bath only once or twice a week, others like to do so twice a day. Whatever the habits, they often become so ingrained that the person may strive to ensure that they can be kept up, for example while staying in a hotel or in lodgings. Nowadays, hospitals are becoming increasingly flexible over the routine of the patients' day and, within reasonable and necessary limits, the continuation of established personal habits in the activities of living is something which is tolerated, if not always actively encouraged.

There is another change too. In describing the days of routinised care, words were deliberately chosen which emphasise the idea that, in relation to cleansing and dressing activities, patients had things done *to* them by nurses. This idea is fast disappearing that the patient is always a passive recipient of nursing care although, of course, sometimes this is the case. Personal cleansing and dressing activities are normally carried out independently on a daily basis. For any adult, the idea of being washed and dressed by another person — unless help is absolutely indispensable — is a very odd one indeed. Most patients who are able to cope with cleansing and dressing activities themselves are likely not only to want to do so, but to obtain pleasure and satisfaction in the process. They may not achieve an end result as clean and tidy as a nurse would wish, but if that causes a problem, it is the nurse's rather than the patient's problem.

If individuality and independence in the AL of personal cleansing and dressing are to be encouraged within the context of individualised nursing, nurses need to have information about the patient's usual routines; what can and cannot be done independently; what previous coping mechanisms have been employed; and what problems exist or may develop. Such information can be obtained through nursing assessment of a patient. Nurses can discuss the AL of personal cleansing and dressing with the patient, using the résumé presented at the end of the preceding section as a guide to relevant topics, and bearing in mind the following questions:

- what are the individual's usual personal cleansing and dressing habits?

- when and how often are the various activities performed?
- what factors influence the individual's personal cleansing and dressing habits?
- what does the individual know about the relationship of personal cleansing and dressing to health?
- what are the individual's attitudes to personal cleansing and dressing?
- does the individual have any longstanding difficulties regarding personal cleansing and dressing activities and, if so, how have these been coped with?
- what problems does the individual have now (or is likely to develop) with the AL of personal cleansing and dressing?

Of course, the nurse may not have to actually *ask* these questions. More often than not the answers are obtained in the course of discussion, or in what the patient chooses to say in response to a general, open-ended question from the nurse. And, of course, all the questions should not come only from the nurse — valuable information can be gleaned from questions the patient asks, and this is something to be encouraged. An assessment, perhaps especially on admission to hospital, has the purpose of *obtaining* information from patients but, equally, it is an opportunity to *give* information to them as well. And, of course, assessment involves much more than use of interview technique only. Use of all the senses, especially observation, is vital and it may be that some patients' problems are self-evident, requiring discussion only for corroboration.

On the basis of information obtained from assessment, the patient's problems will be identified (as perceived by both nurse and patient) and noted. If relevant, priorities among the problems will be determined and then realistic goals will be set. Some of these will be concerned with alleviating or solving actual problems; others with preventing potential problems from becoming actual ones; and others, perhaps, which aim to help the patient to cope with problems which cannot be solved. Maintaining and encouraging the patient's independence in aspects of this AL is more likely to be achieved if the nursing plan contains details of what the patient is able to do without help, in addition to requirements for nursing assistance. Decisions about appropriate interventions to achieve the set goals must be made within the constraints of prevailing circumstances, existing facilities and available resources. Alongside the written plan of intervention is put the date on which evaluation will be carried out to ascertain whether or not the stated goals have been achieved. All of these activities — the various steps of the process of nursing — are necessary in order to carry out individualised nursing.

The problems which a patient may experience in relation

to personal cleansing and dressing are many and varied; recognising and solving them calls for sensitivity, empathy and ingenuity on the part of the nurse. Many of the problems relate to change of environment in the case of hospitalisation; this increases anxiety and when focused on the many activities related to personal cleansing and dressing, the anxiety is mainly centred on loss of independence and autonomy for such an important part of living, and on loss of privacy.

These issues are central to the first section which follows this introduction. Then there is discussion of some circumstances which demand a change in mode of personal cleansing and dressing. The next section considers some causes of dependence in this AL; and patients' dependence on nurses for mouth care, prevention and management of pressure sores and prevention of wound infection. Finally a few specific problems associated with personal cleansing and dressing are discussed.

Neither the problems nor their solutions can be dealt with exhaustively in a book; only guidelines can be given so that nurses can begin to think creatively about nursing activities related to the AL of personal cleansing and dressing.

CHANGE OF ENVIRONMENT AND ROUTINE

Not all patients are nursed in hospital and the discussion later in this section applies to patients regardless of location. However admission to hospital creates particular problems and these will be discussed first.

Unfamiliar ward routine
The newly admitted patient cannot know the ward routine concerning personal cleansing and dressing activities unless information is given. It is common for patients who are to be admitted from a waiting list to receive general information usually in leaflet form; generally this includes advice about toilet articles and night attire which they should bring with them, whether or not they can retain their daytime clothes, and if not, what alternative arrangements they should make.

On arrival, a patient cannot be expected to know the specific routine of time and place for carrying out personal cleansing and dressing activities. This information requires to be provided on admission and a function of the admitting nurse is to give this information and to create an atmosphere in which questions can be asked.

Those people who are admitted from the waiting list and who have had a bath before setting off for the hospital will, to say the least, be surprised to be asked to have a bath as part of the admission procedure. Should the patient be admitted for surgery, the explanation that frequent baths in the preoperative period reduce the number of microorganisms on the skin will be useful. Otherwise this part of the admission procedure should be used selectively, that is for those who have not bathed within the preceding 24 hours.

If all patients must have baths on admission then the objective clearly must be for observation of their skin condition including bruising which is important for several reasons. The patient may subsequently have an accident and claim that it resulted in a bruise, which in fact was present on admission; or the patient may have been subjected to ill-treatment, referred to as 'battering' or 'non-accidental injury'. Any evidence of pressure sores must also be carefully noted, together with the patient's ability to perform the ALs of personal cleansing and dressing. Unless nurses explain that the condition of each patient's skin has to be recorded, a patient is likely to feel disquiet at having to have an admission bath and to infer that the nurses think personal hygiene habits are deficient.

For most people clothes are important symbols of their independence and patients can experience distress when their clothes are sent home or to the hospital store cupboard, in which case the nurse makes a detailed list of each item and asks the patient to check the list and sign it. The patient will feel less distressed if it is understood that the staff would prefer possessions to be kept in the ward and that the only reason for their removal is inadequate ward facilities for safe keeping. It is important that nurses understand the patient's problem: being without their own clothes creates a sense of 'depersonalisation' and also means being deprived of the freedom to decide to leave the hospital, should there be any reason to do so.

Change from usual routine
For most people the ritual of personal hygiene is an essential part of caring for themselves. These hygiene habits are built into a routine which gives a pattern to the day, an important contribution to a feeling of security and stability. But most patients realise that in hospital the routine will differ from their own. The ward routine must accommodate the needs of a group; it must be both expeditious and safe and must not put the patients at any risk. When the nursing workload is heavy, time can be saved by alternative arrangements for personal cleansing and dressing activities; for example, finger wipes before meals if handbasins are difficult to provide; toothpicks and a drink of water after meals as a substitute for teeth cleaning; and a dry shampoo instead of a proper hairwash.

Most people, even those who are housebound, wear daytime clothes and change into night attire. It is most unusual for people to wear night attire during the day. Many newer and upgraded hospitals encourage ambulant patients to wear daytime clothes; this not only improves their self-image but also gives temporal demarcation to being in bed and being 'up', and it also helps to create a sense of normality. In clinical areas where this has not been encouraged, nurses might consider whether wearing daytime clothes could be introduced, even on a trial basis to begin with. Adams (1987) provides evidence, from a study which investigated aspects of clothing in elderly patients in medical and geriatric wards, that patients who were enabled to wear day clothes preferred to do so rather than wear night clothes during the day. She also found that charge nurses, too, supported this policy although some practical difficulties were highlighted.

Presumably, some of the difficulties inherent in the use of personal clothing in hospitals are now easier to overcome than in the past as a result of general improvements in clothing materials and styles. In particular, simple-to-fasten garments, the variety of stockings and tights and easy care underwear are all improvements which could be exploited. It does not take much imagination to appreciate that an elderly lady with long-standing pride in her appearance is likely to lose her sense of dignity if deprived of personal underwear (albeit unseen clothing) and supplied with stockings which wrinkle or, even worse, are rolled down or fall down. Likewise, an elderly man may well wish to wear a collar and tie daily, and what reason is there why he should not? Apart from aiming to preserve self-esteem and dignity, personal clothing also provides the opportunity for patients in long-term care to preserve their autonomy and exercise decision-making skills.

Lessened decision-making

As already noted, most patients have been used to making decisions about the simple activities of personal cleansing and dressing and this is something which should be encouraged as far as possible. There are not many decisions, however, which a bedfast patient can make about personal hygiene. It is therefore important that nurses allow the patients to make the few decisions left available to them, for instance whether or not they want soap on their face, or deodorant applied, what they would like to wear, and so on. It is equally important to recognise when patients are too exhausted or too ill to make decisions, or perhaps unable to make them because of confusion or intellectual impairment.

When all decision-making is removed from patients, particularly in long-term care, they cease to make the effort to consider alternatives thereby losing initiative and accepting imposed routine; they become institutionalised. When routine is rigid, members of staff cease to question and to consider alternatives; decision-making becomes unnecessary; they too lose their initiative, become bored and institutionalised thus compounding the patient's problem of lack of stimulation.

Lack of privacy

Most people prefer privacy when carrying out personal cleansing and dressing activities, as has been noted. Curtained washing cubicles or curtains round the bed do not provide the same security as the locked bathroom door, and some patients feel threatened when using such facilities. Shrunken or incompletely drawn curtains can preclude privacy and some patients, particularly women, fail to attend to perineal toilet because of this. Should a nurse become aware of a patient's difficulties in this area she can arrange for use of a private facility or replacement of shrunken curtains; and at all times nurses should be vigilant in making sure that curtains are completely drawn.

CHANGE IN MODE OF PERSONAL CLEANSING AND DRESSING

Habits of personal cleansing and dressing are integral to a person's lifestyle and are important manifestations of self-image and self-esteem. Enforced change in the mode of carrying out any of the activities involved means that patients have to cope with the change, and nursing activities aim at helping them to do so with minimum discomfort or distress.

Imposed non-bathing

Empathising with patients who are not permitted to bath is easier when one remembers the unpleasant 'grubby' feeling experienced on a long trip. How much worse the feeling must be when for any reason a bath cannot be taken for a long time: for post-radiotherapy patients it can be weeks; for patients with extensive skin destruction it can be many months. Most people's objective when bathing is to feel clean and relaxed and prevent malodour. The nurse can therefore make suggestions as to how these objectives might be achieved during a period of imposed non-bathing. Unless contraindicated, exposed skin areas (e.g. face, neck, hands and feet) and areas where sweat glands are concentrated (e.g. axillae and anogenital area) should be washed frequently. Anti-perspirants/deodorants and perfume/after-shave lotion, unless contraindicated on medical grounds, can help to promote a feeling of freshness and prevent malodour. Frequent changing of clothes and bedlinen would also increase the patient's feeling of cleanliness and comfort.

Some patients, for example those in a plaster cast, though unable to completely immerse themselves in water, might be able to bathe or shower at least some parts of the body if given appropriate help. Other patients, particularly if not mobile and confined to bed, can be bedbathed by the nurse. Provided this procedure is carried out in privacy and adequately (for example, ensuring that the water is warm throughout and that soap is properly rinsed off), it can be both cleansing and soothing for the patient. Greaves (1985), however, found that the patient can be 'micro-biologically dirtier after the (bed)bath than before'; recommendations offered on the basis of this study include supplying patients with their own bowls (which should be washed properly and dried after use), changing the water during the bedbath and using disposable cloths.

Notwithstanding the hazards of the bedbath, Webster et al (1988) were concerned with patients' views on bathing in their exploratory study and, in particular, whether these were in accordance with nurses' views. Interestingly, the results of the study indicate that patients and nurses seem to hold different views on some issues (for example, patients seem to be less embarrassed at being bathed by a nurse than nurses think they will be) and further research in this area would be enlightening.

A nurse's interest in a procedure which seemed superior to the conventional bedbath stimulated her to undertake a clinical trial of this new bathing procedure — the towel bath. Wright (1988) found this to be preferred by patients, quicker for the nurse and cost-effective. She hopes to encourage this procedure in British hospitals in preference to the long-established bedbath.

Infestation

A change in mode of personal cleansing and dressing is required for treatment of infestation. Lice and scabies are the most common forms of infestation. They have become increasingly common and could be eradicated. Mohylnycky (1983) believes that eradication is hampered by general attitudes towards personal infestation and considers that 'blanket campaigns' directed at the whole community are more effective than orthodox detection and eradication techniques.

Infestation is more common among people who, for any reason, have to be crowded together. Schools are notorious for the spread of head lice and, although previously thought to be more common among children from overcrowded, poorer homes, this is no longer the case. Owen (1982), on the basis of cost-effectiveness, argues the case for abandoning routine head inspections by school nurses and health visitors. She considers that the answer lies in educating parents to inspect and treat the hair of their own children; this view is supported in a more recent article (Milne, 1988).

Knowledge of infestation and its treatment can be used by nurses in a wide variety of contexts, hence the following information.

Head lice. The female lays tiny white eggs called 'nits' and cements them to the hairs near the scalp especially behind the ears. These hatch out in 1 week and are fully grown in 3. During a lifetime of 5 weeks they live on human blood. They cause intense irritation with consequent scratching; if this is performed with dirty finger nails infection can result and the resultant dried discharge and matted hair make detection and disinfestation difficult. There is loss of sleep with lowering of vitality; the sores may even give rise to enlarged lymph glands with possible abscess formation.

Head lice are impervious to washing and hair cutting, but a fine comb is effective. Treatment used to be with DDT but lice became resistant to it and, about the same time, its widespread use was banned. Malathion and Carbaryl are two effective insecticides for the treatment of head lice (Roberts, 1987). Lotions are preferred to shampoos because they are more effective and help to delay the emergence of resistance. The lotion should be applied to the scalp and the hair exactly as instructed.

The hair is then tidied — not combed vigorously which would disturb the lice from the scalp. The nits will be killed but not loosened from the hair. There is protection from re-infestation for some weeks after application because malathion bonds to the hair.

Body lice. The female lays her eggs in the seams of clothing; but in dirty conditions and when day clothes are not changed for night clothes, the eggs can be attached to the body hair. They hatch out in one week, become mature in 2 and live for 4–5 weeks. They too live on human blood and their crawling and biting cause intense irritation with consequent scratching and danger of introducing infection.

It is necessary to remove personal clothes into a bag in which they are generously dusted with malathion powder. The bag is securely tied and left for at least 2 hours, after which the clothes are washed or dry-cleaned as appropriate. The infested person takes a cleansing bath, and after drying the skin, sprinkles it with malathion powder. However, Roberts (1987) maintains that insecticides are not necessary because body lice are easy to eradicate; washing in water above 60°C will kill them, although not the eggs, but tumbledrying will kill both lice and eggs (within 15 minutes if the exhaust temperature is over 60°C). The treatment for pubic (crab) lice is similar but with the addition of shaving the pubic and, if necessary, the axillary hair.

Scabies. Infestation can become a social problem in the same way as lice and, like that problem, scabies is recognised as a problem which extends beyond situations in which living conditions are overcrowded or dirty and into all sections of society. The itch mite favours those areas where the skin is thin: between the finger knuckles, around the axillae, round the waist, between the thighs, around and especially on the medial aspects of the ankles.

The female burrows under the skin, and at the end of a tunnel, visible to the naked eye as a tiny black line, lays her eggs then dies. The eggs hatch in a few days, the mites crawl out to the skin surface causing irritation; they mate and the cycle starts again, the males remaining on the surface. The scratching and trauma to the skin leaves a route for infection to occur.

After removal of clothes they are washed immediately. A bath is taken after which an emulsion of benzyl benzoate is applied from the neck to cover the whole of the skin. This is left to dry before the afflicted person puts on clean clothes. The objective is to leave the first application for 48 hours after which a cleansing bath is taken, clean clothes put on, and removed clothes washed immediately.

Alternatives to benzyl benzoate are lindane and mono-sulfiram; lindane, according to Alderman (1988), has become the most popular treatment in recent years and lotions are preferred to creams as they give better coverage. An important part of eradication is to treat people who have been in close contact with the patient, whether or not they have symptoms.

Whatever type of infestation is concerned, it is important that the nurse relates to the patient in a tactful and sympathetic manner. The person's cooperation is essential if treatment is to be effective, and receptiveness to education with a view to prevention of recurrence, is more likely if the nurse establishes a good rapport.

Modification of clothing

Even with a forearm or ankle in plaster, such things as fitted sleeves or narrow trousers are impossible to put on and clothing has to be modified accordingly. Stretch fabrics, and wide sleeves/trousers — whether or not they are in fashion — are easiest to manage. For a short period this is likely to be accepted by the patient and unlikely to cause undue distress.

However, as was mentioned in an earlier part of the chapter (p. 205), there may be reasons why some elderly people cannot manage to cope with conventional clothing: for example, necessitating wearing front rather than back-opening clothes. Similarly, disabled people may require to modify clothing in order to achieve maximum independence in the activity of dressing. Providing suitable clothing for elderly and disabled people is a basic but often neglected need, as Norton (1983) points out. She recalls how she became aware of this when, as a student nurse some 40 years earlier, she had inflicted pain on a crippled elderly patient when trying to dress her in a hospital issue nightgown. Later, in the course of her research into geriatric nursing problems in hospital (Norton et al, 1962), items of night attire were subjected to systematic study for the first time. Norton acknowledges that since then there has been an increasing awareness of clothing problems and the production of all kinds of garments for all manner of disabilities. Much of this in the UK has been due to the work of the Disabled Living Foundation which has undertaken numerous projects on clothing and dressing problems. However, as Norton says (referring to a recent DLF survey), the practical information which exists does not appear to be widely known. She argues that it is essential for care-givers and administrators to become better informed, ' . . . though knowing of the existence of suitable designs of clothing and footwear to meet the needs of the elderly frail and disabled is only one of a great many factors.' There are problems inherent in the supply of clothing, storage and laundering in hospitals: how to overcome these problems and to introduce successfully a personalised clothing service is the subject of a Disabled Living Foundation publication which Norton commends (DLF, 1977). Carr (1988) draws attention to the fact that the DLF has a clothing adviser who can offer advice on all aspects of clothing.

Nurses, by virtue of their first-hand awareness of the problems, can help in this matter by specifying the clothing needs of individual patients. In addition, empathy is necessary so that any patient who has to wear modified clothing can be helped by the nurse to regain confidence and continue to use dressing as a source of self-esteem and a means of communication.

Wearing a prosthesis

There are various types of prostheses which can be worn, almost all of them resulting in some change in mode of personal cleansing and/or dressing.

An increasing number of people are wearing *dentures* at an earlier age; McCord & Stalker (1988) state that 54% of 55–64-year-olds in the UK are edentulous. Some people are very sensitive about being seen without dentures, even for the short time of removal for cleaning. In older people with shrinking gums, dentures can become so loose that they may cause embarrassment in such activities as eating and speaking. Most dentists now advise that dentures are not removed before sleeping, although many older people still remove them. In contrast, those who have a plate with just one or two teeth attached are strongly advised to remove it before sleeping. In addition to denture cleaning, whole mouth brushing (teeth, gums, palate and tongue) is necessary for oral and dental hygiene to be achieved. Some patients will require assistance to achieve this; McCord & Stalker (1988) provide guidance on oral hygiene for elderly handicapped patients.

The term *'artificial limb'* includes everything from what can reasonably be called a 'wooden leg' to a highly sophisticated powered prosthesis with electrodes placed on opposing muscles that transmit a signal to an electronic device which operates the prosthesis. With the latter device a member of the family is usually taught to help the patient with personal cleansing and dressing activities. If the patient has to be admitted to hospital, anxiety can be reduced if the family member is offered the opportunity to continue his helping role. If this is not possible, the patient can teach the nurse the method of coping with bathing and so on.

People who wear an *artificial eye* become adept at caring for the prosthesis with the necessary apparatus and lotions in a hygienic manner. If for any reason a patient cannot continue to do this, a tissue is placed by the nurse at the outer corner of the eye, the artificial eye is removed on to it using an article with a slight curve and the eye is placed in its container and covered with a suitable lotion such as Optrex. The socket is then wiped with swabs wrung out of water or saline solution. Patients are naturally anxious about the safety of such a precious article, and it is re-assuring if the nurse explains exactly what she has done with it and transmits to the patient her mutual desire for its safety.

Various types of *breast prostheses* are available. Mastectomy patients are helped to come to terms with the 'visible' assault on their femininity by discussing and handling these prostheses before operation. Indeed in some hospitals a previous mastectomy patient who has learned to cope with her prosthesis talks with a newly admitted patient who is scheduled for mastectomy. It is increasingly recognised that an important nursing activity is the facilitation of such discussions. Another one is helping the patient to realise that hygiene of the prosthesis is important because it is in contact with the skin, at least during waking hours. Clothes do not usually have to be modified.

Although wearing *a wig* may be indulged in as a 'fun activity', one's perspective may change if a wig has to be worn for medical reasons. Furthermore one of the most common reasons for having to wear a wig is loss of hair (alopecia) from taking cytotoxic drugs, an increasingly common treatment for cancer. In the case of some forms of cytotoxic therapy, hair loss can be prevented by a procedure known as scalp cooling. This involves the application of an 'ice cap' (or other form of head cooling device) and it can be effective (Tierney, 1987) although chemotherapy-induced alopecia remains a problem for many patients. Such patients may already be debilitated in body and spirit, and loss of hair constitutes an extra problem, often perceived as a major one. Nurses can help by taking an interest in the choice of wig and commending the patient's appearance when it is worn. Advice may be needed regarding shampooing and setting the wig. Patients might welcome further advice in the form of a booklet such as the one on 'Coping with hair loss' produced by BACUP (1987).

CHANGE OF DEPENDENCE/INDEPENDENCE STATUS FOR PERSONAL CLEANSING AND DRESSING

Acquisition of the skills for independent performance of the activities related to personal cleansing and dressing requires an adequately functioning nervous system, not only to control movement in the lower limbs and to facilitate precision movements in the upper limbs, but also to enable learning about the rationale of the skills. Integrity of the musculoskeletal system is simultaneously necessary for carrying out the many manual skills involved. Inadequacies in these systems at birth may prevent the child from achieving independence for this AL; any dysfunction in the systems can prevent a person maintaining independence even to the point of rendering him dependent for one or more of the activities which are part of personal cleansing and dressing.

The nature of the problems in achieving and main-taining independence for this AL varies according to whether the impediment is congenital, immediate, or of gradual onset. Gradual onset permits the patient time to become psychologically adjusted to the changes and to develop physical manoeuvres for coping. Similarly there is a difference in the nature of the problems according to whether the impediment is short-or long-term. Personal hygiene problems experienced by patients vary according to whether one or more limbs are involved, whether they are upper or lower ones or an upper and lower limb on the same side.

Causes of dependence

There is no easy method of classifying the numerous impediments to independence in carrying out the many skills involved in personal cleansing and dressing. Partly because there are so many skills and partly because such a variety of factors can affect the nervous, musculoskeletal and integumentary systems, there cannot be an exhaustive classification of causes of dependence. The following headings show how causes are categorised for purposes of discussion here:

- limited mobility
- absence of limbs
- involuntary movements
- sensory deficits
- unconsciousness
- psychological disturbance
- illness

Limited mobility
The sites at which patients experience limitation of movement determine the particular problems which they experience in performing some or all of the skills necessary for personal cleansing and dressing. A person with a frozen shoulder should be encouraged to put garments over the arm on the affected side first. Crippled hands cannot hold conventional articles for cleaning teeth, manicuring nails, combing hair; nor can they manage to fasten small buttons or zips. A stiff spine on the other hand interferes with getting into and out of the bath and applying garments to the lower limbs. Immobility of the jaw renders the patient dependent for mouth care but usually all the other skills of personal cleansing and dressing can be carried out independently.

Absence of limbs
The congenitally deficient child may not feel the absence of limbs to be a problem because a limb-deficient body has become 'normal'. Should admission to hospital be required there will already be an established regime of managing personal hygiene. On the other hand a person who loses one or more limbs, is faced with learning alternative techniques according to which limbs are absent. In the early

stages there is increased risk of accident should the person even momentarily forget the limb deficiency; it is not unusual for the phenomenon of 'phantom' limb to be experienced.

Involuntary movements

It is difficult for those who have achieved coordination of movement brought about by the smooth, sequential contraction and relaxation of various muscle groups to realise the many difficulties that can be experienced by not being able to control movement. To give an example: exaggerated uncontrollable hand movements (such as caused by Parkinson's disease) make such apparently simple tasks as dressing, shaving, putting paste on a toothbrush, and even combing the hair, arduous.

Sensory deficits

When for any reason the brain is not receiving warning stimuli from the skin about the temperature of the water being used for bathing, there is increased risk of scalding. Lack of pressure stimuli can mean that tissues are subjected to increased pressure which may result in pressure sores (p. 218). Many blind people achieve the necessary skills to attend to all aspects of their personal cleansing and dressing; others require some help with some of the activities related to this AL.

Unconsciousness

Unconscious patients are totally dependent on the nurse for preserving their dignity and for ensuring the safety and integrity of the body during all aspects of personal cleansing and dressing. The limbs will probably be stiff and spastic and will need to be supported by one nurse without stretching the muscles and tendons, while the other nurse washes and dries the skin. Prevention of pressure sores is very important (p. 218).

Psychological disturbance

Even after healthy habits of personal cleansing and dressing have been established, these can be disrupted during psychological disturbance, whether this is caused by cognitive impairment or psychiatric illness of one kind or another. There may be a general deterioriation in the standard of personal cleansing skills and an apparent disregard for dirty malodorous clothing. Development of a nursing plan for such patients usually requires goal setting in small gradations to achieve the final goal of regaining healthy personal hygiene habits.

Illness

Illness can interfere with independence in several ways. Sometimes it is sheer exhaustion which prevents patients attending to themselves; sometimes it is breathlessness, when the slightest movement causes further respiratory embarrassment. When the illness dictates that patients are attached to various machines or gadgets, this can be yet another reason for dependence in some or all of the activities related to personal cleansing and dressing.

These are but a few examples of circumstances which can impede the many skills necessary for personal cleansing and dressing. There can be no hard and fast rules for nursing activities in this AL and a high degree of professional judgement is required to enable the development of an individual nursing plan and expertise in carrying it out.

It is obvious that on admission an accurate assessment of each patient's manner of performance of this AL is imperative. Many disabled people have become experts at coping with their condition. Nurses should acknowledge this, listen to them and encourage them to continue to cope where this is permissible. In instances of psychological disturbance, and illness, the nurse may well have to take the lead in development of a nursing plan, and for an unconscious patient it might be advisable to discuss previous hygiene habits with the relatives before devising a nursing plan. Unconscious patients, demented patients and some mentally handicapped people are dependent on the nursing for preserving their right to privacy during personal cleansing and dressing activities.

The nursing plan indicates where the patient's personal cleansing and dressing will take place: in bed or in the bathroom; what activities can be carried out independently and what sort of help is required with the other activities. There are many variables to consider when these decisions are made, and the following are some principles which nurses can bear in mind when helping patients:

- patients are entitled to privacy during the activities of personal cleansing and dressing
- there is a possibility of lack of congruence between the nurses' and patients' concept of privacy and modesty
- activities related to patients' safety, integrity of their body systems, dignity and modesty are a nursing responsibility for which nurses are accountable
- most patients are entitled to make some decisions about aspects of their personal cleansing and dressing, and thus make an important contribution to preventing deterioration of self-image, and institutionalisation
- when patients are experiencing problems in relation to any or all of the activities necessary for personal cleansing and dressing, provision of relevant aids to independence can help both patients and nurses

Aids to independence

Many types of equipment have been developed as aids to independence for personal cleansing and dressing activities. *For bathing and showering.* Although some baths are sufficiently long to accommodate the reclining body it is difficult to lift and lower a person who has to remain in this position into such a bath. Technologists have overcome the problem by providing 'mobile' reclining baths: part of the bath is a 'trolley' on to which the patient is lifted at the bedside, then wheeled over to the bath which is at a comfortable height for the nurse who is assisting. Another version allows the patient to be lifted on to a nylon stretcher at the bedside and then to be transported to a bath system and lowered on the stretcher into the water; there is a 'high/low' mechanism whereby the bath can be raised to a comfortable height for the nurse who is helping.

For those who must remain in the sitting position there are fixed baths with a modelled seat. In more sophisticated versions the patient is helped into the 'seat' portion at the bedside then is wheeled into the bath. Hermetic sealing takes place followed by introduction of water at a controlled temperature. After bathing, the water is drained away before the 'chair' end of the bath can be removed and wheeled out so that the patient's toilet can be completed.

Another alternative for a patient with mobilising difficulties is to bring to the bedside a special bath chair in which the patient is wheeled to the bathroom. Here a hoist fixed near the bath lifts the patient, in the removable 'chair' that has a lavatory type seat, above the level of the bath. A swivel movement puts the chair above the water, then the hoist lowers it into the water. The reverse process takes place after bathing and the patient can be dried and dressed before being lowered into the mobile chair for return to bed.

Similarly a portable shower has been developed for bed patients who must remain in the supine position. The patient is placed on the shower bed and moved into the shower cabinet, a similar idea to putting a patient in a cabinet-type respirator. The hair can be washed while in the cabinet. For those who can maintain the sitting position during showering there are special chairs with shower attachments and a lavatory-type seat so that the perineal area can be attended to.

Bush (1984), examining what the nurse can do to enhance the sense of well-being of residents who are both physically and mentally handicapped, points out that bath aids available to the public can be used to increase independence. For example, 'soap on a rope' can be hung around the neck so that it is not lost in the bath water. Another idea is to put a bar of soap into a towelling bag, thus combining the soap and flannel and making washing easier for residents who lack fine motor movements and co-ordination.

For care of hair. Extra large combs and brushes with modified handles may be helpful for patients who have difficulty in gripping or with above-shoulder movement. Such a simple measure as positioning a mirror at sitting height may enable some patients to brush and comb hair

without help, for example those in a wheelchair or who have difficulty in standing or balancing. The use of dry shampoo is a substitute for wet hairwashing, enabling independence on occasions for patients who require to have their hair washed. Davis (1977) illustrates the type of combs and brushes which are necessary for care of thick curly hair, together with hairgrooming techniques for black patients. Bush (1984) points out that drying of the hair often poses problems for spastic people and suggests use of a towelling hood to make drying easier.

For care of nails. With a total impediment of one hand there is usually no way in which a person can manicure unaided the nails of the other hand, though the person may be able to manicure the toe nails. Some patients dislike filing their nails or having them filed; if unable to use nail scissors they may find that they can use nail clippers.

For care of teeth and mouth. Electric tooth brushes may be more effective for handicapped patients' use. For patients with shoulder deformities or arthritis who are unable to reach their mouths, it is necessary to lengthen the toothbrush handle; McCord & Stalker (1988) explain how this is done simply with polyethylene tubing and they also illustrate other imaginative devices to enable disabled people to cope with teeth and denture care. However a small baby tooth brush is advisable when brushing the teeth of another person; mouth care procedures are discussed in more detail on page 218. When there is a reduced flow of saliva it is usually thick, and if there is mouth breathing it dries and forms sores. Lovelock (1973) recommends the use of an electric toothbrush dipped in a solution of bicarbonate of soda, or toothpaste foams. There is also a foam stick applicator (Copperman, 1977) which appears to be pleasant and efficient when a patient's mouth has to be cleaned by a nurse. For those with dentures who prefer to remove them for sleeping, labelled covered denture baths are provided. It is customary in some hospitals to use denture kits for naming patients' dentures, especially useful where there are confused patients.

The theoretical basis of nurse-administered oral hygiene is discussed at some length in a paper by Roth & Creason (1986).

For dressing. Velcro and long zip fastenings often help frail elderly and disabled people to continue dressing themselves or doing so with minimal help from another person. Where there is impediment of one arm or leg, the limb is put into the garment first so that maximum use can be made of the flexibility of the normal limb. When both upper limbs are disabled it may be that one sleeve can be drawn over one limb, the garment arranged over the front and back of the trunk and Velcro or a zip used along the second side. For those with disabled lower limbs it is usually preferable to put on trousers while lying on the bed. There are several gadgets which help them to be independent at this manoeuvre. Similar gadgets help with putting on pants and stockings.

Dependence for mouth care

Howarth (1977), in a short article based on her research in this area, reviewed mouth care procedures for the very ill and identified many shortcomings of the procedures as practised. Among suggestions offered, Howarth recommends that small toothbrushes (childsize) should be used because for nurses to clean a dependent patient's teeth with an adult's toothbrush is difficult to accomplish without causing discomfort. She also found that, of substances available, sodium bicarbonate — although unpleasant — was an effective cleansing agent if sores and dry encrusted areas were present. Vaseline was preferred as a lubricant for patients with dry and sore mouths as it lasted longer than other agents, such as glycerine.

Gibbons (1983), a dental officer, refers to Howarth's work in his review of the research into mouth care procedures. Reference is also made to a study which showed that twice-daily use of a chlorhexidine mouthwash inhibited the development of dental plaque and gingivitis, and suggested that it was possible that this agent could remove plaque and treat some cases of gingivitis.

Chlorhexidine gels have become available and have been shown to be beneficial in maintaining oral hygiene when applied on a toothbrush. Gibbons summarises the objectives of mouth care procedures as comfort, cleanliness, moistness and prevention of infection. On the basis of available research evidence he suggests that mouth care procedures, in the majority of instances, can be based on the following recommendations:

- use of a small headed, multi-tufted, childsize toothbrush
- use of fluoride toothpaste or, where the patient has particular problems, a chlorhexidine gel
- use of sodium bicarbonate for dry, encrusted mouths
- use of Vaseline for patients with dry mouth and lips
- use of chlorhexidine mouth washes for prophylactic purposes
- whole mouth brushing — which includes gums, palate and tongue as well as teeth (This requires to be stressed for patients who wear dentures and who normally receive assistance only with denture cleaning.)

It is suggested that a regime based on these recommendations will meet the objectives of mouth care procedures and will also be cheaper than use of prepacked mouth care trays, presently used by nurses in many hospital wards.

But despite the availability of useful and clear recommendations concerning oral hygiene, this aspect of basic nursing is still poorly practised according to Shepherd et al (1987). They review various tools and techniques in common use, concluding most to be ineffective and suggest 'we should ask ourselves why we require all of these instead of the toothbrush and toothpaste that the patient would normally use'.

For the particular oral care needs of patients receiving cancer chemotherapy — which has side-effects which harm the oral mucosa — Richardson (1987) provides a rationale for specific oral hygiene measures aimed at preventing and treating stomatitis and oral ulceration/infections with the dual objectives of comfort and safety. Campbell (1987) suggests solutions to mouth care problems in children who have cancer.

Dependence for prevention of pressure sores

Patients who are at risk of developing pressure sores are dependent on nurses either for teaching them how to avoid developing sores or for carrying out the necessary preventive measures. Use of the term 'pressure sores' in place of the previously used term 'bedsores' or 'decubitus ulcers', is indicative of the recognition of the cause, and acknowledgement that there are surfaces other than the bed which can produce pressure sores. It also acknowledges a changed pattern of nursing care, from most patients being confined to bed for the major portion of their hospital stay, to the majority of patients being up for some part or most of the day, as was the case even in the early 1970s (Table 11.1). The changed pattern is referred to as 'early ambulation' and it was instituted as a preventive measure aiming to prevent pressure sores as well as many other possible complications of bedrest.

The objective of prevention of pressure sores is, however, difficult to achieve as is evidenced in their high frequency. In a survey carried out in one area of the UK Clark et al (1978) reported that, in a population of 10 751 patients in hospital and in the community, 8.8% had at least one pressure sore, ranging in severity from superficial to a deep cavity, and in number from 1 to 14. There were more sores on the chairfast than on the bedfast patients, the site of the sore in the chairfast not following the theoretically expected change: from over the sacrum to over the ischial tuberosities. In other words the chairfast patients had more sores over the sacrum than over the ischial tuberosities. Further research is needed to investigate this phenomenon but it could be due to patients sliding forward on the chair seat creating a shearing force in the sacral tissues. The survey showed that age-wise it is the over-70s who, whatever the disease, are at special risk and disease-wise it is those of any age with multiple sclerosis, cerebral palsy, spina bifida or paraplegia.

David (1981) points out that it is difficult to be certain about the precise size of the problem of pressure sores because data obtained from various studies are not directly comparable. She reviews the findings of four studies, including that reported above, and illustrates differences which could account for the range of results found: for

Table 11.1 Percentage of patients in four clinical settings related to in/out of bed status

| In/out of bed | % of patients per clinical section | | | |
	General N 378	Maternity 67	Psychiatric 135	Community 194
Never out of bed	23*	2	—	2
Out of commode, up for toilet only	7	—	—	10
Up for part of day	19	13	4	10
Up for most of the day	47	34	95	77
Does not apply, infants under 1 yr	5	51	1†	2
Total	101	100	100	101

* Percentages rounded; †One infant

Source: Roper, N 1976 Clinical experience in nurse education. Churchill Livingstone, Edinburgh

example, the type of patients included in the populations studied and the method of grading sores. Nevertheless, it is clear that the prevalence increases in parallel with age; and that chairfast patients require just as much attention as those who are bedfast.

In a national survey in England and Wales which was carried out by the Nursing Practice Research Unit, pressure sore prevalence was found to be 6.7% (David et al, 1983). Nyquist & Hawthorn (1987) summarise the results of various surveys, in which the percentage of patients with pressure sores ranged from 3% to 9.4% (the variations arising from sample, method and definition differences). A consistent finding is that incidence increases with age; of the 885 patients reported to have pressure sores in David et al's survey, 85% were over the age of 65. Further, 41% of these patients with pressure sores were receiving sedatives or narcotics which supports the knowledge that suppressed or reduced mobility is a significant feature in the aetiology of pressure sores (Crow, 1988).

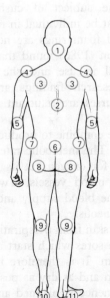

1. Occiput
2. Spinous processes
3. Scapula
4. Shoulder
5. Elbow
6. Sacrum
7. Ischial crest
8. Ischial tuberosity
9. Knee
10. Heel
11. Side of foot

Fig. 11.1 Pressure areas/sites

Pressure areas or sites. These are where body prominences, and the tissues overlying them, support the body weight when sitting or lying (Fig. 11.1).

Factors contributing to pressure sores
In order to understand the rationale of nursing activities which aim to prevent the development of pressure sores, it is essential to know about the various factors, both direct and indirect, which contribute to their development. Pressure sores result from an interruption of the tissue's blood supply, causing a local ischaemia and, if this continues, necrosis of the affected area. There are many predisposing factors but the main factors in pressure sore formation are continuous direct pressure and shearing force.

The various factors contributing to pressure sores are listed in Table 11.2 and hereafter are discussed in turn.

Compression of tissues. Compression of tissues between two hard surfaces is the major cause of pressure sores. Compression of the skin and deeper tissues between the hard, bony skeleton and the unyielding surface of a bed is the most common example, but the same effect can result from the chair seat, stretcher, trolley, operating theatre table or X-ray table. The effect of compression is to reduce the blood supply to the cells so that they receive fewer nutrients and less oxygen, and there is less efficient removal of their waste products. Tissue death results from anoxia, not from mechanical damage to cells. It is understood that pressure evenly distributed over a larger area is less injurious than local 'point pressure'. Prolonged low

Table 11.2 Factors contributing to pressure sores

Compression of tissues
Shearing force
Heat
Moisture
Friction
Poor skin hygiene
Poor general nutrition
Lack of oxygen
Lack of spontaneous body movements

pressure is more hazardous than a short period of high pressure.

On the basis of this knowledge, it is self-evident that relief of pressure is the single most important nursing activity in the prevention of pressure sores. Bearing in mind the particular hazards of localised pressure and prolonged low pressure. it can be deduced that frequent, minor changes of position — which may be accomplished by the patient, if properly instructed — should be incorporated into the nursing plan as well as the more familiar intervention of 'regular turning'. For example, when a patient is bedfast a monkey pole or overhead trapeze is a simple means of achieving frequent relief of pressure by lifting the buttocks off the bed. When they are necessary, turning regimes are usually based on a 2-hourly schedule which to the best of our knowledge is the necessary frequency if those patients particularly at risk are to be adequately protected from developing pressure sores. Lowthian (1979) designed a turning clock to assist nurses in carrying out this preventive measure. The scheme is adaptable to suit each individual's routine and requirements; a list of scheduled times and a signature space accompanies the clock so that there is documentation of the actual implementation of the planned nursing intervention.

Torrance (1983) points out, however, that there are disadvantages in regular turning. First, there is the inconvenience to the patient of regular disturbance, disrupting sleep and perhaps causing pain. Second, it is a time-consuming activity for the nursing staff. In circumstances when regular turning is either undesirable or impossible to accomplish, or indeed as an adjunct to it, pressure-relieving devices can be employed.

Careful positioning and intelligent use of pillows can help to minimise tissue compression. Bed cradles strategically placed relieve the weight of the upper bedclothes from particular parts of the body. Sheepskins and synthetic fleeces used to be favoured as aids to reduce compression but are no longer advocated for that purpose and, in addition, could present a potential source of infection and cross-infection (Jackson, 1983). Devices are also available which alternate the area of body under pressure, the most common example being the alternative pressure mattress or ripple bed. The basic system consists of a cellular air mattress connected to an electrical air pump and the air cells are alternately inflated and deflated. Most pump units can be adjusted to an appropriate weight setting, though in practice the heaviest setting is usually best for most patients. In addition to ripple mattresses, a variety of more recently-developed pressure-relieving beds and mattresses are now available; these include low air loss beds, air-fluidised beds, and the 'Vaperm' mattress.

Although there are many aids of various kinds available, the importance of regular change of position and manual turning where necessary cannot be overemphasised in relation to the prevention of tissue compression, the major cause of pressure sores.

Shearing force. When any part of the supported body is on a gradient, the deeper tissues (mainly muscle) near the bone 'slide' towards the lower gradient while the skin remains at its point of contact with the supporting surface because of friction which is increased in the presence of moisture. The blood vessels in the deeper sheared area are stretched and angulated, thus the deeper tissues become ischaemic with consequent necrosis. Shearing force can be created by badly executed lifting of patients.

Nursing activities to prevent shearing include skilled lifting of patients and positioning which will ensure prevention of sliding in any direction for patients in beds and chairs. Sliding down the bed can be prevented by adjusting the mattress or inserting pillows so that the knees are slightly bent and the thighs supported. A padded footboard is also helpful. It is, of course, important that such measures do not discourage movement and patients should be asked to rotate each foot several times every hour or so. The possibility of shearing in sacral, ischial and heel tissues should not be forgotten when patients spend some part of the day in chairs. The patient is less likely to slump in the chair if the back does not slant too much and if the feet are well supported.

The chair needs to match the patient's physique and be covered with a material which prevents downward sliding. Torrance (1983) identifies a number of factors which contribute to risk of pressure sores in the chairfast patient: slumped posture, badly fitting wheelchairs, or geriatric chairs, and poorly adjusted footrests or footstools. He advocates that patients should be taught to lift free of the chairseat (by hand push-ups) if no pressure-relieving cushions are employed. On the subject of cushions, he emphasises that selection must be individual in relation to size and fit. Air, rubber and foam rings are not recommended. Despite this, Deacon (1986) found that air and foam ring cushions are still in use and she wonders whether this is because research findings are poorly communicated or because nurses are reluctant to accept research findings.

Heat. Friction and pressure combine to produce a localised increase of temperature. The metabolic rate is raised which increases the demand for oxygen yet its supply is lessened by compression of blood vessels. Two hourly relief of pressure increases the blood supply and reduces the local temperature simultaneously.

Moisture. Excessively moist skin from perspiration, urine or faeces encourages pressure sores which start as maceration of devitalised epithelium. It is therefore important to keep patients' skin as clean and as dry as possible. To this end, retraining for continence is planned and implemented for patients who are incontinent of urine.

Immediate washing and changing of patients after incontinence also helps to prevent malodour from decomposing urine and/or faeces.

Friction. The adherence property of friction has already been mentioned. It can also cause injury resulting in the loss of epidermal cells (abrasion). Sometimes the first evidence of a frictional sore is a blister. It can occur on the heels, ankles and knees, especially in restless patients. Maintaining patients in a non-friction position and comforting them are important nursing activities.

Poor skin hygiene. As noted previously skin has a natural flora of microorganisms which are constantly multiplying, so their number is higher if skin is unwashed. Consequently abrasion or maceration of unwashed skin is more likely to become infected.

Poor general nutrition. Poor nutrition results in loss of subcutaneous tissue and muscle bulk, both of which normally act as mechanical padding. Lack of specific nutrients in the blood such as protein and vitamin C render a patient more liable to pressure sores. Particular attention to the dietary intake of patients at risk of developing sores is an important nursing activity.

Lack of oxygen. Localised lack of oxygen due to lessened blood supply caused by compression and shearing has been mentioned. Anaemia is one cause for a generalised reduction in oxygen in the blood (hypoxaemia) and interference with oxygen absorption in the pulmonary membranes is another. Patients with hypoxaemia from any cause are at risk of developing pressure sores. Adequate intake of iron-containing foods such as red meat, egg yolk, green vegetables and salads is useful to maximise the blood's oxygen carrying function.

Lack of spontaneous body movements. People when sitting, lying and sleeping make many small movements in response to sensory stimuli received by the brain. This is a protective physiological phenomenon to avoid excessive pressure on a particular part of the body. In any condition which prevents this protective mechanism, such as frailty, illness, anaesthesia, loss of sensation as in paralysis or being under the influence of alcohol, drugs, and sleeping pills, there is an increased risk of pressure sores.

Types of pressure sores

Various classifications of pressure sores have been suggested but for the purposes of this introductory-level discussion of the subject, types of sores are categorised simply as 'superficial sores' and 'deep sores'.

Superficial sores. In these sores there is destruction of the epidermis with exposure of the dermis which can be caused by such things as creases in the bedclothes and/or personal clothes, crumbs, harsh linen, abrasion from bedpan or commode and persistent scratching. Superficial sores can be precipitated by excessive moisture from fever or incontinence which increases the friction between skin

and the surface supporting it. Friction produces blisters, which may be the first sign of damage. Once the epidermis is removed, the skin's protective function is lost and microorganisms can penetrate the exposed tissue which is moist with lymph. A semi-permeable dressing is applied using aseptic technique and secured in position to prevent entry of microorganisms (p. 224). Relief of pressure is essential until healing has occurred. There can be further destruction including the dermis and the sore is then classified as a deep one.

Deep sores. In these sores there is destruction of the epidermis and dermis exposing deeper tissues which can include muscle and even bone. Unlike the superficial sore the damage can be established in the deep tissues before tracking out to the surface. Deep sores can become infected, discharging an exudate which results in protein and fluid loss so that there has to be reciprocal modification of the AL of eating and drinking. Deep sores can take many weeks, indeed months to heal and can require surgical closure to prevent further debility. The site, whether or not it is surgically dressed (and many new types of dressings and products have become available in recent years), must not be exposed to pressure and meticulous regular relief over the other pressure areas is essential.

Although classification has been discussed here simply in terms of distinguishing between 'superficial' and 'deep' sores, there is an emerging view that a more detailed and standardised classification system would be valuable, not only to guide practice but also as a basis for evaluative research (Lowthian, 1987).

Identifying patients 'at risk'

Knowledge of the factors which contribute to the development of pressure sores leads to an appreciation of those groups of patients who are particularly at risk. The elderly, as already mentioned, constitute the single largest section of the patient population at risk of developing pressure sores. However, any bedfast or chairfast or otherwise immobilised patient should be considered as vulnerable. Crow (1988) mentions that a further condition related to the development of pressure sores is a compromised cardiovascular system. She also comments that, while 'patient characteristics provide general indicators of vulnerability, there are more specific factors leading to irreversible damage in the tissue itself which need to be considered; aspects currently regarded as important concern damaging external loads which close the microcirculation and lymphatic system and intrinsic factors which weaken the tissue or its supporting network.' These various factors have been discussed in the earlier section on 'factors contributing to pressure sores'.

These factors provide the basis for tools which have been developed to identify patients 'at risk'. The Norton scoring system for identifying geriatric patients at risk of

		A	B	C	D	E	
		Physical Condition	Mental Condition	Activity	Mobility	Incontinent	Total score
Name	Date	Good 4 Fair 3 Poor 2 V. bad 1	Alert 4 Apathetic 3 Confused 2 Stuporous 1	Ambulant 4 Walk/help 3 Chairbound 2 Bedfast 1	Full 4 Sl. limited 3 V. limited 2 Immobile 1	Not 4 Occasionally 3 Usually/urine 2 Doubly 1	

Instructions for use

1. Identify the most appropriate description of the patient (4, 3, 2, 1) under each of the five headings (A to E) and total the result.
2. Record the 'score' with its date in the patient's notes or on a chart.
3. Assess weekly and whenever any change in the patient's condition and/or circumstances.

With a 'score' of 14 and below the patient is 'At Risk' denoting need for intensive care, i.e. 1-2 hourly changes of posture and the use of pressure-relieving aids.

Note: When oedema of the sacral area has been present a rise of score above 14 does not indicate less risk of a lesion.

Fig. 11.2 The Norton scoring system

developing pressure sores is illustrated in Figure 11.2. Although it is now many years since the initial publication of the score (Norton et al 1962), widespread knowledge of it and its increasing use in nursing is a relatively recent development. The system is dependent on the subjective judgement of the assessor and, therefore, has limitations as a foolproof tool. The advantage of the Norton score is that it provides at least some means, which is not time-consuming, of assessing patients' risk of developing pressure sores and providing timely warning of the need to implement appropriate preventive nursing activities. Assessments should be repeated regularly (and frequently if the patient's medical condition deteriorates), preferably by the same nurse, and a downward trend in the score is particularly significant.

Since Norton's early work, numerous risk calculators have been devised. Barratt (1987) reviews some of the most commonly used of these and, while recognising their value, warns that 'they should not be used as substitutes for good clinical judgement'.

Prevention of pressure sores

As a summary of the foregoing discussion, which has been based on evidence from research as far as possible, there follows a statement of the principles of prevention of pressure sores:

- assessment of risk (based on knowledge of predisposing factors/use of tools, e.g. Norton score)
- relief of pressure to avoid damage by tissue compression — especially point pressure and

prolonged low pressure (maximal exposure being 2 hours for those at highest risk) avoidance of shearing force (by skilled lifting/positioning in bed or chair to prevent sliding)
- avoidance of excessive heat, moisture and friction
- maintenance of adequate skin hygiene
- maintenance of adequate nutrition
- correction of oxygen lack/anaemia
- avoidance/correction of conditions which decrease spontaneous body movements

The problem of pressure sores is no longer regarded as an indication of poor nursing care. Nevertheless, there is the need for nurses to adopt a more systematic, research-based approach to the prevention of pressure sores. Those patients who are dependent on nurses for prevention of pressure sores have every right to expect that the care which is planned for them is based on available up-to-date knowledge but, as Gould (1986) argues, it would appear that all the research undertaken in the area has not made its proper impact on nursing practice. She believes that one of the reasons for this may be the failure of nurse education programmes to incorporate relevant research. Thus, improved education is one aspect to be tackled in attempting to improve pressure sore prevention.

Livesley (1987), on the other hand, argues that it is time for the introduction of a national policy on the basis that pressure sore prevention is 'not simply a nursing problem but also requires a planned and co-ordinated approach by clinicians and administrators'. At local level, an interesting example of concerted action towards reducing the incidence of pressure sores is provided by Osborne (1987) who describes the efforts of a quality circle and the resulting 50% reduction in pressure sores in the four medical wards concerned. Both local and national coordinated efforts may well be needed if the costly problem of pressure sores is to be tackled seriously for the future.

Dependence for management of pressure sores

If preventive measures are rigorously implemented, many pressure sores can be avoided and those which do occur, if noticed early enough as a result of regular assessment, can usually be treated successfully. When pressure sores do occur, Torrance (1983) suggests that their management can be considered as comprising three aspects:

- removal of pressure (i.e. to keep the ulcerated area free of further pressure)
- treatment of predisposing factors (as described for prevention)
- care of the wound

It is the third aspect — wound care — which remains one of nursing's most controversial issues. Numerous treatments have been invented, advocated, used and later discarded. There seems to be little evidence that any of the many agents which have been used to encourage healing have real proven value. What is needed is rigorous clinical research and that is now only beginning to get underway. As Chapman & Chapman (1986) conclude, from a review of current knowledge of pressure sore treatment, this area 'is at present under-researched so it is not surprising that selection of treatment is often made on an ad-hoc basis'. The authors, involved in David et al's (1983) survey, summarise the findings of that study regarding pressure sore treatment. In the treatment prescribed for the 1506 pressure sores studied (in 885 patients), it was the nursing staff who were solely responsible in 82% of cases, re-inforcing the nurse's pre-eminent role in this area. Cleaning and the application of chemical preparations were the treatments most commonly employed. Findings about the use of chemical preparations are interesting — of the 84 types found to be in use, only 2 were observed on more than 100 occasions and 54% of the sores were treated with preparations used less than 25 times each. Reasons for selection from the array of preparations available were mainly personal, or Sister's preferences, or availability in the lotion cupboard.

Advisedly, Torrance (1983) offers the advice that nurses should choose products and treatments which can be demonstrated to aid healing, and avoid those which have no explanation for their mode of action. From his detailed review of pressure sore management, which should be read in full, Torrance draws a number of conclusions about wound care. Certainly, debridement, treating infection and protecting the sore from dehydration and contamination are important, but what the best methods are for achieving these objectives is not clear-cut. Wound cleansing, frequent dressing changes and wound irrigation may also have some value. An absorption dressing (e.g. Debrisan) which removes bacteria and exudate without drying the wound surface and becoming adherent is effective. Op-Site is appropriate for a clean, superficial wound, if left in place until healing is complete. Torrance emphasises that no single method will suit all patients and, whichever treat-ment is employed, pressure sores should be given the same meticulous attention which is advocated for any surgical wound.

Proper management of the wound is, of course, vital. But perhaps a reminder should be given that management of pressure sores is concerned with patients and not just the sores! Individualised nursing is a vital aspect of the management of pressure sores.

Dependence for prevention of wound infection

In the preceding section, prevention of infection was mentioned in the context of management of pressure sores. This section discusses the subject in a little more detail, with particular reference to surgical wounds. There is no attempt to go into details of available dressings, wound

drains or dressing techniques; these are issues which should be covered in detail at appropriate points in the nursing curriculum. However, it may be useful here to refer readers to short, but helpful, articles by Morison (1987a, b) which outline priorities in wound management and, first, the assessment of wounds which is, of course, a prerequisite to planning appropriate nursing.

For present purposes, the aim of this section is to explain the rationale behind some of the routine nursing activities, pre- and postoperative, which have as their objective the prevention of wound infection. This is an important objective of wound care since infection delays healing (see Torrance 1986 for an account of the physi-ology of wound healing). The signs of wound infection include pyrexia; local pain, erythema and oedema; tachy-cardia; excess exudate and pus; and unpleasant odour. The key principles of preventing wound infection are, as Morison (1987a) outlines, aimed at breaking the chain of infection and include:

- isolating potential sources of infection
- effective cleansing and disinfection of the physical environment
- aseptic wound dressing technique
- protection of the susceptible host

Pre-operatively, the objective of skin preparation is to render the skin as free as possible from pathogenic micro-organisms. It must be remembered that there is no such thing as 'sterile' skin, even after thorough cleansing. Nursing activities to achieve maximum skin cleanliness traditionally have included a 'preoperative bath' for the patient. Some hospitals advocate the addition of a bacteri-cidal agent to the water but the value of this is not proven. Indeed Clarke (1983) states: 'Savlon baths have no effect in reducing skin bacteria.' In the hospital where the study of skin preparation which she reports was carried out, it was routine for all patients to have a Savlon bath on the morning of the operation (and on three mornings pre-operatively for major orthopaedic and cardiac surgery). However, swabs from the skin of patients who did not have a Savlon bath grew no more countable bacteria than those who had.

On the subject of bathing before surgery, Stokes (1984) refers to evidence which points to the ineffectiveness of a single antiseptic bath in reducing skin flora. As the surface of the bath may be contaminated, she recommends that showering is preferable to bathing. Specifically, Stokes states: 'Repeated bathing or showering with 4% chlorhex-idine detergent solution reduced the number of organisms on the skin' (though this has only been shown to reduce the infection rate in a trial relating to vascular surgery). In fact, thorough application of an alcoholic solution or an antiseptic (chlorhexidine or povidone-iodine) at the time of surgery will give a better reduction of skin flora at the operation site. On the basis of the evidence presented by

Stokes, traditional nursing practices regarding preoperative bathing/showering appear to require reconsideration.

Indeed, Morison (1988) mentions the potential hazard of showering or bathing; namely, that it may lead to the transfer of bacteria from areas such as the perineum and nose to other areas previously without colonisation. She cites evidence of the value of whole body disinfectant with an antiseptic solution as an adjunct to preoperative skin cleansing in theatre. Morison also states that Hibiscrub (a detergent solution containing chlorhexidine gluconate) is becoming popular as a preoperative skin agent and that there is evidence of this being effective. On this basis she considers that 'two whole body preoperative washes with Hibiscrub, usually the night before and on the day of the operation, would therefore seem cost effective and beneficial for patients.'

Removal of hair from the skin around the site of incision is another nursing activity carried out in the preoperative period and, again, has prevention of infection as the objective. Customarily this was done by shaving but then there was some evidence (Powis et al, 1976) that the use of depilatory creams results in a lower microorganism count. Certainly, this method is increasingly being advocated, and, indeed, whether hair removal with the purpose of infection control serves any purpose at all has become open to question; for example, Bond (1980) reviewed the evidence with regard to perineovulval shaving before childbirth and concluded that this served no purpose in terms of infection control. In the UK, more and more maternity units now operate a policy of 'no shave' on admission in labour, although the practice is by no means universal yet (Garcia et al, 1986).

It is interesting that in the study previously referred to in connection with preoperative bathing (Clarke, 1983), hair removal was by shaving rather than by use of depilatory cream. In the hospital concerned there was no standard routine regarding time of shaving. However, patients shaved on the morning of operation or in theatre grew more countable bacteria than those who were shaved the day before. On this basis, Clarke states: 'If shaving is to be done it should be the day before surgery.'

However, according to Stokes (1984) there is some evidence that wound infection is higher in patients who are shaved preoperatively than in those who are not. In contradiction to Clarke's statement, Stokes advocates that shaving (if necessary) should be carried out as close to the time of operation as possible because any small abrasions can become colonised with pathogens overnight. For shaving she advocates a disposable razor (or sterilised razor with a clean blade) and foam (rather than soap), or an electric razor (with removable head which can be immersed in 70% alcohol). But, according to Pettersson (1986), all of the research evidence points to one fact — that shaving ought to be avoided. The author, a Danish nurse, explains that nurses and doctors in Denmark have changed their attitude towards preoperative hair removal, considering it to be unnecessary unless hair around the operation site is copious, coarse or very long. If removal is necessary, shaving is being replaced by depilation or clipping using electric hair clippers. Morison (1988) refers to evidence that clippers can nip the skin creases and, for this reason — and because of the hazard of cutting the skin when a safety razor is used — she favours the use of depilatory creams. If shaving of the operation site is requested by the surgeon, Morison recommends that this is performed as near as possible to the time of operation and certainly not the night before surgery.

As will be apparent from the foregoing discussion, the issue of preoperative skin preparation is a complex and controversial one. Nurses should try to keep abreast with new knowledge arising from research in this area and perhaps encouragement could be given to their local Control of Infection Committee or Infection Control Nurse to supply up-to-date advice on the procedures which should be adopted on the basis of the best information available.

In addition to preparation of the skin, further protection is afforded by the provision of special clothing for the patient's transfer to theatre. Morison (1988) recommends that there is a complete change of bedlinen after the second Hibiscrub preoperative bath, before the patient is dressed in a theatre gown. To decrease the possibility of microorganisms being shed from the hair, a theatre cap is also provided. These necessary modifications in the AL of personal cleansing and dressing can add to the normally raised anxiety level of the patient who requires surgery. Adequate explanation of the rationale helps to allay fears.

When the patient returns to the ward after surgery the wound will be protected from invasion by microorganisms with a dressing. Usually the theatre dressing is left undisturbed for 24–48 hours unless gross seepage occurs, in which case it is replaced with a film dressing such as Opsite.

Whenever wounds are exposed, precautions are necessary to ensure that the air contains minimal microorganisms. Sometimes a treatment room with special ventilation is available. If not, the wound is dressed in the ward; domestic and nursing 'dust-producing' activities such as sweeping and bedmaking should have ceased at least 1 hour previously, during which time the 'dust' will have settled out of the atmosphere. Every hospital has its particular regime of 'aseptic technique' to prevent microorganisms gaining access to wounds, equipment and lotions. Thomlinson (1987), however, questions whether conventional methods of cleaning wounds are actually effective in reducing the number of pathogenic organisms, and suggests that this question should be further researched. Some useful, up-to-date guidance on wound cleansing (in particular the use of cleansing agents) is provided in a recent paper by Morison (1989). The same author, in an earlier publication, summarised the key nursing aspects of postoperative prevention of wound infection as follows:

- unless requested to do otherwise, or where there is gross seepage of exudate from the wound, the theatre dressing should be left intact for at least 24 hours
- remove the wound dressing in a well-ventilated treatment room — if the dressing must be changed at the bedside, then this should be done at least 1 hour after bedmaking and cleaning are completed
- maintain high standards in aseptic technique — this includes care of intravenous lines, wound drains and catheters (Morison, 1988)

Nursing activities such as these have an important part to play in the prevention of wound infection. There is no doubt that efforts to improve the effectiveness of prevention are required when one remembers the prevalence of hospital-acquired infection, surgical wound infection accounting for over 18% of the total (p. 94). The incidence of wound infection after surgery, according to Westaby (1982), ranges from 1% for 'clean' operations after elective surgery not involving the gastrointestinal or urinary tract to 30% after frank bacteriological contamination of the operative field by faeces or pus. Westaby points out that although bacteria are the basic cause of wound infection, other factors such as host resistance to infection should not be ignored. The fact is that every operation site is contaminated to some extent by airborne or other microorganisms, but not every patient develops a wound infection.

Observation of signs of infection in a wound is an important nursing activity and prompt reporting will enable the doctor to prescribe appropriate treatment. Inflammation, pain and tenderness at the site of the incision, usually accompanied by an increased body temperature, are the classic signs of wound infection. In the absence of other signs, elevated temperature does not necessarily indicate wound infection. Sometimes pus may be produced around the sutures or drain site or along the incision. Bacteriological analysis of a specimen of exudate from the wound will identify the organism responsible and permit a decision to be made about the most appropriate therapy. Antibiotic therapy now is normally only recommended in cases of severe infection where a systemic antibiotic may be indicated. The use of topical antiseptics and other measures for infected wounds are discussed by Morison (1987b).

As will be apparent from this discussion, prevention of wound infection is an excellent example of the interdependence of nurses and doctors in their daily work. Indeed, as was pointed out earlier in the book in a general discussion of this subject (p. 95), infection control can only be accomplished on a teamwork basis. And, of course, although in a position of dependence, the patient must be seen as a member of that team.

Before ending this discussion of prevention of wound infection, some comment should be made regarding the need for additional precautions in view of the increasing problem of HIV infection and AIDS. First, there is the need to protect the patient with a wound from the possibility of inadvertent infection by the nurse or doctor; therefore, staff involved in surgery or wound care should ensure that any skin abrasion or cut is covered by a waterproof dressing and Smith (1988) maintains, in a comment on 'surgeons and others and HIV', that 'health care workers with exudative lesions or weeping dermatitis must refrain from all direct patient care and from handling patient care equipment'. Secondly, there is the need for staff to protect themselves against inadvertent infection by an HIV seropositive patient. Smith, on this issue, states that 'the basic rule is that our health care workers must take precautions to prevent exposure to skin and mucous membranes when contact with blood or other body fluids of any patient may occur.' In practice, this means that surgical gloves and protective plastic aprons will be used more often than in the past and blood (and other body fluid) splashes must be dealt with properly and promptly. Theatre staff constitute a group in special need of protection; Sadler (1987) outlines guidelines which should be followed, while emphasising that panic is unwarranted whereas precautions are.

SOME SPECIFIC PROBLEMS ASSOCIATED WITH PERSONAL CLEANSING AND DRESSING

The total surface area covered with skin is extensive and it is therefore not surprising that anything which causes 'difference' can produce problems for the person. The minimum areas of the skin which are exposed in most cultures and climates during the day are the face, neck and hands and they are customarily mutually observed when a person is in the company of others. Some people have extensive birthmarks (naevi) and if they are on a part of the body normally covered by clothing during the day, they do not cause undue distress. Yet if they are on the face and neck they can be a source of psychological trauma. Nurses can help by having a positive not a discriminating attitude toward people with visible birthmarks or other disfigurement of the skin.

Psychological problems

Any visible stigma can produce psychological reaction in the person bearing the stigma and in the observer. Either of them can react by being self-conscious, embarrassed, anxious, fearful, shocked and even repulsed if the sight is of extensive skin trauma.

Most children experience self-consciousness and embarrassment in response to loss of the front milk teeth. People react differently to wearing dentures; most suffer initial self-consciousness and embarrassment and thereafter go to great lengths so that they are never seen without their dentures, perhaps not even by their spouse. Naturally for such people, admission to hospital presents them with a very special personal problem. Nurses need to be sensitive when caring for patients who have such idiosyncrasies.

Idiopathic loss of hair can sometimes be accepted by cancer patients because they hope that the cytotoxic drugs will improve their condition. Shock and anxiety can be precipitating factors in causing patchy baldness which the patient finds disconcerting. If the condition can be accepted as a temporary one it will be remedied, but continuing anxiety can result in increasing baldness. Encouraging the patient to talk about the anxiety and helping to identify its cause is an important part of treatment. Wearing a wig might be a helpful solution if baldness is severe.

People with skin disease can become very depressed; indeed some skin diseases are a somatic expression of a psychological disturbance. Attending to the afflicted areas can be time-consuming and healing can be slow. Also in periods of excessive stress the condition can exacerbate which is disappointing to all concerned. If patients with visible skin disease experience avoiding actions by others, they naturally feel uncomfortable and discriminated against. Nurses can help by positive behaviour towards patients with skin disease.

Skin disorders in a child can be very distressing for parents; Cutler (1988) describes some of the more common conditions, many of which can be treated successfully.

Scars

The formation of scars, an inevitable sequel to wound healing after trauma, disease or surgery, has both physical and psychological implications for the patient. Dowding & Horn (1986) describe some of the effects of scars on the sufferer, pointing out that disfiguring facial scars have particularly profound effects as do those which affect sexuality in a direct way; for example, scars on the breasts or genital area. They suggest that it is especially important for patients to be realistically prepared in advance of surgery for what the scar will look like since research has indicated a relationship between expectations and adaptation.

Burns

Burn injuries can have an equally profound physical and psychological effect on the victim and Wilding (1986) considers that it is vital for nurses to fully understand the effect a scald or burn injury has on the skin and on the person. The area of body surface burned is assessed on a percentage basis and, initially, it is the extent of the burn which determines the severity of the injury and the threat to life; the depth of injury is also important in terms of the treatment plan. Prevention of infection and pain control are vital aspects of treatment, along with wound care and nutrition.

In the long-term, many burns victims suffer psychological problems such as depression and anxiety; Wallace (1988) reports that this was the case in 30–40% of adult patients who had been treated in a regional burns unit. She advocates that professional counselling services should be available for burns victims to help them come to terms with the effects of their injuries.

Excessive sweating (hyperhidrosis)

There are changes in a patient's internal environment in response to such states as anxiety and fear. At whatever point they contact the health care system, whether at a doctor's surgery, clinic, health centre or hospital, and on going to such places as the X-ray department and the operating theatre, they will experience some degree of anxiety. One of the body's reactions is increased secretion of sweat. There may be added embarrassment at wet patches on clothing in the axillary region and damp footwear. A constant readiness on the nurse's part to give adequate preparatory explanation; to listen to the patient, and to observe non-verbal behaviour for clues as to the cause of anxiety is necessary. Arranging for a daily change of clothing will help to prevent odour which could cause further embarrassment. The patient may benefit from knowledge about more effective anti-perspirants and deodorants.

Generalised hyperhidrosis, according to Alderman (1988a), can be a symptom of many conditions (including thyrotoxicosis, chronic infection, diabetes, acromegaly and gout) and so careful investigation is necessary if excessive sweating appears to be more than a temporary concomitant of fear, anxiety or increased metabolic rate!

Itching (pruritus)

Itching is not a disease per se but can be symptomatic of many diseases. The patient's problem is that he/she is cross, irritable and cannot sleep because of the discomfort. A natural reaction is to scratch an itching part of the body; scratching can induce more itching and more scratching can break the skin so that there is a portal of entry for microorganisms. The sight of the broken skin may make the patient feel guilty and this can add to the misery.

The nurse can help in a general way by offering suggestions that short clean nails will lessen trauma and risk of infection. Cotton gloves may help, especially if scratching during sleep is a problem. Use of bland non-perfumed talcum powder and soap is helpful; soap should be well rinsed off before drying the skin, and the addition of bath oil to the water is undesirable. Over-spiced food and hot baths are best avoided. Overheating from any cause is undesirable. Loose clothing made of non-irritant material is advisable especially for night clothes. If the patient's mental activity can be diverted to other interests, so much the better.

When itching may indicate the presence of a disorder which should be medically treated, the appropriate action should be taken; an example is the case of a mole which becomes itchy since this may be indicative of malignant melanoma.

Causes of itching
- Allergic reaction to
    topical application
    ingestion of specific drugs or food
- Infectious disease
    German measles
    chicken pox
- Skin disease
    impetigo
    eczema
    dermatitis
    skin cancer
- Other disease
    obstructive jaundice
    diabetes
- Infestation
    head lice
    body lice
    scabies
- Discharge
    vaginal

When itching from skin disease is severe, particularly in children, arm constraint is sometimes necessary to prevent further skin damage from scratching, but wherever possible patients are taught the reasons for self-restraint and should be praised for compliance.

Individualising nursing

The first part of this chapter reflects the Roper, Logan and Tierney model for nursing — the nature of the AL of personal cleansing and dressing; the relationship of the lifespan to the AL; the effect of the individual's dependence/independence status; the influence of physical, psychological, sociocultural, environmental and politico-economic factors on the AL. In the second part of the chapter, a selection of problems and discomforts which are experienced by people in relation to the AL have been described. With this background of *general* knowledge about the AL, it should be possible to incorporate such

information in an individualised nursing plan when such information is relevant to the person's current circumstances.

While describing the Roper, Logan and Tierney model for nursing, *general* information was provided about Individualising nursing (p. 51) which in fact is synonymous with the concept of the nursing process.

Out of this background of *general* knowledge about the AL of personal cleansing and dressing and about Individualising nursing, it should then be possible to extract the issues which are relevant to an individual's current circumstances (whether in a health or an illness setting), i.e. to make an assessment of relevant issues according to the individual's stage on the lifespan; according to current level of dependence/independence; and take into account the relevant physical, psychological, sociocultural (including ethical, spiritual and religious), environmental and politicoeconomic (including legal) factors. Collectively, this information would provide a profile of the person's individuality in relation to this AL.

As indicated earlier in the text, this assessment would be achieved by various means such as observing the person; acquiring information about the individual's usual habits in relation to this AL partly by asking appropriate questions, partly by listening to the patient and/or relatives, and using relevant information from available records including medical records. The collected information could then be examined to identify any actual problems being experienced with the AL and these could be arranged in some order of priority. The nurse might also recognise some potential problems — not all possible potential problems but those which are relevant. Realistic goals, mutually agreed with the patient when this is possible, could then be set to prevent potential problems from becoming actual ones; to alleviate or solve the actual problems; or to help the person cope with those which cannot be alleviated or solved.

Keeping in mind what the person can and cannot do unaided, the nursing interventions to achieve the mutually set goals could then be selected according to local circumstances and available resources.

Following implementation of the interventions, their effects could be evaluated in relation to the goals set, and if goals were not reached, they would then be revised or re-scheduled, or even discarded. It is worth repeating here that although discussed in four phases — assessing, planning, implementing and evaluating — individualising nursing is not a linear progression; it assumes a built-in responsiveness to feedback at any of the phases, with ample allowance for change within the overall framework.

This chapter has been concerned with the AL of personal cleansing and dressing. However, as stated previously, it is only for the purpose of discussion that any AL can be considered on its own; in reality the various activities are so closely related and do not have distinct boundaries. Figure 11.3 is a reminder that the AL of

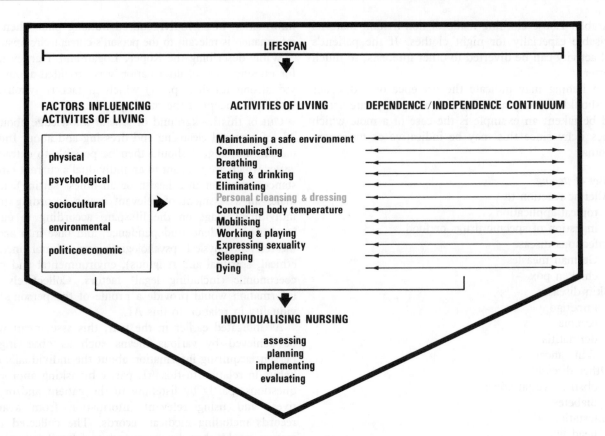

Fig. 11.3   The AL of personal cleansing and dressing within the model for nursing

personal cleansing and dressing is related to the other ALs and also to the various components of the model for nursing. However, it must be repeated that it may not be relevant to consider this particular AL for every patient in every circumstance. Professional judgement is required to assess its relevance to any one patient.

Acknowledgements
Thanks are extended to Dr M. Clark of the Nursing Practice Research Unit, University of Surrey and to Mrs M. Morison, Forth Valley Health Board for their helpful suggestions towards the revision of this chapter's discussion of pressure sores and wound management respectively.

REFERENCES

Adams S 1987 The relationship of clothing to self-esteem of elderly patients. Nursing Times Occasional Paper 83 (5): 41–45
Alderman C 1988a Honest sweat. Nursing Standard 2 (38) June 25: 35
Alderman C 1988b Scabies: no respect. Nursing Standard 10 (3) December 3: 24
Barratt E 1987 Pressure sores: Putting risk calculators in their place. Nursing Times 83 (7) February 18: 65–70
Bond S 1980 Shave it . . . or save it? Nursing Times 76 (9) February 28: 362–363

British Association of Cancer United Patients — BACUP 1987 Coping with hair loss. Published by BACUP, 121/123 Charterhouse Street, London, EC1M 6AA
Bush T 1984 The sense of well-being. Nursing Times 80 (1) January 4: 31–32
Campbell S 1987 Mouth care in cancer patients. Nursing Times 83 (29) July 22: 59–60
Carr E 1988 Research can solve the problem of getting dressed. The Professional Nurse 3 (9) June: 369
Casey N 1988 Malignant melanomas. Nursing Standard 2 (21) February 27: 31
Chapman E J, Chapman R 1986 Treatment of pressure sores: the state of the art. In: Tierney A J (ed) Recent advances in clinical nursing practice. Churchill Livingstone, Edinburgh, ch 5, p 105–124
Clark M O, Barbanel J C, Jordan M M, Nicol S M 1978 Pressure sores. Nursing Times 74 (9) March 2: 363–366
Clarke J 1983 The effectiveness of surgical skin preparations. Nursing Times Theatre nursing supplement September 28: 8–17
Copperman H 1977 Foam stick applicators. Nursing Times 73 (13) March 31: 459
Cormack J F 1983 Dentistry. Nursing (April) 2nd Series 12: 329
Crow R 1988 The challenge of pressure sores. Nursing Times 84(38) September 21: 68–73
Cutler T 1988 Problems that are skin deep (skin disorders in childhood). Nursing Times Community Outlook May: 16–19
David J 1981 The size of the problem of pressure sores. Journal of the Society for Tissue Viability and the Wessex Special Interest Groups 1 (1) July: 10–13
David J A, Chapman R G, Chapman E J, Lockett B 1983 An investigation of the current methods used in nursing for the care of patients with established pressure sores. Nursing Practice Research Unit, Northwick Park Hospital and Clinical Research Unit, Harrow, UK
Davis M 1977 Getting to the root of the problem: hair grooming for black patients. Nursing 77 (7): 60–65

Deacon L 1986 Pressure sores: Does anyone read research? Nursing Times 82 (32) August 6: 57–59

Disabled Living Foundation 1977 Dressing for disabled people. A manual for nurses and others. Disabled Living Foundation, London

Donaldson R J 1977 Head infestation. Nursing Mirror 144 (3) January 20: 56–57

Dowding C M, Horn S 1986 Scars: formation and effects. Nursing 3 (6) June: 200–202

Garcia J, Garforth S, Ayres S 1986 The policy and practice in midwifery study — Progress Report, MIDIRS Information Pack No. 2, July

Geissler P, McCord F 1986 Dental care for the elderly. Nursing Times 82 (20) May 14: 53–54

Gibbons D E 1983 Mouth care procedures. Nursing Times 79 (7) February 16: 30

Gidley C 1987 Now, wash your hands! Nursing Times 83 (29) July 22: 40–42

Gould D 1986 Pressure sore prevention and treatment: an example of nurses' failure to implement research findings. Journal of Advanced Nursing 11 (4) July: 389–394

Greaves A 1985 We'll just freshen you up, dear . . . (on bedbathing). Nursing Times 27 March 6: 3–8

Howarth H 1977 Mouth care procedures for the very ill. Nursing Times 73 (10) March 10: 354–355

Jackson J 1983 Sheepskins — a potential hazard? Nursing Times 79 (18) May 4: 41–45

Livesley B 1987 Pressure sores: an expensive epidemic. Nursing Times 83 (6) February 18: 79

Lovelock D J 1973 Oral hygiene for patients in hospital. Nursing Mirror 137 (42) October 12: 39

Lowthian P 1979 Turning clocks system to prevent pressure sores. Nursing Mirror 148 (21) May 24: 30–31

Lowthian P 1987 The classification and grading of pressure sores. CARE (The British Journal of Rehabilitation and Tissue Viability) 51 March: 5–9

McCord F, Stalker A 1988 Brushing up on oral care. Nursing Times 84 (13) March 30: 40–41

Milne C 1988 Nit picking. Nursing Standard 2 (38) June 25: 25

Mohylnycky N 1983 Parasitic skin infections. Nursing 2nd series No. 9 (January): 246–248

Morison M 1987a Wound assessment. The Professional Nurse 2 (10) July: 315–317

Morison M M 1987b Priorities in wound management. The Professional Nurse 2 (11) August: 352–355; 2 (12) September: 402–411

Morison M J 1988 How can the incidence of surgical wound infection be reduced? The Professional Nurse December: 122–125

Morison M J 1989 Wound cleansing — which solution? The Professional Nurse February: 220–225

Nichols S 1988 Beware of the mid-day sun. Nursing Times 84 (23) June 8: 38–39

Norton D 1983 Clothes sense. Nursing Times 79 (44) November 2: 12–14

Norton D, McLaren R, Exton-Smith A 1962 An investigation of geriatric nursing problems in hospital. Churchill Livingstone, Edinburgh (Reissued in 1975)

Nyquist R, Hawthorn P J 1987 The prevalence of pressure sores within an area health authority. Journal of Advanced Nursing 12: 183–187

Osborne S 1987 Pressure sores: a quality circle investigation. Nursing Times 83 (6) February 18: 73–76

Owen C M 1982 Too much nit-picking? Nursing Times 78 (15) April 14: 632–634

Pettersson E 1986 Preoperative hair removal and infection control. In: Tierney A J (ed) Recent advances in clinical nursing practice. Churchill Livingstone, Edinburgh, p 169–175

Powis S, Waterworth T, Arkell D 1976 Preoperative skin preparation: clinical evaluation of depilatory cream. British Medical Journal 2: 1166–1168

Pritchard V, Hathaway C 1988 Patient handwashing practice. Nursing Times 84 (36) September 7: 68–72

Richardson A 1987 A process standard for oral care (in cancer chemotherapy). Nursing Times 83 (32) August 12: 38–40

Roberts C 1987 A lousy life. Nursing Times Community Outlook August: 16–19

Roth P T, Creason N S 1986 Nurse administered oral hygiene: is there a scientific basis? Journal of Advanced Nursing 11 (3): 323–331

Sadler C 1987 Who's at risk? (Theatre staff and AIDS). Nursing Times 83 (45) November 11: 16–17

Shepherd G, Page C, Sammon P 1987 Oral hygiene: the mouth trap. Nursing Times 83 (19) May 13: 24–27

Smith M B 1988 Surgeons and others and HIV. British Medical Journal 296 February 13: 497–498

Steward M 1988 Teething troubles. Nursing Times Community Outlook May: 27–28

Stokes E 1984 Showering before surgery. Shaving before surgery. Nursing Times 80 (20) May 16: 71

Thomlinson D 1987 To clean or not to clean? Nursing Times 83 (9) March 14: 73–75

Tierney A J 1987 Preventing chemotherapy-induced alopecia in cancer patients: is scalp cooling worthwhile? Journal of Advanced Nursing 12: 303–310

Torrance C 1983 Pressure sores: aetiology, treatment and prevention. Croom Helm, London

Torrance C 1986 The physiology of wound healing. Nursing 3 (5) May: 162–168

Wallace L 1988 Abandoned to a 'social death'? (Burns victims). Nursing Times 84 (10) March 9: 34–37

Webster R, Thompson D, Bowman G, Sutton T 1988 Patients' and nurses' opinions about bathing. Nursing Times Occasional Paper 84 (7) September 14: 54–57

Westaby S 1982 Wound care (9): Wound infection-treatment. Nursing Times 78(20) May 19: Centre supplement

Wilding P A 1986 Burns. Nursing 3 (5) May: 184–187

Wright L 1988 It's hard making history (the introduction of a new patient bathing procedure — the towel bath — in a District General Hospital). Unpublished paper. Royal Hallamshire Hospital, Sheffield, England

12
Controlling body temperature

The activity of controlling body temperature

Unlike the cold-blooded animals whose temperature fluctuates according to the changing temperature of their external environment, man is able to maintain body temperature at a constant level, independent of the degree of heat or cold in the surrounding environment.

THE NATURE OF CONTROLLING BODY TEMPERATURE

For most of the time man is unaware of his body temperature and this is because it remains constantly at a comfortable level. This control of temperature is accomplished because a special regulating centre in the brain carefully balances the amount of heat produced and lost by the body.

When the body temperature rises or falls outside the range of normal, a person is aware of feeling too hot or too cold. In either circumstance, the individual must perform certain activities to assist the physiological process of body temperature control. If people feel too hot when indoors, they can cease being active if that is the cause; or they can turn down heating appliances, open windows, draw curtains to keep out the sun, remove some clothing, take a cool shower or bath, or have a cold drink. If they are outside doing manual work they can remove some layers of clothing or can rest for a while until they cool down; if they are in direct sunshine they can move into the shade and, perhaps, use any suitable article such as a fan to move the surrounding air thereby cooling themselves further.

When people feel too cold indoors or outdoors, they can perform various activities which are the converse of those indulged in by people when they are too hot. Physical activity quickly generates body heat and additional items of clothing provide extra warmth and protection from the chill of a wind. Materials made of fibres which entrap air are warmer since air, being a poor conductor, preserves body heat. Use can also be made of the fact that dark colours absorb heat from the sun and so help to keep the body warm whereas light colours reflect heat.

Regulating the temperature of the atmosphere in homes and buildings is another activity which must be performed if body temperature is to be controlled satisfactorily. Any householder knows how expensive it is to equip a home so that it is capable of being cool in hot weather and warm in cold weather. Coal, electricity, gas and oil are all expensive commodities and, in addition, many countries are experiencing a shortage of energy resources. Some governments, in an attempt to minimise wastage of these important and scarce resources provide financial aid to householders for double-glazing windows and insulating walls and roofs. Special publicity campaigns are also common to remind the public to save these particular resources. When the temperature outdoors is low it is essential for health and comfort that homes are kept especially warm; this is particularly important for the very young and the elderly.

In man, maintenance of a constant body temperature is essential. Most of the numerous biochemical processes occurring within the body can only take place if the temperature of the body remains at a fairly constant level and within a relatively narrow range. The functioning of the nervous system is easily disturbed by temperatures outwith that narrow range of normal and, at the same time, many other systems of the body are adversely affected. Eventually, if the body temperature rises or falls excessively, there is permanent damage to body cells and the possibility of death.

In addition, the fact that body temperature remains constant within a relatively narrow range of normal, irrespective of the temperature of the external environment, enables man to adapt not only to very different climates but also to daily and seasonal variations in the environmental temperature. If this adaptation were not possible, the scope of human activity would be severely limited and the individual would suffer such discomfort from extremes of heat and cold that everyday living would be disrupted and miserable.

So, to summarise, controlling body temperature is an activity which relies on both the behaviour of the individual and the body's own thermoregulation. In terms of the latter, the key factors are the temperature regulating centre, heat production and heat loss; these are outlined briefly below.

Temperature-regulating centre. An area of nerve tissue in the anterior part of the hypothalamus of the brain acts as a centre which regulates body temperature. Nerve cells in this area respond to changes in the temperature of circulating blood. It is thought that the centre also responds to impulses from the temperature sensitive receptors in the skin, muscles, blood vessels, the abdominal cavity and various areas of the central nervous system.

The centre's function is to balance the amount of heat produced by the body and the amount of heat lost by the body. It works just like a thermostat; there is a constant 'set' temperature which is maintained as the centre responds by balancing heat production and heat loss. To achieve this the centre has two control mechanisms: its *heat-promoting centre* activates processes which increase heat production and reduce heat loss; conversely its *heat-losing centre* stimulates actions which reduce heat production and increase heat loss. These two centres work reciprocally; when one is activated, the other is depressed.

Heat production. All the metabolic processes continuously proceeding in the human body produce heat. At rest and during sleep the body is kept warm enough by the amount of energy produced at the basal metabolic rate. Additional heat production results mainly from skeletal muscle movement and, if this is not sufficient, the body initiates reflex muscular activity — shivering — which increases the rate of heat production up to fourfold. At the same time, stimulation of the sympathetic nervous system speeds up the process of cellular metabolism and raises the hairs on the skin, a vestigial mechanism in humans, which in hairier mammals traps the warm air next to the body, thereby insulating it.

The prevention of unnecessary heat loss is an important way of conserving body heat. Most heat loss occurs through the skin by evaporation, conduction, convection and radiation. Vasoconstriction, the constriction of blood vessels, minimises this heat loss because less warm blood circulates in the subcutaneous tissue. At the same time sweating is greatly diminished, reducing heat loss by evaporation.

Heat loss. A variety of means are used by the human body to lose heat. Heat is lost from skin which is in direct contact with cooler air by the process called conduction; this is assisted by convection currents of air circulating around the body. Heat is also lost by evaporation of moisture from the skin surface, naturally increased by sweating. There is some loss of heat by radiation from the body into the cooler atmosphere. Vasodilation enhances loss of heat through the skin by bringing more blood to the surface of the body. Panting, more common in animals though it does occur in man, aids heat loss by increasing evaporative heat loss from the moist respiratory tract. At the same time the heat-losing centre depresses the mechanisms which result in heat production, metabolism is slowed down and muscular activity is decreased.

It is the balance between heat production and heat loss

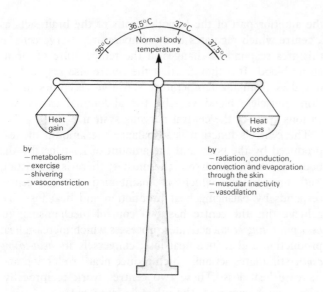

Fig. 12.1   Heat loss/heat gain balance

which must constantly be regulated to keep the body temperature within the limits of the range of normal. This concept of temperature control by balance is illustrated in Figure 12.1.

LIFESPAN: EFFECT ON CONTROLLING BODY TEMPERATURE

The lifespan component of the model of living is especially relevant to the AL of controlling body temperature. As long ago as 1900 a French neonatologist observed that the survival rate in the postnatal period was only 10% for infants whose body temperatures were 32.5 to 34°C and that survival rose to 77% when the infants were kept at 36 to 37°C (Drummond, 1979). Survival rates have improved among preterm and low birth weight babies and this is partly attributable to a better understanding of body temperature control.

The newborn baby requires to have the skin dried immediately to prevent loss of heat by evaporation, and to be wrapped in warm clothing to prevent further loss of heat through conduction, convection and radiation. An infant's body weight comprises 2–6% brown fat (Drummond, 1979). This is richly supplied with blood and has many nerve endings: these provide the stimulus for increased metabolism when the baby is exposed to cold, but prolonged exposure depletes the store of brown fat and this is undesirable. The heat receptors in the face are particularly sensitive and it is especially important that a baby is kept free from draughts. In the first few months and indeed years of life, the heat regulating system continues to be highly sensitive to stimuli which cause heat production, for example, even the exertion of prolonged crying can raise the body temperature above the range of normal. Until the young child learns to associate for instance the discomfort of being hot and sweaty with the relief obtained by taking off a garment and sitting still for a while, parents need to be vigilant on the child's behalf to avoid unpleasant excessive rises in body temperature. The same principle applies to falls in body temperature.

Throughout a woman's fertile life there is a slight rise in temperature just after ovulation and until 2 days before menstruation but many women are not aware of it. Some women have hot flushes as part of the menopause caused by the hormonal imbalance which occurs at this time. They usually manage to cope by wearing a jacket or cardigan which is easily removed when they are too hot.

Towards the end of the lifespan too, thermoregulation is less efficient due to impaired temperature discrimination, a reduction in the ability to constrict peripheral blood vessels, and a possible reduction in the shivering threshold (Collins et al, 1977; Macmillan et al, 1967). Older people can quickly suffer from the ill-effects of extreme heat or extreme cold. At the same time they may be less active and take less food so that it becomes important to provide extra environmental warmth for them, to prevent the potential problem of hypothermia becoming an actual one.

DEPENDENCE/INDEPENDENCE IN CONTROLLING BODY TEMPERATURE

The concept of a dependent/independent continuum as a component of the model has relevance to the stages of the lifespan when considering the AL of controlling body temperature. As well as children's physiological control being highly sensitive to stimuli, the many behavioural aspects of this AL have to be learned, as well as the perception of when they are necessary. In the later years of life, some degree of dependence on others may return in terms of carrying out the various activities required for controlling body temperature.

However at any stage a person can have an infection when the body's response is to increase its temperature and make the person dependent on drugs such as aspirin or antibiotics to reduce it, or on people to carry out cooling activities until normal temperature is regained. Conversely the body can respond to inadequate food, clothing and heating by lowering its temperature to dangerously low levels, rendering such a person dependent on others for gradually warming the body to restore it to normal temperature.

FACTORS INFLUENCING CONTROLLING BODY TEMPERATURE

The factors influencing controlling body temperature will now be considered. The objective of this component of the model is to encourage consideration of how the five factors — physical, psychological, sociocultural, environmental and politicoeconomic — influence the way a person develops individuality in carrying out the AL of controlling body temperature.

Physical factors

The mechanisms of thermoregulation have already been outlined in the section describing the nature of body temperature control. A number of physical factors influence the process of thermoregulation and also the individual's ability to assist with controlling body temperature. There are several factors in this category and they will be discussed under the headings of exercise, hormones, social drugs, food intake and time of day.

Exercise. Body heat is produced by skeletal movement and so the body temperature is related to a person's activity level. It is because heat production increases with activity that, on feeling cold, people spontaneously begin to move about more, rubbing their hands together and stamping their feet. Conversely, the sensible thing to do when feeling too warm is to reduce activity because this reduces heat production. The body temperature is highest during periods of great activity and lowest during periods of sleep.

Exercise, if overdone, can cause overheating and 'exertion-induced heat illness is now a recognised disorder which occurs in basically healthy individuals during or following prolonged strenuous exercise' (Walker, 1986). Heat cramps, heat exhaustion and heat stroke are now not uncommon occurrences at events such as fun-runs, marathons and athletic meetings and, given the potential danger of severe overheating, caution should be observed and proper precautions taken.

Hormones. During the female fertility cycle some temperature variations occur due to the influences of the female sex hormones. In the menstrual cycle there is an abrupt slight rise in temperature just after ovulation; a couple of days before menstruation the temperature falls again. This naturally occurring variation of temperature is the basis of the 'rhythm method' of birth control in which abstinence from sexual intercourse is practised during the fertile phase of the monthly cycle, the time of which is ascertained from the temperature variation.

There is a hormonal reason for the slight rise in a woman's temperature during the first trimester of pregnancy; it falls in the second and third trimesters and returns to normal level after delivery.

An excess production of the hormone thyroxine results from over-activity of the thyroid gland and this increases the body's metabolic rate, thus raising the body temperature. Conversely with an underactive thyroid gland less thyroxin is produced and body temperature is lower than normal.

Social drugs. Caffeine increases the metabolic rate, although how it does so is not fully understood. Smoking cigarettes has a similar effect since nicotine stimulates the sympathetic nervous system. Alcohol can increase cooling since it causes vasodilatation of the blood vessels in the skin, resulting in a greater loss of heat from the body surface.

Food intake. Body heat is generated by the metabolism of food and the body's metabolic rate is increased directly as a result of ingestion of food. This is particularly so when the food eaten is high in protein and the stimulatory effect may last as long as 6 hours. Mothers who encourage their children to take a nourishing protein breakfast in order to keep warm in cold weather are therefore, albeit unknowingly, encouraging a practice which is based on sound knowledge of factors which influence body temperature.

Time of day. Variations in body temperature which are related to time of day are obviously influenced by the day and night pattern of activity and sleep. Body temperature is highest in the evening (1700 to 2000 hours GMT) and lowest in the early morning (0200 to 0800 hours GMT). The converse is true for people who regularly work at night and sleep during the day.

Psychological factors

Extremes of emotion sometimes affect the body's metabolic rate causing slight increase or decrease in body temperature. Excitement, excessive anxiety or anger may cause an elevation of temperature and, indeed, this fact is reflected in such phrases as 'flushed with excitement' and 'hot with rage'. On the other hand, apathy or depression may cause the body temperature to fall.

Knowledge acquired in the formative years about the sort of precautions to be taken when the outdoor temperature is very high or low will influence how a person carries out this dimension of the AL of controlling body temperature. Similarly the value which a person attaches to making the home capable of being cool in hot weather and warm in cold weather will be reflected in efforts to achieve this. A person's temperament and personality traits will have an effect on whether or not a person takes sensible precautions, or risks exposure to the potential problems of heatstroke or frostbite. Current mood will influence how a person carries out this AL; for example, when advised to wear a coat, a child may resent this and may react by going outdoors inadequately clad.

Sociocultural factors

The sociocultural factors which can have an effect on the AL of controlling body temperature are fairly limited but customs concerning clothes are certainly pertinent. Some religions, for example, dictate the wearing of a head cover at all times, regardless of the environmental temperature. Similarly, ceremonial occasions which are part of a certain culture may demand elaborate dress which is uncomfortably hot in summer weather; or, conversely, not warm enough on a cold day, as any British winter bride will testify! Everyone, too, no matter where in the world, is socialised into acceptance of norms regarding the extent to which clothing can be shed in the hottest weather; this varies between countries, and sometimes between the sexes, and is socioculturally determined rather than by the need for comfort and body temperature control.

Environmental factors

As previously mentioned, changes or extremes of environmental temperature can cause the body temperature to vary and the person to feel warm or cold. In any extreme climate there can be dramatic temperature variations: for example, in parts of North Africa it can be bitterly cold during the night but as hot as 40°C in the mid-afternoon of the same day. Even in the so-called temperate climate of the UK there are considerable seasonal variations; the temperature can fall to −10°C or lower in winter and reach 40°C in summer. But heat waves in countries such as the UK, much as they are welcomed, catch the public unaware of the risks as Feinmann (1986) describes, mentioning hyperthermia in children and the elderly as one of the undesirable consequences. It is only by the process called acclimatisation that the human body is capable of adaptation to very hot, very cold or very extreme climates. There is no chance for acclimatisation to occur in sudden, short-term change of climate as happens in a heat wave or a brief summer holiday abroad. It is the popularity of such holidays which has increased the population's exposure to the problems of hyperthermia particularly; and, of course, also to the risk of skin cancer from excessive exposure to the sun's rays although that is not directly related to body temperature as such.

The body's ability to tolerate extremely high temperatures is closely related to the humidity of the atmosphere. A hot day which is dry and breezy, as opposed to one which is humid and still, is less uncomfortable because body heat is readily lost by convection and evaporation of sweat. Similarly, cold, dry weather is less chilling than cold, damp weather.

The availability of hot/cold baths and showers will determine whether or not a person can take advantage of these facilities in controlling body temperature. Likewise, whether or not a house has central heating, air conditioning and double glazing will influence the other activities which the occupants need to carry out to help control their body temperature.

Politicoeconomic factors

Many of the activities which individuals carry out in relation to the AL of controlling body temperature need money — to buy clothes, bedding and food; to heat a house and prevent loss of heat from it by excluding draughts, installing double glazing and insulating lofts. Inadequate provisions of this kind may mean that a person

is vulnerable to the adverse effects of cold; the two most vulnerable groups in terms of the resultant condition of hypothermia are the young and the elderly.

A national survey of hospital admissions carried out by the Royal College of Physicians in 1965 showed that 0.68% of all patients admitted had temperatures below 35°C. Of these the highest incidence was in children aged 0–1 years which worked out at 82.2 cases per 1000 admissions. It has to be pointed out that hypothermia was not the reason for admission nor did the patients have clinical signs and symptoms of hypothermia; nevertheless they had an unacceptably low body temperature (Millard, 1977). In 1972 the DHSS recommended a temperature of 70°F for a living room when the temperature outside is 30°F. Yet in the early 1980s the Electricity Consumer Council's annual reports stated that some elderly people were attempting to heat their homes on less than £1 per week, the inference being that such homes were inadequately heated.

Age Concern, a voluntary organisation, is seeking a better deal for the elderly to prevent the 700 deaths annually from hypothermia recorded on the death certificate (Taylor, 1982), and to reduce other such cold-related deaths as coronary heart disease, stroke and chest infections. Much the same point is made in a more recent reference (Hillman, 1987); although less than 1000 deaths a year in the UK are certified as hypothermia, many more patients are seen in casualty departments with this diagnosis. Further, there are about 70 000 more deaths in Britain in winter than in summer — many believed to be the result of diseases exacerbated by cold. There is no doubt that prevention of hypothermia (p. 238) is essentially a politicoeconomic issue, at least in the UK situation.

INDIVIDUALITY IN CONTROLLING BODY TEMPERATURE

From the foregoing discussion it is evident that there are many dimensions of each component of the model which help us to describe how a particular person develops individuality in the AL of controlling body temperature. The following is a résumé of these dimensions:

Lifespan: effect on controlling body temperature
- Infants: maintenance of body temperature at 36–37°C by being kept dry, warm and out of draughts
- Young children: parental vigilance to avoid excessive rise/fall in temperature
- Adults: avoidance of adverse effects of excessive heat or cold
- Elderly people: requirement for adequate heating, clothing, exercise and nutrition to avoid hypothermia

Dependence/independence in controlling body temperature
- Infants/children dependent on adults for maintenance of temperature
- Elderly may be dependent on others for maintenance of temperature/prevention of hypothermia

Factors influencing controlling body temperature

- Physical
  - — exercise
  - — hormones
  - — social drugs
  - — food intake
  - — time of day

- Psychological
  - — knowledge about precautions in high or low outdoor temperature.
  - — value in making home appropriately warm/cool
  - — temperament
  - — personality traits ⎫ does/ does not take sensible precautions ⎭

- Sociocultural
  - — choice of clothing

- Environmental
  - — extremes of environmental temperature
  - — high/low humidity
  - — air velocity

- Politicoeconomic
  - — vulnerability of young, elderly
  - — availability of money for heating, insulation, clothing, bedding, food
  - — public education to prevent hypothermia

Controlling body temperature: patients' problems and related nursing

Knowledge about the person's individual habits in carrying out the AL of controlling body temperature is absolutely crucial for planning individualised nursing. The discussion so far will have given an idea of what nurses should keep in mind when carrying out the initial assessment. The following questions will help the nurse to focus on the sort of information being sought:

- does the individual perceive body temperature to be comfortable, too high or too low?
- what factors influence the way the individual carries out the AL of controlling body temperature?
- what does the individual know about controlling body temperature?
- are sensible precautions taken to avoid excessive rise or fall in body temperature, or does the individual take risks relating to, for example, the potential problems of hyperthermia (hyperpyrexia/heatstroke), hypothermia and frostbite?
- what value does the individual put on adequate food, clothing, bedding, heating and insulation in order to assist in controlling body temperature?
- is there any financial hardship which prevents the individual from attending to the AL of controlling body temperature?
- has the individual any longstanding problems with the AL of controlling body temperature and, if so, how have these been coped with?
- what problems, if any, does the individual have at present with controlling body temperature and/or are any likely to develop?

The information obtained will be examined to identify, in collaboration with the patient whenever possible, any actual or potential problems. The nurse may recognise from the information that the ward temperature is higher than the one to which the patient is accustomed and can verify this, and make suggestions about how it can be coped with. Many patients in hospital and in the community do not have a changed body temperature but if there is evidence of an increased or decreased body temperature then the goal will be a return to that person's normal body temperature. The nursing interventions to achieve the set goals will be selected according to local circumstances and available resources. The interventions will be written on the nursing plan together with the date on which the evaluation will be carried out to discern whether or not they are achieving the set goals. All these activities are necessary in order to carry out individualised nursing related to the AL of controlling body temperature.

However, before nurses can begin to think in terms of individualised nursing they need to have a generalised idea of the kind of problems which patients can experience in carrying out the AL of controlling body temperature and the kind of nursing activities which may be appropriate. Discussion is arranged under three headings:

- change of environment
- change in controlling body temperature
- change of dependence/independence status for controlling body temperature

CHANGE OF ENVIRONMENT

When people are confined to bed at home, whether it is for a short or long time the problem may well be that they exchange the atmosphere of the living room for the cooler atmosphere of most bedrooms, unless of course the central heating extends there or another form of heating is affordable. Those patients who are admitted to hospital almost invariably find the atmosphere warmer than that at home and this, equally, can be a problem. When people are ill, they become less tolerant of minor discomforts and are more quickly prone to feel miserable if the environment is too cold or too hot, draughty or stuffy, or changeable. Some people like to wear a lot of clothing and have the room well ventilated; others prefer to have the room well heated and wear less. In an open hospital ward, it is impossible to cater for each patient's particular preference.

However, it is essential for the nurse to find out from assessment each patient's usual habits. If any patient is feeling very uncomfortable, the nurse can help by adjusting the heating and ventilation for the majority, and advising extra or less clothing for individuals according to their needs and wishes. Elderly and immobile patients feel the cold more readily and may appreciate the extra warmth of a blanket around the shoulders or over the knees. Electric blankets and heating pads can also be employed; hot water bottles now tend to be discouraged due to their dangers.

Body temperature falls during the night and patients should be encouraged to express their preference as to the amount of bedclothes they require in order to keep warm during sleep. In helping to maintain a comfortable environmental temperature, nurses should always give first consideration to the patients' needs and remember that, being active in their work, they are less likely to appreciate that it may be cold for the patients when it seems warm to them.

CHANGE IN CONTROLLING BODY TEMPERATURE

For healthy adults the range of normal (oral) temperature is 36–37.5°C. Therefore, if a person's temperature goes higher than 37.5°C or lower than 36°C it can be regarded as abnormal, suggesting a problem has arisen with the AL of controlling body temperature. An abnormally high body temperature is referred to as *pyrexia*; the name given to describe the condition of an abnormally low temperature is *hypothermia*. The upper and lower limits of survival are not known exactly but are thought to be at temperatures of above 43°C and below 25°C (Edholm, 1978) respectively. Figure 12.2 illustrates these temperature ranges.

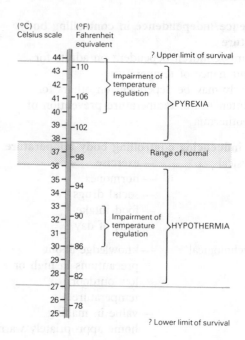

Fig. 12.2 Range of normal/abnormal body temperature (oral)

Pyrexia

The condition of pyrexia exists when the body temperature rises above the upper limit of the range of normal, that is above 37.5°C. It is one of the cardinal signs of physical illness, often the first indication that there is some disturbance of body function. Most commonly, pyrexia is a manifestation of infections, neoplasms, trauma (accidental and surgical), diseases of the nervous system, and metabolic disorders. There is reason to believe that pyrexia actually helps the body to combat infection because bacteria survive less readily, and production of immune bodies increases, when body temperature is raised above normal.

Pyrexia itself is a very debilitating condition and a dangerous one for young children, even if the associated disease condition is not particularly serious. The abnormally high body temperature is a source of discomfort and anxiety for the patient and it places considerable strain on the body. These consequences are particularly undesirable in some instances, for example postoperatively when the excessive demands on body systems may impede recovery and wound healing. (A slight postoperative pyrexia is the normal response to surgical trauma but it may also be a warning sign of such diverse complications as infection of the wound, respiratory tract or urinary tract; or of formation of a blood clot in a vein, or deep venous thrombosis.)

Onset of pyrexia. Although the onset of pyrexia is sometimes sudden, more often it is gradual and the problem is a feeling of unwellness. The person may complain of a headache, loss of appetite, lethargy and tiredness and, usually fairly quickly begins to feel cold and shivery. This is what is referred to as *chill* and it can last for a few minutes or even an hour, depending on the speed of onset of the pyrexia.

Chill can be explained — the infection or causative factor raises the 'set' point of the body temperature and to cope with this, heat production increases due to shivering and the metabolic rate increases; there is vasoconstriction and reduced sweating. The patient feels cold and often lies curled up, a position which reduces excess heat loss by conduction, convection and radiation. Once the body temperature is raised, the balancing mechanism keeps it at the new 'set' level.

Features of pyrexia. Once the temperature stabilises at the higher than normal level, the patient has the problem of feeling uncomfortably hot. In an attempt to lower the temperature again, heat loss mechanisms are activated; vasodilation makes the skin warm and flushed and sweating increases which creates another problem. At this stage the hot patient desperately tries to get cool by removing clothing and keeping as still as possible. Usually the patient will feel thirsty due to excess fluid loss through the skin, and dehydration can result quite quickly. Loss of appetite turns into loss of weight, contributing to the person's overall feeling of lethargy and weakness which are further problems.

There are also mental changes associated with pyrexia. The person becomes irritable and restless and this is very obvious in children, who cry, refuse to be comforted and toss and turn in bed. Sometimes severe headache, photophobia (sensitivity to light) and drowsiness may add to the patient's problems: sometimes disorientation ensues and it is known, for example that 'speeded time' perception can be caused by a high body temperature. The problem for the patient is that time seems to drag because the 'internal clock' runs more quickly than the watch. Sometimes mental processes are upset to such an extent that hallucinations may occur and delirium may result. Not infrequently convulsions (p. 330) occur in young children.

During the course of a fever, body temperature may fluctuate quite dramatically as there is continual adjustment to reduce the raised temperature. Alternating episodes of fever and chill are characteristic of pyrexia until the reduction of the 'set' level is permanently achieved. Usually the return of the body temperature to normal occurs gradually. A typical temperature chart of a pyrexial patient is shown in Figure 12.3.

Nursing a pyrexial patient. If a raised body temperature is not lowered, it tends to get higher and higher; eventually the regulating mechanisms become impaired, damage to cells occurs and death ensues. The aims of nursing intervention are threefold:

- to prevent any further increase of body temperature
- to reduce body temperature to the patient's normal level

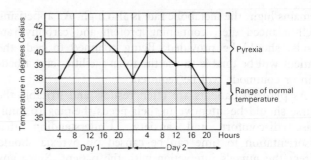

Fig. 12.3 Example of a typical temperature chart of a pyrexial patient

- to alleviate the discomforts associated with pyrexia

The nursing activities that are carried out are based on the principles involved in the body's heat production and heat loss mechanisms. Which activities are appropriate depend on the stage and severity of the pyrexia and are decided on the basis of ongoing nursing assessment. Regular assessment of the patient is necessary as the condition changes and as the outcome of nursing intervention is ascertained by evaluation. Measurement of body temperature (p. 239) is an important part of evaluation and it is essential that accuracy is ensured so that the progress of the fever is recorded and effectiveness of treatment ascertained.

Promotion of heat loss by radiation is encouraged by removing excess clothing, and heat loss by convection by using fans to circulate air. Body heat can be dispersed utilising the principles of conduction and evaporation as when tepid sponging or applying cold wet sheets or ice packs. Cold water or ice should be applied with caution since they are likely to cause localised vasoconstriction; this would then reduce heat loss, the opposite of the desired effect. Although it seems radical, and in contradiction to a mother's instinct, a tepid immersion bath may be the most effective way of quickly reducing severe pyrexia in a child.

Additional heat gain can be prevented by limiting the patient's activity and encouraging as much relaxation, rest and sleep as possible. For this reason, patients with pyrexia are usually nursed in bed; body temperature is lowest during periods of inactivity and sleep.

Alleviating discomforts associated with pyrexia involves a variety of nursing activities. Special help may be required with personal cleansing and dressing because with excessive sweating, the patient will need to wash more frequently than usual. It is important to pay special attention to the skin folds and the genitalia, and to change the nightclothes and bedclothes when they are damp with perspiration.

To prevent dehydration, and the discomfort of a dry mouth, frequent drinks should be encouraged and opportunities made for cleaning teeth and rinsing the mouth. Although unlikely to have a good appetite, the patient should continue to eat because while the temperature remains high, the metabolic rate is also high. An appetising well-balanced diet, containing protein and carbohydrate foods, should be provided. Being confined to bed, the patient will be unable to use the toilet facilities and a bed-pan or commode will be required.

As pyrexial patients are often restless and irritable the nurse should be attentive to their needs, helping to minimise discomfort and anxiety. Understanding that disorientation to time can be caused by pyrexia should direct the nurse's interaction with the patient. Since any period of waiting, when there is speeded time perception, is likely to seem longer than it actually is, the nurse must try to be punctual in time-related activities, such as meals, and continually assist the patient in time estimation (Alderson, 1974).

Hyperpyrexia

An extremely high fever, hyperpyrexia, is a feature of the condition of *heatstroke* which results from prolonged exposure to a very high environmental temperature. Heatstroke is a life-threatening condition and usually there is partial or total loss of consciousness. The heat regulating centre loses control and as a result of the physical effect of heat on brain tissue and that of other large organs, various injurious processes are triggered off. The most important of these is clotting of blood in the capillaries which, in turn, reduces oxygenation of vital organs, such as the heart and liver. Without immediate treatment to cool the body and maintain functioning of the large organs the person affected by heatstroke will die (Davies, 1977).

Illness or death from heatstroke are not unusual in parts of the world where the temperature is very high during the hot season. But even in temperate climates a heatwave may cause some people (particularly the very young and the elderly) to succumb to heat exhaustion. The affected person becomes pale, complains of nausea and headache and shows signs of shock. Usually moving the person to a cool place and providing a cold drink are sufficient to relieve the discomfort.

When heat exhaustion turns to heatstroke there are signs of very high temperature: the skin is flushed, hot and dry, and there is impaired consciousness. Sometimes if the person has been exposed to excessive direct sunlight, there is accompanying sunburn which is extremely painful as well as hazardous. As a result of excessive loss of body fluid in perspiration, causing salt depletion, heat cramps may occur. These are severe muscle cramps and they are often accompanied by extreme thirst, nausea and dizziness. A long salt-containing drink usually gives relief.

Lack of acclimatisation plays a major role in people's intolerance of heat, and illness due to heat is most likely to occur when there is excessive physical activity while working or playing in exceptionally hot or humid conditions. The nurse concerned with industrial health services, or with health education for the young and the elderly, can contribute to the prevention of illness due to heat by advising those at risk to limit activity, keep as cool as possible and maintain hydration when exposed to heat for any length of time.

Hypothermia

The problem of hypothermia has already been mentioned in relation to the lifespan (the susceptibility of the young and the old) and in terms of related politicoeconomic factors. Interestingly, hypothermia has only been a recognised clinical condition internationally since the 1970s (Hillman, 1987).

Literally, 'hypothermia' means lower than normal body temperature. In 1966 the Royal College of Physicians (UK) defined hypothermia as a 'deep body' or 'core' temperature of 35°C or under, measured either rectally or in freshly passed urine (Taylor, 1982).

The most common cause of hypothermia is prolonged exposure to a cold and damp environment. It is well-known that exposure in cold water or winter blizzard conditions can cause hypothermia to develop rapidly. Fishermen, sailors, farmers, skiers, climbers, yachtsmen and motorists are a few of the many people who, in the course of working or playing, are exposed to cold, wet and windy conditions. Without wearing special clothing and taking safety precautions they have little chance of staying alive when the weather conditions are severe.

However, within the walls of a house, people can succumb to the dangerous effects of cold and dampness and recently, as already pointed out, it has been recognised that the elderly constitute a group particularly at risk of hypothermia. On low income they are often forced to live without adequate heating or warm clothing; in addition, they are less active physically and tend to eat less well so that body heat production is lowered. Sometimes an elderly person, who lives alone, falls or suffers a stroke and, having lain on a cold floor all night, when discovered, is found to be hypothermic.

The risk is also great for those at the opposite end of the lifespan. Without stability of body temperature or the ability to increase heat production voluntarily very young babies are susceptible to hypothermia unless at all times they are kept warm, dry and out of draughts. Premature babies, or others considered to be at risk, may be nursed in an incubator so that a constant warm environment can be provided, thus preventing hypothermia.

Hypothermia may also occur as a consequence of routine surgery (Goldberg & Roe, 1966), particularly when large body cavities are exposed and when the patient receives substantial volumes of blood and other intravenous fluids. In addition, hypothermia is deliberately induced during specific types of operation such as cardiac surgery, when the body's oxygen requirements are reduced by lowering its temperature. Careful monitoring of body temperature during the immediate postoperative period is therefore of considerable importance in these situations.

Features of hypothermia. The most significant feature of hypothermia is that even parts of the body well covered with clothing feel extremely cold to the touch. (If, in addition to exposure to a cold atmosphere, parts of the person's body actually come directly into contact with extreme cold, hypothermia is likely to be accompanied by frostbite.) As the body temperature falls, the whole of the body becomes cold to the touch, looks waxy and the face appears swollen. As the metabolic rate lowers, breathing becomes slower and more shallow and there is a progressive fall in heart rate, cardiac output and blood pressure. The onset is often insidious; this is why people affected often have failed to recognise the serious cause of their feeling of lethargy and extreme tiredness. All they want to do is to lie down and go to sleep which is the worst possible course of action. Quickly their drowsiness increases and eventually coma results. Then the body temperature falls even more rapidly and, if the condition remains untreated, death will occur.

In summary, Hillman (1987) lists the stages of hypothermia as:

1. Feeling of cold and shivering
2. Fall of body temperature to 35°C or below
3. Confusion
4. Dyspnoea
5. Irregular heart beat
6. Respiratory arrest
7. Cardiac arrest
8. Death

Nursing a hypothermic patient. A nurse (or anyone else) who comes across a person who appears to be suffering from hypothermia should summon the assistance of a doctor or the emergency services. In the worst conditions resuscitation may be necessary and, in such circumstances, the priorities are (in order) respiration, circulation and warming (Hillman, 1987). Rapid re-warming, however tempting, is dangerous because it may cause circulatory collapse. The aim should be slow re-warming of the body to return it to normal/usual temperature. Direct heat is inadvisable too, as this causes peripheral vasodilation which draws heat away from the vital organs in the core of the body. Slow re-warming, a rise of 0.5°C/hour, can best be achieved by putting the patient to bed, covered with lightweight blankets or a metal impregnated space blanket and warming the environmental temperature to 26–29°C (79–84°F), if possible. Regular measurement of body temperature using a special low-reading thermometer (p. 240) is the method of evaluating the effectiveness of intervention.

As the body temperature gradually rises (Fig. 12.4) and consciousness is regained, the patient can be encouraged to increase mobilising and, by taking warm drinks and

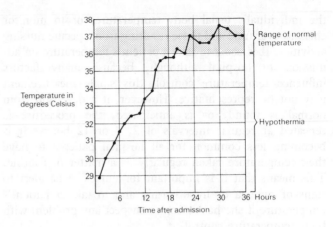

Fig. 12.4 Example of a typical temperature chart of patient with hypothermia

nourishing food, increase heat production further until the temperature reaches normal levels.

Preventing hypothermia. There is scope for all nurses, in their role as health educators — whether in community or hospital settings — to attempt to educate people about how to prevent hypothermia and to detect those at risk. Key target groups are those who care for the young and the old, and independent elderly people themselves. The elderly in the community must be helped to understand and implement the principles involved in prevention. A room temperature of 21°C (70°F) is recommended; it may be most economical if one room of a house is kept warm and used throughout the day and night. It must be remembered that the coldest time is just before daybreak. The amount and type of clothing worn are also important. Several layers of light but warm material provide more warmth and protection from cold than one heavy garment; heat is conducted away from the body when clothing is damp and so dryness of material is essential as well as warmth. For this reason, old people should be advised to dry themselves thoroughly after a bath. Warming the bed with a hot water bottle or electric blanket can help, as can wearing bedsocks and even a head cover of some sort (Professional Nurse, 1986).

MEASURING BODY TEMPERATURE

It is clear that being able to measure body temperature objectively is extremely helpful in the identification of an abnormal body temperature and in the evaluation of the outcomes of related nursing intervention. While it may not be possible to measure body temperature with complete accuracy in the clinical situation, for reasons discussed below, careful measurements will provide the nurse with a useful assessment and evaluative tool.

The aim of measuring body temperature is to identify deviations from the range of normal (and, in particular, from the individual's usual body temperature) or to monitor changes over time and those resulting from specific nursing activities. It is usual to take a patient's temperature on admission to hospital although, because many factors influence temperature control, this single measurement may not be representative. However, if a deviation from normal is found, or is anticipated, the procedure is repeated at regular intervals of 2, 4 or 12 hours. It is becoming less common for all hospital patients to have their temperature taken regularly as a matter of routine. This means that it is important for nurses to be alert to signs of pyrexia or hypothermia and to take a patient's temperature if she has reason to suspect any problem with body temperature control.

The clinical glass thermometer is the instrument still most commonly used for measuring body temperature. It is a simple, inexpensive instrument containing mercury which expands with heat. The amount of expansion, as indicated by calibrations marked on the glass, gives the measure of body temperature. The Celsius scale is now in use (1° Celsius = 1°Centigrade) and the standard thermometer registers temperatures between 35°C and 43.5°C. The low-reading thermometer, for use with patients at risk of or suffering from hypothermia, registers down to 21°C. All clinical thermometers have a constriction above the bulb so that when the mercury has risen it remains at the level reached until forcibly shaken down. The special thermometer for use in the rectal site only has a short, blunt bulb to prevent injury to the anal mucous membrane; it is coloured to distinguish it from those used in the oral or axillary sites (Fig. 12.5).

Accurate measurement of body temperature is essential if the exercise is to be useful. To achieve this the nurse must use a reliable instrument, select an appropriate site, leave the instrument in situ for the necessary length of time and, finally, read the thermometer accurately. While all thermometers with the British Standard Kitemark are virtually guaranteed to be accurate, the site of the body used should be carefully considered since environmental influences can produce inaccurate readings.

Most nurses consider taking temperatures to be a simple basic procedure requiring little skill or knowledge, but the findings of some research projects suggest that traditional practice is far from accurate and is being continued in ignorance of the facts. Excellent reviews of the relevant literature have been provided by Sims-Williams (1976) and, more recently, Erickson (1980); and, on the basis of evidence, guidance can be given on the procedure which should be followed.

The oral site is most commonly selected because it is convenient and is considered to be the most sensitive to changes in the temperature of the blood in the arteries. It is certainly the most appropriate site in the case of the fully conscious adult.

The exact placement of the bulb of the thermometer is

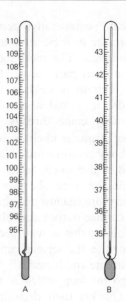

Fig. 12.5   Clinical glass thermometer (A) oral F (B) rectal C

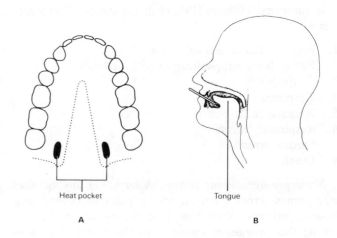

Fig. 12.6   The oral site (A) position of heat pockets on mouth floor (B) thermometer in position in a heat pocket

important. This should not go just anywhere in the sublingual cavity (under the tongue); the exact place where the maximum mouth temperature is ascertained is at the junction of the base of the tongue and the floor of the mouth either to the left or to the right of the frenulum. Areas of the mouth other than these two 'heat pockets' (Fig. 12.6) are lower in temperature and, therefore, are not an accurate reflection of the actual body temperature.

Still further precautions must be taken to ensure an accurate measurement. If the patient has taken a hot drink, a time lapse of 6 minutes is needed prior to inserting the thermometer and 15 minutes if the drink is an iced one. A hot bath may raise body temperature and the effect can last up to 45 minutes; strenuous exercise has a similar effect. People who wear lower dentures require relatively longer to return to a stable oral temperature after such activities. Contrary to most people's expectations, smoking does not appear to affect recordings.

To ensure statistically reliable recordings, the optimum placement time is 8 minutes for men, and 9 minutes for women in room temperatures of 18–24°C (65–75°F). However, Pugh Davies et al (1986) showed that no clinical advantage was gained when using a measurement time longer than 3 minutes. A 3-minute reading should therefore be regarded as the minimum.

The axillary site provides a measure of skin temperature. It is difficult to obtain a reading which accurately reflects deep body temperature due to variations in both the temperature of the air and the blood flow to the skin. Values obtained therefore tend to be lower than those from the sublingual cavity or the rectum. The axillary site is, however, useful for babies, children or patients who are confused, breathless or unconscious. The thermometer must be maintained in a secure underarm position for about 9 minutes in adults and 4–8 minutes in babies and children.

The rectal site is traditionally reserved for babies and those adults, particularly the elderly, whose temperature is highly variable, or suspected of being abnormally low. It is considered to be the site best able to provide a recording which is an accurate reflection of the temperature of the core of the body, although it is slower to respond to changes. The thermometer should be inserted to a depth of at least 4 cm past the anal sphincter in adults and 2–3 cm in babies. The thermometer should be left in place for 3 minutes to obtain an optimal rectal temperature. However, the procedure does subject the patient to considerable embarrassment and so should not be used unless essential. There is, in addition, the hazard of cross-infection when a thermometer is coming in contact with faeces.

The reason for using this site with babies is that environmental temperatures alter axillary temperatures more than anal temperatures. However, as Eoff et al (1974) are able to point out, the environmental temperature of the nursery is usually kept stable and, in fact, the very small differences between recordings taken in the two sites do not pose any risk to the baby. Given this, use of the axillary site avoids two risks associated with the rectal site; firstly, reflex defaecation and secondly, there is no chance of accidental injury to the mucous membrane of the anus.

Measuring body temperature is an important aspect of nursing assessment, and of evaluation of the effectiveness of nursing activities related to the AL of controlling body temperature. It is clear that traditional practice which does not take account of all relevant knowledge is unsatisfactory; it is essential that nurses apply research findings about this particular nursing activity to their practice.

Alternative temperature-recording instruments to the clinical glass thermometer are becoming increasingly popular. This is not surprising as entrepreneurs in business are aware that many queries still remain about the satisfactory use of glass thermometers. The electronic thermometer is an example of this new technology, favoured because it is said to be accurate, quicker to register and easier to read the result. Stronge & Newton (1980) carried out a clinical trial to compare another electronic thermometer, the IVAC 821 with the current system of glass thermometers in performance and cost. They concluded that the time saved using an electronic thermometer on the surgical ward equalled one extra nurse a week.

New technology in the form of infra-red thermometers are currently being developed (Shinozaki et al, 1988). These are accurate and give a reading within 2 seconds. Depending on cost, these may become available in clinical areas in the future. Both electronic and British Standard glass and mercury thermometers are acceptably accurate for clinical use (Closs, 1987). Most inaccuracies in practice are due to difficulties encountered in using the sites generally favoured for temperature measurement. The mercury thermometer is a safe, simple and inexpensive instrument but it is easily broken. This fact alone makes investing in expensive electronic thermometers a viable proposition.

Measuring body temperature is the most frequently carried out nursing activity in relation to the AL of controlling body temperature. From the foregoing discussion, readers will realise the importance of basing nursing activities on the best available knowledge; and that this can change in the light of information as it becomes available from new research.

CHANGE OF DEPENDENCE/INDEPENDENCE STATUS FOR CONTROLLING BODY TEMPERATURE

In the model of living the dependence/independence continuum for the AL of controlling body temperature is closely related to the lifespan, a greater level of dependence being a characteristic of those people at either end. This is also the case in a nursing context; many of the patients who have problems which change their dependence/independence status are children or are elderly. But people can have a change in status when they are at any stage on the lifespan, and the sort of change in status will be different according to the problem causing the change. Some of these will now be discussed.

As already mentioned many adult patients do not have an abnormal body temperature. The minority who do have problems associated with an increase/decrease of body temperature may well be dependent on the nurse for measuring and monitoring the increase/decrease: for administering the prescribed drugs, in the prescribed dose, at the prescribed time, by the prescribed route; and monitoring the effect not only on the temperature but also

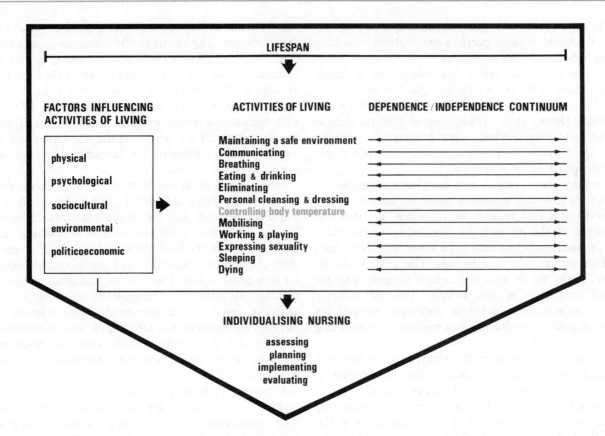

Fig. 12.7   The AL of controlling body temperature within the model for nursing

the general effect, for example the extent of sweating and restlessness, return of appetite and a moist mouth. Should the prescribed treatment be tepid/warm sponging, exposure of the body to air currents produced by a fan, or to ice packs, or to cold/warm immersion baths, then the patient is dependent on the nurse's knowledge and efficient method of carrying out these intimate procedures in such a way that the anxiety level is not increased and hopefully is decreased. When the stated goal of return to that particular patient's normal body temperature has been achieved, the patient is dependent on the nurse for encouraging return to the previous status of independence with (when appropriate) adequate knowledge to prevent recurrence of the condition which caused a change in status, particularly important in the case of hypothermia.

Individualising nursing

The first part of this chapter reflects the Roper, Logan and Tierney model for nursing — the nature of the AL of controlling body temperature; the relationship of the lifespan to the AL; the effect of the individual's dependence/independence status; the influence of physical, psychological, sociocultural, environmental and politicoeconomic factors on the AL. In the second part of the chapter, a selection of problems and discomforts which are experienced by people in relation to the AL have been described. With this background of *general* knowledge about the AL, it should be possible to incorporate such information in an individualised nursing plan when such information is relevant to the person's current circumstances.

While describing the Roper, Logan and Tierney model for nursing, *general* information was provided about Individualising nursing (p. 51) which in fact is synonymous with the concept of the process of nursing.

Out of this background of *general* knowledge about the AL of controlling body temperature and about Individualising nursing, it should then be possible to extract the issues which are relevant to an individual's current circumstances (whether in a health or an illness setting), i.e. to make an assessment of relevant issues according to the individual's stage on the lifespan; according to current level of dependence/independence; and take into account the relevant physical, psychological, sociocultural (including ethical, spiritual and religous), environmental and politicoeconomic (including legal) factors. Collectively, this information would provide a profile of the person's individuality in relation to this AL.

As indicated earlier in the text, this assessment would be achieved by various means such as observing the person; acquiring information about the individual's usual habits in relation to this AL, partly by asking appropriate questions, partly by listening to the patient and/or relatives; and using relevant information from available records including medical records. The collected information could then be examined to identify any actual problems being experienced with the AL and these could be arranged in some order of priority. The nurse might also recognise some potential problems — not all possible potential problems but those which are relevant. Realistic goals, mutually agreed with the patient when this is possible, could then be set to prevent potential problems from becoming actual ones; to alleviate or solve the actual problems; or to help the person cope with those which cannot be alleviated or solved.

Keeping in mind what the person can and cannot do unaided, the nursing interventions to achieve the mutually set goals could then be selected according to local circumstances and available resources.

Following implementation of the interventions, their effects could be evaluated in relation to the goals set, and if goals were not reached, they would then be revised or rescheduled, or even discarded. It is worth repeating here that although discussed in four phases — assessing, planning, implementing and evaluating — individualising nursing is not a linear progression; it assumes a built-in responsiveness to feedback at any of the phases, with ample allowance for change within the overall framework.

This chapter has been concerned with the AL of controlling body temperature. However, as stated previously, it is only for the purpose of discussion that any AL can be considered on its own; in reality the various activities are so closely related and do not have distinct boundaries. Figure 12.7 is a reminder that the AL of controlling body temperature is related to the other ALs and also to the various components of the model for nursing. However, it must be repeated that it may not be relevant to consider this particular AL for every patient in every circumstance. Professional judgement is required to assess its relevance to any one patient.

Acknowledgement
Thanks are extended to José Closs of the Nursing Research Unit, Department of Nursing Studies, University of Edinburgh for her helpful suggestions towards the revision of this chapter.

REFERENCES

Alderson M J 1974 The effect of increased body temperature on the perception of time. Nursing Research 23(1) January/February: 42–49
Closs S J 1987 Oral temperature measurement. Nursing Times 83(1) January 7: 36–39
Collins K J, Dore C, Exton-Smith A N 1977 Accidental hypothermia and impaired temperature homeostasis in the elderly. British Medical Journal 1: 353–356
Davies A G 1977 Illness due to heat. Nursing Mirror 144(25) June 23: 13–14
DHSS 1972 Keeping warm in winter. Simple guidance notes for those engaged in helping old people. DHSS, London
Drummond G 1979 Hypothermia: its causes, effects and treatment in the very young and the very old. Nursing Times 75(49) December 6: 2115–2116
Edholm O G 1978 Man — hot and cold. Edward Arnold, London
Eoff M J, Meier R S, Miller C 1974 Temperature measurement in infants. Nursing Research 23(6) November/December: 457–460
Erickson R 1980 A sourcebook for temperature taking. IVAC Corporation
Feinmann 1986 Some don't like it hot. Nursing Times 82(29) 16 July: 21–24
Goldberg M J, Roe C F 1966 Temperature changes during anaesthesia and operations. Archives of Surgery 93: 365–369
Hillman H 1987 Hypothermia: the cold that kills. Nursing Times 83(4) 28 January: 19–20
Macmillan A L, Corbett J L, Johnson R H, Crampton-Smith A, Spalding J M K, Wollner L 1967 Temperature regulation in survivors of accidental hypothermia of the elderly. Lancet 22 July: 165–169
Millard P H 1977 Hypothermia in the elderly. Nursing Mirror 145(18) November 3: 23–25
Professional Nurse 1986 Hypothermia: one of winter's threats to the elderly. Professional Nurse 1(5) February: 136–137
Pugh Davies S, Kassab J Y, Thrush A J, Smith P H S 1986 A comparison of mercury and digital clinical thermometers. Journal of Advanced Nursing 11(5): 535–543
Shinozaki T, Deane R, Perkins F M 1988 Infrared tympanic thermometer: evaluation of a new clinical thermometer. Critical Care Medicine 16(2): 148–150
Sims-Williams A J 1976 Temperature taking with glass thermometers; a review. Journal of Advanced Nursing 1 November: 481–493
Stronge J L, Newton G 1980 Electronic thermometers. A costly rise in efficiency? Nursing Mirror 151(8) August 21:29
Taylor G 1982 Cold comfort. Nursing Times 78(5) February 3:181
Walker M 1986 When the going gets hot. Nursing Times 83(32) 6 August: 44–47

ADDITIONAL READING

Barrus D H 1983 A comparison of rectal and axillary temperatures by electronic thermometer measurement in preschool children. Pediatric Nursing 9(6) November/December: 424–425
Closs S J, Macdonald I A, Hawthorn P J 1986 Factors affecting perioperative body temperature. Journal of Advanced Nursing 11: 739–744
Holloway A M 1988 Monitoring and controlling temperature. Anaesthesia and Intensive Care 16: 44–47
Takacs K M, Valenti W M 1982 Temperature measurement in a clinical setting. Nursing Research 31(6) November/December: 368–370
Yonkman C A 1982 Cool and heated aerosol and the mesurement of oral temperature. Nursing Research 31(6) November/December: 354–357

13

Mobilising

The activity of mobilising

The reason for selecting the word 'mobilising' for this AL has already been discussed (p. 24). By its very nature it is closely associated with most of the other Activities of Living. The ability to move the body freely is taken for granted by the majority of people. To push, to pull and lift; to walk, run, jog; or indeed just to maintain posture, various groups of large voluntary muscles surrounding the trunk and limbs are used. Other groups of smaller muscles are constantly in use to bring about movement of the hands and feet. It is well known that muscles which are used regularly are kept at a desirable tension which makes them firm to touch, and this usually results in a feeling of well-being which can be recognised in the person's appearance. Conversely, muscles which are used infrequently lose tone, become soft and flabby and are inadequate at maintaining the body in a desirable posture so that the person looks dejected, and this is not conducive to a feeling of well-being.

THE NATURE OF MOBILISING

Physical activity is a basic human drive and is important throughout life, even into old age. When awake, healthy children are constantly on the move; most adolescents seem to have boundless energy; for adults, work and recreational activities involve overt movement; the cherished independence of the older person is impossible without some degree of mobility.

The acquisition of motor skills is, however, a very complicated process. At birth the nervous system is not sufficiently developed to permit coordinated movement and even when the nervous system is in a state of readiness for

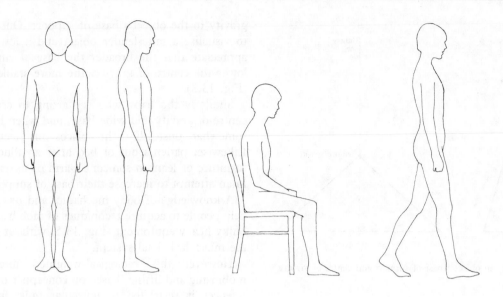

Fig. 13.1 Effective standing, sitting and walking positions

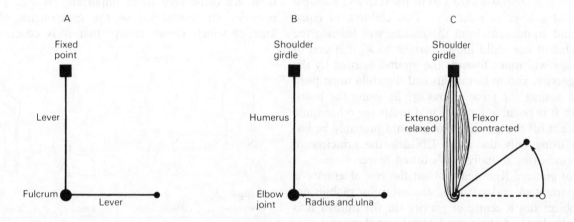

Fig. 13.2 Principles of muscle movement at the elbow joint

learning to take place, human infants, if compared to young animals and birds, are relatively slow to adopt independent coordinated movement. Observation of a baby trying to walk will indicate how many failures there are before there is management of standing and walking unsupported and even then, the sense of balance is unpredictable.

Good walking, standing and sitting positions (Fig. 13.1), as well as being aesthetically pleasing to the onlooker, conserve energy and are cultivated for everyday activities at home, at work and at play; and many recreational activities such as gymnastics, ice-skating and dancing encourage good posture. To achieve some understanding about the nature of mobilising there are several physical principles which are helpful, for example, those of contraction and relaxation, leverage and gravity.

Contraction and relaxation (extension). In health, all muscles fibres are in a state of what is called muscle tone, ready for instant, smooth movement. Muscles contract to produce action and are often arranged in pairs associated with two or more bones and a joint, such that the pair have opposing functions; as one muscle (the flexor) contracts and flexes, the other (the extensor) relaxes and extends to allow movement in the desired direction. When, for example, the flexor muscles on the anterior aspect of the upper arm contract to bring the forearm up towards the shoulder, the extensors on the posterior aspect relax to allow movement in the desired direction (Fig. 13.2). This diagram is a simplification of the highly sophisticated muscle activity in the human body, indeed muscles usually work not only in pairs but in groups and Figure 13.2 merely demonstrates one of the principles of muscle action.

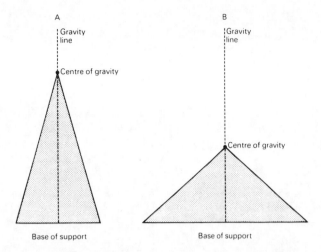

Fig. 13.3   Stability in objects: base of support and centre of gravity

Leverage. The principle of leverage is also useful in understanding the nature of mobilising. A lever is a rigid bar which revolves around a fixed axis or fulcrum and a simple example of a lever is a see-saw. Two children of equal weight and equidistant from the middle will balance the see-saw but if one child moves further back, that end of the see-saw will move towards the ground assisted by the pull of gravity, and to elevate his end the child must push upwards against the force of gravity. By using the board as a lever it is possible for one child to lift the other quite some height off the ground, which would probably be impossible using only the arms. Utilising the principle of leverage increases an individual's lifting power.

Law of gravity. Knowledge about the law of gravity is also important in understanding the nature of mobilising. Every object has a centre of gravity (in the human it is around the level of the second sacral vertebra) and it is possible to draw an imaginary line through the centre of

gravity to the object's base of support. One merely needs to visualise a tall slender object and a low squat one to appreciate that the broader the base of support and the lower the centre of gravity, the more stable is the object (Fig. 13.3).

Similarly the baby who is starting to crawl has a low centre of gravity and wide base, and when he first stands, somewhat unsteadily, he places his feet wide apart. Likewise, patients out of bed after an illness hold on to furniture or lean on someone's arm or use a walking stick in an attempt to increase their base of support (Fig. 13.4).

A knowledge of body mechanics and its application can help people to acquire techniques of mobilising: and lifting bulky heavy equipment (Fig. 13.5) without compromising the musculoskeletal system.

However this biological-weighted interpretation of mobilising and lifting, based on concepts from the physical sciences is restricted to muscular bulk and contracting power. In the concept of human kinetics, elasticity of body tissues, together with accuracy and speed of muscular reactions are considered more important (Walsh, 1988). He provides an illustration of the components of human kinetics which shows clearly that it is concerned with

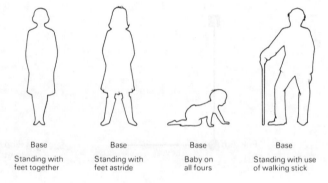

| Base | Base | Base | Base |
| Standing with feet together | Standing with feet astride | Baby on all fours | Standing with use of walking stick |

Fig. 13.4   Stability in the human frame

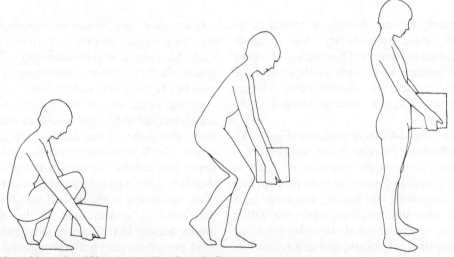

Fig. 13.5   Desirable body positions when lifting a heavy object from the floor.

'physical, social and mental' aspects of living: consequently functional as well as physical analysis is necessary because it contributes to 'skill, happiness and health' which the writer calls 'functional efficiency'.

The illustrated 'Fatigue posture chart' details the possible ill-effects from specific aspects of particular dimensions of undesirable posture, and these are described in the article. Walsh contends that beginning students and clinical nurses, can, through instruction and practice, become totally conversant with healthy movement as a natural feature of their daily lives; they are then equipped with the required practical skills to observe faulty movements in others and can help to correct them, which is a natural extension of the nurses' role into health education.

A consequence of compromising any of the many structures forming 'the back' is 'low back pain', a term which is not only in the medical domain but also in the public one. Bryan (1988) in an article in the *Observer Magazine* wrote that back pain costs the National Health Service £150 million, and industry 33 million working days each year. It itemises 'The Back Facts' which were compiled from the publication *Back Pain: The Facts* (Jayson, 1988) published in association with the Open University, the Back Pain Association and the Office of Health Economics. Whereas bedrest was usually prescribed in the early stages of the attack of low back pain, some clinics are now recommending exercise rather than rest in the treatment of an attack (Bryan, 1988).

The many dimensions of the AL of mobilising will be encapsulated for the beginning student under the following headings — exploring the environment, enjoying rhythmic movement, channelling emotional energy, promoting well-being, and transferring man and goods.

Exploring the environment. It is the capacity for movement which first allows the infant to explore himself and his environment. If the child's movement is restricted or if he is deprived of opportunities to respond to stimuli in his surroundings, his physical and psychosocial growth may be impeded. Intellectual development too may be curtailed if the growing child is denied exposure to new experiences beyond the home environment, with people other than the immediate family. The capacity for physical movement to explore the environment is critical to many aspects of the individual's development, and lack of or loss of mobility, or reduced mobility, can have a devastating effect on the person's image of himself, perhaps ultimately affecting his capacity to take his place effectively in society.

Enjoying rhythmic movement. Young children seem intuitively and uninhibitedly to engage in body movement as a response to music and in time with the rhythm. Many adults too seem to enjoy rhythmic body movement, almost subconsciously, and when sitting alone or in company can be observed tapping a foot or a hand, or swinging a leg. Recreations such as dancing, ice-skating and even gymnastics are frequently performed to the accompaniment of music, probably enhancing the pleasure derived by both performers and spectators. At work too, long before the advent of piped music, artisans were known to sing while busy with the weaving frame, or hauling in the fishing nets, and many well-known songs reflect this rhythmic association.

Channelling emotional energy. Some people use physical activity as an outlet for emotions, for reasons as diverse as boredom and aggression. Many 'normal' teenagers and young adults who engage in strenuous activities say that they do so to 'let off steam' and many admit that by so doing they experience relaxation and recreation. In a similar vein, physical activities are deliberately encouraged in social clubs for young offenders, so that energies may be expended in a way which is pleasurable to the individual, rather than in uncontrolled, and sometimes violent, types of behaviour.

Promoting well-being. It is well known that not only the musculoskeletal system benefits from regular exercise but the function of all the other systems is enhanced. Currently the media extol the benefits, both physiological and psychological, of exercise for all age groups and deplore the sedentary lifestyle of people in most industrialised countries; a lifestyle which is considered to be a major contributing factor to conditions such as hypertension, coronary heart disease and obesity. All of these have increased in incidence in the last few decades, indeed coronary heart disease is a major cause of death in most countries in the Western world.

Transferring man and goods. In industrialised countries the capacity for personal physical movement from place to place is greatly enhanced by machines. In the initial stages of man's existence on this planet he had to rely on his own body's energy to move himself and his goods from place to place, but as he learned to domesticate animals, he came to conserve his own energy by riding a horse or a bullock or an elephant. With the advent of the wheel, he was able to construct a carrier of sorts which could be drawn by animals. Making an immense chronological leap down to the industrial and technological revolutions, he was able to harness other forms of energy in devising fuel-powered vehicles such as cars, trains, ships and planes for rapid transit of people and vast quantities of goods.

It is interesting that man is now showing concern about the dwindling natural energy sources in the world and there is a drive to conserve existing supplies. There is also considerable activity in the development of nuclear power, and exploration of the possibilities for utilising solar and wave energy to man's advantage so that he can continue to augment his own capacity for physical mobility. Hopefully man will find the appropriate balance between exploiting the mobilising power of machines, and maintaining a personal exercise level which is conducive to health and the enjoyment of everyday living. In the ensuing text, the AL of mobilising will be focused to the other four components of the model of living, namely lifespan, dependence/independence continuum, factors influencing mobilising, and, ending the first part of the chapter, to individuality in mobilising.

LIFESPAN: EFFECT ON MOBILISING

Mobilising is an intrinsic part of living as evidenced by the first movements of the baby's hands and feet. The kicking and arm waving continue as older babies lie awake for periods during the day and these become more active when they are changed and bathed. Crawling is the next experiment; standing, walking, jumping and running are achieved sequentially. From the second year onwards the mobilising dimension of eliminating is mastered; and for most children the many skills (requiring dexterity as well as mobilising) required for carrying out personal cleansing and dressing are acquired by 4–5 years of age. The majority of adults make decisions about mobilising while working and playing and the words 'sedentary' and 'physically demanding' can be applied to leisure activities as well as income-generating work. Pregnancy can affect mobilising and many people recognise the changed gait of a pregnant woman, and low back pain may be experienced. In the postmenopausal phase, women are prone to develop osteoporosis (softening of bone) which can result in fracture from application of a force which would not break normal bone. It can also cause abnormal curvature of the spine, and hormone replacement therapy can be used to help to prevent the condition. Attitudes to old age and old people need to change in a positive direction, since the expected lifespan in the West has increased. However, for most ageing people, there comes a time when they lose body weight, have less energy and shrink in height. Not only will this directly affect the AL of mobilising but also the mobilising dimensions of for example, personal cleansing and dressing; eliminating, and eating and drinking.

DEPENDENCE/INDEPENDENCE IN MOBILISING

It is relevant here to point out that with regard to the AL of mobilising, the dependence/independence component of the model is closely related to the lifespan component. For the majority of people, after a period of dependence in infancy, there is increasing independence in childhood. At the other end of the lifespan, the majority of old people experience a gradual decrease in the level of independence until many of them become dependent on some type of aid, often a walking stick, to broaden the base and take some of the body weight when walking.

However there are some people who at birth do not have adequate body structure and function to achieve independence in mobilising, as they progress through the stages of the lifespan. There are others, who having achieved independence, are deprived of it at a further stage on the lifespan, perhaps due to accident or disease. Aided independence may be a possibility by learning to use such external aids as walking frames, crutches, leg calipers, and artificial limbs which may be body worn aids. There may be dependence on another person for help with applying the aid. For those who cannot stand, mobilising has to be achieved by dependence on a wheelchair and possibly another person to push it; some are able to use a self-propelled or a battery operated wheelchair. Some can also manage to drive a modified car and indeed become independent as they use a hoist to transfer from wheelchair to car.

FACTORS INFLUENCING MOBILISING

An important part of the model of living is how five factors — physical, psychological, sociocultural, environmental and politicoeconomic — influence the way in which individuality in mobilising develops, and they will now be discussed in turn.

Physical factors

A fully functioning musculoskeletal system is essential for acquisition of the skills related to mobilising. It is not the purpose of this book to provide biological detail of the human body systems. The capacity for unaided physical mobility is affected by any circumstances which interfere with any part of the musculoskeletal system and its associated nerve pathways. The adverse circumstances may be congenital in origin but good obstetric care aims at prevention of birth injuries and disabling conditions occurring in the neonatal period.

Fractured or diseased bones can interfere with mobilising in many different ways. Joints too may become diseased and so painful that movement is impeded. Should the hips, knees or ankles be affected, walking becomes difficult; when the small joints of the hands are involved there can be interference with many aspects of mobilising for example those used in domestic activities, personal cleansing and dressing, and working and playing. A muscle sprain may cause swelling and thereby reduce movement. Any form of paralysis such as hemiplegia caused by a stroke, or paraplegia caused by accident, severely restricts mobilising.

For those who have a permanent physical impairment which reduces mobility, the aim is to help them to enjoy everyday living to the optimum level. If physically impaired from birth, the goal will be the achievement of a lifestyle where they will have the maximum possible mobility. For those who succumb to an immobilising disease or injury, it may mean adapting to a lifestyle which is less physically active but just as personally fulfilling, and the adaptation may be merely temporary or it may require to be a lifelong adjustment.

Psychological factors

A minimum level of intelligence is necessary to learn the skills necessary for safe mobilising. Temperament also influences this AL; there are people who are constantly curious and characteristically active and their mobilising is often of an adventurous nature. There are others whose curiosity relates to acquiring knowledge; they are usually less active in mobilising and may be described as 'thinkers rather than doers'. A person's values and beliefs may provide the motivation to exercise in order to keep fit, and indeed they may provide a driving ambition so that daily practice for many hours can be sustained. People also display different attitudes to safety while mobilising, for example complying with speed regulations and the wearing of seat belts.

Sociocultural factors

Some sociocultural factors were mentioned on page 247 — artisans' songs to bring rhythm to the movements involved in weaving and fishing. Most countries of the world have national dances which are a much valued expression of national pride and patriotic fervour, and have been handed down from generation to generation. On the other hand members of some religious and cultural groups exclude, for example, dancing as a form of pleasurable exercise. Social class may well determine how this AL is carried out, for example whether a person travels on foot or public transport, by car or in private plane or yacht. There are also sports and other leisure activities which are characteristic of the higher and lower social classes; children from the former may go skiing abroad while those from the latter play football on a piece of waste ground near their home. Of course social class undoubtedly dictates the mobilising component of the working day; the majority of people in the higher classes have sedentary jobs although they may involve worldwide travel, while many in the lower group are manual workers.

Cultural factors make their contribution to the sort of sport which is characteristic of countries. The names of many famous tennis and cricket clubs, and rugby leagues are indicative of the strong tradition attached to the sport in that part of the world. At international gatherings, too, the influence of culture can be observed in for example the style of dress and the music chosen to accompany the movement, as in gymnastics and ice skating.

Environmental factors

The type of residence is an important determinant of optimal achievement in mobilising.

High rise flats are not conducive to children's optimal development of the AL of mobilising. A third-floor flat which is not serviced by a lift may deter a frail elderly person from taking a daily walk. Available space within the home is another influencing factor; the type of furniture for toddlers and frail people to use as a support while walking is also important. Ergonomists pay special attention to the design of furniture, particularly chairs so that for example a desirable sitting posture is maintained. There are many other environmental factors which influence the AL of mobilising particularly for those with impaired vision, hearing or agility. These include having to cross busy streets, having to climb a gradient when setting out from or returning to the house, or lack of parks and open spaces in which to take exercise in an unhurried manner.

One should not forget that local climate and terrain can affect mobilising. The majority of people do not exercise strenuously in a hot and humid atmosphere, and where facilities are available are much more likely to go swimming for example. People who have a tendency to breathlessness fare badly in a windy climate and may not get sufficient outdoor exercise. Those brought up in hilly districts may be influenced to take up fell walking as a hobby and the adventurous ones may be attracted to mountaineering.

Politicoeconomic factors

It is said that every city has its slums and areas of substandard housing and these are usually owned by the local council, or administrative body. The environs of such areas are often in bad repair and poorly lit, so that there are restrictions on young children in terms of possibilities for physically active pursuits. Councils vary in the provisions of parks and open spaces, children's playgrounds, playing fields, swimming baths, sports arenas and leisure centres and all these can directly influence the mobilising habits of the population.

The local council is of course responsible for the state schools in which physical education is available. The range of sports can vary from one city to another, but if for instance the school does not have facilities for swimming, tuition arrangements can usually be made with the municipal swimming pool so that pupils are not deprived of this sport which is such a healthy form of mobilising.

The council is also responsible for the state of city pavements so that pedestrians can walk safely. There is usually a kerb of several inches between pavement and street and these can be hazardous for both adult and child when a pushchair is being used. Such kerbs also present problems to those of all ages whose form of transport is a wheelchair whether it is manually wheeled by another person, or is self-propelled or battery driven. In some countries it is now mandatory to provide suitably placed ramps when new pavements are being constructed in order to cater for the special needs of these groups of people.

The central government in the UK encourages local councils to provide wheelchair access to public buildings and shops so that the users of this form of mobilising are not deprived of entry. A transport allowance is available to disabled people and if their cars display the necessary sticker, they can park in areas which are normally forbidden to private vehicles, or restricted in some way.

Pedestrian crossings are usually sited at traffic lights but where these are absent on a long straight street or road, many campaigners have succeeded in getting the council to instal a pedestrian-controlled crossing so that particularly those with some impediment in walking can take time to cross safely.

INDIVIDUALITY IN MOBILISING

Considering the effect on mobilising of the lifespan, the dependence/independence continuum, and the factors influencing the ALs, it is not surprising that by the time people have reached adulthood, they have developed highly individualised mobilising habits. Sometimes those who have a physically active work pattern also choose to have strenuous play activities. On the other hand they may deliberately engage in more sedentary recreation in order to balance the daily energy output. There are many variations on the theme and they provide an interesting diversity in the life of a community. When describing a particular person's individuality in mobilising the nurse will find the foregoing description of this AL in the context of the model useful, and the following résumé helpful:

Lifespan: effect on mobilising
- Infancy and childhood — increasing skills in mobilising
- Adolescence and young adulthood — peak performance in mobilising
- Later years — decreasing agility

Dependence/independence in mobilising
- Increasing independence in childhood
- Dependence on another person
- Body worn aids } for aided independence
- External aids }
- Transport

Factors influencing mobilising
- Physical — fully functioning musculoskeletal system
  — congenital interference with function
  — trauma, disease
- Psychological — intelligence; temperament; values, beliefs, motivation, ambition; attitudes
- Sociocultural — rhythm of mobilising; dancing; religious constraints; social class; tradition
- Environmental — type and place of residence; local climate and terrain; influence on hobbies
- Politicoeconomic — substandard housing
  — kerbs and pavements
  — access to buildings
  — safe street crossings
  — exercise facilities

Mobilising: patients' problems and related nursing

Health visitors and school nurses help children to prevent potential problems with mobilising from becoming actual ones. They will also encounter a minority who have actual problems with mobilising, perhaps because they have some disability, probably congenital; but may be acquired from accident or disease, and the nurse as a member of a multidisciplinary team will seek to maximise the person's compromised ability to mobilise. The majority of people entering the health care service at any point, will not have an actual problem with mobilising but the changed circumstances may provide some potential problems.

If the newly admitted patient already has a problem with mobilising — whether it is in using upper and/or lower limbs — then at the initial assessment whether it is carried out in the home or in hospital, information about the home environment is collected. It is useful for planning rehabilitation, with its goal of discharging the person from the health service with maximum mobilising ability, according to the particular circumstances. The proforma on page 55 has a space for such information. To minimise problems nurses need to know about the patient's previous habits and at least some of this information will be gained at the initial assessment. The following questions will help the nurse to collect the required information:

- how much exercise does the individual take daily/weekly?
- when does the individual exercise?
- what factors influence the way the individual mobilises?
- what does the individual know about mobilising, particularly with regard to health?
- what is the individual's attitude to mobilising?
- has the individual any longstanding problems with

mobilising and if so, how have these been coped with?

- what problems, if any, does the individual have at present with mobilising, and are any likely to develop?

It will probably be unnecessary to ask all the questions; answers to some of them may be evident from observation of the patient. There may be relevant information in the medical records and some might be revealed when patients talk about their occupation; the nurse could ask for example, how far the workplace is from home, and what form of transport is used. Indeed the ALs of working and playing, and mobilising are so closely related that it may be advisable to collect information about them simultaneously. The collected information will then be examined, in collaboration with the patient whenever possible, to discover what the patient can/cannot do independently and to identify any actual problems with the AL of mobilising. There may be potential problems and these too will be discussed with the patient. For each actual and potential problem a realistic and achievable goal will be set, again in discussion with the patient and where appropriate with the physiotherapist.

The goals may well be to prevent potential problems becoming actual ones; or to alleviate or solve the actual problems; or help the patient to cope with those which cannot be alleviated or solved. The nursing interventions to achieve the goals will take into account the local circumstances and the available resources: they will be written on the nursing plan together with any activities which the patient has agreed to carry out, for example foot exercises to prevent the potential problem of foot drop. A date for evaluation will also be written on the nursing plan to discover whether or not the interventions are achieving or have achieved the stated goals. These activities incorporate the four phases of the process of nursing and they are necessary to carry out *individualised nursing* related to the AL of mobilising.

However before nurses can begin to think in terms of individualised nursing they need to have some idea of the kinds of problems which patients can experience in carrying out the AL of mobilising. They will be discussed under the following headings.

- change of environment and routine
- change of mobilising habit
- change of dependence/independence status for mobilising
- some specific problems associated with mobilising

CHANGE OF ENVIRONMENT AND ROUTINE

Some people who have both actual and potential problems related to the AL of mobilising are cared for in their homes; for those who are in the terminal phase of an illness, the problems arise from either being chairbound for most of the day, or being totally bedbound. The main potential problem from decreased mobilising is pressure sores (p. 218); therefore the changed 'environment' in contact with the pressure areas includes cushions and beds described by David (1986) and Clements (1987). Some local authorities provide a loan service for such items. On the other hand, admission to hospital is an obvious change of environment and will be discussed as change in mobilising routine, and lack of specific knowledge about mobilising routine.

Change in mobilising routine

In order to prepare an individualised plan related to the patient's AL of mobilising it is important to collect information about previous routines at the initial assessment. As mentioned previously, this AL is, for many people, so closely related to working and playing that it may be advisable to seek information about them, either together or in sequence. Knowledge about the previous pattern of the patient's day will help the nurse to help the patient to adapt accordingly. The help, of course, will be different according to whether the patient is mobile, bedfast or chairfast.

Mobile patients. Inevitably there is a degree of restriction in activities, even for mobile patients although some hospitals have amenities which permit them to exercise in the attractive grounds. Nowadays an increasing number of hospitals, particularly those providing long stay treatment for psychiatric and elderly patients, acknowledge the important part mobilising plays in daily living and make arrangements to ensure that patients continue this AL.

Admission to hospital almost always causes a patient distress and anxiety of some sort. The anxiety may be exacerbated, however, for the person with a long-standing mobility impairment which has been present perhaps from birth and who may have learned to cope adequately in his home surroundings. Admission to hospital may be for some quite unrelated reason and disrupts his daily mobilising routine. Activities which he managed at home perhaps independently, perhaps with family help in the privacy of his bedroom or bathroom, may become a problem in an unfamiliar setting which does not have his accustomed aids and fixtures. In these circumstances, the nurse must be sensitive to his need for privacy and appreciate that, for example, he may require a longer time for dressing/ undressing or for feeding. Help from the nurse may be interpreted as an intrusion and a threat to personal dignity and independence, so it is of paramount importance to assess what the patient can/cannot do, so that he can control the situation without having to struggle unnecessarily.

Bedfast and chairfast patients. Those patients who are confined to bed are deprived of many of their mobilising routines and may well feel angry and distressed at their predicament. On the other hand they may be so ill that they are glad to regress and hand over control to the nursing staff. They may have difficulty maintaining the sitting position which (unless contra-indicated) is desirable for eating purposes and to facilitate breathing, and is usually preferred by the patient during waking hours.

Bedfast patients may require assistance to maintain the sitting position and there are specific techniques for lifting patients which are effective, cause minimum upset to the patient, and are crucial for the nurse to know and perfect if she is to avoid back injury (Figs 13.6 and 13.7). The same lifting principles are used to help patients out of bed into a chair and vice versa (Figs 13.8 and 13.9) and to help a seated patient into the standing position (Fig. 13.10).

Those patients who are chairfast for most of the day are frequently adapting to change in their mobilising routines. They usually require the help of a nurse to rise from the chair and to walk whatever distance they are capable of walking, supported by another person; and usually the walking exercise is organised to include a visit to the toilet.

Whether in bed or seated in a chair, the patient with reduced capacity for movement must be assisted to feel as independent as possible and it is the nurse's responsibility to ensure that a glass of water, the call-bell, and articles such as spectacles, paper tissues, books and newspapers are within reach; that an immobilised arm or leg is adequately supported by pads and pillows in a desirable position; that the patient is not exposed to chill; that the patient is not left in one position for too long a period (this maxim is just as important when the patient is sitting in a chair). When conscious patients with reduced capacity for mobility are left in one position for too long a period, they will almost certainly experience discomfort; even if there is loss of sensation in the impaired part, other parts of the body may be strained in maintaining that position.

Lack of specific knowledge about mobilising routine
It is important for patients to know what they can, and what they should not do in relation to mobilising. Newly admitted but mobile patients may feel insecure about continuing the AL of mobilising unless they are told where it is permissible for them to walk; whether or not there are specific times when they require to be in bed or at the bedside; whether it is customary for patients to leave the ward, for example, to go the hospital shop, the public telephone booths or for a walk in the grounds.

Patients who are on 'early ambulation' programmes need to understand exactly how much and what type of activity they carry out each day; and the increasing activity should be clearly described in the patient's nursing plan. It is interesting to note that Lelean (1973) found eight different interpretations among nurses of the phrase 'up and about' written in the nursing Kardex, and this highlights the importance of careful and concise recording.

All patients are exposed to potential problems because of their reduction in mobilising. However they can, whether they are ambulant, chairfast or bedfast help to prevent the potential problems becoming actual ones if they are given adequate information, encouragement and supervision.

One important purpose in exercising is to assist return of blood against gravity to the heart by the 'massage' action of active muscle on blood vessels, particularly in the legs. This is further assisted when the increased 'suction' from deep breathing draws blood along the large vessels back to the heart. Both these actions help to prevent stagnation of blood in the leg vessels. With reduction in mobilising there is a danger of stagnant blood clotting (thrombosis). A portion of the clot can become detached (embolus) and flow in the blood until it impacts in a vessel too narrow to permit its passage, usually in the lungs. The condition, called pulmonary embolism, may be fatal and it was to help to prevent this condition that 'early ambulation' was introduced in the 1950s. Patients should therefore be taught to do deep breathing exercises and instructed about moving their feet and toes in a circular direction at regular times throughout waking hours.

CHANGE IN MOBILISING HABIT

Although it is difficult to describe, most people have some idea of what constitutes normal or average activity in relation to the human body. Comment may be passed when a person's activity level changes from busy and bustling to lethargy and relative inactivity. There are gradations of activity/inactivity, but when appearing in an extreme form both over-activity and under-activity are pathological.

Hyperactivity and hypoactivity
A change to generalised hyperactivity and hypoactivity is found, for example, where there are defects in the function of the thyroid gland, part of the endocrine system. Hyperthyroidism occurs when there is oversecretion of the gland and the person has problems because of hyperactivity, breathlessness on exertion, increased pulse rate, and may be palpitations; there is tiredness yet constant restlessness. On the other hand hypothyroidism occurs when there is undersecretion of the gland and in extreme cases the patient's problem is that there is a gradual slowing down to a state of almost complete inertia. Due to the hormone deficiency, energy is not being produced in the body. Usually drugs can be prescribed to achieve hormonal balance and counteract the hyperactivity/hypoactivity.

Muscular hyperactivity in the form of spasticity is a problem for some congenitally brain-damaged people. The sinuous, writhing, purposeless movements interfere with manual dexterity and if the muscles in the lower limbs are affected, they dictate the strange and uncoordinated movement of the legs, while walking. Writhing, purposeless movement along with a shuffling gait is characteristic also of Parkinson's disease, currently of particular interest because it can be a side-effect of some antidepressant drugs. Muscular hyperactivity occurs too, though usually transiently, during an epileptic fit (p. 330).

Some psychiatric illnesses have physical manifestations which include change in the normal level of activity. The patient with a neurotic disorder has a problem because of difficulty with emotional adaptation to circumstances. In a florid anxiety state, patients may be acutely distressed because they experience intense feelings of anxiety. One manifestation of the condition is an increased output of energy indicated by general restlessness and sometimes uncontrollable tremors. Some patients reduce the anxiety level by the use of a mechanism called a conversion reaction. The mechanism is always unconscious and it produces physical impairment in a part of the body which would

normally be under voluntary control. Motor symptoms include paralysis of the limbs, twitchings, tics and fits and there may also be sensory symptoms including numbness and pain. A description of the symptoms is often a reflection of the person's own idea of anatomical structure and when examined medically, there is no indication of organic disease. But such people have an emotional and a physical problem and until effective psychiatric treatment is given, they will not part with this physical mobility/immobility impairment.

Another example of a psychiatric condition which has motor manifestations is called catatonic schizophrenia. Schizophrenia is characterised by a withdrawal of interest from everyday affairs and an emotional coldness. In extreme forms of catatonic schizophrenia, behaviour may range from stupor to excessive excitement and hyperactivity. In complete stupor, patients often lie in an unusual position in bed, completely rigid. They may passively allow

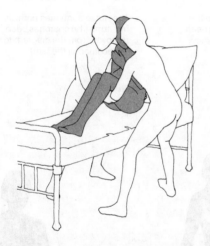

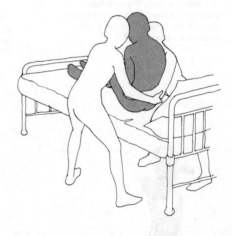

Fig. 13.6   Two nurses lifting a patient in bed: orthodox lift

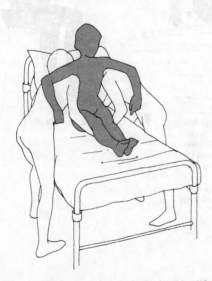

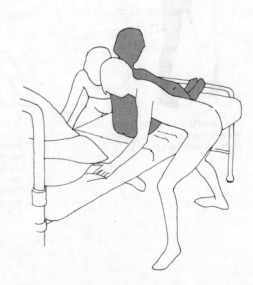

Fig. 13.7   Two nurses lifting a patient in bed: shoulder lift

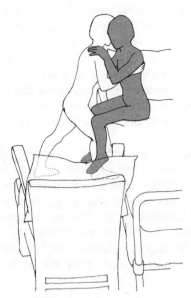

The nurse is standing with her weight over her front foot and keeps close to the patient; her arms are under the patient's arms.

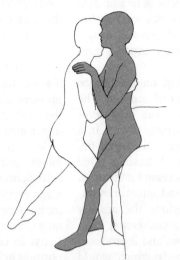

The nurse's weight is transferred to the back foot as she thrusts upwards with her arms.

The patient slides his feet on to the floor, wide apart (the chair has been removed from the diagram to show the position of the feet).

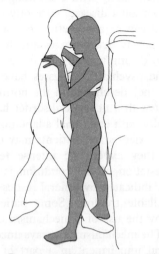

The patient and nurse stand upright, each with their weight central over their own base of support.

The nurse continues upthrust with her arms (the chair has been removed from the diagram to show the position of the feet).

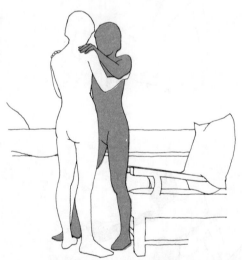

The nurse takes a walking step and swivels the patient, maintaining upthrust with her arms.

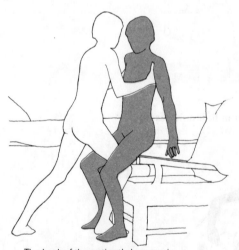

The back of the patient's legs are in contact with the chair. The nurse, maintaining a straight back, takes her weight forward and starts to lower the patient by bending her front knee.
The patient bends his knees and stretches the hands backwards to hold the chair.

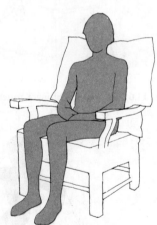

The patient is seated on the chair.

Fig. 13.8 One nurse helping a patient from the bed to a chair

the position to be altered or may resist and can maintain the unusual position for hours; some patients are known to have held their heads a few inches above the pillow for many hours or to have remained standing on one leg until their position is physically altered by one of the staff.

These are examples of mobilising problems experienced by patients who have neurotic and psychotic conditions involving physical hyperactivity or hypoactivity. As a result, apart from their emotional imbalance which requires expert psychiatric care, problems arise related to almost all the activities of everyday living, since mobilisation is a part of most ALs.

Over the last few decades the problem of hyperactivity in children has assumed the title of 'hyperkinesis' and the relevant literature describes a 'hyperkinetic syndrome' which occurs predominantly in first-born males in the age range of 6–12 years. Many of these children have behaviour problems; mealtimes are difficult and there are usually learning disabilities. Parents seek help when home life becomes intolerable (Raper, 1985). Health visitors and school nurses may encounter such children, and of course they can be admitted to hospital for a reason other than hyper-

kinesis. However, when considering changes in mobilising habit, some of the obvious examples are related to people who have a physical (locomotor) impairment, disability or handicap and these words are defined by the World Health Organization (1980):

- *impairment* is any loss or abnormality of psychological, physiological or anatomical structure or function
- *disability* is any restriction or lack of ability (resulting from an impairment) to perform an activity in the manner or within the range considered normal for a human being
- *handicap* is a disadvantage for a given individual, resulting from an impairment or a disability, that limits or prevents the fulfilment of a role that is normal (depending on age, sex, social and cultural factors) for that individual

Physical disability/handicap
Where available, a multidisciplinary team including nurses is necessary to help to prevent those diseases and accidents

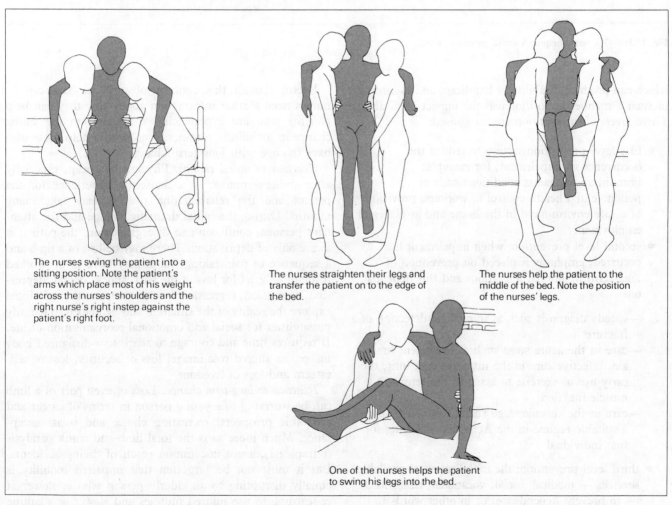

The nurses swing the patient into a sitting position. Note the patient's arms which place most of his weight across the nurses' shoulders and the right nurse's right instep against the patient's right foot.

The nurses straighten their legs and transfer the patient on to the edge of the bed.

The nurses help the patient to the middle of the bed. Note the position of the nurses' legs.

One of the nurses helps the patient to swing his legs into the bed.

Fig. 13.9 Two nurses helping a standing patient into bed

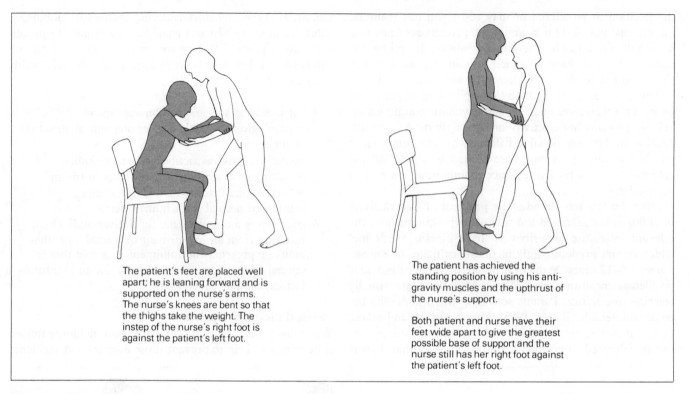

The patient's feet are placed well apart; he is leaning forward and is supported on the nurse's arms. The nurse's knees are bent so that the thighs take the weight. The instep of the nurse's right foot is against the patient's left foot.

The patient has achieved the standing position by using his anti-gravity muscles and the upthrust of the nurse's support.

Both patient and nurse have their feet wide apart to give the greatest possible base of support and the nurse still has her right foot against the patient's left foot.

Fig. 13.10   One nurse helping a seated patient to stand

which can produce disability or handicap; and to intervene in such a manner as to diminish the impact of disability. Three levels of intervention are recognised:

- first level prevention: action to reduce the occurrence of impairment; for example, immunisation against conditions such as poliomyelitis; health control of workers; provision of a safe environment in the home and at places of employment
- second level prevention: when impairment has occurred, emphasis is placed on prevention of long-term functional limitations and this depends on:

  —speedy diagnosis such as immediate detection of a fracture
  —care in the acute stage such as intelligent first aid, effective care in the intensive care unit, the early use of exercise to assist in the return of muscle function
  —care in the chronic stage such as establishment of a suitable regime in the Activities of Living for that individual

- third level prevention: the mobilisation of available services — medical, social, vocational, educational — to prevent dependence, or in other words to encourage self-care and economic independence

Useful though this concept of physical handicap is, nurses need further information about how they can help patients who are experiencing a reaction to the initial change in mobilising routines, then how to help those who have to cope with long-term change.

Reaction to initial change. Physical handicap, especially after sudden trauma, is a shattering experience for the patient and the rehabilitation process may take many months. During the initial dramatic change and the attendant personal confusion and disorganisation, the patient is aware only of deprivation. There may be loss of a limb and a sequence of painstaking stages may have to be worked through — grief for loss of the part, shock, denial, depression, aggression, regression — only then can the individual explore the reality of the situation and be helped to identify possibilities for social and emotional reorganisation of life. It requires time and courage to adapt to a disfigured body image, an altered role image, loss of security, loss of self-esteem and loss of freedom.

Reaction to long-term change. Loss of even part of a limb can be worrying to a young person in terms of career and economic prospects, recreation choice and social acceptance. Much more so is the total limb and trunk paralysis (tetraplegia), a not uncommon result of diving accidents. But it must not be forgotten that impaired mobility is equally disrupting to an elderly person who is slower at re-learning to use injured muscles and slower at adapting to changed circumstances especially when other faculties such as sight and hearing may also be failing.

Even in the protective environment of the hospital, patients keep on discovering just how much mobilising impairment affects the other Activities of Living. After all, one can do very little without moving some part of the body. But if it is a long-term disability further adaptation is required to the harsh realities of 20th century living when faced with discharge and coping in the outside world. Sometimes a patient will progress through a rehabilitation unit to ease the transition, but whether or not, a team of health and social service professionals is usually involved in the patient's care and adaptation — doctors, nurses, physiotherapists, occupational therapists, social workers, rehabilitation officers, educationists, employment officers, employers, housing officials — and the chaplain and voluntary agencies may also make an invaluable contribution.

The most important members of the team however are the patients and their families. The patients' motivation to help is critical to successful rehabilitation, so it is imperative to include them in the planning process and the decision making about their future mode of living. Rehabilitation implies restoration to the fullest physical, mental and social capability for that individual. Families, too, must be convinced that their efforts are worthwhile and be helped to understand that it is not always in the interests of disabled people to have things done for them, because they find them difficult to do. For the nurse and the family, it is important to learn when to give assistance and when to withdraw.

CHANGE OF DEPENDENCE/INDEPENDENCE STATUS FOR MOBILISING

It is important to remember that change of dependence/independence status for mobilising can be in either direction along the continuum. For example after a Colles' fracture of the radius, the forearm, wrist and upper hand are encased in plaster, which has to be kept dry, so the person at first is unable to carry out some activities. The early dependence is greater when the preferred hand is involved, but with ingenuity, some tasks can be carried out using the unpreferred hand, so the person becomes less dependent and more independent for particular tasks. After amputation of an upper limb, similar changes in the dependence/independence continuum occur. Even with the availability of technologically improved prostheses, many upper limb amputees continue to require help with placement and removal of the prosthesis.

Fracture of the lower limb is less frequently treated by encasing the leg in plaster. After thorough drying of the plaster, the patient learns to walk with crutches, so again, there is movement towards the dependent pole, then a gradual movement towards the independent pole of the continuum. Fractures are more commonly treated by surgical insertion of various biotechnical plates, screws and nails to immobilise the ends of the broken bone in approximation so that they can heal. The initial pre- and postoperative periods involve greater dependence, but there is a shortened period of regaining independence. Fractures and disease of the bones of the lower limb can be treated by traction. It is applied by passing a wire through the ankle bones to which weights are attached; with the foot of the bed raised, the weight of the supine body provides counter-traction to bring the bone ends into alignment ready for healing. Patients requiring such treatment are bedfast and dependent on having services brought to the bedside. Most patients have full mobility in the upper limbs, and the level of dependence/independence for eating and drinking, personal cleansing and dressing, eliminating, and preventing boredom which is part of the AL of working and playing, will depend on assessment of each individual.

There are some conditions which are still treated by enclosure of the trunk and one or both lower limbs in plaster — a simple or double spica — creating almost total dependence for as long as 12 weeks. Regaining independence for mobilising depends on the rate at which the unused muscles regain their tone by exercising them. Hip and knee replacement surgery is now so successful that many people can mobilise independently without aids, in contrast to previous mobilisation which was painful because of arthritic joints and required the use of walking aids. There are people who are afflicted with one of the muscular dystrophies which renders them increasingly dependent for any activity which involves even minimal mobilising. Some technologists have become interested in their plight and have devised such things as computers, and electronic apparatus which can be operated by such minimal movement as a blink of the eyelid, or an expiratory 'puff'. 'Biomedical' is now a special branch of 'engineering' so that people who are dependent for mobilising will increasingly be able to regain 'aided independence'. But for a variety of reasons these facilities are not available to all the people who have limb defects, so a few of the ways in which people have achieved optimal independence by overcoming the problem will be mentioned.

Upper limb defects. Many actions carried out by the two hands can be performed by one hand. Often the second hand is merely used to hold an object steady. In principle therefore, if some other means can be used for 'steadying', for example securing vegetables on a spiked board, the good hand can be used to carry out the activity of peeling the vegetable. Similarly bread can be steadied ready for buttering; a grater can be fixed to the wall in a suitable position; a hot water bottle can be placed securely in a specially adapted wall fixture and the kettle held in the good hand; clothes can be washed using one hand then wrung out by twisting them round the tap. When eating, a rubber pad under the plate will hold it securely, a guard on the plate will prevent food sliding on to the table and a fork with a cutting edge allows manipulation of food by one hand.

It is possible to surmount the problem of upper limb mobility at work too, and also for leisure activities. A paper-weight can secure writing paper and allow handwritten correspondence; a typewriter can be manipulated with one hand; various aids have been devised to facilitate, for example, manual skills at the place of employment and for hobbies such as knitting, sewing and gardening.

Lower limb defects. If the mobilising problem is associated with one of the lower limbs, a walking stick with a rubber tip or a quadruped (light metal stick with four small feet) can increase the base of support and help to maintain balance. It is crucial that the stick is of the correct length for that person and it is useful to have a loop of elastic attached to the handle so that the person is free to grasp door knobs and open doors himself without dropping the stick.

On stairs there should be rails on both sides to assist ascending and descending and until patients gain confidence, helpers should always stand below patients, that is behind them when going up, and in front of them when they are coming down. When ascending, the patient should use the good leg first and when coming down, the affected leg first. Manipulation of stairways may be particularly difficult for an elderly person who has a plaster of Paris bandage on a lower limb. For the young as well as the old, the plaster is heavy and unwieldy resulting in another problem — fatigue.

At home in the kitchen, a re-arrangement of storage space and adjustment of working heights can help to increase the patient's independence, and articles such as long-handled dustpans can make floor cleaning relatively simple. A trolley can be used for transporting articles from one place to another.

Some people have a lower limb incapacity which necessitates use of a wheelchair. In the UK a wheelchair can be provided free, under the national health service arrangements, indeed more than one may be supplied if medically recommended: a transit chair to take in a car and another for use in the house. It is almost impossible to get all the desired features in one model and it is important to assess individual needs: width (important in relation to size of doorways, corridors, lifts, public toilets), depth, seat height, position of foot support, angle of back, wheel diameter, type of tyre, weight, fixed or detachable arm rests and so on. When choosing a wheelchair for long-term use it is imperative to see the home surroundings. It will almost certainly be necessary to rearrange furniture and carpets, and it may be necessary to widen doorways or provide ramps, modifications which may qualify for a local authority grant in the UK.

Problems related to dependence in the AL of eliminating were discussed in Chapter 10, those related to personal cleansing and dressing in Chapter 11, and those related to incapacity because of body paralysis were discussed in Chapter 7. They are all associated with mobilising, yet another instance of the relatedness of the ALs.

Attitudes to dependence

For many people, their concept of 'dependence' in a health context is of physical and/or mental handicap. And in the not too distant past, many such dependent people were segregated from the general public and were cared for in large, old fashioned institutions. Ordinary people therefore did not have an opportunity to develop a positive attitude to dependent people. Attempts to encourage a more positive approach were given international publicity when the World Health Organization designated 1981 as 'The Year of the Disabled Person'. People were made more aware of the many hobbies and sports in which disabled people can take part; these include shooting, bowling, archery, fencing, field and track events, snooker and weight lifting.

The Year of the Disabled Person also drew people's attention to the types of work which can be accomplished by disabled people. In the work context, disabled people have fared less well, but some of the opportunities open to them are mentioned in the chapter on working and playing under the headings 'Physical disability (p. 280), 'Mental handicap' (p. 281), 'Mental illness' (p. 282) and 'Sensory loss/impairment' (p. 284).

Dependent people can be distressed by the public's attitude to their dependence. Some members of the public show their discomfort by using 'distancing' techniques which make disabled people feel uncomfortable; some may be embarrassingly over-solicitous; yet others manage a mature interaction, conveying that the disabled person is valued as a 'person', yet acknowledging, probably by non-verbal communications, the reality of the dependence.

It is desirable that ordinary people should become more aware of the ways in which handicapped people can be helped to achieve a satisfactory life-style in work, leisure, recreation and family situations. Adequate provision for their needs will overcome their disadvantages to some extent and help them to make a positive contribution to the life of the community in which they live.

The idea still persists that disabled people should be protected from the rigours of everyday living. It is becoming more accepted, however, that instead of a passive role, it is preferable to assist them to face the stress of active participation in the life of the community. To help them to do this, a wide range of facilities must be available from health and social services, from housing agencies, from education and employment departments and from voluntary organisations (Fig. 13.11). Different organisations offer help of various kinds related to disability. It is obvious that coordination of these services is needed in the UK if the disabled person is to have maximum benefit. In an ideal world no one would be dependent, but in the real world there will always be a reservoir of dependent people.

Professional attitudes to dependence. Nurses, like members of any other professional group, have a variety of attitudes to dependence, fashioned by their previous experience and current knowledge. In the acute hospital wards they gain considerable experience with patients who are temporarily dependent for some aspect of the AL of mobilising. However, they must be on their guard against expecting patients to be independent for mobilising before they can comfortably be so. For example, when can a patient after extensive abdominal surgery reasonably be expected to get in and out of bed independently? Nurses need to develop professional judgement of patients' individuality in readiness for regaining independence for this AL. Roper (1988) discusses the reasons for and the meaning of 'early ambulation' which is not a licence for patients to be up and about all day in the early postoperative days.

Dependent people have usually developed mechanisms for coping with their condition and when they have to be admitted to a general ward can experience undue anxiety and vulnerability. They are not sure if the nurses will be available to give the necessary help when needed and whether they will give it willingly or grudgingly. It is therefore especially important for nurses to collect adequate data about the patient's mobilising dependence/independence and to write on the nursing plan exactly what sort of help is required, and when, so that nurses on different shifts will offer the same sort of help. The physiotherapist's advice may be necessary to reinforce the nurses' professional judgement of 'optimal' independence for a particular patient.

Nurses may find that handicapped people are putting up with practical difficulties in mobilising which need not exist. Usually successful adjustments can be made if first of all the problem is identified, then possible solutions sought, then the most feasible solution implemented and the result evaluated. If the implemented solution is not effective for the disabled individual, it may need modification, or perhaps the original idea abandoned and a different solution sought.

Thinking through this type of problem requires the same logical thought sequence as is used for the process of nursing. Probably the nurse will not seek to solve this kind of patient's problem alone, however. All members of the health team should combine their knowledge and expertise to provide what is best for the individual patient and help to achieve an optimal level of mobilising.

Some specific problems associated with mobilising

The body structures associated with mobilising are extensive and it is understandable that patients can experience a wide variety of problems related to this AL which involve many of the other ALs. Prolonged bedrest in the home or in hospital, for example, causes reduced activity in all the body systems and can create discomfort related to almost every facet of daily life.

The problems mentioned in this section, however, will refer essentially to the musculoskeletal system itself.

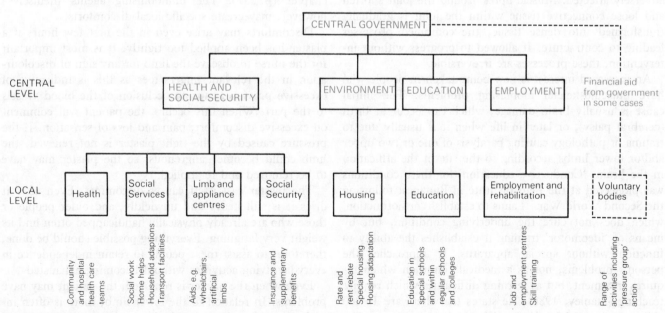

Fig. 13.11 Some of the services available to handicapped people

Musculoskeletal problems

When muscles are inactive, atrophy (wasting) commences and this muscle degeneration in turn depletes the capacity for movement and leads to further impairment and so the cycle continues. Exercises may be performed by the patient (active) or by the nurse helping the patient (passive or assisted). The muscle contraction involved not only increases muscle strength, it improves circulation and the movement preserves muscle tone and helps to prevent contracture (Fig. 13.12). In the bones too, lack of muscle action contributes to degenerative changes — a complication; release of calcium from the bones begins (osteoporosis); and even if halted, it may take months for the bone to return to normal. However, osteoporosis is a metabolic bone disease, which in the last few decades has become recognised in postmenopausal women in Western society. As the postmenopausal population is on the increase there is a need for preventive treatment and, as Brockie (1987) writes, this includes educating the medical and nursing professions. It is helpful if postmenopausal women take adequate calcium in the diet and continue to exercise, including a walk of 1–3+ miles daily. But the experts say that these preventive actions are not enough and should be accompanied by oral hormone replacement therapy immediately after the menopause and for a further 10 years. Pownall (1987) reports an international meeting of experts who reached consensus about the need for hormone treatment. Nulliparous women are particularly at risk and also those who have a family history of osteoporosis. It can be asymptomatic, its presence only being discovered when the older woman arrives in hospital with a fractured neck of femur.

Understandably, if joints are left in one position due to immobilisation over a prolonged period, they too become adversely affected. Muscle fibres around the joint shorten and loose connective tissue within the joint is gradually transformed into dense tissue, the combined processes leading to contracture. If allowed to progress without intervention, these processes are irreversible.

An increased interest is now being taken in people who have musculoskeletal mobilising problems. The initial cause is usually brain damage, which can occur at birth (cerebral palsy), or later in life when it is usually due to trauma or pathology causing paralysis of one or two upper and/or lower limbs according to the site of the affliction in the brain. 'Conductive education' for these conditions was pioneered at the Peto Institute in Budapest following the Second World War. It aims to establish 'orthofunction' which does not cure the underlying condition, but by means of 'ideomotor' training it establishes the ability to function without special apparatus. It approaches the person's problems, not as a medical condition which requires treatment, but as learning difficulties which require teaching (Stanley, 1988). He states that there are 16 000 children of school age in the UK who have cerebral palsy, and their parents are increasingly demanding 'conductive education' for them.

The Bobath technique is similar in some ways and is used for people who have had a stroke. The main principle is to move the damaged body symmetrically so that it is retrained in natural patterns of movement; it needs to be encouraged to develop new nerve pathways to accomplish the movements independently. Another principle is to break the automatic pattern of spasticity which is characterised by the clawed hand and the stiff bent elbow; the straightened knee and pointed foot. In a bid to become independent stroke patients are often encouraged to learn ways 'around problems' by using the unaffected side of the body, so the affected side is not rehabilitated. Because nurses are with patients round the clock, their support and involvement is crucial to the success of rehabilitation using the Bobath technique (Holmes, 1988).

Therapeutic immobilising procedures

After injury which results in one or more broken bones, most commonly the long ones in the upper and/or lower limbs, the bone ends need to be immobilised in alignment so that they can heal. The joint above and below the broken bone may need to be immobilised and in the case of a fractured femur it may mean application of a hip spica which confines the person to bed. Because of the hazards of bedrest (Roper, 1988) the older women mentioned previously, can die from one of these complications, rather than from the fracture per se. To avoid this, intramedullary fixation can be achieved by the surgical insertion of a nail, plate or screw (p. 257), so that early ambulation becomes a realistic goal. Some of the general problems experienced by the patient due to immobility/reduced mobility of the upper or lower limbs have already been discussed in this chapter (p. 257). The immobilising agents themselves however, may create specific local discomforts.

Discomforts may arise even in the first few hours if a plaster has been applied too tightly. It is most important for the nurse to observe the limb for any sign of discolouration in the relevant fingers/toes as this is indicative of excessive pressure, causing occlusion of the blood vessels to the part. When this occurs, the patient will comment on excessive discomfort, pain and loss of sensation. If the pressure caused by the tight plaster is not relieved, the limb could become gangrenous, so the plaster may have to be removed and re-applied.

The plaster cast itself causes discomfort. Even after it dries it is still heavy and unwieldly, and older people or those who are already physically handicapped often find its weight very fatiguing. Everything possible should be done, therefore, to assist these people to retain independence in everyday living activities without becoming exhausted.

Even when the plaster is removed, the patient may have problems. In relation to the lower limb, there is often initial discomfort in rising and exercising the joints and

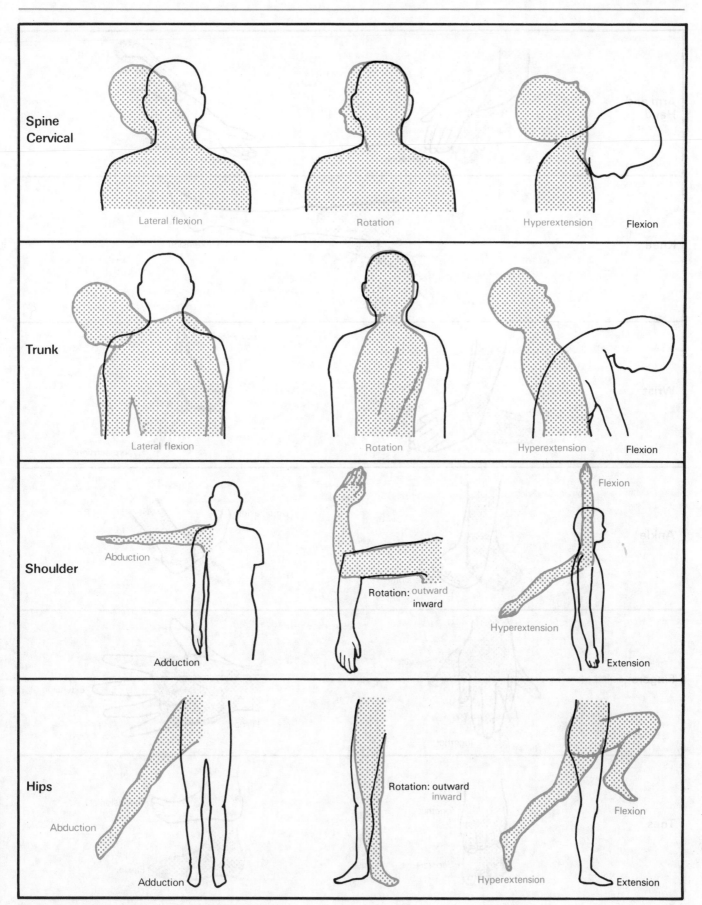

Fig. 13.12 Assisted (passive) exercises for bedfast patients

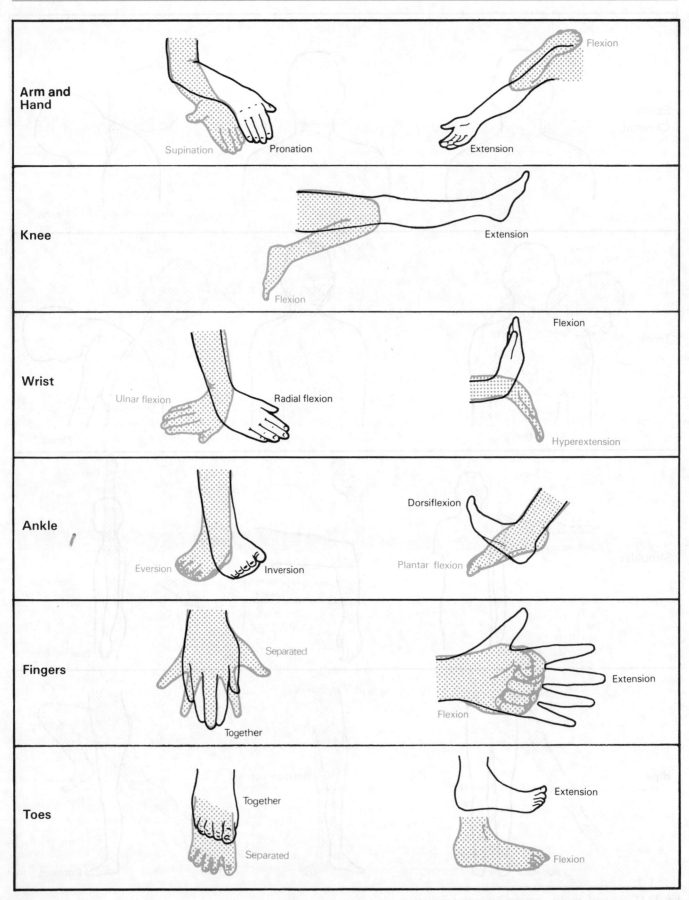

Fig. 13.12 (contd)

muscles which have been relatively immobile during the time when the plaster was in position. In addition the affected limb may look discoloured and it may be covered with scales of dead skin. These discomforts are usually rectified within a few days, however, as the limb is exercised and the circulation is improved. The scales of skin, too, gradually become detached if gently bathed. They should not be removed forcibly and sometimes an emollient is helpful.

The technique called skeletal traction involves passing as specially-designed, sterile pin through a fragment of the bone distal to the fracture, and maintaining the bone's position once it has been aligned, by a system of pulleys and weights attached to a special bed-frame. Countertraction (a force in the opposite direction) is necessary and is provided, in the case of a lower limb, by elevating the foot of the bed.

The same effect is achieved by applying adhesive tape to the skin in the area of the fracture (skin traction) and attaching the adhesive bandaging to a similar system of pulleys and weights. In both instances, there may be discomfort due to irritation of the skin and in the former, the small wounds where the pin protrudes may cause discomfort unless carefully tended.

After an initial period of awkwardness in manipulation, people who have a plaster of Paris bandage applied to a limb are usually ambulant and can carry out the AL of mobilising without too much discomfort; when the traction methods are used, however, bedrest is needed, with all the attendant discomforts of restriction on freedom and independence. Patients in traction usually require to remain in the supine position, and ingenuity is needed to help them to be as comfortable as possible, to make activities such as eating, drinking and eliminating as easy as possible, to prevent the formation of pressure sores and to reduce boredom and frustration. Another problem which requires thought is the positioning of bedclothes such that the traction ropes are unimpeded yet the patient is protected from draughts and loss of modesty. Small blankets can be strategically placed to provide warmth and adequate cover and the patient will usually wish to wear bedsocks. Especially for the older patient on traction, it is important to be on the alert for indications of hypostatic pneumonia and encouragement of regular, deep breathing exercises will help to prevent this distressing complication.

Pain

Pain is a subjective experience and for that reason was discussed in the AL of communicating on page 121. It is pertinent to remind readers that there is discussion about the use of a painometer for assessment and monitoring of the pain experience. However, because the prime purpose of the musculoskeletal system is to produce movement, it is not unnatural to expect that many of the dysfunctions produce pain on movement, and information gained at the initial assessment can be documented at this AL. And different kinds of pain can be experienced in relation to mobilising.

Sudden severe pain. The pain experienced by a person when a limb is fractured is certainly sudden and usually severe. It results from muscle spasm and tissue damage; it produces deformity and shortening of the limb, impaired mobility and loss of function. The immobility continues until the person can have specialist treatment usually in hospital, to align the bone ends and immobilise the limb. An analgesic is needed and as, in all probability, an anaesthetic will be required to undertake the bone alignment, the drug is not give orally but by injection. It is important that a written note of the drug, dose, time and route is sent with the person to the hospital.

Chronic pain. Many people experience chronic pain associated with the musculoskeletal system variously referred to as muscular rheumatism (fibrositis), low-back pain (lumbago) and joint pain (arthritis). These dysfunctions are responsible for much temporary and permanent disablement and are the cause of much absenteeism from work.

Precise information about the number of people suffering low back pain is impossible as some do not report it. Horgan (1985) states that 1 in 20 adults will see their GP each year, and gives the most common reasons for low back pain as:

- soft tissue rheumatism
- degenerative disease of the spine
- prolapsed intervertebral disc
- nerve entrapment syndrome

Horgan states that low back pain costs the health service between 1 and 2 million pounds annually, and it is responsible for over 30 million lost working days each year. Howie (1986) summarises a 5-year project carried out at the University of Surrey's Ergonomics Department into back pain in nurses. The data showed that every year nearly one-tenth of the UK's 470 000 practising nurses suffer some degree of back pain, and that 764 000 working days are lost to the National Health Service as a result. With a problem of this magnitude in the general population, and the nursing population in particular, nurses require detailed knowledge, and practise at manoeuvres to prevent low back pain. It is being increasingly recognised that efficient patient handling techniques alone, are not sufficient; employers need to take an ergonomic approach (p. 247) to the problem by which the work is made to fit the worker (Harvey, 1987).

As pain is the main reason for seeking medical aid, much of the treatment is aimed at relieving this distressing symptom. The measures used involve, for example, rest of the involved joints, physiotherapy, use of anti-inflammatory drugs, analgesics and corticosteroids, surgery to restructure affected joints with prostheses and rehabilitation programmes to restore maximum function.

District nurses, particularly those 'attached' to a family doctor's surgery, can help these patients by assessing whether or not they protect themselves from chill, take reasonable exercise outdoors according to their disability, get the best advantage from their drug regime and so on. As excessive weight usually exacerbates the pain, those who are overweight can be encouraged to reduce their kilojoule intake. Some patients obtain relief by the application of dry or moist heat to the painful area and they can be taught to do this safely. Others find the application of liniment useful. There is a wide range of age in people who experience chronic pain related to mobilising. Whitwan (1989) reports ongoing work at the Leeds Rheumatism and Rehabilitation Research Unit into the emotional and physical stresses on arthritic mothers with young children. The unit includes a regular 'Still's clinic' for children with juvenile rheumatoid arthritis. The article states that an estimated 8 million people in the UK are being actively treated for arthritis.

Sharp shooting pain. Even a tiny protrusion from a compromised intervertebral disc can touch a nerve root causing a sharp shooting pain which is experienced along the pathway of the nerve. In the case of the sciatic nerve the pain is experienced in the buttock and along the back of the leg and control by oral analgesics is necessary until the fragment shrinks. The patient may or may not be on bedrest but most people with an acute attack of sciatica find rest in bed helpful.

The nurse needs to discover whether or not these patients do heavy lifting at work or at home and what knowledge they have about safe lifting methods. Again being overweight is not advisable for people with a disc lesion and the nurse can discuss accordingly.

Deep boring pain. Pain in bone is often described as excruciating. Since bone is a relatively dense structure it has little space to accommodate the swelling caused by inflammation or the extra tissue from a new growth like a cancer. The nurse can help by careful positioning and supporting of the part relative to the rest of the body and by giving analgesics, anti-inflammatory and any other prescribed drugs promptly and safely.

Phantom pain. A discomfort which is particularly disturbing to patients who have had an amputation is 'phantom limb pain'; there is a sensation of pain in the amputated part of the limb. The mechanism of this type of 'referred' pain is not clearly understood but it is probably related to previously established body image. Pain is a subjective experience and as such it is a psychological event, not a physical one. The concept of pain must involve location in the body for the experience, even when there is not a physical cause. So phantom limb pain is peculiarly distressing to patients, because they can see that, physically, the amputated part is no longer there. Such patients require special care and attention from the nurse, to help them with this manifestation of pain which is very real to them. Dernham (1986) describes a project which identified some common characteristics that provide a framework for assessing the risk of occurrence of phantom pain. Nursing can then be planned to minimise the risk, and postoperatively the patient can learn particular muscle relaxation techniques as well as phantom limb and stump exercises. Warm baths, massage and distraction were all found to be useful.

Social and emotional problems

When there is interference with mobilising there is emotional discomfort and upset because of loss of freedom, loss of independence and loss of personal dignity. In addition there is anxiety about the state of immobility and its cause. There may also be a change in social role related to family, and to work and leisure activities which can be destructive to the individual's self-image. Together these assaults on personal identity may manifest themselves as aggressive behaviour or as apathy, or frustration or regression.

Nurses must therefore learn to listen to patients and help them to work through these stages so that they can restore their image of personal worth and dignity. In these circumstances, it is necessary to support the relatives by, among other things, encouraging them to express their feelings in response to behaviour of this type. Aggression or apathy may be quite atypical of the person's usual behaviour and can cause extreme discomfort, distress and bewilderment to the family.

Falls

Because the population in the UK is ageing the problem of falls and accidents among the elderly has been highlighted. 'The majority occur in females of 75 years or over who have poor vision and restricted mobility' (Williams, 1989) and elderly people who express a fear of falling may be expressing a loss of confidence. Estimates of the size of the problem state that at least 3 million elderly people fall in Britain each year. Williams' article (1989) is entitled 'Did she fall or was she pushed?' acknowledging the increasing problem of abuse of elderly people. Abuse by professional carers is discussed and a profile of an abused person is given; it is based on several research reports and the implications for nursing practice are described. It is a well referenced article, thereby providing further information. *Nursing Times* (1989) provides data about the size of the problem of falls among the elderly in Scotland. It is customary for an 'accident form' to be filled in as soon as possible after an accident to any person on hospital premises. Nurses need to be familiar with the form used, and the practice of accident reporting required by the hospitals in which they work.

Individualising nursing

To individualise nursing, nurses need to know about the person's individuality in mobilising which is discussed in the first half of this chapter. While describing the model for nursing, general information was given about individualising nursing (p. 51) which in fact is synonymous with the concept of the process of nursing. The assessment would be achieved by various means such as observing the person, acquiring information about usual habits, partly by asking appropriate questions; partly by listening to the person and/or relatives; and partly by using relevant information from available records, including medical ones. The collected information could then be examined to identify any actual problems being experienced with mobilising and these could be arranged in an order of priority. The nurse might also recognise some potential problems — not all possible potential problems but those which are relevant. Mutually agreed realistic goals could then be set to prevent potential problems from becoming actual ones; to alleviate or solve the actual problems; or to help the person cope with those which cannot be alleviated or solved.

Keeping in mind what the person can and cannot do unaided, the nursing interventions to achieve the mutually set goals could then be selected according to local circumstances and available resources.

Following implementation of the interventions, their effects could be evaluated in relation to the set goals, and if goals were not reached, they would then be revised or rescheduled, or even discarded. It is worth repeating that although discussed in four phases — assessing, planning, implementing and evaluating — individualising nursing is not a linear progression; it assumes a built-in responsiveness to feedback at any of the phases, with ample allowance for change within the overall framework.

During an illness episode, an important consideration is rehabilitation of the individual, and planning for this could commence almost as soon as the person enters the health system. Another important feature is the professional judgement needed to discontinue the nurse/patient relationship when it is no longer relevant.

This chapter has been concerned with the AL of mobilising. However, as stated previously, it is only for the purpose of discussion that any AL can be considered on its own; in reality the various activities are so closely related and do not have distinct boundaries. Figure 13.11 is a reminder that the AL of mobilising is related to the other ALs and also to the various components of the model for nursing.

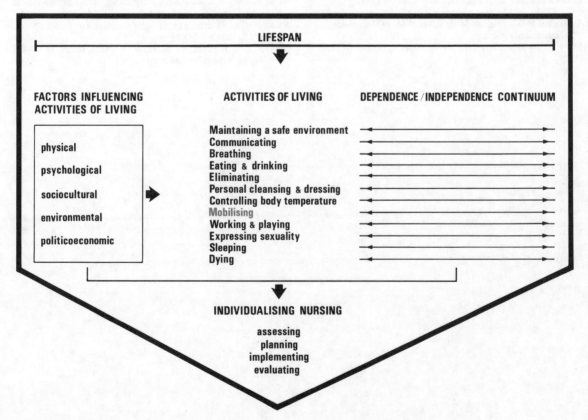

Fig. 13.13 The AL of mobilising within the model for nursing

REFERENCES

Brockie J 1987 Preventive treatment for bone loss. Nursing Times 83 (19) May 13: 56–57

Bryan J 1988 Backs and beyond. Observer Magazine July 3 (3): 32–39

Clements S 1987 And so to bed. Community Outlook September: 16–17

David J A 1986 Additions to the bed. Nursing: The Add-On Journal of Clinical Nursing 3 (3) March: 112–114

Dernham P 1986 Phantom limb pain. Geriatric Nursing 7 (1): 34–37

General and Municipal Workers' Union (GMBATU) 1984 Hazards in the health service — an A to Z guide. GMBATU, London

Harvey J 1987 Back to the drawing board. Nursing Times 83 (7) February 18: 47–48 (ergonomics approach)

Holmes P 1988 A world turned upside down. Nursing Times 84 (6) February 10: 42 (Bobath technique)

Horgan M G 1985 Low back pain and its management. Nursing: The Add-On Journal of Clinical Nursing 2 (44) December: 1298–1300

Howie C 1986 Back to basics. Nursing Times 82 (39) September 24: 18–19 (résumé of report from research at the University of Surrey)

Jayson M 1988 Back pain: the facts. Open University, Back Pain Association, Office of Health Economics

Nursing Times 1989 Elderly Scots more prone to fatal falls. Nursing Times 85 (5) February 1: 9

Pownall M 1987 Consensus on osteoporosis. Nursing Times 83 (45) November 11: 23

Raper M M 1985 Hyperactive children: play therapy. Nursing Mirror 160 (12) March 20: 19–21

Roper N 1988 The principles of nursing in process context. Churchill Livingstone, Edinburgh (p 40: hazards of bedrest; p 155–156: early ambulation)

Simpson G 1984 Ergonomic problems and solutions. In: Brothwood J (ed) Occupational aspects of back disorders. Society of Occupational Medicine, London

Stanley R 1988 Conducive to change. Nursing Times 84 (45) November 9: 37–39 (conductive education)

Stubbs D A, Buckel P W, Hudson M P, River P M 1983 Ergonomics 26: 767–779 (job design)

Walsh R 1988 Human kinetics: on the move. Nursing Times 84 (35) August 31: 26–28, 30

Whitwam L 1989 Arthritis: social problems and practical solutions. Nursing Times 85 (5) February 1: 36–39

Williams G 1989 Did she fall or was she pushed? Nursing Standard 19 (3) February 4: 22–24 (falls, abuse)

World Health Organization 1980 International classification of impairments, disabilities and handicaps: a manual of classification relating to the consequences of disease. WHO, Geneva

ADDITIONAL READING

Ansell B, Lawton S (undated) Your home and your rheumatism. Arthritis and Rheumatism Council, London

Boyle A M 1984 The adult hemiplegic patient — a functional approach. Nursing: The Add-On Journal of Clinical Nursing 2 (32) December: 952–954 (Bobath technique)

Devlin R 1984 The painful isolation of the district nurse. Nursing Times Community Outlook October 10: 356, 358 (staff shortages, lack of hoists)

Lambert J 1985 Adjusting to tetraplegia. Nursing Times 81 (6) February 6: 32–33

Lloyd P, Tarling C, Troup J D G, Wright B, Charlesworth D 1987 The handling of patients. Back Pain Association and the Royal College of Nursing, London

Maycock J 1985 Towards pain relief. Nursing Mirror 160 (3) January 16: 40–41 (methods of non-drug pain relief for rheumatic disease)

Price B 1986 Giving the patient control. Nursing Times 82 (20) May 14: 28–30 (a model of rehabilitation)

Rafferty A M 1988 Postoperative backache. Nursing Times 84 (46) November 16: 32–35

Tarling C 1984 Assessing mobility needs of the dependent person. Nursing: The Add-On Journal of Clinical Nursing 2 (32) December: 947–950 (mobility aids)

Walsh R 1988 Human kinetics: conflicting ideas of movement. Nursing Times 84 (36) September 7: 51–53

Walsh R 1988 Human kinetics: good movement habits. Nursing Times 84 (37) September 14: 59–61

Wood P 1987 A repetitive problem. Nursing Times 84 (7) February 17: 41–43 (repetition strain injury)

14

Working and playing

The activities of working and playing

Broadly speaking, most people spend about one-third of the day sleeping. For the remainder, a major portion of the day is used for 'working' and the free time left over is available for 'playing'. Work and play are complementary, and both are fundamental aspects of living. As the following discussion shows, the activities of working and playing have many dimensions and, according to the different stages of the lifespan, their nature and purpose are open to various interpretations.

THE NATURE OF WORKING AND PLAYING

Working is the word most commonly used to describe an individual's main daily activity and tends to be thought of first in terms of gainful employment. People work to earn an income in order to provide for the necessities of living, for themselves and their dependants. Because work is necessary, it is often thought of in a rather negative way. However, it is worth remembering that a job not only provides an income: it is also an important part of a person's identity and provides a sense of purpose and accomplishment, a structure to each day and the year, a source of company and a certain status in the family and in society. In these times of high unemployment, it is vital to recognise that many people are being deprived of these benefits as well as being denied the right to earn their living. Nevertheless, they — like others, such as schoolchildren, students, mothers at home, housewives, voluntary workers and retired people — would still describe much of their daily activity as 'work'. So, although discussion of the nature of the activity of 'working' inevitably focuses on gainful employment, the broader interpretation of the term should not be forgotten.

Even when work is for financial gain, remuneration is not the only consideration when choosing a job or career. For example, nursing is frequently chosen by those who wish to find a job which allows them 'to work with people'. Others pursue their jobs as an opportunity to use their hands or their intellect or particular qualifications; to be able to travel; or to become powerful. People who choose to do voluntary work see their purpose as giving service to the community. Women who choose to stay at home to look after children would describe their purpose in terms of their children's well-being. Whatever the job, be it paid or unpaid, prevention of boredom and meaningful use of time are basic reasons for working.

Work does not only affect the individual and the community; it also has national implications. All work involved in commercially producing goods or services represents the Gross National Product (GNP) of a country; and by implication, the more economically wealthy the nation, the more services it can provide, although which services and in what quantity and to whom is a political decision.

Playing is the term being used to describe what a person does in 'non-work' time. It is a convenient term because it emphasises that, by nature, 'playing' is the opposite of 'working' and it is an all-inclusive term which covers many other words such as leisure, relaxation, recreation, hobby, exercise, sport and holiday. In recent years as unemployment has grown, as retirement has come at an earlier age and as working hours have become shorter, so there has been increased interest in the use of leisure. Enjoyment and occupation are prime objectives in all forms of playing. However, for children, playing is also essentially a means of learning and development.

Playing is a universal activity of children and is absent only in conditions of extreme deprivation (Bateman, 1987). Through play the child learns about the surrounding physical and social environment and acquires many of the physical, psychological and social skills which are necessary to cope with independent, adult life. Adults pursue different types of leisure activities with different purposes — outdoor activities to breathe fresh air; sporting activities for exercise, slimming or competition; group activities for company; reading, theatre or musical activities for relaxation and enlightenment. Whatever the choice, enjoyment and prevention of boredom are the basic purposes of playing.

For some people, play becomes work: for example, there are sportsmen and women who earn their income as 'professionals'. Indeed, there are many examples of activities which can be one man's work and another man's play, illustrating that work and play are relative terms.

LIFESPAN: EFFECTS ON WORKING AND PLAYING

The inclusion of the lifespan in the model serves as a reminder that the way an individual carries out any Activity of Living varies throughout the stages of life. This is certainly true of the AL of working and playing and there is a change in the balance between the two activities at different stages of the lifespan.

In infancy and early childhood it is the activity of playing which assumes priority. The importance of purposeful playing in the development of physical, intellectual, interpersonal and social skills is undisputed. Play begins spontaneously and there is general agreement that its satisfactory development depends on continuing adult encouragement and the provision of suitable toys and play equipment. Four provisions are of primary importance — playthings, playspace, playtime and play fellows. There are many different types of play — ranging from the exploratory finger play of the young infant to imitative play, constructive play, make-believe play, games with rules, and hobbies. These different types of play emerge in sequence as the child first learns to use the five senses and body movement and then, later, the ability to communicate, interact with others and use creativity and imagination (Bateman, 1987).

Toys are the tools of play. They should be fun but should also present the child with some sort of challenge, while at the same time allowing a degree of success. Toys allow practice in object discrimination and exploration of shape, and a balance can be found between visual manipulation and intellectual function. By means of imaginative play, the child transforms objects and people into entities which best fit the existing structures of his thinking, . . . giving him a sense of mastery (Swanwick, 1985). Persistent day-dreaming and resort to a fantasy world, however, may be a form of escape from a stressful situation and may even be pathological.

Recognition of the importance of playing in early life has resulted in widespread provision of playgroups and nurseries for children of pre-school age. In primary school, there is little distinction nowadays between working and playing, for much of what is traditionally described as school 'work' is accomplished through 'play' activities. However, most people's perception of secondary school would include a clearer differentiation between 'working' and 'playing' activities. In the past, the emphasis was very much on preparation for work and acquiring qualifications for employment. However, in the context of high unemployment and with an increasing awareness of the need for preparation for all aspects of adult life, school education has taken on a broader perspective.

Nevertheless, the choice of, and establishment in, an occupation must be regarded as a central task of young adulthood. As Barnard (1981) points out:

The process of choosing a career and the period of adaptation to work or vocational training can be stressful. For many young people the transition from school to work is extremely uncomfortable. Their general education, at home and at school, may have been inadequate to prepare them for the world of work.

And in recent years, there have been increasing opportunities at school for what is termed work orientation; senior pupils spend time as observers in local factories, banks and other workplaces as part of the school curriculum.

In both the activities of working and playing, peak performance is usually reached in the years of adulthood. However, whereas young athletes may be past their peak by their 30s, at the other extreme there are people, such as judges and politicians, who do not reach their peak until an age when many people are retiring from work. The effects of the process of ageing on working and playing vary greatly according to the nature of the work and play, and the person's health and psychological outlook. Hammond (1981) highlights some of the different effects in relation to unskilled, semi-skilled, skilled and professional workers.

With retirement from work, there is more time for activities which fall into the category of 'playing'. Society now recognises the importance of providing suitable and varied leisure activities for older people so that mental and physical health is maintained. *Preparation for a healthy retirement* is now regarded as extremely important in view of the increased life expectancy. It is now accepted that people need to be educated about measures which can be taken to maintain health and prevent illness in retirement. Psychological readiness for retirement is also important and, increasingly, employers see it as a responsibility to provide pre-retirement courses so that people can prepare themselves to cope with the changes involved.

Garrett (1983) observes that withdrawal from gainful employment is a relatively new phenomenon. Although there is now an almost universal acceptance of the principle of retirement, in pre-industrial society the worker was expected to continue at his job just as long as he remained physically able. Garret says that for working class men, retirement is often associated with four 'losses' — the loss of social status and role; of companionship; of income; and of a meaningful lifestyle. Seen this way, it is not surprising that retirement is viewed as a negative event.

However, all 'work' is not necessarily linked to paid employment and there are many non-financial benefits of work which can be obtained in other ways in the post-retirement period.

So, it can be seen that the AL of working and playing undergoes considerable change as a person progresses through the stages of the lifespan. For most people, the lifespan is punctuated by significant work-related events — starting school, leaving school, starting work, changing jobs, gaining promotion and, ultimately, retiring. Though 'working' predominates in the adult years and 'playing' in the early years, both activities are an integral and important aspect at every stage of the lifespan, indeed especially in the working years, an imbalance can be detrimental to health.

DEPENDENCE/INDEPENDENCE IN WORKING AND PLAYING

The inclusion of the dependence/independence continuum in the model draws attention to the fact that there are periods in life when 'dependence' is to be expected and, at other times, 'independence' is the expectation, and this principle applies to the AL of working and playing. Children are dependent on adults for the development of skills in playing and the provision of playthings and, at a later stage, they are dependent on the education system for the acquisition of skills to equip them for working.

The so-called 'independence' of adulthood is largely due to the adult's ability to be financially independent, a state which is possible through income from working. By definition, a 'dependant' is a person who is not financially self-sufficient: a child is dependent on parents and an unemployed person may be dependent on state aid. Independence in playing allows the adult to make choices about leisure activities, including the choice to give up previously compulsory school sport and perhaps thus to jeopardise health through lack of exercise!

To a great extent, independent control of working and playing activities continues throughout the rest of the lifespan. Whereas some people would say that there is a loss of independence on retirement from work, others might argue that independence is actually increased. However, frailty and ill-health in old age may cause some loss of independence and necessitate dependence on others or on aids.

There are a number of reasons why people, at any stage of the lifespan, might be unable to achieve or maintain independence in the activities of working and playing. The main reasons — physical disability, mental handicap, mental illness and sensory loss/impairment — are discussed later in this chapter.

FACTORS INFLUENCING WORKING AND PLAYING

The nature of the AL of working and playing is multi-faceted, and as described earlier, there is variation in both of these activities in the course of the human lifespan. However, there is great variation in working and playing even among individuals of similar age because many factors can influence this AL. In keeping with the relevant component of the model, this section is subdivided into physical, psychological, sociocultural, environmental and politicoeconomic factors. The last of these is discussed in some detail in view of its importance to the subject of this chapter.

Physical factors

In infancy and childhood, the development of increasingly complex and varied play is closely related to physical growth and the maturation of the neuromuscular system.

Physique enters into the suitability of a person for some occupations, examples being a minimum height for policemen and a maximum weight for jockeys. Some jobs — such as those in heavy industry, those which are concerned with sport and others like nursing — require considerable physical fitness and energy while others do not, notably sedentary jobs such as working in a bank. People who work in the physically demanding occupations may experience considerable tiredness towards the end of their working lives, when physical fitness and energy decline in the process of ageing.

The capacity for both working and playing, at any stage of the lifespan, is obviously influenced by a person's state of physical health. Athletes and those who participate in physically demanding sport, either as professionals or amateurs, are considered to have reached a pinnacle of physical fitness, although it is a sad indictment on the concept of sport that so many instances are currently being identified where competitors are resorting to the use of steroids and hormones in an attempt to gain, for example, Olympic glory. Apart from the 'cheating element', continued use of such drugs can lead to 'bodybuilder's psychoses', mood disturbances and violent behaviour (Monmaney & Robins, 1988).

Any physical dysfunction in the form of, for example, obesity, heart disease, respiratory problems, musculoskeletal disorders and certain specific conditions, such as diabetes mellitus, may dictate that certain types of work and play are impossible or undesirable or necessary to regulate within certain limits. Physical disability or impairment of the senses, too, are important factors which influence this AL. Physically disabled people may need to be retrained for work within their physical capacity. Similarly the blind and the deaf need to choose work which is compatible with their disability. What disabled people choose to do in non-work time is influenced by the special facilities available to them. In recent years the scope of playing activities for the physically and visually disabled have increased, for example, riding, swimming, and cycling on tandem bicycles, though deaf people have fared less well and many are frustrated by inadequate leisure time activities.

Because of the many physical variables involved in working and playing, no specific biological system is aligned with this AL in the Roper, Logan and Tierney model.

Psychological factors

As described in the section on the lifespan, both purposeful playing in childhood and productive work in adulthood contribute to an individual's intellectual and emotional development and, indeed, to the development of their total personality. There are many different kinds of psychological factors which can influence a person's working and playing habits and preferences.

Level of intelligence is usually one factor in the type of occupation which the individual can satisfactorily follow, as are temperament and personality traits. These traits range from patience to impatience, from gregariousness to being a loner. No one is patient all the time but an impatient person is unlikely to enjoy working at intricate tasks or with ill people. Similarly a gregarious person usually enjoys being alone sometimes and a loner sometimes seeks the company of others, but a loner is unlikely to enjoy working with a number of people in the same room or constantly meeting new people as in nursing. It is hoped that career counselling will help people choose occupations suited to their particular attributes. Some occupations devise and use entrance tests in an attempt to reduce malplacement of new staff.

Level of intelligence, temperament and personality traits also play an important part in choosing leisure time activities. There is now a wide range of activities available, catering for most skills and tastes. If the desired choice is not available in the locality in which a person lives, it is usually possible to travel to a nearby centre offering the facilities at weekends and in holiday periods.

At work, lack of development in self-discipline can result in difficulties. Workers may fail to take adequate precautions in hazardous occupations, for instance construction staff not wearing safety helmets and nurses not using well-defined lifting skills and not taking adequate preventive measures in relation to infection.

Safety at work is a phrase which immediately conjures up the idea of physical safety but is also includes the less tangible but potentially harmful risk of working in an environment which is too demanding emotionally. Rogers & Salvage (1988) maintain that stress is a major occupational hazard, responsible for more time off work than accidents — in the UK, an estimated 37 million working days per year. The problems caused, they say, are not only the obvious ones such as headache or depression; heart disease, asthma, diabetes, peptic ulcer and many other 'physical' illnesses have been linked to stress. The word stress, say Rogers & Salvage, is normally used to describe an unpleasant feeling of too much pressure and a subsequent inability to cope; although those who have studied the subject in depth are usually careful to distinguish between 'stress' and 'dis-stress' — the associated harmful effects when stress is in excess of the optimum. As a rule, stress is associated with excessive pressure and overstimulation but it can also be caused by understimulation, and they quote Bond (1986) who makes a distinction between stress, stimulation and rest. Bond gives a working description of stress as 'the experience of unpleasant over- or under-stimulation, as defined by the individual in question, that actually or potentially leads to ill-health'.

Stress can occur in any occupation but Rogers & Salvage (1988) suggest some issues which contribute to stress in nursing and categorise them as *societal* stressors (domestic commitments, childcare, caring for dependants/relatives or neighbours, sexual harrassment, racism, homophobia); *employer-induced* stressors (workload, shiftwork, home/work conflicts, pay and conditions); *professional* stressors (daily contact with illness/death/disability/pain, lack of attention to individual development, inadequate role preparation, lack of professional autonomy, the speed of change socially and in the profession). They go on to suggest how personal coping strategies can help as suggested by Bond (1986), and how peer group support as well as counselling and education can contribute to alleviation of stress. Learning how to manage stress is immediately important, but the long-term strategy, of course, is to deal with the cause. However, some of the stress at work may be induced by non-work causes — a family crisis or incipient disease. Whatever the cause, the personnel officer and the occupational health nurse can often identify people at risk, and if the occupational health service does not have the necessary facilities or expertise, individuals can be referred to a suitable resource or advised to consult their own general practitioner. Gough & Hingley (1988) estimate that in the UK, 30 – 40 million working days are lost each year because of psychiatric and psychosomatic disorders, many of them resulting from stress.

So far, discussion of psychological factors has concentrated on people in work, but the absence of work has equally important psychological considerations. Unemployment can have severe consequences for the individual and the family. Not only is there the loss of financial independence, but also the loss of self-esteem and self-confidence; there are threatening and humiliating experiences when they apply for a job and are rejected, and there is a decline in social standing. The person is denied the opportunity to use existing skills and to develop new ones; and there is, too, the loss of social contacts. These losses can lead to feelings of frustration and anger, or to depression and a feeling of worthlessness, even to the point of contemplating suicide. Robertson (1986) talks of the 'learned helplessness' associated with unemployment — an identifiable syndrome in humans (and animals) when they cannot control the things which happen to them. It affects for example motivation, causing passivity, intellectual slowness and social impairment; it affects thinking, causing difficulty in relearning that actions can control the outcome; it affects emotion, causing depression and hopelessness.

Reviewing a series of 14 articles on unemployment in the British Medical Journal, Laurance (1986) summed up the findings — there are strong indications that unemployed people die earlier, especially by suicide, and suffer more mental and physical ill-health than those in work. In most surveys, about one-fifth of the unemployed report a deterioration in mental health since losing jobs (more anxiety, insomnia, depression, irritability and so on) and the longer unemployment lasts, the worse the health becomes. Families suffer too. Apart from the increased mortality among their wives, the evidence points to increases in divorce, domestic violence, abortions, unwanted pregnancies, and perinatal mortality.

Redundancy, too, or even the fear of it can have dramatic effects. Beale & Nethercott (1988) found that workers fearing job loss reported more illness, and their periods of absence were significantly longer, especially for men who had previously consulted their general practitioner infrequently. Discussing redundancy for over-55s, Laurance (1986) comments that for many, it seemed like an early death. However, the scene is not totally negative because Laurance indicates that 5% of unemployed people said their health had improved — some because they said they had escaped from miserable jobs, but others because they found positive aspects to unemployment. And Megranahan (1985) even refers to redundancy, for some people, as being 'a time when previously prohibited areas may be explored . . . perhaps revealing new areas of interest which may ultimately result in a new job.'

Although a different situation, retirement from work may cause reactions which are similar to the 'worthlessness' of unemployment (Moores, 1987). The syndrome is now well recognised to the extent that pre- and post-retirement assistance is available from statutory and voluntary sources although industry also now contributes; and there are many pre-retirement courses, services, benefits, workshops, and social and leisure activities available. They are planned to help people disengage from work and re-engage in leisure. Retirement from work can, undoubtedly, offer opportunities for self-development and continuing happiness well into old age, but coming to terms with the absence of work requires considerable psychological adjustment and, in turn, a new attitude towards playing.

Sociocultural factors

When the structure of society was less complex, both working and playing were centred round small, self-sufficient communities of families. For all members there was no differentiation between those people comprising the work, play and family groups. As society grew more complex, communities began to exchange different commodities and goods by the bartering method. Later money was used as the mode of exchange. The realisation that the commodities produced by one community were 'desired' by another created supply and demand which encouraged more organised trading systems resulting in intercommunity dependence.

These changes had significant effects on the activity of working. It often became necessary to leave the community to pursue one's work, thus the work group was differentiated from the family and play groups. The long process of industrialisation brought the gradual changeover from handmade to mass-produced goods, and from intercommunity to international trading systems, resulting in even further differentiation of the play, work and family groups, the basic groups from which a person obtains support and recognition. In most cultures the sex of an individual affects choice of work. There are preconceived ideas about the kind of work which only men and only women can do, not just as an occupation but also in the home. However, these attitudes are changing rapidly in many countries, and for example in the USA and the UK, it is illegal for advertisements to state the sex of the person required for the work. Also the current trend for both wife and husband to follow their occupations and the gradual acceptance of shared parental responsibility is changing the expectations of a man's 'work' in the home.

Similarly in many cultures there are games which are usually played by boys and others which are usually played by girls. However, it is likely that the currently changing attitudes toward adult work will have their effect on the games children (as opposed to boys and girls) will play in the future. Play is often an imitation of adult life and as the distinctions break down for adults so will they for children.

Religious factors can influence work and play; beliefs may preclude some activities in both. There are religions which do not permit drinking or gambling and adherents would not choose to work in industries associated with such pursuits. Followers of some religions, and some people because of secular beliefs, do not countenance for example abortion and would not therefore work in jobs connected with it. Some communities will not permit local factories to function on a Sunday. There are still some religious sects which forbid their members to dance, to visit cinemas and theatres, to listen to radio, to watch television and to read any book other than the Bible on Sundays.

In industrialised countries in general, there seems to be an increase in the incidence of violent crime and this was discussed in the chapter about Maintaining a Safe Environment. A feature which is relatively new to the social scene in the UK is the increase in the amount of violence at work. Hay (1987) makes the comment that one might expect it in banks, but not towards a housing estate caretaker, a nurse, a teacher or an unemployment benefits clerk. A Report by the Health & Safety Commission 1987 indicated that 1 in 2000 health service workers have been assaulted. Discussing possible reasons for such violence, Hay makes the point that, currently, people are bombarded with pressure to conform. If one is successful, there is no problem; if one is poor, then violence can become the way of taking things you need, as well as avenging yourself on a society which has deprived you of work or money.

The significance of work has come to be a crucial feature in industrialised countries and although it may seem a crude yardstick, the nature of the work contributed by each person is used by many governments to define social class. An example of this, as used in the UK, is given in Table 14.1.

Table 14.1 Social class by occupation

Social class	
I	Professional occupations
II	Intermediate occupations
III (N)	Skilled occupations: non-manual
III (M)	Skilled occupations: manual
IV	Partly skilled occupations
V	Unskilled occupations

Source: Registrar General's classification

Environmental factors

An infinite variety of environmental, including climatic factors, can affect working conditions. In fact to ensure that the workplace is as healthy as possible, legal requirements under the Health & Safety at Work Act (1974) place a duty on employers to protect the health and safety of the workforce, and on employees to comply with the various regulations. There are conditions which employers must provide and others which they are advised to provide for both indoor and outdoor workers. Examples are protective clothing for dirty work; pads for kneeling; gloves for handling hot materials; goggles to prevent not only strain from glare but also injury from sparks, hot metals and corrosive liquids; filters and masks in dusty industries and for the prevention of spread of infection; and the provision of a fluorescent garment wherever it is important for workers to be easily visible, for example on highways. And with the current heightened publicity about AIDS/HIV, there are specific guidelines (RCN, 1986) about maintaining a safe environment in the workplace, especially in relation to health care personnel.

Following the evidence of recent research, there are now also requirements to have 'no smoking' areas at work so that employees are not subjected to breathing smoke-laden air which, it has been proved, is injurious to health, and this topic is discussed in more detail in the chapter on the AL of breathing. In relation to the use of specific hazardous substances in the workplace, more recent legislation (Control of Substances Hazardous to Health, 1988) requires all employers to make, and usually record, a comprehensive assessment of all the risks of using such substances. In addition, there must be subsequent monitoring of concentrations of the substances in the air, and medical surveillance of the workforce. From January 1990, any work with such substances is prohibited unless as assessment has been made (Seaton, 1989).

The noise level, too, is subjected to control, for example noise associated with construction work, loudspeakers and equipment. Noise in the workplace — defined as unwanted sound — can cause stress, fatigue, loss of concentration, hypertension, and insomnia when it is prolonged or excessive, and a recent European Community directive has reduced the limit above which ear protection is compulsory (Rogers & Salvage, 1988). Payment of compensation for loss of hearing may be enforced by law when an employer can be proved to have been negligent.

Excessive heat at the workplace, whether climatic or environmental, increases sweating; salted fruit drinks may be needed to maintain the body's fluid balance. Although all workers are entitled to a morning and an afternoon break, a more frequent rest period helps to offset excessive fatigue and stress due to heat, both of which can increase the risk of accident.

Outdoor weather conditions can from time to time adversely affect indoor working conditions. For example large expanses of window can cause excessive cold in winter and excessive heat in summer as well as glare from the sun, resulting in a slower pace of working and potentially less tolerance of irritation. Icy roads increase risk of accident and injury for many, in particular transport drivers.

The effect of the work environment on women in the reproductive age group merits particular mention in view of the fact that, according to a UK government report (Martin & Roberts, 1984), women spend more of their lives in paid employment than ever before. It is difficult to assess the proportion of reproductive problems caused by occupational hazards — agents such as chemicals and radiation, and working conditions such as stress and heavy manual work — say Roger & Salvage (1988) but adverse effects can result in infertility, stillbirth, miscarriage, congenital abnormality and childhood cancer. Such environmental hazards may be relevant in a number of occupations but they go on to say that health workers are at greater risk because the majority are women. However, men, too, are at risk and lowered sperm counts, damaged sperm, loss of libido, and impotence have all been ascribed to adverse environmental conditions in the workplace.

Leisure time activities, too, reflect a region's climate and environment, sailing and hill walking being examples. Swimming is traditionally associated with hot weather and the sea, but nowadays swimming facilities are available in all weather conditions even thousands of miles from the sea. Similarly ski-ing was once dependent on the availability of snow-covered slopes but there are now artificial ski slopes in the environs of many large cities.

The importance of maintaining a safe environment for the activities of working and playing is discussed in some detail in Chapter 6, particularly in the section on 'preventing accidents at work' (p. 70) and 'preventing accidents at play' (p. 71).

Politicoeconomic factors

This section concentrates almost entirely on the 'working' aspect of this AL, with only a comparatively brief mention of 'playing'.

Work is the means by which an individual earns an income and the level of that income is a very important factor which influences many aspects of living. Social class is determined by the nature of a person's occupation (Table 14.1) and this, in turn, determines economic status.

Collectively, work is the basis of a nation's wealth. In the Western world, the process of industrialisation has been the main factor in creating wealth and currently contributes to the highly complex national and international economic systems. However, although industrialisation has been conducive to economic improvement, it has also helped to create poor working conditions and numerous social problems. In most industrialised countries therefore, over the course of many years, health and social systems have been developed to deal with the social ills, and employment legislation has been introduced to establish protective measures, for example:

- the minimum age at which a person can be gainfully employed
- the maximum number of hours to be worked per week in certain jobs
- alternative remuneration during unemployment or absence from work due to illness, injury or maternity leave
- the number of weeks of paid holiday
- the age at which there can be retirement from work on a pension

In any national economy which provides employment, health and social services, the relative numbers of certain population groups are of critical importance: children, workers, unemployed, workers absent because of illness/pregnancy and pensioners. These people are financially dependent, and the services have to be paid for by the earners.

For work a person receives remuneration in the form of a wage or salary, exceptions being voluntary work and the occupation of housewife/mother. In the UK, national insurance paid by the workers, and income tax paid by those with an income above a stipulated amount contribute to the total national income, part of which is used to finance services such as the National Health Service, unemployment and sickness benefit, and the retirement pension. There is great disparity, some would say inequity, in the level of income accorded to different occupations. The way in which income is determined is largely historical and any changes in pay structure, and any pay increases, are introduced by agreement of the employers, government and trade unions.

Contrary to the impression which may be created by the media, trades unions are not only interested in pay negotiations but, in various ways, act to safeguard the rights of employees. From a health and safety point of view unions are particularly interested in:

- identification of health hazards
- provision of a safe work environment
- provision of education for workers in an attempt to prevent accident and minimise risk
- surveillance of the workers' health
- collection of data to monitor the effect of health on work and vice versa

In the UK, the Health & Safety at Work Act (1974) and its subsequent amendments are important pieces of legislation which aim to secure the health and safety of workers, and various applications are mentioned in the chapter on the AL of maintaining a safe environment (p. 71). And in many countries, there is an occupational health service, employing nurses and doctors, which also plays a vital role in the promotion of health and safety at work. The nurses' role is essentially preventive and educational, though occupational health nurses deal with any accidents which occur and with certain treatment regimes; and they are also concerned with rehabilitation and resettlement at work after an extended absence due to injury or illness.

Resettlement of physically disabled people in work is a subject discussed in more detail later in this chapter (p. 280) but it is appropriate here to mention the role of the government in relation to this matter. There is a wide range of facilities provided to help disabled people to find and keep suitable work and, in the UK, these are mainly provided under the Disabled Persons Employment Acts of 1944 and 1958, and their subsequent amendments. From the individual's point of view, a key figure in the complex system is the Disablement Resettlement Officer who works closely with members of the health care professions. Another aspect of the Acts is the provision of a quota scheme whereby firms of a certain size are required to employ a percentage (presently 3%) of disabled people.

Help with deployment and re-employment is available, too, to the nonhandicapped and in many countries advice on employment is offered by guidance units sponsored by the government. Technological advances may mean that some workers in future will need to be trained for a second and possibly a third type of employment in a lifetime. High unemployment in certain occupations, and mid-career redundancy, are other reasons why more people nowadays may need to retrain in the course of their working lives. New attitudes towards working are becoming essential in these times. The age of retirement is reducing; the working week is shorter; more women are working outside the home than before; part-time work is becoming increasingly com-

mon; and the concept of job-sharing is gaining ground. Part-time work and job-sharing are ways of spreading the increasingly limited work available more equitably. As long ago as 1983, Tierney argued that nursing was one profession which appeared to have tremendous potential for a widescale introduction of job-sharing as already a substantial proportion of practising nurses worked part-time, a fact not surprising because the majority are married women; and Davies & Richardson (1988) describe a successful exercise in job-sharing in a community setting.

There is no doubt, however, that although decreasing, unemployment is a crucial politicoeconomic issue of our time. In the UK, the number of unemployed people is still high (just under 2 million in March, 1989) and many other Western countries too have high levels of unemployment. The way in which governments attempt to deal with the problem, and the way societies react to it and cope with it, will determine the nature of the activity of working for future generations.

High unemployment and, for others, reduced working hours and longer retirement, means however that people increasingly have more time for the activity which complements working — playing.

All schools encourage physical education and the foundation for enjoying leisure-time activities in adult life is also laid in various school classes, such as needlework, woodwork and music. Social reforms have resulted in provision by local government for community recreation and this includes adventure playgrounds for children and a range of sports and arts facilities to cater for people of all ages.

Although in relative terms more people nowadays have more time for leisure and more money, many recreational pursuits are expensive and this can be a problem for the lowest paid workers, parents with several children, single-parent families, students, the unemployed and pensioners. This fact is recognised for these groups who are often offered reduced rates for travelling, and for attendance at theatres and cinemas.

There is no doubt that, with less work, there will be greater emphasis on play. Education for leisure and the provision of adequate recreation facilities will therefore assume even greater political importance in the future since a bored society can so easily become a troubled and rebellious society.

However, in some developing countries, there is no question of seeking leisure; even the children cannot indulge in play. In 'Children of the dust' Jackman (1988) describes how in the brickworks of India, boys become men at 8 years of age, and die early. These children carry on their heads, about three tons of bricks over the course of a day. Despite a Child Labour Act 1986, which forbids the employment of children under 14 years in potentially hazardous occupations such as building and construction, these boys are literally 'beasts of burden for a few chapatis and a handful of rice' but the pittance they earn is vital to keep the family alive. These children will never know school or the luxury of playing; the family's survival depends on their working.

INDIVIDUALITY IN WORKING AND PLAYING

The model of living places great emphasis on the idea of *individuality*. A person's individuality in the AL of working and playing is the result of many different circumstances and influences. In attempting to draw up a profile of one individual's working and playing habits, consideration would have to be given to a vast array of topics. The list below draws together the range of topics which have entered into the discussion of the various components of the model and which are relevant in considering the idea of individuality in the AL of working and playing.

Lifespan: effect on working and playing

- Infancy   — type of play/playthings
- Childhood   — play and work in school/out of school
- Adolescence   — preparation for work
- Adulthood   — type of occupation and recreation
- Old age   — retirement

Dependence/independence in working and playing

- Dependence on others (e.g. children, disabled)
- Dependence on aids (e.g. disabled)
- Financial dependence (e.g. unemployed)

Factors influencing working and playing

- Physical   — physique
                   — physical fitness/energy level
                   — state of health/ill-health
                   — physical/sensory disability
- Psychological   — intelligence
                   — self-discipline and attitude to safety
                   — temperament and personality, reaction to stress
                   — fulfilment/boredom/motivation
                   — reaction to unemployment/ redundancy
                   — reaction to retirement
                   — balanced attitude to work/play
- Sociocultural   — sex differences
                   — cultural factors
                   — religious factors, secular beliefs
                   — social pressures at work
                   — social class by occupation
- Environmental   — climate and milieu for work/play
                   — hazards to health and safety at work/play
- Politicoeconomic — personal economic status
                   — health and safety at work acts
                   — employment of disabled people
                   — unemployment

Working and playing: patients' problems and related nursing

The time at which the day's work — whatever kind of work it is — begins and ends, are the two points around which the rest of the day is organised. During waking hours, when people are not 'working', they are 'playing'. These two activities then are an integral part of people's lives. However, the nature of the activities and their relation to one another varies at different stages of the lifespan and each person develops individuality in the AL of working and playing.

If individualised nursing is to take account of this aspect of a person's lifestyle, nurses need information about individual working and playing habits. Such information can be obtained in the course of nursing assessment by discussing with the person, in the detail and manner appropriate to the circumstances, topics along the lines summarised in the preceding section. While discussing relevant topics with the individual, the nurse might bear in mind the following questions:

- what kind of working/playing activities does the individual usually engage in?
- how much time does the individual spend working/playing, and when?
- where does the individual work/play, and with whom?
- what factors influence the individual's working/playing?
- what does the individual know about the relationship of working/playing to health?
- what is the individual's attitude to working/playing?
- has the individual any longstanding problems with working/playing and, if so, how have these been coped with?
- what problems, if any, does the individual have at present with working/playing or seem likely to develop?

The objective in collecting this information is to discover the person's usual working and playing routines; what can and cannot be done independently; previous coping mechanisms; and current problems.

Taking account of what is relevant, the information obtained about the person's working and playing habits is then recorded on the nursing assessment form. The information is examined to identify, in collaboration with the patient whenever possible, any problems with the AL of working and playing. The nurse may well recognise potential problems and these too will be discussed with the patient. Some patients' problems with this AL, although identified from nursing assessment, may well lie outwith the scope of nursing intervention. In such cases, after discussion with the patient, those problems may be referred to other members of the health care team, such as the doctor or social worker.

For those actual and potential problems with which nurses can assist, realistic goals can be set and nursing interventions to achieve these can be decided. The problems, goals and interventions are written on the patient's nursing plan, together with the date on which evaluation will be carried out. The steps described are those of the process of nursing, and all the activities mentioned are necessary if effective *individualised nursing* is to be achieved.

This systematic approach to nursing has already been applied to each of the eight preceding Activities of Living. But how important is it with respect to the AL of working and playing? Clearly there are circumstances, such as acute illness, when this AL assumes a low priority compared to others, such as the ALs of breathing, eating and drinking, and eliminating. However, in other circumstances, the AL of working and playing assumes considerable importance. Nurses who work in the fields of psychiatry and mental handicap do seem to have developed a better understanding of the significance of the AL of working and playing, both in terms of the structure of the patients' day and in terms of the therapeutic value of work and play activities as an integral part of treatment and rehabilitation. And, certainly, the importance of play is now widely recognised by nurses who work with children, whether in the hospital setting or in the community.

Yet in most general hospitals, the AL of working and playing is generally accorded a very low priority and it would seem to merit more attention than sometimes it appears to receive from nurses.

It is usual for nurses to know something about a patient's job and leisure interests. This knowledge is frequently used to initiate social conversation, thus indicating to patients an interest in them as individuals. The perceptive nurse is likely to realise too that events such as starting work, being made redundant and retiring from work constitute significant life events. Patients who have recently experienced these events may well be anxious or depressed and welcome additional emotional support from the nursing staff.

What may be less widely recognised is that enforced absence from usual working and playing routines can simply in itself be distressing for patients. Wilson-Barnett made this point as long ago as 1978 in a report of her study about the feelings and opinions of a group of patients in hospital. Many of the patients expressed negative comments on being away from their family and work, ranging from 'wondering what was going on without me' to 'being very bored without work' and 'missing my friends'. A reduction in income affected many self-employed men and fear of actually losing their jobs affected many, especially men over 40 years of age. Research findings like these are not really any revelation but, nevertheless, should help to remind nurses that patients do worry about work, and do feel sadness because of separation from family and friends.

There is also the problem of boredom. In most general hospitals there are few special facilities for patients to occupy that part of the day when they are not undergoing treatment. Gooch (1984) writing about anxiety and stress in surgical care, comments:

The anxiety of how to fill the time when one is denied the normal work or leisure activities can be very real. Boredom and frustration result in greater problems . . . A day-room with books, games and television can provide diversion for a short stay but more needs to be done for the long-stay patients.

It would seem to be important for all nurses to try to understand what absence from work and separation from friends mean to patients, and to use ingenuity in helping them to avoid feeling unduly bored and lonely.

Further discussion along these lines is developed in the section below which, as in previous chapters, considers some patients' problems which arise from the change of environment and routine imposed by the hospital setting. Following that, there is a section which considers some of the main causes of change of dependence/independence status in relation to the AL of working and playing. The final section of the chapter looks at the change in working and playing habit which results from drug/substance abuse and unemployment.

These three sections by no means cover the entire range of patients' potential and actual problems with working and playing, but should go some way towards helping readers to see how an understanding of these activities of everyday living can be applied in the context of nursing.

CHANGE OF ENVIRONMENT AND ROUTINE

A hospital is a very different environment from the surroundings in which people normally spend their day, working and playing. Although it may be true for some elderly or disabled people, it is unusual to spend all day in one place and people seldom sleep in the same place as they spend the day. So, it is not surprising that patients who are confined to a hospital ward for days, and sometimes weeks, may become tired by the monotony of their surroundings and bored by lack of the stimulation of variety. It is no wonder that patients often take an intense interest in the goings on around them, for they have little else by way of distraction. Another problem for patients in hospital, or indeed for people who are ill in bed at home, is that they are confined indoors.

Confinement to indoor environment

Most children are accustomed to playing out of doors for at least part of the time, and for them it is unnatural to be indoors all day in a confined space in hospital (Fradd, 1986). Similarly those adults whose working and playing activities take them outside for much of the time are likely to find confinement to a hospital ward particularly irksome. Whatever their occupation, there are few people who do not go outdoors for some part of each day, even if it is just travelling to and from work or going to the local shops or collecting children from school. Such outings have a specific purpose, but they also provide diversion, fresh air, physical exercise and the opportunity to meet and talk to people.

If nurses are to help patients to cope with the change of environment which results from hospitalisation, they must have information about the patients' usual working and playing habits in order to appreciate the results of deprivation and if appropriate, to plan suitable alternative activities. The day room is intended to provide an alternative and a more relaxing environment than the bedside area and is often equipped with television, books and games. In some wards, nurses and/or physiotherapists organise daily exercise sessions to compensate to some extent for the sedentary lifestyle which patients lead. Sometimes patients are able to walk about the hospital and if there are facilities for patients, such as a canteen or shop or library, nurses should make sure that patients know about them and where they are situated. Some hospitals have attractive grounds in which, health and weather permitting, patients can walk and sit at leisure and enjoy a change from the environment of the ward. Hospitals for psychiatric and mentally handicapped patients tend to have more spacious grounds but even in a built-up area area Fradd (1986) describes the effectiveness, for children, of a converted roof space at the top of the hospital which can be used both in winter and summer as an alternative to the ward.

Altered daily routine

It has already been mentioned that the activities of working and playing are important in that they provide a structure to each person's day. According to a person's occupation, the time at which work begins and ends each day determines the time of rising and going to bed, and the amount of time left for pursuing leisure interests. Hospital routine has become more flexible in recent years, but in some health care settings there could be good practical reasons for patients being expected to conform to regular times for example for rising, going to bed, and having meals. For the majority of patients this routine, even though different from their norm, is unlikely to cause undue upset, indeed for children and some elderly people, it may provide a reassuring framework for their day.

Nevertheless, everyone becomes anxious when faced with uncertainty so nurses should inform patients and relatives about the ward routine — other patients will doubtless inform newcomers about the flexibility or otherwise of the 'official' routine! On the subject of information-giving, Gooch (1984) writes:

To feel secure in their environment people must understand it and the part they themselves are expected to play in it. Patients are unlikely to ask directly for information about the ward environment so should be told what is to happen and when it is to happen, what they will be expected to do and when to do it. If they can discuss these things, they may feel more in command of the new situation.

Being encouraged and enabled to exercise control over their own lives is important to patients. In their everyday lives, adults make decisions and exercise choice as an integral part of working and playing. How difficult then, if, as patients, they are treated by nurses as though incapable of making decisions and taking initiatives. Nurses who have been patients may well have experienced the loss of self-esteem which results from such insensitivity. Male patients, especially those whose job gives them authority over others, may resent being dominated by young female nurses. Female patients who, as mothers, are accustomed to running a home and attending to the ceaseless demands of a family, might equally well be demoralised by being made to feel incapable of continuing to do as much as possible for themselves. Nurses not only create unnecessary distress by failing to recognise that patients have a need to cling to their accustomed roles and routines, but they do patients a disservice. After all, their established working and playing routines will hopefully be resumed and so, the less disruption there is, the easier rehabilitation will be and the more confident the patient.

How can patients be helped to incorporate their work and play interests into the daily routine of the hospital ward? For many people, having a daily newspaper, reading, watching the news or a favourite programme on television, listening to the radio or making telephone calls are regular daily activities. In hospital, the sale of daily papers, a trolley library service, television facilities, radio earphones and portable telephones are provided to help patients to continue with these activities.

There is no reason either, providing it is not detrimental to health and does not interfere with treatment, why patients should not continue with work activities if that is possible. Students might keep up with reading and writing essays; teachers might do marking; businessmen and women might be able to keep abreast with correspondence; and mothers might want to make shopping lists and menus, or continue to help with homework when children visit. Not all patients would be able to continue with work in this way, either because of the nature of their job or the severity of their illness. Some patients may need to be convinced that doing work or even worrying about it may jeopardise their recovery, and others may welcome the opportunity of 'doing nothing' for a change. Encouraging patients to do something to occupy the time may not always be in their best interest. However, skilled judgement is needed to assess when patients are ready and indeed should be encouraged to start occupying their time. Thoughtful yet simple acts can be helpful, such as introducing those patients with similar interests. Patients do appreciate the nurse who conveys a concern to prevent their day from being long and boring.

For children in hospital, an altered daily routine can be just as disturbing. Arrangements can be made for children of school age to have homework brought in so that the effects of absence from school are minimised, and also to provide purposeful occupation. In fact in long-stay paediatric units, school lessons may be available within the hospital and even, says Fradd (1986), in intensive care units. Links with local schools for ambulant patients are also mentioned by Fradd, who describes how school teachers will even accept children with intravenous infusions and drains in situ. She extols the value of schooling as one of the normal activities which should be encouraged in an otherwise unusual and unnatural routine.

The value of play to the sick child has long been recognised, says Belson (1987):

Play is not just a way of passing the time or keeping the young from being a nuisance. It is a vital factor in the intellectual, social and emotional development of every child . . . and the hospital must provide suitable play facilities supervised by a trained member of staff as an integral part of the treatment plan . . . the enjoyment counteracts in no small way the unavoidable and inevitable discomfort, pain and misery a child may have to endure.

Belson quotes the DHSS Report (1984) which indicates that children do not play with concentration or enjoyment when left to their own devices. Without assistance, many young children may become increasingly passive, or helpless in play. They may even stop playing altogether or do tasks well below their developmental level — a clear sign of an inability to cope. Recognising the significance of these findings, play coordinators and play therapists are now employed by many paediatric units but this does not mean that nurses have abdicated that part of their role; indeed, experience has shown that they become more skilled at helping children to play purposefully when a therapist is available. The child's feelings of fear, anger, hope and love can often be safely expressed in play. In special circumstances, even a visiting pet may have a part to play in assisting the child to keep in touch with normality (Fradd, 1986).

Absence from work and play groups

It is not only the loss of a familiar working and playing *routine* which patients find difficult but, equally, their absence from the *people* with whom they work and play. Apart from the family group (which is discussed separately below), work and play groups make up a major part of an adult's network of social relationships. Absence from work and play groups may cause emotional problems for a patient in that there is a lack of the day-to-day feedback which is so important as a source of feelings of acceptance and belonging. Since membership of one's play groups is from choice, they are probably chosen by most people to enhance self-esteem and self-confidence. Membership of the work group may result less from choice than necessity, and may be more or less rewarding. Furthermore when things are going badly in the work group, a person may rely more on the play group for reinforcement of self-esteem, and vice versa. The patient in hospital is thus denied the usual sources of company and emotional support and has to rely on staff and fellow patients instead. It is important that new patients are helped to feel a part of the ward group so that feelings of insecurity and isolation are decreased, and those of acceptance and support are increased.

The importance of the patient group as a source of mutual support is highlighted by Rowden & Jones (1983) in an article describing a nurse-initiated programme of diversional activities for patients with cancer. They wrote:

Patients in hospital are often bombarded with information by doctors, nurses and other clinical staff. On many occasions, we have seen interactions between patients which have eased anxieties about treatment, prognosis, investigations and a host of other subjects. However hard staff try to break down barriers between them and their patients, there will always be an intrinsic value in patient-to-patient contact. We believe our programme allows us to maximise the benefits of that contact in a positive and controlled environment.

The programme itself, for patients with cancer who were no longer receiving active treatment for their disease, was designed to divert the patients' attention in a positive way, and to provide entertainment and relaxation.

The variety of activities — video, concerts, sport, games and relaxation techniques — enabled both individual and collective needs to be taken into account, as did the flexible timing of the programme. The more traditional activities, such as basket weaving and carpentry, were also available to the patients and the occupational therapy department and other service departments within the hospital collaborated with the nurses on a team-work basis. Concluding their article, the authors commented:

Through our programme . . . we believe we can begin to offer choices which reinforce the importance of individuality as a hospital inpatient. That process is as important as every investigation or drug that we give our patients in determining the quality of his return to a healthy life outside hospital, independent of others.

This example shows that the effects of absence from work and play groups can, to some extent at least, be lessened if the patient group is seen as a means of providing companionship, occupation and support during the period of hospitalisation.

Absence from family group

Play is certainly important in the child's life, but even more so is the family. An understanding of the adverse effects of separation of children from their parents has resulted in open visiting being the norm, with parent care much in evidence (Sawley, 1987). In fact Fradd (1986) considers that families should be involved not only in the ward but in all departments of the hospital where children have treatment including casualty, intensive care and the anaesthetic and recovery rooms. Fradd describes the success, in one unit, of appointing an auxiliary to be responsible for the needs of resident parents — arranging the sleeping accommodation, providing meal vouchers, organising a tour of the hospital, and, in general, befriending the parents. Visits from siblings should not be forgotten; the separation can sometimes inflict on them as much anxiety as it causes the patient.

Children can also be very distressed when an adult member of the family is being taken to hospital. This is now recognised and it is government policy in the UK that children should be allowed to visit adults and relieve the nagging fear that the person has gone away and left them (p. 337). As long ago as 1859 Florence Nightingale wrote:

There is no better society than babies and sick people for one another. Of course you must manage this so that neither shall suffer from it which is perfectly possible. If you think the 'air of the sick room' bad for baby, why it is bad for the invalid too, and therefore, you will of course correct it for both. It freshens up a sick person's whole mind to see 'the baby'. And a very young child, if unspoiled, will generally adapt itself wonderfully to the ways of the sick person, if the time they spend together is not too long.

Notes on Nursing

Visiting, and being visited, is very important in the case of children and so it is for adults. For any patient who belongs to a family, absence from it on account of being in hospital can be a distressing and traumatic experience. Though using the term 'family' here, it needs to be remembered that not all patients have a family and, even if they have, it should not be assumed that members of the family are necessarily the most important people to the patient.

For these reasons, the nurses should find out who are the 'significant others' for each individual patient. It is also important for nurses to appreciate that the separation not only affects the patient, but equally those who have been left at home. Sometimes they may experience considerable difficulties while the patient is in hospital: for example, the young husband who has to take over running the house and looking after the children when his wife is admitted; or the elderly woman in poor health who, deprived of her husband's help, is trying to cope on her own. These are just two examples but serve to illustrate the general point that absence from the family group during hospitalisation does affect the patient, but also affects the rest of the family. Hospital visiting is, therefore, a facility which is important to both parties — the patient being visited and the family members and others who are the visitors. In some circumstances, it may not be possible to visit, of course, and a phone call may be a good substitute. Being visited in hospital can, however, be a rather strange experience. At home, the person has some control over who visits, when and for how long. When a patient is in hospital, this control is usually forfeited. The visitors can also find the experience somewhat strange because, after all, a hospital ward does not afford either privacy or comfort; it is busy and often noisy; and to some people it is an intimidating, even frightening environment. For both parties then, hospital visiting may be somewhat stressful but it is an important means of minimising the effects of the patient's absence from the family group.

The norm was for hospitals to have specific daily visiting hours and often a rule that there may be only two visitors per patient at any given time, but the trend now favours more liberal and more flexible visiting hours.

Discussing visiting, Darbyshire (1987) makes the point that separating patients from their families is a feature of our culture; in many parts of the world, it would be considered a strange practice. The authority of the hospital to exclude visitors has, of course, been more stridently questioned with the growth of consumerism. Tracing the visiting practices of relatives over several decades, Darbyshire notes the advent of a more enlightened attitude in children's hospitals, and in psychiatric and mental handicap hospitals some time before more liberal and flexible arrangements were made in general hospitals. Current concepts of health care are moving closer to accepting the basic notion of patient autonomy, about visiting as in several other issues, yet in a survey of general medical and surgical wards, when 404 out of 430 hospitals answered, the mean number of visiting hours per day was 4.2, ranging from 1.7–6.1 (Griffith, 1988).

Highlighting the significance of visiting, Ralphs (1988) refers to a study where patients' views about hospital life were sought; it was found that 'visiting hours, along with meal-times, were the most important and looked-forward-to part of the day'. However, the point is made that some people are naturally good at visiting and are enjoyed by the patient, whereas others made their visits tiresome to all concerned. He provides a table featuring the attributes of 'good' and 'bad' visitors and goes on to quote Grollman — 'visiting is like a medicine; useful and pleasant at certain times, but can become toxic at higher levels'. Ralphs suggests that nurses can prevent visiting times from becoming 'toxic', and that they have a role to play in ensuring that patients can derive maximum benefit from such important events.

For a flexible policy to succeed, however, there has to be adequate extensive preparation of the staff and the public. It was not intended that visitors (even near relatives) should visit continuously from early morning till late at night. Some relatives who interpreted 'free visiting' in this way felt guilty if they did not stay, and if they did, they found it a marathon task. It was merely intended that patients and their relatives could have mutual choice about the time and duration of visits, subject to staff approval. It was hoped that this would spread the number of visitors in a ward at any one time and the staff could continue their ministrations to those patients who were not being visited at that time.

Also with visitors spread over a longer period it could afford both visitors and staff a much better opportunity to communicate with each other. For each ill person there are anxious relatives and friends who need information, not only to keep their anxiety within reasonable limits, but also to teach them how they can help their ill relative to recover or to die peacefully. Each dying patient has special visiting needs; if conscious the patient's wishes should be granted; if unconscious, it is the relatives who need information and consideration about whether or not to stay at the bedside.

There are a few occasions when a patient may need to be 'protected' from large numbers of visitors, for example a patient who is breathless and distressed, but while acknowledging that there can be problems associated with liberal hospital visiting Gooch (1984) argues in favour of this system. She writes:

Why are families considered to be 'visitors' merely because one of their number has become a patient . . .? Relatives are part of the patient's care and therefore *belong* in the ward whenever they wish to be there.

There are of course some patients whose family may not be able to visit and for them, communication by phone and letter may help to compensate for lack of visiting. Other patients, for instance the elderly, may no longer have a family group and nurses can help by discussing with them whether they would like to take advantage of any of the voluntary visitors' schemes, should these be available in the area.

In conclusion, the objectives of hospital visiting are to enable contact to be maintained between members of the family group; to make the patient's day more meaningful; and to provide mutual benefit and pleasure for both patients and their visitors. Nurses are in a strategic position to help in the achievement of these objectives, whatever visiting policy is adopted by the institution.

CHANGE OF DEPENDENCE/INDEPENDENCE STATUS

Independence in the activities of working and playing is regarded as the desirable norm for adults. Clearly, then, those who are unable to achieve or retain independence are disadvantaged members of society. In any country there are some people who are unable to work and, therefore, are financially dependent on their families and/or the state. There are many different reasons for lack or loss of independence and here these are categorised as physical disability, mental handicap, mental illness and sensory loss/impairment. An understanding of the causes and effects of dependence in the activities of working and playing is a relevant part of nursing knowledge. There are many different circumstances in which nurses can contribute to helping people to achieve their optimal level of independence in work and play activities.

Physical disability

Obviously there will be a difference in the difficulties experienced in gaining or maintaining independence for working and playing depending on the nature of the disability and the body systems affected. Disease of the cardiopulmonary system can render a person so breathless and short of oxygen that 'work' is impossible and entertainment only of the passive variety is possible. On the other hand, many of the chronic disabling diseases affect the nervous system and the musculoskeletal system, and the patient's work and play problems are in fact mobilising problems. Depending on the person's previous working and playing activities, the degree of dependence caused by the disability will vary and there will need to be more or less adaptation. The outdoor worker and the active sports enthusiast may well find it difficult to settle for sedentary work and more passive leisure time activities. If the sedentary workers can be rehabilitated to an 'independent' wheelchair life, they are more likely to be able to resume their previous work.

Prior to the 1970s there was legislation in the UK about people disabled when in the armed services or following industrial accidents, but legislation affecting the so-called 'civilian' population was extremely limited; the single factor which influenced provisions for improving their daily lives dramatically was the Chronically Sick & Disabled Persons Bill of 1970 (Greaves, 1981). Thereafter, in fact, all legislation affecting the general population has been scrutinised to ensure that equality of opportunity is provided for disabled people, for example in relation to education, housing, transport and employment. Further publicity was given, worldwide, to the plight of disabled people when the United Nations Organization launched the International Year of Disabled People in 1981 and great emphasis was given to their rights including the right to secure and retain employment, and the right to enjoy recreation.

Discussing the employment of disabled people, Darnbrough & Kinrade (1981) maintain that many disabled people are additionally handicapped by prejudice, discrimination, lack of opportunity and sheer callousness. In fact, they say, disabled people are only too well aware of their disability and will often prove far more conscientious and hard-working than their able-bodied counterparts. They quote research which shows they are less likely to be absent from work, less likely to have accidents, and are just as productive or more so. The Chronically Sick & Disabled Persons (Amendment) Act 1976 further improved matters with regard to access to work (both to and within premises), parking facilities and sanitary arrangements.

An individual may be disabled from birth, or may become disabled because of disease or injury, and for the latter, following a period of rehabilitation, the Disablement Resettlement Service and the contact of the Disablement Resettlement Officer (DRO) are important factors on the road to re-employment. With the advances in electronics and technology, it is possible to place even severely disabled people in open employment but some may only be able to function in sheltered employment. Sheltered workshops may be operated by a voluntary organisation, a local authority or a government-sponsored, non-profit-making company.

Physical disablement not only changes a person's independence status for working, but also affects playing. Increasing awareness of the needs of disabled people in this respect has led to the development of special sports facilities and international sports events are now organised in just the same way as they are for able-bodied sportsmen and women. Cotton (1983), in his book *Outdoor Adventure for Handicapped People*, makes the point that the only difference between the handicapped and the normal person is their degree of ability, and that 'adventure' does not need to involve climbing mountains. Swimming, sailing, canoeing, fishing, riding, camping, and snow sports such as tobogganing, are all possible and all offer the excitement and stimulation which result from the challenge of adventure. Other handicapped people, again no different from normal people, may prefer to choose more passive, indoor leisure pursuits. Nowadays, theatres, cinemas, art galleries, restaurants and hotels are becoming better equipped — and in new buildings, intentionally designed especially in relation to physical access, and access to toilet accommodation — to enable physically disabled people to make use of and enjoy these facilities.

In a UK survey conducted for the government by Martin et al (1988) it was estimated that 6.2 million people suffer from some disability, the definition being 'any restriction or lack of ability in performance of activities arising from an impairment'. The comparatively low threshold of disability used in the survey means, says the report, that sweeping conclusions must be avoided, for instance that all those included 'are unable to support themselves, or are unable to lead normal lives, or are necessarily dependent on services or social security benefits'. Among the main findings were that over 1 million adults are in the lowest severity category of the 10 defined, and only 200 000 in the highest category; and almost 70% of the disabled adults were aged 60 years or over. This is the first part of a series of national surveys which will provide information about people in the population who are disabled, and will include up-to-date data about issues such as employment.

Mental handicap

By definition, mentally handicapped people may be expected to be less independent in the AL of working and playing than others within society, but they too have the need for the satisfaction and occupation of time which are obtained from working and playing. In industralised societies, 'work' has become so complex that there has tended to be an almost unquestioned assumption that someone who is mentally handicapped is incapable of working. However, this can be seen to be a false notion if a logical view is taken. All but the most severely handicapped are quite capable of work which does not necessarily demand a high level of intellectual capacity. Domestic work, work with animals, gardening and horticulture, farming and repetitive industrial jobs are examples of the kind of work which many mentally handicapped people are perfectly capable of doing. And contrary to many expectations, some have talent in areas such as writing and art which tend to be viewed as more intellectual than physical.

Working is part of normal adult life and the principle of 'normalisation' for mentally handicapped people is based on the argument that they too have the right and the need to work. To cope with the demands of work in contemporary society, this means that they require education and training for work. In the UK, where the emphasis is shifting from institutional care to community care, there has been an increase in the provision for mentally handicapped people of what are called 'adult training centres', and also of 'sheltered workshops'. Opportunities for the more able mentally handicapped person to be employed under normal working conditions are still limited but are being actively pursued. The 'eternal child' adult image still prevails so they become the victims of overprotection, for example, they are not allowed to take the normal risks involved in using machinery, working in a kitchen, and crossing roads. As a consequence, they are effectively denied many of the activities of normal living, made to feel more dependent than necessary, and segregated from the rest of society. Mental handicap is a social handicap. However, even when employers adopt a more enlightened attitude, mentally handicapped people are unlikely to fare well in the competitiveness which a state of high unemployment has created in many industrialised countries.

For people who are so severely mentally handicapped as to be unable to achieve sufficient independence to live in the community, countries vary as to the type of residential provision which is made for them. Some utilise the model of a village with a group of houses, a workshop, shops and a village hall for sports and entertainment. Other countries care for the mentally handicapped in hospitals, the system which has operated in the UK. Nowadays, in mental handicap hospitals considerable emphasis is placed on the residents' need for productive occupation. Hence, there are occupational therapy and industrial therapy units in most hospitals with the aim of giving a sense of purpose and satisfaction, and providing a small monetary income. Much attention has always been paid to the social side of life, and sports and entertainment of increasing diversity provide the opportunity for regular playing. However, more recently there has developed an awareness that play can be exploited to therapeutic advantage too.

Roberts (1984) looks at the impact of play on communicating with mentally handicapped children. After discussing the value of play for all children, he goes on to say that for those with a mental handicap, it has two special functions—training in coping skills, and as a preparation and neutralisation for anxiety-provoking experiences. He explains that while, as a rule, play is spontaneous, one of the features of mental handicap is that the spontaneity is reduced or absent. So when playing with these children it is important to choose a topic which the individual can enjoy; ensure that the enjoyment span is not exceeded (it is shorter than the attention span); give the child the opportunity to join in the fun and interact with others; and allow play to involve small groups.

Children who are mentally handicapped can enjoy the same types of play as other children — exploratory, energetic, skilful, social, imaginative, puzzle-it-out play—although the last two may be reduced or absent in children who are severely handicapped. Different media can be used such as water play, sand play, music, painting, rough and tumble play, large ball games, adventure playground, and short tricycle journeys under supervision. Some units for mentally handicapped people have a toy library although quite ingenious toys can be created often at low cost. Roberts (1984) describes a game he devised, using the Makaton language which he called Makatony and he outlines the materials required, the rules, and the positive reactions of some staff and children who used the game. Toys and games of course are only an aid to play and Benicki & Leslie (1983) write:

Surrounding the child or handicapped adult with play equipment is not sufficient; the impetus must come from the staff to encourage and demonstrate the use of the toy, and reward must be given when interest is shown. Play . . . fosters communication, intellectual development and social interaction.

Toys can be said to be tools to aid this development; the right toys at the correct moment can improve and extend these skills.

In relation to adult mentally handicapped patients, Benicki & Leslie comment that nurses often seem to be uncertain as to the appropriateness of play as an activity and again they emphasise:

Toys alone are insufficient; to offer them to a mentally handicapped adult who has no concept of play will only cause frustration and subsequent rejection of the equipment. Staff must be willing to show interest, understanding, and patience to motivate and develop play skills . . . Play can help to overcome many of the secondary handicaps or problem areas projected by the residents; lack of motivation, poor concentration, difficulties in hand-eye co-ordination, balance and movement difficulties, or general lack of physical co-ordination.

Nowadays, play and recreation for handicapped people is not only recognised at local and national levels. Teams from several countries attended a special Olympic Games held in the UK in 1986. Vousden (1986) describes how nearly 1000 contestants who had a mental handicap competed over 4 days, watched by 15 000–20 000 spectators. The games included track and field athletics, gymnastics, swimming, football, hockey and bowls. He maintained that participants derived exactly the same sort of enjoyment and sense of achievement as any others involved in sport, and makes the point that the spectators were helped to overcome some of their prejudices about people with a mental handicap. It is expected that these Games will become a regular event.

Playing, then, is a means of increasing independence and it, like working, is an important dimension of the lives of people who are mentally handicapped.

Mental illness

Some people experience difficulty in gaining or maintaining independence for working and playing because of mental illness. Among the more commonly occurring features of mental illness are excessive anxiety, depression, phobias, obsessional thoughts or behaviour, delusions, confusion, overactivity or apathy, aggression, loss of confidence, forgetfulness, dependence on alcohol and disturbed personal relationships. It is not difficult to appreciate that these kinds of psychological difficulties can diminish a person's independence for the activities of working and playing.

In fact, it is a characteristic of mental illness that the person is unable to plan or enjoy leisure, and leisure activities which include social contacts are unsuccessful because the individual is not at ease in the company of others. Discussing the problem, Altschul & McGovern (1985) describe various ways of re-introducing the mentally ill person to enjoyment of leisure. In some hospitals, for example, volunteer groups and patient groups, along with nursing staff, organise social activities such as imitation of radio and television games, amateur dramatics, keep fit classes, and dancing. Associated with such social events, the patients can be encouraged to dress carefully and take time with their general appearance — the AL of personal cleansing and dressing and the AL of expressing sexuality — which assists them to recover a sense of personal dignity and boosts morale. According to the patient's usual interests and inclinations, of course, it could be more appropriate to indulge in less vigorous leisure pursuits such as games of draughts, chess and cards, or listening to records, or watching television.

Assisting patients to recover an interest in leisure is, however, a considerable art. It is not helpful if the staff are too organising; the patient should be involved at every stage of the planning and deciding (Altschul & McGovern, 1985). The degree of organisation by staff and the degree of participation by the patient can be graded starting with spectator activities which the patient can share passively, then on perhaps to community singing where the person is one of a crowd, then eventually to personal performance, for example in a theatre group. And as recovery progresses, it is desirable to make provision for more unorganised time involving activities such as reading the newspaper or a book, writing letters, conversing with others and enjoying more privacy — as occurs in everyday living. Psychiatric hospitals now operate, as far as possible, like a normal community with a shop, hairdressing salon, coffee bar so that the patient can have practice in decision-making and community living, including leisure and work activities.

Some patients, however, have spent many years in psychiatric hospitals and many of these institutions are old, large and cut off from the local community — a most abnormal environment for a member of society whose basic social unit is the nuclear family. The adverse effects of 'institutionalisation' were first noticed in long-term psychiatric wards. At first it was thought that the patient's tendency to become so apathetic, withdrawn and dependent was a result of the psychiatric illness itself. Then it was realised that the behaviour was actually the effect of the patient's resignation to the unchallenging and unchanging institutional environment. The syndrome was described by Barton in 1966 as institutional neurosis, characterised by a stooping gait, vacant facial expression, little interest in personal appearance and general inactivity. Such people appeared so uninterested that staff were unaware of the individual's abilities and mistakenly, answered and acted for them. It is now realised, of course, that a realistic programme of rehabilitation, including work and leisure, is needed.

The cooperation of family and visitors is an important facet of such rehabilitation, the patient going out with them to practise living in the community. They often need to relearn how to use money; they have become unfamiliar with the price of food, the cost of a bus or train fare, how much it takes to buy clothes, or purchase a gift.

Valuing money is associated with work, and Altschul & McGovern (1985) consider work to be an essential therapeutic tool, especially if the person is paid. As well as helping the patient to cope with financial affairs, it helps to restore self-esteem. Some hospitals provide occupational therapy departments with craftsmen to grade and supervise the work undertaken, thus helping to ensure that the patient adopts realistic aims because, initially, it is necessary to protect such patients from the consequences of failure. A number of hospitals provide industrial training, have their own workshops, and negotiate contracts related to industrial assignments for which patients receive normal rates of pay. By so doing, the patients develop work habits; clock in and out; have rest pauses; observe trades union practices and work organisation; accept correction and may have to give orders to subordinates — all of which contribute to a realisation of self as opposed to the submission of being a patient. Work is highly regarded in the West and unemployment causes distress (p. 286) so assisting mentally ill people to resume work practices can contribute considerably to their rehabilitation in the community. Some such patients are not so able, however, and it may be possible for a hospital in a rural area to organise gardening or farming work.

In the UK, the trend in the 1980s has been to encourage the rehabilitation of long-stay patients into the community (Corke, 1989). Group homes are often used where, with some supervision, such people can become accustomed to housekeeping, cleaning, shopping, cooking, and entertaining friends in a normal setting. Eventually some people graduate from these group homes to live unaided in the community. Some may acquire employment on their own merit or qualify for retraining at Employment Rehabilitation Centres; others may be employed under the Disabled Persons (Employment) Act of 1944 which makes it compulsory for certain employers to engage a percentage of registered disabled people, and psychiatric disabilities qualify. On the other hand, they may work in sheltered workshops, or they may live outside but come back to the hospital to work. Whatever method is used, the objective is to help the long-term patient to become as independent as possible. Doing this utilises the concept of each individual having a dependence/independence continuum for each AL as described in the model of living and the model for nursing.

Of course, finding suitable employment after discharge depends on the current economic state of the country as well as the labour market, and psychiatric patients may be particularly vulnerable. Mental illness is likely to lessen an individual's ability to secure a job and, if employed, to continue to function satisfactorily at work.

Quite apart from the type of rehabilitation programme just described, the treatment and care of mentally ill people has changed considerably over the years; for those who are newly diagnosed and for those who have acute episodes.

The availability of treatment by tranquilliser drugs and anti-depressants has meant that many people can be helped, or at least the symptoms sufficiently controlled, without the necessity for admission to a psychiatric hospital or even much time off work. Behaviour therapy can be provided on an out-patient basis, as can psychotherapy and counselling, and being encouraged to continue with regular working and playing activities may in itself be therapeutic.

Sensory loss/impairment

In the chapter dealing with the AL of communicating, some of the difficulties encountered by people who have dysfunctions related to speech, hearing and sight are discussed (p. 117–119). For most people so affected, these difficulties are reflected in their capacity for work and play.

Most people who become *blind* are faced with changing their occupation. Those who have the necessary ability and aptitude can be encouraged to take special training courses, for example in typing, machine sewing and physiotherapy. There are also various craft courses which can be undertaken in the workshops for the blind. Most people with acquired blindness will be able to continue independently some of their playing habits, and with help from the various organisations for the blind, can continue others in a modified form, for example reading journals in Braille, listening to tape recordings of books, using Braille playing cards, and take advantage of new facilities made available because of the computer age (p. 119).

Gradual onset of *deafness* may permit a person to learn to lip read and to make preparation for future working. Some can continue with their previous employment, but there are many types of work which require a person with adequate hearing. When it is possible, there should be preparation for enjoying leisure time when eventually all hearing is lost. Nurses can encourage patients to develop suitable physical activities in which they are interested and help them to decide about visual activities which can be pursued by deaf people.

Impairment of *speech* will cause considerable problems since for most people verbal communication is an essential part of working and playing. The problem of aphasia commonly results, in addition to paralysis, from a cerebrovascular accident. Whether it is mainly expressive or receptive (p. 117), or a mixture of the two, it will interfere with their ability to communicate. Nurses can be guided by speech therapists as to the ways in which they can help these patients to improve or regain their ability to communicate while working and playing.

CHANGE IN WORKING AND PLAYING HABIT

A change in dependence/independence status for the activities of working and playing often results, as is apparent in the foregoing section, in a change in habit. For example,

chronic disabling disease which causes physical disability is very likely to necessitate a change in both working and playing habits. In this section, the two problems discussed — drug substance abuse and unemployment — do have links with the concept of dependence/independence. However, primarily they result in change of working and playing *habit* and for that reason are placed here.

Change due to drug/substance abuse

Experimentation with drugs and various substances which can be abused usually starts in relation to leisure time activities. In many countries it seems to be part of present day culture and indeed some people look on it as part of growing up. Adolescents claim that the selected 'substance' makes them feel excited and allows them to experience heightened awareness. It could be argued that no one has the right to deprive another of such experience which is a precious part of living, but many people experience the full impact of their emotions in heightened awareness without resorting to such activities.

However, if adolescents start abusing these substances as leisure time experimentation it can, perhaps insidiously, have an effect on working habits. Perhaps they find that they cannot discipline themselves to arrive on time, to take the necessary precautions while at work and to complete the scheduled amount of work before leaving. So they continue to resort to these substances.

Yet another group who indulge in substance abuse do so as a reaction to stress at work. For some reason, perhaps too heavy a work load, members of this group are not managing and work piles up to the extent that it becomes unmanageable. One way of tackling the problem would be by adjusting the work load but conscientious people often find it difficult to admit to those in authority that they are not managing. To gain some respite they indulge in substance abuse, only to find it does not solve the problem but brings others in its wake.

This complex problem is something about which nurses should have knowledge as they, along with other health care professionals, have a part to play in prevention through health education of the public, especially youngsters.

Substance abuse is not new. Cameron (1987) reminds us that down through the ages, man has experimented with a variety of substances. The Ancient Greeks used incense for religious ceremonies, for example, and chloroform has an interesting history of recreational usage. During this century, substances such as amyl-nitrate and transmission fluid have been abused in the USA, as has glue-butane gas in the UK, and coca leaves in some South American countries.

Nowadays, a staggering number of substances are being abused, continues Cameron. These include aspirin combined with Coca Cola; banana skins, generally grilled and smoked in a cigarette; table tennis balls, bin liners and plastic containers, often burned over a smoking fire and sniffed; and inhalation of fumes from substances such as hair lacquer and shoe polish. Over-the-counter drugs, too, can be abused, for example cough expectorants, codeine, and travel sickness pills. When these or more potent drugs are not available, youngsters gravitate to the use of solvents and every shop, home, handbag and jacket is a source of solvents. Moreover, they are cheaper than drugs, so infinitely more accessible. To provide an overview of the problem, a few of the main groups of 'abused' substances are mentioned below.

Solvent abuse. The term solvent abuse has come to be used in place of 'glue sniffing' or 'fume sniffing'. Cameron describes how a solvent intoxication session may last only an hour, although for chronic abusers it may extend over 48 hours, when they will inhale, then sleep, then resume inhaling. The method of inhalation varies according to the substance. Glue is usually put into an empty crisp bag, placed over the nose and mouth, then sniffed; butane gas is often inhaled from a gas lighter refill cannister, the nozzle of which is put against the teeth and pressed, thereby spraying the back of the throat; hair lacquers and sprays are inhaled after several cans have been sprayed into a small room, where gaps in windows and doors have been sealed.

Headache and nausea are two common complaints after a solvent intoxication session but more serious complications can occur such as damage to cardiac muscle, respiratory failure, convulsive disorders, memory failure, renal failure and psychotic disorders. More immediate damage may occur, too, because while under the influence of the solvent, abusers can be asphyxiated; some have been known to indulge in bizarre and dangerous behaviour such as jumping out of windows or trying to climb high walls; and following a severe reaction, instances of sudden death have been recorded in a number of countries. Pointers to solvent abuse include a lingering smell of solvent on hair and clothes and possession of glue and bags. Staggering walk, slurred speech, violent behaviour, dilated pupils, and spots around the mouth and nose are other signs of solvent abuse. Many cities now have treatment centres which offer guidance and counselling, and involvement of the parents is considered to be vital to the success of treatment of habitual solvent abusers.

Marijuana. Other terms used are cannabis, pot, joint, reefer, weed or grass. The source is the hemp plant which can be found in many parts of the world, and the cannabis can be eaten in the form of 'hash cookies', or can be smoked as a cigarette which can affect pulmonary function. In general it can cause euphoria and hallucinations and is associated with mood swings, so its use can have an effect on both working and playing.

There is a possibility that the use of cannabis (a soft drug) can lead to a *life of dependence* on hard drugs so there are those who are for, and those who are against the legal use of cannabis. Currently there are many countries in which the use of cannabis is illegal and possession of the drug is a punishable offence.

Amphetamines. These are the much talked about 'pep' pills; they can be obtained in tablet or capsule form and have a variety of street names — black bombers, French blues, purple hearts, uppers, wake-ups, jelly beans and copilots. After ingestion the pupils dilate and behaviour can be described as boisterous. When the effects wear off, there is usually lethargy, irritability and unsociability. This psychological see-saw is an indication to members of the family, and to work and play groups that an individual might be using amphetamines for other than medicinal purposes. Loss of appetite with consequent loss of weight and sleeplessness can also result from taking this drug, and constant users may become mentally ill.

As with other drugs, desire for the next dose can become compulsive, and as money is spent acquiring it often to the exclusion of food and clothing, the person may resort to stealing. In many countries amphetamines are only obtainable on a doctor's prescription and doctors are discouraged from prescribing them.

Heroin, cocaine and morphine. Heroin is a narcotic derived from the opium poppy and has street names including skag, horse and smoke. It can be smoked (chasing the dragon) or injected. Cocaine comes from the leaves of the coca bush and has street names such as coke, snow, toot and blow. Heroin, cocaine and morphine all have a useful though small part to play in medical therapy. 'Hard drugs' is the term used when they are peddled for illicit purposes and they are often introduced in a social setting when the uninitiated are invited to experiment with 'just one injection'. Unfortunately for some personalities however, even after just one injection, abstinence is not possible. Such people find themselves on the road to a gradual decline in health and loss of independence which eventually rules their lives (McLennan, 1986). They become 'drop-outs' from work because obtaining the next dose ('fix') takes precedence over any other activity. Eventually they may have to be injected up to several times daily, the dose getting higher and higher to satisfy the craving. In addition there is always the danger that infected syringes will cause hepatitis B, AIDS, local sepsis or fatal septicaemia. Other common accompaniments of drug taking are loss of interest in personal appearance and lack of appetite to the extent of causing malnutrition with a consequent lowered resistance to infection.

LSD/Lysergic acid diethylamide. LSD is a hallucinogen which has street names including acid and pearly gates, and according to Cameron (1987) it is not so commonly used now as solvents, marijuana, amphetamines, and heroin. It is a transparent liquid, effective in minute quantities so can be dropped on to sugar cubes or the back of postage stamps both of which are common means of distribution. It can also be made in tablet form and is usually taken orally but may also be injected. It has the effect of raising the blood pressure and increasing the heart rate and may also cause insomnia, convulsions and hallucinations which are false perceptions occurring without any sensory stimulus. Coping with the torrent of psychological experience released by the drug can be difficult and dangerous without medical supervision. In most countries lysergic acid is not legally for sale, and to possess it is an offence.

Writing about drug abuse and the controversy over the use of methadone as a treatment, Atkinson (1988) quotes Home Office statistics which indicate that drug misuse is increasing. He briefly outlines methods of treatment down through the years including the use of maintenance programmes. However, he says, treatment centres have now moved away from maintenance regimes, and any detoxification programme is usually supplemented with intense therapy aimed at giving back power and control to the person, while coaxing them through other changes in their lifestyle. Wood (1988) also emphasises lifestyle change. He mentions four different fashions in drug education and advocates the cultural approach which involves education for life skills and an understanding of drug use in social and working life. To contribute to such therapies requires adequate staff preparation and Cameron (1987) describes a UK clinic staffed by a multidisciplinary team. As well as providing a comprehensive assessment and management programme for young solvent and drug abusers, it offers inservice training for professional and non-professional staff, and also participates in educational programmes for schools and colleges.

However, a penetrating comment by Salmon (1987) pinpoints an important problem when she describes the confused feelings, voiced by many youngsters, about society's rules; society allows smoking tobacco (p. 135) and drinking alcohol (p. 159) yet bans solvents and drugs.

As already mentioned, substance abuse often arises in relation to leisure time activities. When addiction develops, however, the adverse effects are so pervasive that not only the enjoyment of playing is reduced, work is also affected perhaps causing absenteeism, accidents and poor performance. And this deterioration of the self spills over to affect many other activities of living.

Change due to unemployment

It is not difficult to appreciate that having been part of the workforce, becoming unemployed necessitates tremendous change in a person's established working and playing habits. Loss of work is a problem in its own right, denying the person a whole range of benefits: personal, social and financial. But having no job to go to also obviates the purpose of many daily living habits which are primarily work-related: for example, habitual time of rising; usual daily dress; regular exercise obtained getting to and from work; and the type and timing of meals. Being without work means that there is unlimited time for playing. For some resourceful people this may not pose a problem but for most it does. Almost all leisure activities cost money. Deprived of income from work, established playing habits may be impossible to continue. Apart from that, the person's motivation to seek enjoyment and diversion may be lost and the inevitable stress and gloom which unemployment brings may cause such apathy and depression of mood that there is no enthusiasm or energy for playing. There is little incentive to get up in the morning and sleeping longer is one way of passing the time and obliterating worries. Watching television, smoking and drinking are other ways of coping with boredom and anxiety. None of these habits in excess is conducive to health and some can lead to further financial difficulties.

There is increasing concern that unemployment has deleterious effects on health and it seems reasonable to conjecture that the enforced change in working and playing habits contributes to this. Stress-related health problems, such as high blood pressure and heart disease, have been cited in discussion linking ill-health and unemployment, as have psychiatric illness, alcohol-related problems and parasuicide.

In 1987, Smith updated his previous intensive review of data, still seeking for the links, and concluded that the evidence linking unemployment with poor mental health was stronger than links with poor physical health. Studies which have measured the mental health of the unemployed, using standardised questionnaires countenanced in psychological and psychiatric research, show consistently that the mental health of those out of work is poorer than that of the employed. The unemployed tend to be more anxious, repressed, unhappy, dissatisfied, neurotic and worried; they have lower confidence and self-esteem; and they sleep worse than the employed. However, Smith maintains the evidence does not prove that unemployment, on its own, is the cause of deterioration; it may be that people with poorer mental health are more likely to become unemployed.

As far as physical health is concerned, there were also pointers to associate unemployment with deteriorating health but, again, there were no conclusive data. Admittedly consultation rates in a general practice in the UK did rise 20%, compared to a control group, when staff in a neighbouring factory were threatened with redundancy which eventually materialised; and similar studies in the USA and Canada have shown that the unemployed use health services more than the employed. In the large Canadian study, examination by the doctor showed that the unemployed had significantly more heart trouble, pain in the heart and chest, spells of fainting and dizziness, high blood pressure, and bone and joint problems.

Unemployment is also associated with high divorce rates, child abuse and neglect, wife battering, unwanted pregnancies, abortion, reduced birth weights of babies, increased prenatal and infant mortality rates, reduced growth in children, and increased morbidity in wives and children. Yet from his research, Smith concluded that it was not possible to be confident that only unemployment was the cause.

More than anything else, quotes Smith, poverty may be the link between unemployment and poor health, and he goes on to suggest that raising the living standards of the unemployed may be one of the most effective ways of improving their health.

In the UK the Manpower Services Commission (since 1988 called The Employment Department Training Agency) which was created at the time of the Employment & Training Services Act, 1973, has done something to provide work and training for the unemployed, particularly the young. Two of its aims are 'to promote a more efficient labour market and competitive workforce' and 'to help those at a disadvantage in the labour market to overcome their employment problems'. The Youth Training Scheme is the largest single item on its budget and it has many critics, some labelling it as slave labour, but undoubtedly it has provided work experience as well as training for thousands of young people. The Agency has other schemes such as a community programme, essentially for the long-term unemployed; an enterprise allowance scheme which helps unemployed people to start their own businesses; a voluntary projects scheme which allows the young unemployed to undertake voluntary work without their state benefits being affected; and in certain areas, there is in-depth counselling at Job Centres for long-term unemployed people.

Of course this unemployment problem is not peculiar to the UK, it is affecting many countries; and on a regional basis, as long ago as 1985, the WHO Office for Europe published a strategy for counteracting the health damage caused by unemployment (Westcott et al, 1985). However, not only governments are attempting to grapple with the problem; industry, trades unions, employers, voluntary organisations and individuals all have a part to play. The provision of work is not the only goal for the unemployed; there are many examples of free or subsidised entry to entertainment, sport and leisure facilities; free travel; and free entry to educational facilities. Thus recognition is being given to the importance of working and playing habits in the lives of people who have the misfortune to be unemployed.

Like many aspects of the AL of working and playing, it is not easy to be precise about the nature of nursing activities which are directly related to the problem of unemployment. After all, the problem of a person's joblessness cannot be solved by nurses. On the other hand, an understanding of this problem — especially its links with ill-health — is relevant in nursing. So, too, is a sympathetic attitude to those who have the misfortune to be unemployed, for many suffer from feelings of shame and desolation.

Thinking in more specific terms, the knowledge that unemployment can affect the health of the whole family is obviously of relevance to those nurses who are concerned with health surveillance and health promotion in the community. Families in which there are young children, and one or both parents are unemployed, might be visited more frequently, thus allowing them an opportunity to discuss their problems and feelings. Assessment of what changes have been made to compensate for lack of working, and to fill the unlimited time available for playing, might reveal some actual and potential health problems. The member of the family might welcome the opportunity to review their changed lifestyle in this way and to be helped to plan activities which would maintain, rather than endanger, their health.

This might also be very relevant in the context of hospital nursing and, indeed in that setting, patients might be highly receptive to education about health problems to which they may be vulnerable because they are unemployed. Actual and potential problems might be identified from nursing assessment on admission and the fact that the patient is unemployed should be borne in mind when assessing all the Activities of Living. When finding out about usual habits and routines, it might be revealing to find out whether these have changed since unemployment. If problems identified, such as excessive alcohol intake or insomnia, do appear to have resulted from unemployment then planning to deal with them would have to take that into account. Indeed, the fact of a person's joblessness is relevant to much of the nursing plan which, after all, is geared towards rehabilitation and discharge. The needs of a patient who is returning to work are different from those of the person who has no job to go back to. This would certainly be a major preoccupation of treatment and rehabilitation of patients in the context of psychiatric nursing.

There are, therefore, implications of unemployment for individualised nursing, both in hospitals and in the community. In direct contact with families and sick people, the nurse may be able to help constructively with some of the adverse consequences of joblessness.

Some would say that nurses have another responsibility too — to become involved politically in the matter of unemployment. Seabrook (1982) writing about suffering of the unemployed says:

the consequences of unemployment in the eighties remain essentially secret: part of an individual burden, contained within families for the most part . . . This means that those, including health visitors, who actually penetrate the outer defences, those who have access to people's homes, carry a heavy responsibility in that it is up to them to assess the extent of the harm that is done inside the privacy of those despairing and demoralised homes, and to make sure that the rest of us understand exactly what it is we are asking of people.

He ends the article:

The caring professions are uniquely placed, in their privileged access to people's lives, to make sense of some of the remorseless pressures and to raise their voice against them. If they don't, nobody else will.

Individualising nursing

The first part of this chapter reflects the Roper, Logan and Tierney model — the nature of the AL of working and playing; the relationship of the lifespan to the AL; the effect of an individual's dependence/independence status; and the influence of physical, psychological, sociocultural, environmental and politicoeconomic factors on the AL. Mainly, the first part provides examples of potential problems occurring in everyday living, and what might be done to prevent them from becoming actual problems. In the second part of the chapter, a selection of actual problems and discomforts which can be experienced by people in relation to the AL have been described. This provides a background of general knowledge about the AL as such.

While describing the Roper, Logan and Tierney model for nursing, general information was provided about in-

dividualising nursing (p. 51) which, in fact, is synonymous with the concept of the process of nursing.

Out of this background of general knowledge about the AL of working and playing, and about individualising nursing, it should then be possible to extract the issues which are relevant to one individual's current circumstances (whether in a health or an illness setting), i.e. make an assessment of relevant issues according to the individual's stage on the lifespan; according to current level of dependence/independence; and take into account the relevant physical, psychological, sociocultural, environmental and politicoeconomic factors. Collectively, this information would provide a profile of the person's individuality in living for this AL, and therefore guides the nurse in devising a plan for individualising nursing.

As indicated earlier in the text, this assessment would be achieved by various means such as observing the person; acquiring information about the person's usual habits in relation to this AL partly by asking appropriate questions, partly by listening to the patient and/or relatives; and using relevant information from available records, including medical records. The collected information could then be examined to identify any actual problems being experienced with the AL and these could be arranged in some order of priority. The nurse might also recognise some potential problems — not all possible potential problems but those which are relevant. Realistic goals,

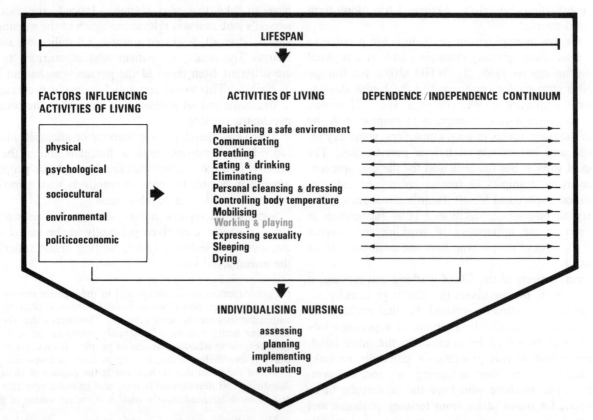

Fig. 14.1   The AL of working and playing within the model for nursing

mutually agreed with the patient when this is possible, could then be set to prevent potential problems from becoming actual ones; to alleviate or solve the actual problems; or to help the person cope with those which cannot be alleviated or solved. Of course, some of the patient's problems with this AL, although identified from the nursing assessment, may well be outwith the scope of nursing intervention. In such instances, after discussion with the patient when appropriate, these problems may be referred to other members of the health care team such as medical staff, dietitians, physiotherapists or social workers.

Keeping in mind what the person can and cannot do unaided, the nursing interventions to achieve the mutually set goals could then be selected according to local circumstances and available resources.

Following implementation of the interventions, their effects could be evaluated in relation to the goals set, and if goals were not reached, they could be revised or rescheduled, or even discarded.

It is worth repeating here that although discussed in four phases — assessing, planning, implementing and evaluating — individualising nursing is not a linear progression; it assumes a built-in responsiveness to feedback at any of the phases, giving ample allowance for change within the overall framework. Also, during an illness episode, an important consideration is rehabilitation of the individual, and planning for this could commence as soon as the person enters the health care system. Another important features is the professional judgement needed to discontinue the nurse/patient relationship when it is no longer relevant.

This chapter has been concerned with the AL of working and playing. However, as stated previously, it is only for the purposes of discussion that any AL can be considered on its own; in reality, the various activities are closely related and do not have distinct boundaries. Figure 14.1 is a reminder that the AL of working and playing is related to the other ALs and also to the other components of the model for nursing.

REFERENCES

Altschul A, McGovern M 1985 Psychiatric nursing. Baillière Tindall, London, p 247–257
Atkinson A 1988 Addictive treatment. Nursing Times 84 (17) April 27: 42–47
Barnard J 1981 The young adult and work. Nursing 1 (25) May: 1076–1078
Bateman H 1987 Fun and games. Community Outlook in Nursing Times 83 (14) April: 12–17
Beale N, Nethercott S 1988 Certified sickness absence in individual employees threatened with redundancy. British Medical Journal 296 (6635) May 28: 1508–1510
Belson P 1987 A plea for play. Nursing Times 83 (26) July 1: 16–18
Benicki A, Leslie F 1983 The mental handicap nurse's special role. In: Tierney A (ed) Nurses and the mentally handicapped. Wiley, Bristol, ch 5
Bond M 1986 Stress and self-awareness: a guide for nurses. Heinemann, London, p 52, 67, 48, 133
Burns D 1979 Resettlement and employment of psychiatric patients. Nursing Times 75 (19) May 10: 799–801
Cameron J 1987 Hidden dangers. Nursing Times 83 (11) March 18: 59–60
Corke P 1989 Resettlement of long-stay psychiatric patients. Nursing Times Occasional Paper 85 (9) March 1: 44–46
Cotton J 1983 Outdoor adventure for handicapped people. Souvenir Press, London
Darbyshire P 1987 Sour grapes. Nursing Times 83 (37) September 16: 23–25
Darnbrough A, Kinrade D 1981 The disabled person and employment. In: Guthrie D (ed) Disability; legislation and practice. Macmillan, London
Davies J, Richardson S 1988 Two's company. Community Outlook in Nursing Times 84 (45) November 9: 16–18
Fradd E 1986 It's child's play. Nursing Times 82 (41) October 8: 40–42
Garrett G 1983 Health needs of the elderly (The essentials of nursing series). Macmillan, London, p 15
Gooch J 1984 The other side of surgery. Macmillan, London, p 3, 21, 60
Gough P, Hingley P 1988 Combatting the pressure. Nursing Times 82 (2) January 13: 43–45

Greaves M 1981 The disabled person looks at legislation. In: Guthrie D (ed) Disability: legislation and practice. Macmillan, London
Griffith D 1988 Hospital visiting hours: time for improvement. British Medical Journal 296 (6632) May 7: 1303–1304
Hammond G 1981 Effects of ageing on work performance. Nursing 1 (25) May: 1079–1080
Hay P 1987 Violence at work. The Listener 118 (3043) December 31: 10–11
Jackman B 1988 Children of the dust. Sunday Times Supplement November 13: 24–31
Laurance J 1986 Unemployment: health hazards. New Society 75 (1212) March 21: 492–493
McLennan A 1986 Taken over by heroin. Nursing Times 82 (7) February 12: 45–47
Martin J, Roberts C 1984 Women and employment: a life time perspective. HMSO, London
Martin J, Meltzer H, Elliott D 1988 The prevalence of disability. HMSO, London
Megranahan M 1985 On the scrap-heap? Nursing Times 81 (34) August 21: 24–27
Monmaney T, Robins K 1988 The insanity of steroid abuse. Newsweek CX1 (24) June 13: 47
Moores A 1987 Walking back to happiness. Nursing Times 83 (42) October 21: 55–57
Nightingale F 1859 Notes on nursing. Duckworth, London, (reprinted 1952) p 108
Ralphs J 1988 Visiting: should you be more involved? The Professional Nurse 2 (30) May: 315–317
Roberts M 1984 It's more than child's play. Nursing Times 80 (22) May 30: 48–50
Robertson I 1986 Learned helplessness. Nursing Times 82 (51) December 17: 28–30
Rogers R, Salvage J 1988 Nurses at risk. Heinemann, London, p 50, 54–56, 48, 132–133
Rowden R, Jones L 1983 A diversional programme for patients with cancer. Nursing Times 79 (11) March 16: 25–27
Royal College of Nursing 1986 AIDS: nursing guidelines. RCN, London
Salmon R 1987 Ganging up against glue. Community Outlook in Nursing Times December: 11–14
Sawley L 1987 Visiting time. Nursing Times 83 (1) January 7: 46
Seabrook J 1982 The human cost of unemployment. Nursing Mirror 155 (18) November 3: 30–31

Seaton A 1989 Control of substances hazardous to health. British Medical Journal 298 April 1(6677): 846–847

Smith R 1987 Unemployment and health. Oxford University Press, Oxford

Swanwick M 1985 Play as a coping mechanism. Nursing 2 (39) July 1154–1156

Tierney A 1983 Married women in nursing. Nursing Times Occasional Paper 79 (24) September 7: 30–33

Vousden M 1986 Every one a winner. Nursing Times 82 (38) September 17: 24–25

Westcott G, Svensson P, Zollner H (eds) 1985 Health policy implications of unemployment. WHO, Copenhagen

Wilson-Barnett J 1978 In hospital: patient's feelings and opinions. Nursing Times Occasional Paper 74 (8) March 16: 29–32

Wood J 1988 Young offenders. Nursing Times 82 (2) January 13: 46–47

ADDITIONAL READING

Chudley P 1988 Second time around (re-using disposable equipment). Nursing Times 84 (39) September 28: 18–19

Copp G 1988 The reality behind stress. Nursing Times 84 (45) November 9: 50–53

Devlin R 1989 Helping disabled mothers. Community Outlook in Nursing Times 85 (15) April 12: 4–10

Disability Alliance Educational and Research Foundation. The Disability Rights Handbook. Produced annually

Health Services Advisory Committee 1987 Violence to staff in the health services. HMSO, London

International Labour Organization 1985 Convention 161 and Convention 171 on Occupational Health Services. ILO, Geneva

Symington I 1987 Hepatitis B — an avoidable hazard? Nursing Times 83 (2) January 14: 50–51

15

Expressing sexuality

The activity of expressing sexuality

'It's a boy' or 'It's a girl' is almost always the very first thing which parents are told about their newly-delivered baby. As the basic body structure of males and females is distinctly different even at birth, identification of the baby's sex is almost instantaneous. Interestingly, scientists have long been puzzled by exactly what determines whether a baby is a boy or a girl. Geneticists now think that sex seems to be fixed by a single gene called testis determining factor (TDF) on the Y chromosome; this triggers male sexual development, and without this gene the embryo becomes female (Lemonick, 1988). Whatever the mechanism, a person's sex is determined at conception and, throughout the entire lifespan, sexuality is a significant dimension of personality and interpersonal behaviour.

Each human being is a 'sexual' human being and has a sexual identity, that is, there is a perception of 'self' as boy or girl, then as man or woman. The ways in which sexuality is expressed vary according to culture but, in any given society, males and females tend to show differentiation in a variety of ways other than simply those determined by biological difference. Invariably, men and women adopt different styles of dress; and, traditionally, males and females occupy different roles, both domestically and socially. In many parts of the Western world, however, long-established differences between the sexes are fast disappearing. There is generally a more egalitarian view and, at the same time, social mores have become more liberal in terms of the ways in which sexuality may be expressed. There is a less rigid interpretation of activities, attitudes, beliefs and values associated with expressing sexuality as 'good' or 'bad', 'normal' or 'abnormal'. The subject of sex is increasingly being aired by the media so that people are becoming more aware of the many dimensions of the AL of expressing sexuality, not least in terms of its relationship to health and illness.

Perhaps this relationship has never been more to the fore than it is now as a result of the AIDS epidemic which is posing a major health threat throughout the world. The global scale of this problem has already been outlined in the chapter on the AL of maintaining a safe environment (Ch. 6). It bears repeating that AIDS is a worldwide problem, and one of enormous magnitude. The first epidemic, which began in the 1970s and continues still, is what is described in a WHO (1988) booklet for nurses as 'the silent pandemic of HIV infection'. It is estimated that, in 1988, between 5 and 10 million people throughout the world were infected with HIV (the human immuno-deficiency virus). The second epidemic is that of the disease caused by HIV — AIDS (i.e. acquired immunodeficiency syndrome) and it is estimated that 10–30% of the 5–10 million HIV-infected people will develop AIDS within the next 5 years. Not everyone, therefore, with the HIV infection appears necessarily to develop AIDS. But for those who do, there is as yet no cure. It is for this reason that preventing the further spread of HIV infection is vital. There is no means of prevention other than education aimed at modifying risk behaviour and reducing the risk of exposure and transmission. Since sexual transmission of HIV is the most important mode of spread of the disease, the target of education is sexual behaviour. So, the AL of expressing sexuality has to be considered in a new light and the subject of AIDS will be touched on time and again throughout this chapter.

THE NATURE OF EXPRESSING SEXUALITY

Human beings have an innate sensuality; being cuddled, rocked and stroked are pleasurable experiences for even the very young infant. It is not long before children discover how to create enjoyable sensations themselves by, for example, mouthing objects, body rocking and touching particular parts of the body, including the genitals and, indeed, baby boys can have penile erections. From the child's point of view there is nothing explicitly sexual about these activities at this stage.

However, a little later on, the child's increasing curiosity about body structure and function manifests itself in constant questioning of the parents, not least of all, the age-old questions about sex and reproduction. All of this is quite natural and normal; the child is expressing an interest in sex in general and, in particular, about his/her sexuality.

Children experiment with the concept of sexuality in their everyday play and in their private fantasy world.

They act out the ways in which masculinity and femininity can be conveyed in gait, mode of dress, make-up and choice of working and playing activities. Children's play characters can be the stereotype of the strong, aggressive male or the seductive, submissive female. Inevitably, families feature prominently in children's play and this allows them to act out their view of the roles of men and women as fathers and mothers.

From these learning opportunities, the growing child becomes increasingly aware of the complexities of human sexuality and the different ways in which men and women express their masculinity and femininity. This growing awareness helps the adolescent at puberty to understand his/her own sexual feelings and how he/she is expected to behave as a sexually mature person. There is a great deal of experimentation going on in the adolescent's ways of expressing sexuality. In private, masturbation enables the youngster to try out and enjoy the physical pleasure of sex; in friendships with members of their own and the opposite sex, adolescents begin to learn how human sexuality influences at a fundamental level how adult men and women relate to each other.

Relating to each other in an explicitly sexual way is central to intimate adult relationships and especially in the husband-wife relationship of marriage. Many different ways of expressing sexuality are involved in adult sexual relationships in addition to sexual intercourse although this is, of course, the ultimate form of sexual behaviour. It is interesting that in most lower mammals, sexual behaviour tends to occur only when fertilisation can take place and courting and mating activities are inextricably linked to reproduction. In contrast, human sexual behaviour serves both reproductive and non-reproductive functions and, indeed is much more frequently performed for non-reproductive reasons than for the purpose of procreation.

LIFESPAN: EFFECT ON EXPRESSING SEXUALITY

The lifespan component of the model of living, as already will be apparent, is intimately connected with the AL of expressing sexuality. Through infancy, childhood, adolescence, adulthood and old age there is a continual adjustment in terms of the ways in which sexuality is expressed. To a great extent, variations at different stages of the lifespan are determined by physical sexual development; key features of this are noted in Table 15.1 which provides a summary of aspects of sexuality throughout the lifespan. More is said about physical factors which affect the AL of expressing sexuality a little later in the chapter (p. 294).

Adolescence and adulthood are perhaps the stages of the lifespan during which the AL of expressing sexuality assumes most significance. Puberty (in males) and the

Stages in the life-span

	Pre-natal	INFANCY (0-5 years)	CHILDHOOD (6-12 years)	ADOLESCENCE (13-18 years)	YOUNG ADULTHOOD (19-30 years)	MIDDLE YEARS (31-44 years)	LATE ADULTHOOD (45-64 years)	OLD AGE (65+)
PHYSICAL SEXUAL DEVELOPMENT	DETERMIN- ATION OF SEX	Growth of sex organs. Sex differences in body build, appearance and rate of growth		♂ PUBERTY ♀ MENARCHE	Continuing sex differences in body build and strength Completion of development of secondary sex characteristics	Changes of pregnancy ♀	MENOPAUSE ♀	Physical and hormonal changes may cause decline in libido and potency
PSYCHO-SEXUAL DEVELOPMENT		Establishment of sexual orientation (masculine/ feminine)		Consolidation of sexual self-image	Development and modification of sexual self-image and attitudes towards sex, sexual relationships, sexual behaviour and sex-related roles and functions			
SEXUALITY and SOCIAL ROLES			Sex differences in roles and functions within family, school and community settings.		Sex differences in family roles: Sex differences in social roles Sex differences in occupational roles	♂ as FATHER ♀ as MOTHER	Decreasing differentiation of role and function according to sex	
INTERPERSONAL/ SEXUAL RELATIONSHIPS		Mainly confined to FAMILY relationships	Friendships with same and opposite sex	Homosexual liaisons Heterosexual friendship and partnerships	ESTABLISHMENT AND DEVELOPMENT OF ADULT SEXUAL PARTNERSHIPS:— Temporary liaisons or long-term mateship/marriage (heterosexual or homosexual)		Possible loss of sexual partner through death	
SEXUAL BEHAVIOUR		EARLY SELF-STIMULATORY SEX PLAY		MASTURBATION Various forms of non-coital behaviour with same and opposite sex	ADULT SEXUAL BEHAVIOUR PATTERNS Attracting/courting behaviours Self-stimulatory activities Sexual intercourse			Possible decline in sexual behaviour and in libido
SEXUAL REPRODUCTION				CAPABILITY FOR EJACULATION AND FERTILISATION ♂ CAPABILITY TO CONCEIVE ♀	♂ CAPABILITY FOR EJACULATION AND FERTILISATION OF FEMALE ♀ CAPABILITY FOR CONCEPTION AND REPRODUCTION (i.e. FERTILE)		♀ incapable of conception after menopause

Table 15.1 Summary of aspects of the development of sexuality throughout the lifespan

menarche (in females) result in the capability for fertilisation/conception. With the onset of the menarche, around 13 years of age, female menstruation occurs periodically (the 'normal' menstrual cycle described as a 28-day cycle, from the first day of one period to the first day of the next) until ceasing, usually only except with pregnancy, with the menopause. Learning to cope with menstruation, and any mood fluctuations which result from the hormonal variations, is an important developmental task for girls.

For both girls and boys adolescence is a critical period of emotional as well as physical development; and it is a time of experimentation in friendships and partnerships. Added to all the usual anxieties and uncertainties which accompany sexual development, today's adolescents have to cope with the very serious threat of AIDS. The sexual lives of adults are equally affected by this new and enormous problem. 'Safe sex' and only safe sex is the message now, and this requires a degree of thought and care about sexual partners and sexual behaviour which, in recent times of sexual permissiveness, has not been considered necessary (whether or not it was desirable).

That apart, adulthood can be a particularly satisfying stage of the lifespan in terms of sex and reproduction before the onset of the menopause which, although technically a female condition, also affects males. Although libido and sexual function may decrease, couples can still continue to enjoy sexual pleasure throughout their old age, provided their health remains good.

DEPENDENCE/INDEPENDENCE IN EXPRESSING SEXUALITY

In relation to all of the Activities of Living, the lifespan is closely linked with another component of the model — the dependence/independence continuum. Children's dependence is for guidance in development; for knowledge — not only to understand their current individual development but also to anticipate what they can expect will happen in their development at later stages of the lifespan. They are dependent on protection from sexual abuse and need to understand the undesirability of going with strangers without impeding the development of friendliness. *It's OK to say No* is the title of a book, designed to put across that message to children, which is reviewed by Holmes (1986) who notes that a number of publishers have released similar books, all aiming to make children more aware of the problem of child sex abuse. This is a problem which has attracted considerable publicity in recent years. In the UK it is estimated that some 1500 children are sexually abused each year. The father, or father substitute, is the most likely perpetrator of the crime which often, alas, goes unreported. There are often long-term effects; people who have been abused as children often are confused about sexuality in later years and

may not develop the sexual confidence which rightly should be enjoyed by independent adults.

Independence can only be achieved by having adequate knowledge and experience; only then can adults trust young people to behave independently and responsibly in relation to aspects of the AL of expressing sexuality according to the attitudes, knowledge and beliefs acquired in the early years.

By definition, the mentally handicapped are slow to learn and therefore may not be able to achieve independence in some aspects of this AL, as one would expect of people with greater intellectual ability. For example, adolescent girls who are mentally handicapped may not be able to be independent in relation to coping with menstruation, and young adults may be unable to make independent decisions about the appropriateness of a marriage or about the need for, and type of, contraception. More is said later (p. 305) about ways in which mentally handicapped people can be helped to achieve optimal independence in these and other aspects of this AL.

For different reasons, some people who are physically handicapped may not achieve independence for all aspects of this AL. They have the intellectual ability to understand their situation, but lack the physical ability to carry out what they wish to do: for example, to manage a date or accomplish sexual relations or use contraceptives in the way able-bodied people can. Again, further discussion of problems which physically handicapped people may experience comes later (p. 305), along with suggestions about ways in which they can be helped to enjoy the AL of expressing sexuality.

FACTORS INFLUENCING EXPRESSING SEXUALITY

In the model of living, factors which influence each AL were considered (p. 27) and they are particularly applicable to expressing sexuality. The five factors — physical, psychological, sociocultural, environmental and politico-economic — will now be considered.

Physical factors
The stage on the lifespan is obviously important in terms of the influence which physical factors exert on the AL of expressing sexuality. The main features of physical sexual development were outlined in the preceding section concerned with the lifespan component of the model in relation to this AL, and are contained in the summary provided in Table 15.1.

In adulthood, following puberty and the menarche, the reproductive system is fully developed and the physical capability established for sexual function and reproduction. Although the reproductive system is the body structure and function most obviously associated with sex and reproduction, equally important is a fully functioning nervous system, sensory system and musculoskeletal system for the carrying out of the many activities which are included in the AL of expressing sexuality. A detailed knowledge of the human reproductive system is, of course, particularly important for an informed understanding of the processes and problems of sexual function and reproduction. Knowledge of the differences between the male and female reproductive systems is, of course, especially relevant to an understanding of how physical factors influence the AL of expressing sexuality.

Gender differences in body structure and function

The male and female reproductive systems differ, both in terms of structure and function. The organs which comprise the male reproductive system are the testes (glands which produce the spermatozoa capable of fertilising the female ova and the male sex hormone testosterone, responsible for the secondary sex characteristics); the mechanisms for transfer of semen, containing the spermatozoa, to the exterior (i.e. the epididymis, vas deferens, seminal vesicle, ejaculatory duct, prostate gland and urethra); and the penis, the most sensitive part being the glans which is covered by the prepuce or foreskin (which is not present if the man has been circumcised). This brief mention of the names of the organs of the male reproductive system will remind readers of this knowledge, covered in biology in the curriculum. A reminder of the fact that the reproductive system is linked with other systems of the body, a point made a little earlier, is evident in relation to male erection and ejaculation. Penile erection is the male's response to sexual excitement; it results from a spinal reflex, but is also influenced by impulses from higher centres in the brain. Ejaculation (by which the male achieves orgasm) occurs as a spinal reflex, triggered by friction which, in penetrative sexual intercourse, can make considerable demands on the musculoskeletal and cardiopulmonary sytems of the body.

Sexual intercourse can be just as physically energetic for women although the form of activity and orgasm is different, for reasons determined by the body structure and function of the female reproductive system. Again, by way of reminder — and because these anatomical terms will be used later in the text without definition — mention is made here of the female sex organs. These are the external genitalia (the mons veneris, labia majora, labia minora, clitoris, vaginal orifice, Skene's and Bartholin's lubricating glands and the hymen); the internal genitalia which are contained within the pelvic cavity (and consist of the vagina, cervix, uterus, uterine tubes and ovaries); and the breasts (which are accessory organs). The vagina, which is penetrated by the penis in heterosexual intercourse, lies between the bladder and urethra in front and the rectum and anus behind. The close physical proximity of the reproductive organs and those of the urinary/defaecatory systems means that either system can be readily affected by dysfunction or infection of the other. Vaginal fluid, being acid, inhibits the growth of invading pathogenic microorganisms. However, before puberty and after the menopause, this mechanism is not so effective and the vagina is more susceptible to infection at these stages of the lifespan, as well as during pregnancy.

Physical changes in pregnancy

Pregnancy is most often suspected on the basis of a missed menstrual period. Although some 350 ripened ova are produced during a woman's fertile years, only two or three on average become fertilised to result in pregnancy. Pregnancy lasts about 40 weeks and the expected date of delivery is calculated as 9 calender months and 1 week from the first day of the last normal menstrual period.

In the early weeks of pregnancy, breast tenderness and enlargement, nausea and vomiting, and fatigue are commonly experienced by the woman. Pregnancy tests can be done to confirm the diagnosis of pregnancy. These are based on the fact that human chorionic gonadotrophin (HCG) is produced by the placenta and excreted in the mother's urine.

Later, positive signs of pregnancy become established. Fetal heart sounds can be heard on auscultation and fetal parts felt by examination from about the 24th week.

After the 12th week the enlarging uterus becomes palpable abdominally. The growth of the uterus is the most overt sign of pregnancy, along with changes which occur in the breasts. The nipples and areolae darken in colour and the sebaceous glands (Montgomery's tubercles) become more noticeable. From the 16th week or so, small amounts of colostrum sometimes can be expressed from the breasts.

In addition to changes within the reproductive organs, many other systems of the body alter in adaptation to pregnancy. The cardiovascular system increases its capacity, a 30% increase in blood volume occurring by the 30th week. With this the haemoglobin concentration may fall and iron and folic acid supplements to prevent anaemia may be prescribed. Due to the action of progesterone the veins become relaxed and varicose veins and haemorrhoids may develop. Extra oxygen is needed for the fetus and pregnant women breathe more deeply to obtain this. It is now established that cigarette smoking can diminish the oxygen supply to the fetus via the placenta and so smoking is strongly discouraged (p. 131). Black (1984) in her report of a small study said that individual support was essential to help pregnant women to stop smoking. From other research she reports that the risk of spontaneous abortion was doubled in smokers, but the most common consequence was a lower birth weight of the babies compared to those of non-smokers. The urinary system has to cope with the increased volume of fluid and so the rate of glomerular filtration rises. Increased frequency of micturition is common in the first and last trimester of pregnancy. Progesterone acts on the digestive tract to relax smooth muscle and this can cause the discomforts of heartburn, indigestion, nausea and constipation.

There is no need to increase greatly the amount of food taken but a balanced diet is essential for the health of the mother and the growth of the fetus. Protein, calcium and vitamins are important constituents of the diet at this time. Alcohol is discouraged — for it is now known that even moderate drinking in pregnancy may adversely affect the fetus (Wright, 1986) — as is any form of substance abuse; the increasing problem of drug abuse in society and one of its consequences — neonatal drug addiction — is discussed by Phillips (1986).

As the body shape alters during pregnancy, posture and gait change and the tendency to exaggerate the lumbar curve often results in backache. The skin also shows changes with pigmentation occurring on the areola of the breasts, the linea nigra (midline of the lower abdomen) and sometimes the face (called chloasma, 'the mask of pregnancy'). The skin of the abdomen and breasts becomes stretched and marks (striae gravidarum) appear on these areas.

All pregnant women are advised to have regular prenatal care to help them maintain good health and to enable the early detection and treatment of complications. Perhaps, however, it should be noted that sexual intercourse (including orgasm) has no ill-effects during pregnancy. Thomson (1987) considers that this, and other advice on sexuality during pregnancy, is something which many couples would welcome. Equally, there is a need for advice on postnatal sexuality; Yates (1987) explains some of the changes and problems which occur (such as pain during intercourse) and suggests ways in which couples can be better informed to cope with and prevent such difficulties.

After pregnancy the reproductive organs gradually return to their non-pregnant state and regular menstruation recommences within 3 months or so of delivery. Because the time of the first ovulation cannot be predicted, contraception should be practised whenever sexual relations are resumed as a further early pregnancy is undesirable.

Physical control of fertility
The availability of contraceptive techniques — which are mainly by physical or chemical control of fertility — is considered to be an important advance of modern times. Contraception allows women to exercise control over their lives as well as making it possible for the problem of overpopulation to be dealt with. This, for some countries, poses a major threat to economic and social survival. In many developing countries, governments are active in promoting family planning services and educating people about the importance of birth control.

A wide variety of contraceptive methods is available and some of the most commonly used are described below. Many factors enter into the choice of a particular method of contraception for a particular couple at a particular time; Shapiro (1984) provides a useful discussion of the factors involved, along with a brief description of common contraceptive methods, similar to the following account.

The pill is a hormonal method of contraception. The 'combined pill' (oestrogen and progesterone) works by inhibiting ovulation. It is taken orally and is the most reliable method of contraception available today. There is a small risk of thrombosis associated with prolonged use, and it is now thought that the degree of risk increases with age and in women who smoke.

Patch hormone (oestrogen) contraceptives are a recent innovation and, according to a London gynaecologist, could prove to be safer than the pill for women over 35 years of age (Nursing Times, 1988).

A morning-after pill can be used by those who have had unprotected sexual intercourse but this form of contraception must be supervised by a doctor or a family planning clinic. One pill is taken as soon as possible and the other 12 hours later and they must be taken within 72 hours of the intercourse before the fertilised ovum has had a chance to implant in the uterus. Such treatment is useful in cases of rape.

An injectable long-term contraceptive. Depo-provera, which is one of the long-acting progestins given by intramuscular injection, has been the cause of much controversy about its safeness. Wigington (1981) reviewed the research findings on its action, side-effects, and use in 65 countries — many of them in the Third World. Some governments have reconsidered their ban on this contraceptive and in the UK the position in 1984 was that it could be used as a 'last resort contraceptive' (Sadler, 1984), as long as the laid-down precautions, which are given in the article, are observed. Depo-provera is sometimes recommended for lactating women and this appears to be safe for a 3–6 month period (Pernoll & Benson, 1987).

The diaphragm is a barrier method used by the woman and is a rubber cap which covers the cervix and thereby creates a mechanical barrier between ova and spermatozoa. It is inserted into the vagina before intercourse and removed not less than 6 hours afterwards. There are no harmful side-effects to consider, although some women find the diaphragm a distasteful and bothersome method. However, it has become more popular since other more recent methods of contraception (notably the pill and the IUD) have been associated with hazards, as Spencer (1986) notes in her article on the diaphragm and cervical cap.

The condom is a male barrier method and is a cover fitted over the penis to prevent the semen entering the vagina. It is a reliable method if the sheath is put on prior to any genital contact and if care is taken to prevent leakage on removal. Reliability can be improved if used in conjunction with a spermicide and the sheath may give some protection to the partner if one of them suffers from a sexually transmitted disease. Use of a condom is currently being promoted as the most effective protection against HIV infection and AIDS. Recently, the development of a female condom has been reported (Ernsberger & Jones, 1988), one advantage of this in terms of protection against AIDS and other sexually-transmitted diseases being that women would not need to depend on their partner's prudency.

The intra-uterine device (IUD) is a device inserted (by a doctor) into the uterine cavity through the cervix. In situ it prevents the successful implantation of a fertilised ovum in the endometrium. It is a reliable method and requires no special preparation by either partner prior to intercourse, although for a variety of reasons it may not be the most suitable method for some women to use. There can be complications such as bleeding, pain, infection and uterine perforation. But these are steadily being reduced with improvements in the shape of IUDs and in techniques of insertion (Beischer & Mackay, 1986).

The 'rhythm' method, also called the calendar method, involves abstinence from intercourse during the female's fertile time of the menstrual cycle. The time of ovulation is estimated from records of the woman's menstrual cycle or, more accurately, from recordings of body temperature. The temperature rises after ovulation and there should be abstention from intercourse for 7 days prior to the earliest recorded temperature rise and for 5 days afterwards. The method requires high motivation on the part of both partners and is not reliable because the time of ovulation can vary unpredictably and as Torrance & Milligan (1986) point out, there is the relative imprecision inherent in both the use of thermometers and the detection of the small temperature shifts.

Sterilisation is a permanent method of contraception, completely reliable in the majority of cases, and often the ideal method after a couple have completed their family or do not wish to have any children. Male sterilisation is called *vasectomy* and involves the division of the vas deferens to prevent spermatozoa reaching the urethra. The operation is performed under local anaesthetic and has no adverse effects on the production of semen or on sexual sensation and performance. It takes some time for the semen to become completely void of spermatozoa and another contraceptive method must always be used until tests of the ejaculate indicate that it is clear. Female sterilisation, *tubal ligation*, is usually performed under general anaesthetic and is effective immediately. It involves the division of the uterine tubes to prevent ova reaching the uterus. More men and women each year choose sterilisation as their preferred method of controlling fertility; Shapiro (1986) examines this trend and discusses factors which nurses should bear in mind when involved with people who are deciding on sterilisation.

The effectiveness of a particular method, apart from the IUD and sterilisation, depends largely on the correctness of its use. Choice of method must be based not only on the degree of reliability ensured but also on the couple's preference about which method is most appropriate to them and their needs. People's feelings about contraception can be very complex indeed. Their decision to use contraception and which method to choose is influenced by the nature of their relationship, attitude to sex, desire to have or not to have children, knowledge about sex and contraception, family upbringing and religion.

Abortion is the termination of a pregnancy and it can be accidental or induced. Many pregnancies terminate spontaneously during the first trimester, most of these due to fetal malformation or some abnormality in the mother. Vaginal bleeding during pregnancy is the cardinal sign of a threatened abortion.

In the UK the 1967 Abortion Act permits termination of pregnancy up to the time (the 28th week) when the fetus becomes viable. Due to improved neonatal intensive care, some infants born before this date have survived so, if possible, induced abortion is carried out before the 12th week of pregnancy. As well as medical reasons for carrying out abortion, there may be social and psychological reasons. The politicoeconomic aspects of abortion are discussed on page 301.

Physical changes with the menopause
The menopause most commonly happens around the 50th year of life, but can occur at any time between the ages of 45 and 55. The menopause marks the cessation of ovarian function and the loss of the capability to conceive and reproduce. Discontinuation of the monthly periods is sometimes sudden but more often is gradual with a lengthening of the intervals between periods.

Like puberty, this is a time of hormonal change and imbalance and there are often temporary emotional and physical disturbances. Symptoms can be experienced such as hot flushes, insomnia, palpitations, sweating, vertigo, headache, depression and fatigue; these result from the decrease in the levels of the sex hormones. Loss of libido at the menopause is not uncommon but the physical changes which occur do not in fact reduce a woman's potential to experience normal sexual feelings and to achieve orgasm and sexual satisfaction.

The very wide range of symptoms experienced by menopausal women is illustrated in the report of a survey by Masling (1988). Apart from asking the women about their symptoms, Masling wanted to know what sources of information they found useful and what sources of help and support are available. She concluded that information provision needs to be improved and women made more aware of help available, particularly in the context of well-women clinics. It is not only physical changes and problems which make the menopause a tiresome thing for women, but also the accompanying emotional and psychological stresses; these are mentioned in the next section which discusses 'psychological factors'.

Physical contact in communication/interaction

Much of the discussion so far has concentrated on physical factors affecting the AL of expressing sexuality which are directly linked to sexual function and reproduction. There are, of course, many other more subtle ways in which physical factors relate to sexual expression. An example of this is the way in which sexual expression is conveyed by physical contact which occurs in the course of everyday interpersonal communication and interaction. The extent to which bodily contact occurs between individuals depends very much on the nature of their relationship. The mother-infant relationship involves very close physical contact, perhaps the closest being in breast feeding. However, as the child grows, the mother engages in less and less direct bodily contact especially towards adolescence when the child's awareness of sexuality is developing. There is a certain amount of physical contact between children of the same sex, but little between adults of the same sex. It is extensive in the husband-wife relationship but, in contrast, very limited between adults of the opposite sex who are not in any close relationship.

As long ago as 1966, Jourard published his observations on patterns of physical contact occurring between people in different kinds of relationships. He showed that the amount of bodily contact is closely related to the degree to which the relationship involves sexual affiliation. Clearly there is a taboo on touching areas of the body which have a sexual connotation when the individuals concerned are not in a sexual relationship. Understanding this 'taboo on touch' is especially important in the context of health care where, of course, patients and professionals sometimes have to violate the taboo and this can be an uncomfortable experience on both sides. A little more is said on that issue in the second section of this chapter.

Physical disability/disfigurement

As so many systems are involved in the AL of expressing sexuality, it is not surprising that some people do not have the necessary physical attributes required for expressing sexuality in the usual ways, whether the condition is congenital or acquired. More is said in the second part of this chapter about how people with physical disabilities or disfigurement can be helped to express sexuality, which, it must be stressed again, is much more than sexual intercourse and permeates all aspects of everyday living.

Psychological factors

The intellectual and emotional development as discussed in Chapter 4 in relation to the various stages of the lifespan is clearly relevant to the AL of expressing sexuality.

Developmental aspects

A certain level of intelligence is necessary for learning about the body and how it functions; the changes that can be expected at puberty and how to cope with them; human relationships; close relationships with people of the same and opposite sex; the social norms concerning courting; contraception; pregnancy; childbirth and rearing a family.

Attitudes to expressing sexuality are established during the early years. Children who are reprimanded, for example for touching the genital area or masturbating, may develop a negative attitude to this aspect of expressing sexuality. As Deakin (1988) points out, as learning is so central to the development of an individual's sexuality, maladaptive learning can occur relatively easily. Preferences for unusual or inappropriate sexual behaviour are not uncommon, he says, appearing to result from reinforced learning in the course of development. The development of male sexuality is, according to Deakin, particularly complicated by the multiple pressures of contemporary society through changes in the role of women, employment and media pressure.

Sexual orientation

Although modes of sexual behaviour are shaped as well as restricted by social pressure, individuals can still exercise considerable control over the ways in which they wish to express their sexuality.

Preference for heterosexuality is the norm for the majority of adults. For those who are involved in a heterosexual relationship, various factors influence how the partners express their sexual drives and achieve a mutually satisfying sexual relationship. There is now much greater understanding of the nature of sexual relationships as a result of research investigation, notably the work of Masters & Johnson (1966, 1970). Such work has helped to clarify what constitutes 'normal' sexual behaviour.

For example, in Western societies, married couples engage in intercourse about two or three times a week on average, although individual variation is great. The age of the husband tends to influence the frequency, a decrease being common from several times a week in the early 20s to once a week in the 60s. With advancing age there is a progressive increase in the length of time and amount of stimulation necessary to produce an erection, a decrease in the duration of complete erection and in the capacity for multiple orgasms. Sexual responsiveness varies with changes in physiological condition and, for example, extreme physical tiredness inhibits libido and potency.

Many women experience cycles of increased sexual desire according to their pattern of menstruation. There may be decreased libido during the menopause and in later life. Some societies prohibit sexual intercourse during menstruation, pregnancy and lactation.

Sexual attraction to a person of the same sex —

homosexuality — has existed through the ages and is found in all societies. It has been treated in different ways at different times, ranging from acceptance and understanding to hostility, ignorance and sometimes imprisonment. In Western countries today there is a trend towards a greater enlightenment and acceptance of the right of consenting adults to have a homosexual relationship if that is their wish. Preference for homosexuality is much more common than many people imagine. Fong (1978) notes that the Kinsey Report indicated that as many as 37% of men and 13% of women had had a homosexual experience leading to orgasm by the age of 45, that probably up to 10% of the adult population remain exclusively homosexual and that about half of all unmarried men over the age of 35 are homosexual. Many homosexuals are also heterosexual (i.e. bisexual) and often married and have children; homosexuality is not an absolute state but a sexual orientation on the continuum which ranges from exclusively heterosexual to exclusively homosexual.

There are a few people who, even in childhood, feel that they have been mysteriously born into the sex opposite their actual body structure, a condition described as transsexuality (Bradshaw & Issa, 1981). Transsexualism has as its central feature disturbed gender identity and the transsexual not only dresses and acts like a person of the opposite sex but usually wants to have surgery and treatment to make the body like that of the opposite sex, although this may not be possible. Transvestites, on the other hand, although they dress in clothes of the opposite sex for sexual gratification, do not generally wish to belong to the opposite sex. Whereas unconventional forms of sexual behaviour (sometimes called sexual deviations) need not be viewed as problems, there is another group of conditions called sexual dysfunctions which are problems as such. Deakin & Kirkpatrick (1987) state: 'A sexual problem where impairment of pleasure, both giving or receiving, and the inability to participate in and perform adequately with another person in sexual activity is reduced, is termed a sexual dysfunction.' Deakin & Kirkpatrick comment that these difficulties are common and a significant factor in marital breakdown. Treatment of sexual dysfunction has developed rapidly in recent years and the main approaches of sex therapy/counselling are described in this article.

Among adults who experience sexual problems are those who experienced sexual abuse in childhood. This problem has been mentioned previously (p. 294 and in Chapter 6 on the AL of maintaining safe environment) in terms of children's dependence on adults for protection. For those who do experience sexual/incestuous assault, there can be long-term effects; Lowery (1987) calls for better detection and support of these 'adult survivors of childhood incest'. Further discussion of child abuse, including incest, is contained in articles by Vousden (1987) and McAree (1987).

Pyschological aspects of pregnancy and childbirth

In the previous section, on physical factors affecting the AL of expressing sexuality, physical changes which occur in pregnancy were described. Pregnancy is also a time of emotional and psychological adaptation. Increasingly, prenatal education and support is taking account of this fact and includes the emotional preparation of the mother and her partner for the birth and the postnatal period too.

This appreciation of the support which the partner needs, as well as provides, is reflected in the positive management which is now given for fathers to be involved in prenatal classes and to be present at the birth. The presence of the father at the birth was something almost unheard of in the UK even 20 years ago and is just one of the indications of major changes which are occurring in the fatherhood role. Bozett & Hanson (1986) describe some of the changes taking place and advocate nurses' encouragement of paternal participation in childrearing and family life.

The stresses of parenting and family life are increasingly being better recognised. An example of this is the growing awareness of the problem of postnatal depression. It is thought that about 10% of women are affected. Early detection currently is being stressed since, untreated, the depression can have profound effects, not only on the new mother but the family as a whole (Williams, 1986). Holden (1987) outlines the findings of research which suggests that health visitors can successfully intervene in the treatment of mothers with postnatal depression, using non-directive counselling techniques.

Psychological difficulties at the menopause

As was noted earlier (p. 297), it is not only the physical effects of the menopause which women find difficult, but also the emotional and psychological difficulties which seem to characterise these 'middle years'. Pownall (1987) notes the need for attention to both aspects. He describes the work of a special menopause clinic in London and sees this as a reflection of an increasing concern to help women with menopausal problems which, in the past, have tended to be dealt with somewhat unsympathetically by doctors. Currently, there is considerable interest in the use of hormone replacement therapy (HRT) which not only seems to alleviate distressing symptoms of the menopause but also protects women against osteoporosis. Masling (1988) mentions this in her article on the menopause, noting that HRT remains a controversial issue.

Sociocultural factors

Like all of the Activities of Living, the AL of expressing sexuality is universal and it is both interesting and important to understand the way in which this AL is influenced by sociocultural factors.

Socialisation

Individuals learn to adopt the norms and mores of their society through the process of socialisation. Parents influence the child's sexual development from an early age; femininity or masculinity can be encouraged by the particular choice of clothes and games, and demonstrated by the sexual behaviour of the parents themselves. School education further shapes the child's developing concept of sexuality by reinforcing the attitudes of society towards sex and the respective roles and functions of men and women. Gradually the child begins to learn society's expectations of how men and women should behave and what overt expressions of sexuality are permissible.

Sociocultural similarities and differences

While forms of sexual expression vary considerably from one society to another, similar forms of behaviour to attract a sexual partner are universal. Physical appearance is of considerable importance in this, although there are no uniform standards of sexual attractiveness.

Some religious rites and some cultural customs reinforce in members a positive perception of themselves as man/woman. To give but a few examples, all orthodox male Jews are circumcised shortly after birth; female circumcision is still practised in some parts of the world (p. 308), and some cultures have a rite-de-passage to demarcate childhood from adulthood; this usually coinciding with the time when the individual becomes physically capable of reproduction.

Each society has its own code of sexual behaviour based on cultural values, norms, attitudes, morals and laws. While universal regulations prohibit some particularly undesirable sexual relationships such as incest and adult sexual intercourse with children, most societies have their own laws delineating the forms of sexual partnerships which are acceptable. In Western civilisation the monogamous marriage is the norm whereas in other parts of the world, polygamy (two or more females married to one male) is practised.

But, gradually, these long-established norms are disappearing and there is almost more variety than there is uniformity in the so-called 'social permissiveness' of the present time.

Social permissiveness and resultant problems

Social permissiveness has brought about a so-called 'sexual revolution' in this century; and, while there are no doubt real benefits, it is also clear that there are many problems as a result. Never before has Western society, at least, seen in such large numbers people suffering from dissatisfaction about sexual adequacy, from marital stress, from the difficulties which follow separation and divorce, from the strains of single-parenting and from the perpetration of sexual abuse in the form of incest, rape and sexual assault. The growing invasion of pornography is another unsavoury

trend, an issue particularly commented on by Orr (1988).

Social permissiveness towards sex has removed the stigma which used to be attached to multiple sexual partnerships and such behaviour, made more possible by more available and reliable contraception and by free travel around the world, has resulted in the ever-increasing problem of sexually-transmitted disease (STD). According to Panja (1988), over the last decade in the UK the number of patients attending STD clinics has increased at the rate of 10% annually. Data collected by that author at one clinic over a year on 1000 consecutive female patients showed that the majority were young (61% below the age of 25) and single (72%); 28% of these women had regular sexual contact before the legal consent age of 16 and 86% had casual partners within the last 12 months (while 38% had 1–5 sexual partners during that time, the remainder had more and some 17% had 16 or above). Of the group, 92% were regular alcohol drinkers and drugs were very frequently used.

Although these data cannot necessarily be generalised, they do support a general picture which is one of young people in society today as being sexually active and, as a result — compounded by the effects of alcohol and drugs — at risk of contracting sexually-transmitted diseases. Added to the problem of infection with chlamydia, warts and herpes is the threat of HIV infection and AIDS.

Society threatened by AIDS

Virtually no sector of society is immune from the threat of AIDS. Although the problem of HIV infection first affected the homosexual community, it was not long before a quite unrelated group became involved — those haemophiliacs and others who received infected blood by transfusion — and now it is clear that the disease has spread more and more widely throughout society. More babies are being born with AIDS than ever before (Hicks, 1987; Snell, 1988); more and more intravenous drug users are succumbing to the infection (Gafoor, 1988); and, increasingly, the disease is spreading into the heterosexual population. In terms of heterosexual transmission of HIV, female prostitutes have been identified recently as a potentially significant group but, according to Day et al (1988), there are indications that these women recognise the risk and are increasing their use of condoms.

The distribution of HIV infection shows sociocultural variations and, even in any one country, there are differences, for example, in the UK, while the problem remains largely one affecting the homosexual community in England, in parts of Scotland the picture is quite different. Greenwood (1988) provides statistics for Lothian Region which includes Scotland's capital city; here, there is the highest known rate of HIV infection in the UK, with 111 per 100 000 people known to be seropositive (compared with 61 per 100 000 in N.W. Thames), and this means that approximately 1 in 250 adults here are already known to be affected (excluding children and the elderly). Of these, the main proportion are young (average age 24), in a ratio of 2:1 male/female, heterosexual, and past or current drug abusers who have not changed their lifestyles.

Changes in sexual behaviour, however, have certainly taken place in the UK among homosexual men and there is some evidence of a similarly positive trend among other groups, notably heterosexual women. Kenn & Goorney (1988) attempted to assess changes in behaviour and attitudes with respect to AIDS in a group of 559 new attenders at a sexually transmitted disease clinic; 56% of females, 51% of males and 78% of homo/bisexual males stated that their attitudes to sex had changed in the light of increased awareness of AIDS; and 74% of homo/bisexual males (compared to 7% two years before), 44% of females (6% previously) and 47% of heterosexual males (0% previously) reported discussing the risk of AIDS with their partners prior to sexual intercourse.

Such evidence of positive change in response to the threat of AIDS is encouraging for, while the disease has no cure, the only hope lies in prevention arising from social change.

Environmental factors
Environmental factors which influence the AL of expressing sexuality include availability of things which individuals perceive to be necessary for them to express their sexuality, as well as surroundings which are conducive for aspects of this activity of living.

Influences at home
The provision of toys and games, for example, in the child's environment will exert some influence on how sexuality is expressed. Even although there is a move away from 'sexist' toys in many cultures, there are still toys and games and adult encouragement which promote a perhaps unnecessary degree of gender stereotyping.

Similar criticism might be made of the mass media; certainly, the dominance of the TV in some homes means that children (and adults) are greatly influenced through this medium, and particularly its advertising. There is increasing criticism of the way in which sexuality is expressed by influential others, often portraying unrealistic and unhelpful images of women.

Influences at school and work
School and work environment also exert their influence, both positively and negatively. While a healthy, balanced mixed-sex environment is likely to provide social benefits all round, a situation of single-sex domination may be of disadvantage to the minority. Women are increasingly complaining of the problem of sexual harassment at work.

Conduciveness of surroundings is certainly important in relation to sexual intimacy. It is usually the case that sexual intercourse is expected to take place in the privacy of a bedroom, at least in the Western world. When the parents and children have separate bedrooms, children can become curious on hearing sounds coming from the parents' bedroom. Whether or not they voice this curiosity, and if they do, how the parents deal with it may well influence developing attitudes to expressing sexuality. Separate bedrooms for the children, or at least separate beds can influence masturbating habits. However, sometimes from choice and sometimes because there is no alternative, all members of the family may sleep in one room, either separately or huddled together. It is thought that huddling together can predispose to incest (Young, 1981).

Politicoeconomic factors
At first thought, it may seem strange to accept that the AL of expressing sexuality is influenced by politicoeconomic factors. But, it certainly is the case that even sex is subject to the influence of politics, economics (both personal and national), the law and ethics. The case of AIDS, essentially a sexually-transmitted disease, perhaps provides the most obvious confirmation of this.

AIDS aside for the moment, what other examples are there of politicoeconomic influence on the AL of expressing sexuality?

Economic factors
Taking economic factors first, there are obvious examples in relation to personal finances (such as being able to afford clothes and other adornments which enhance sexuality) and also others on the level of national economy. Contraceptives are subsidised in many countries, and in some are provided free; and, in some of those countries where overpopulation is a problem, surgical sterilisation is offered free. Even something as basic as sanitary protection can be a problem for women in poor countries, as Milligan (1987) points out, and advocates the need for assistance and health education about menstruation. On a larger scale, and affecting all countries, is the economic cost of AIDS; this not only in terms of the cost of education and care, but also the loss of a vital sector of a nation's workforce.

Legal factors
Now considering legal factors, again there are obvious examples of the influence of the law (and, often, inextricably-linked ethical issues) on aspects of the AL of expressing sexuality. In many countries there are laws regarding permissible sexual relations. Homosexuality has been mentioned and in this context it is fair to say that in many countries it is no longer a criminal offence to have a sexual relationship with a consenting adult of the same sex. Incest on the other hand is usually a criminal offence which may well be a reason for under-reporting its occurrence, a point made earlier (p. 294). The most usual form is between father and daughter but it can be between an adult male family member and a boy, and more rarely between

a mother and son. Low socioeconomic class, poverty, over-crowding and unemployment are all factors which have been linked with child abuse (McAree, 1987). Rape is also deemed a criminal offence but, like incest, the number of victims who report the occurrence to the police is thought to be many less than the number of offenders. Some local authorities contribute financially to special centres or-ganised by women to give help to rape victims; the role of rape crisis centres is discussed by Moore (1985) and she attributes women's reluctance about contacting official authorities to their fear of an unsympathetic reaction, as-suming blame will be directed at the woman rather than at her assailant.

Legislation also exists in relation to termination of preg-nancy; the term 'legal abortion' is used in contrast to 'illegal abortion' which is a punishable offence in many countries. Recently in the UK, the abortion law came under review and there is controversy about the current limits set on the period during which an abortion may be performed.

The 'politics' of AIDS

Controversy has also raged about some aspects of what has been called 'the politics of AIDS', although Warden (1987) argues that 'the politics of AIDS is not primarily about either money or law . . . it is to do with morals, ethics, individual freedom, and communication.' The contro-versies, such as the issue of HIV testing, are an inevitable consequence of a world-wide disease epidemic which, without a cure, raises questions of the balance between the public health and personal freedom. On one point at least, all governments are agreed; namely, that the only way for-ward is through health education. Glenister (1988) reviews how the American and Canadian governments have tackled this health education task and Kay (1988) describes WHO's strategy world-wide through the WHO Special Programme on AIDS. (This was discussed in Chapter 6 on maintaining a safe environment.) Reflecting on the brief history of global AIDS, it is said there have been three periods — of silence, of discovery and of mobilization. The question now is whether 'mobilisation' can halt the pan-demic spread of this deadly disease.

The cost already is enormous in terms of death and suf-fering. On the 1988 World AIDS day (1st Dec.), the total number of AIDS cases reported to the WHO from 142 countries (since 1979) stood at 129 385. But the real figure is said to be two or three times that, with 5 million people infected with HIV now said to be the conservative es-timate. Based on that figure, at least 1 million new AIDS cases may be expected during the next 5 years; beyond that, if unaverted, the projected toll is almost incalculable and certainly unthinkable.

INDIVIDUALITY IN EXPRESSING SEXUALITY

It can be seen from the discussion so far that there are several dimensions to each of the components of the model of living which can influence individuality in expressing sexuality. Since the purpose of the model is to describe how a particular person develops individuality in relation to expressing sexuality, what follows is a résumé of topics discussed in relation to the components of the model of living.

Lifespan: effect on expressing sexuality
* Development of sexual self-image in childhood
* Puberty/menarche in adolescence
* Sexual/reproductive roles in adulthood
* Menopause in middle years
* Decreasing sexual function in old age

Dependence/independence status in expressing sexuality
* Knowledge/guidance needed in childhood
* Dependence for protection from sexual abuse
* Dependence arising from mental/physical handicap in some activities

Factors influencing expressing sexuality

● Physical	— stage of physical sexual development
	— gender differences in body structure and function
	— physical changes in pregnancy
	— physical control of fertility
	— physical changes with the menopause
	— physical contact in communication/interaction
● Psychological	— intellectual/emotional development
	— attitudes to sexuality
	— sexual orientation
	— aspects of pregnancy/childbirth
	— difficulties at the menopause
● Sociocultural	— socialisation process
	— sociocultural similarities/differences
	— social permissiveness and resultant problems
	— society threatened by AIDS
● Environmental	— influences at home (e.g. toys, TV)
	— influences at school and work
	— milieu for sexual intimacy

- Politicoeconomic — economic factors
  — legal factors
  — the 'politics' of AIDS

Expressing sexuality: patients' problems and related nursing

In society at large, sex is no longer such a taboo subject. In the field of health care the subject of human sexuality is at last being introduced into the core curriculum of education programmes for nurses, doctors and other health care workers. When this book was published in 1980, it was one of the first British nursing texts to take account of the dimension of expressing sexuality as an integral aspect of individualised nursing. Webb (1985, 1988) has since done much to promote the importance and relevance of this topic, recognising from her research in gynaecological nursing that both patients and nurses had low levels of knowledge about sexual matters, which included misinformation and folk-myths.

But even though doctors and nurses are beginning to acknowledge that illness and hospitalisation may cause sex-related problems, some are still reticent about discussing them openly with patients. Acknowledging this area of difficulty, the WHO European Regional Office is encouraging the development of educational materials and, in the introduction to one of the volumes, it is noted: 'People working in (the) helping professions often feel incapable of giving help, partly because they do not have the information and skills, and often because they are affected, like their clients, by taboos and constraints which make it difficult to talk about sexuality' (WHO, 1987).

Talking with patients about sexual problems requires tact, sensitivity, tolerance and knowledge. Perhaps most important, it requires a nurse to be comfortable about his/her own sexuality and at ease when discussing sex-related topics with others. Those nurses who do experience anxiety and embarrassment when discussing explicit sexual matters such as homosexuality and masturbation, can be helped to overcome these difficulties. Two articles describe the sexual attitude restructuring (SAR) process, which can be used to accomplish change from a negative to a positive attitude towards sex and sexuality (Linken et al, 1980; Llewelyn & Fielding, 1983).

Certainly, it is important that the nurse is tolerant of a patient's sexuality, whether or not it is akin to her/his own sexual orientation. Jones (1988) argues that the assumption everyone is heterosexual can affect the standard of care offered to those who are not and, in particular, she refers to the problems experienced in health care by lesbian women.

Homosexual men have doubtless experienced similar problems and now, because of AIDS and the homosexual community, are particularly at risk of being unsympathetically cared for unless nurses come to terms with their own prejudices (and, sometimes, mistaken fears) about homosexuality. 'Isolate the disease, not the patient' is perhaps the single most important message for nurses in relation to caring for people with HIV infection and AIDS (Holmes, 1985).

But, as Parker (1988) points out, health professionals continue to react fearfully when confronted with an AIDS patient whereas, in fact, it is the patient who is fearful and in need of support. For nurses to provide this, they need sound information and education about HIV infection and AIDS; the fact that knowledge is lacking has been shown up in surveys, such as Stanford's study in the UK (Stanford, 1988) and Neill's (1988) survey in the USA. The latter, involving 1194 health care workers (including 343 responding nurses), produced some startling findings: negative attitudes towards AIDS patients were reflected in the fact that 44% of respondents believed that most AIDS patients had their disease 'through their own fault', and 34% felt that hospital employees should be allowed to refuse to care for patients with AIDS. Much needs to be done to improve this situation for, by all predictions, there will be many people with AIDS in years to come and the nurse's concern with the AL of expressing sexuality will assume even greater significance than it has in the past.

Most Activities of Living continue to be performed even if in a modified way after admission to hospital. The patient continues breathing, and eating and drinking; and perhaps with more emphasis than usual he performs personal cleansing activities. Communicating, a two-way process between nurse and patient, becomes a most important activity in orientation to the new and unfamiliar environment; the AL of maintaining a safe environment becomes crucial. But what happens to the AL of expressing sexuality? A patient does not cease to be 'male' or 'female' but the significance of this characteristic is not always acknowledged in the context of a hospital ward and this may result in problems for the patient.

The purpose of the process of nursing, an integral part of our model for nursing, is to provide a method whereby nurses can carry out an individualised nursing plan of those activities which are nurse-initiated and related to the patient's activities of living; and this includes the AL of expressing sexuality when it is relevant to the person's current circumstances. The initial assessment is the means by which the patient's individuality is first identified. It involves collecting certain biographical and health details as well as information about the patient's ALs; by observing the patient, family and friends and asking relevant questions. This is supplemented by appropriate information already written on health records, and when applicable, from other members of the health team. From all this information the nurse will become aware of the patient's previous routines in the many activities which make up the AL of expressing sexuality; what can and cannot be done independently in expressing sexuality, and if there is a longstanding problem such as physical disability, how expressing sexuality has been coped with.

While collecting this information nurses will find the résumé under the heading 'Individuality in expressing sexuality' (p. 302) useful, and it will be helpful to bear in mind the following questions:

- what factors influence the way in which the individual expresses sexuality?
- what does the individual know about expressing sexuality?
- what is the individual's attitude to expressing sexuality?
- has the individual any longstanding problems with expressing sexuality and if so, how have these been coped with?
- what current problems (if any) does the individual have with expressing sexuality, and are any likely to develop?

When the reason for admission directly concerns the reproductive system, explicit information about several intimate aspects of this AL will need to be collected at the initial assessment. After this the nurse will, in discussion with the patient (and partner where appropriate), identify and agree about the current problems and their priority for which realistic and achievable short- and long-term goals will be set. A date will also be written for evaluating whether or not the goals are being or have been achieved.

There then has to be discussion about the necessary nursing interventions and any activities which the patient agrees to do to achieve the goals and these are written on the nursing plan in sufficient detail for a nurse reading them to be able to carry out the planned nursing. A large part of daily nursing consists of implementing the plan, together with further assessing and evaluating of the patient. Evaluation can only be as good as the goal setting, so it is imperative that the goals are set out clearly and in unambiguous terms. All these activities take into account the patient's individuality which is the basis for individualised nursing.

Before nurses can begin to think about individualised nursing they need to have a generalised idea of the sort of problems which can be experienced by patients with regard to the AL of expressing sexuality. These, as already mentioned, are likely to be more or less significant according to whether or not the patient's reason for admission is directly related to this AL. Some relevant problems will now be discussed.

CHANGE OF ENVIRONMENT

In normal life people have developed individual ways of expressing sexuality and it is only when faced with change that they might realise the inappropriateness of continuing some of these in a hospital ward. For example, a person may enjoy sleeping in the nude and even changing such a simple habit adds yet another difficulty in getting off to sleep. But by far the biggest problem for most patients is embarrassment concerning aspects of sexuality and there are many ways in which, if the patient's individuality is appreciated, nurses can help to prevent or minimise embarrassment.

This is particularly important in instances where there is violation of the normal social taboos on touching which are closely associated with patterns of sexual affiliation (p. 298). The intimate nature of many medical and nursing procedures can cause much embarrassment and confusion for both patients and staff. In helping patients with the ALs of personal cleansing and dressing, and eliminating, nurses see patients' bodies exposed, and they handle body parts normally kept discreetly covered. If, for example, a young female nurse is bedbathing a middle-aged man both parties may experience a sense of embarrassment. Understanding that embarrassment is a natural reaction to being in a relationship which disregards normal social taboos can help to ease the uncomfortable feelings experienced. The patient will be reassured if the nurse deals with such situations tactfully and sensibly, acknowledging the mutual embarrassment and helping the patient to maintain dignity and privacy. Nurses soon become accustomed to this aspect of their professional role, but should never forget that patients may find intimate procedures disarming and embarrassing.

The vaginal examination is an example of an intimate medical procedure which few women manage to undergo without some anxiety and embarrassment. The woman's genitals are exposed and handled in a way which totally violates the usual codes of allowed physical contact. She may be confused by the sexual overtones of the examination and Moyes (1977), in an article discussing women's reactions to the internal examination given at the prenatal booking clinic, emphasises that such confusion need not arise if the encounter is not seen in sexual terms. However, as she points out, this means that the medical reason for the procedure must be explained clearly to the patient. Sometimes the anxiety is because the woman is afraid she may be unable to allow entry of the speculum (the instrument used to open the vagina) or that the procedure may be painful or damaging. Recognising these natural fears should help the doctor and nurse to prevent undue embarrassment. In preparation for the procedure nurses should appreciate the importance of an explicit explanation concerning its nature and the reason for it being done.

During the procedure nurses can convey their empathy by such acts as keeping the patient covered as much as possible. Couch-Hockedy (1989) provides a very apt description of the nurse's role in this context as 'to support the doctor by providing a running explanation of what is being done and to encourage the patient to ask any questions and express any fears.' She outlines the reasons why women 'dread pelvic examinations and smears' in terms of the following (after Settlage, 1975):

- Exposure and manipulation of the genitals is intimate and usually in a relationship of mutual trust and closeness
- Violation of body privacy
- Fear of showing signs of sexual arousal
- Physical discomfort
- Fear of finding some pathology

It is important for nurses to recognise these fears and help women to overcome them so that pelvic examinations and smears are not dreaded. The need for women in certain age groups to have smear tests regularly is of increasing importance as the problem of cervical cancer in the UK becomes worse and, therefore, early detection all the more important.

Change of environment also poses a problem for patients in terms of the restriction which hospitalisation places on normal sexual expression, a matter which must be seriously considered when long-term care is necessary. A child in hospital for a considerable length of time will be less able to master sexual development if not given opportunities to express normal sexual feelings of childhood and to engage in the usual sex-related games and roles. An adolescent may experience frustration at being cut off from peers and unable to satisfy sexual desires by normal self-stimulatory activities such as masturbation, unless given opportunities for privacy.

Long-term hospitalisation for an adult can seriously disrupt the continuity of a sexual relationship. The patient and partner may suffer from loneliness and, if abstinence from sexual intercourse is prolonged, loss of libido and even severe dysfunction may result. If appropriate, such patients should be given opportunities to go home from time to time so that social and sexual relationships can be resumed and sustained.

Attitudes towards the sexual needs of the mentally ill and the mentally handicapped in the past have been most restrictive and, in institutions for those people, the practice was to deny patients any opportunity for expressing sexuality. Somehow it was thought that 'madness' and 'imbecility' rendered a person 'sexless' or sexually dangerous. Gradually it is being realised that it is desirable to allow sexual expression and that mental impairment does not preclude achieving enjoyment from sexuality. Indeed, it is being realised that expressing sexuality is a right for people with mental handicap, just as it is for anyone else (Bunyan et al, 1986; Behi & Edwards-Behi, 1987).

Helping patients to cope with their sexuality and behave in a socially acceptable way is, therefore, an important aspect of care of the mentally handicapped. These people, like all others, need to be helped to understand how their bodies work and that changes in their bodies and emotions are a normal part of sexual development. For example, instead of being punitive towards patients who masturbate openly in the ward, the nurse can teach them that this is a normal form of sexual behaviour, but should be done in private. And teaching is certainly needed to help mentally handicapped young women to learn to cope with the practical aspects of menstruation, as Fraser & Ross (1986) point out in their article which describes a health education programme with this purpose.

Like all human beings, mentally handicapped people are capable of forming and maintaining relationships with others. More and more hospitals now encourage male and female patients to mix together in occupational and recreational activities. This requires nurses to help them to learn about normal social patterns of interaction and it is obvious that the patients enjoy opportunities to behave as adult males and females do in everyday life. It is becoming common practice in hospitals for the mentally handicapped to ensure that female patients are protected from unwanted pregnancy by teaching them about sex and, if appropriate, providing contraception. This removes the anxiety that social integration of patients may have undesirable consequences and encourages the patients themselves to appreciate that adult sexual behaviour carries with it serious responsibilities.

Mentally handicapped people are not the only group to have been neglected in terms of the need for long-term care environments to accommodate their sexuality and sexual needs; much the same neglect has occurred in relation to the elderly. Griffiths (1988) calls for a more enlightened understanding of elderly patients' sexuality and, in particular, of the problems of the confused elderly.

CHANGE IN MODE OF EXPRESSING SEXUALITY

A person may encounter difficulties associated with expressing sexuality at any stage of the lifespan and for a great variety of reasons. However, the majority of disabled people and many of those who suffer certain kinds of physical disease or disfigurement are particularly prone to experience sexual difficulty.

Physical disability
People can be disabled in many different ways. It is

probably true to say that most people's perception of disability is associated with musculoskeletal conditions, or people who are chairfast from whatever cause. Here, disability will be discussed under the headings, Sexuality and disablement; Attitudes to sexuality and disablement; and Helping disabled people who have sexual difficulties.

Sexuality and disablement

Wells (1982) gives an extended review of a book by Bullard & Knight (see Additional reading) in which several disabled people express their views on their sexuality needs, the problems which they have in satisfying these because of disability, and how they have achieved satisfaction by physical and psychological adaptation. Contributors include a blind person, a deaf person, an arthritic person, a young nurse of 22 who had a radical vaginectomy; and people with spinal cord injuries, cerebral palsy, head injuries, stoma formation and many other conditions. This list is a useful introduction to the wide range of disabling conditions.

All the contributors to the book viewed themselves not only as human beings but as sexual human beings with the same needs as those who are not disabled. They describe their struggle to maintain or achieve a sexual identity; and emphasise that the issue of a normal sex life is much more complex than erection, penetration and orgasm. These aspects of sexuality assume secondary importance to touch, closeness, alternative methods of satisfying a partner and establishing a lasting relationship thus making it clear that sexual intercourse is only a small part of the whole AL of expressing sexuality. The book states emphatically that society has no right to 'de-sexualise' individuals just because they are disabled, and that it has a duty to think in terms of 'sexualisation' for those with disabilities from birth, and of 're-sexualisation for those whose disabilities occur after satisfactory sexualisation has been achieved. There is advice on how to make sexual intimacy a meaningful part of the love-making ritual, for example removal of a leg caliper, or the clothes of a paraplegic person, by the partner.

With such a wealth of information about first-hand experience of problems encountered by people with very diverse physical disabilities, nurses will be challenged to be creative in helping patients to achieve alternative ways of participating in relationships so that they not only express their love, but also feel loved.

Campling (1980) thinks that female sexuality as such is less well attended to in the literature. She says that sexuality exists for everyone and cannot be dismissed because of crutches, wheelchairs, scars or spasms. She quotes Anna Freud: 'Sex is something we do, sexuality is something we are', and an unnamed woman as saying 'Sex may end in the penis, but it starts in the mind.' Campling thinks that the need to be more open and experimental can lead disabled couples to discover a range of touching, positions and pleasures which able-bodied couples might never discover. Disability can have the effect of forcing a couple to be completely honest with themselves and with each other, leading to that 'exchange of mutual vulnerabilities' which Masters & Johnson saw as central in loving relationships.

Attitudes to sexuality and disablement

Sometimes, however, able-bodied people feel repulsed by the idea of the physically handicapped wanting to have sexual relations and even wishing to have children, or by the notion that unconventional modes of sexual activity may need to be used for sexual satisfaction. Anyone with such thoughts would do well to read the book so aptly called *Entitled to Love* (Greengross, 1976) in which the sexual needs and problems of disabled people are discussed with frankness and sympathy, making it clear that many of the problems would be alleviated by a more humane and informed attitude of society.

Helping disabled people who have sexual difficulties

Difficulties of children. A child disabled from birth needs the help of his parents and the encouragement of others to allow sexuality to develop as naturally as possible and to find ways of sexual expression compatible with the handicap. Difficulties will almost certainly arise if the child's sexuality is ignored and, in the course of answering questions and giving information about sex and reproduction, it may be helpful for the special difficulties and needs of the child to be acknowledged and openly discussed. A girl who has to wear an artificial limb may be helped to feel feminine despite this if special attention is paid to her personal appearance; and once she begins to menstruate, she may need advice to help her cope realistically with anxieties about the effect of her disability on relationships and reproductive function.

For an adolescent boy confined to a wheelchair, masturbation will provide an outlet for sexual frustration and he should be reassured, if anxious, that this is an absolutely normal activity. Throughout adolescence it is essential for girls and boys who are physically disabled to have opportunities to mix with able-bodied people of the opposite sex and as far as possible, like them, learn to enjoy and come to terms with their own sexuality.

Difficulties of adults. People who become physically disabled in adulthood may have major readjustments to make in the sphere of sexuality depending on their previous level of sexual activity and feelings about how physical disability may affect sexual function. The disability may be the result of a sudden event, such as a road traffic accident causing the loss of a leg, or the result of a stroke causing paralysis or it may signify the onset of a chronic disabling illness such as multiple sclerosis or rheumatoid arthritis.

The person's sexual difficulty may be the direct result

of the physical disablement, perhaps difficulty in coping physically with sexual intercourse, or it may be predominantly psychological, for example a feeling of worthlessness or fear of rejection by the partner. The disability does affect both the person and the partner, sometimes drastically altering their relationship if, for example, the person affected is forced to give up work. Many people too find it difficult to be both nurse and lover to a disabled spouse. A man may, as a result of direct damage to the central nervous system, have difficulties associated with erection or ejaculation or both. If the disability is accompanied by recurring or persistent pain this can cause loss of libido for a person of either sex.

If pain is a cause of difficulty, as for example the pain affecting joints in rheumatoid arthritis, the person could be advised to take analgesics prior to attempting intercourse. Sometimes, too, a warm bath in advance may add to relief of pain. Adopting a comfortable position is essential. For full sexual satisfaction the glans penis and the clitoris must rub against each other. The conventional 'man-on-top' position may not be the most comfortable or effective and very practical help can be given to couples about alternative positions for intercourse. A complete erection and full penetration of the penis are not essential for ejaculation and a great deal of exertion is not necessary for the achievement of an orgasm. If erection is impossible, a man may wish to try using a penile prosthesis, one of the many available sex aids. There is nothing weird or wrong about people trying out any of these possibilities. The important thing is that the solution to difficulties must be acceptable to both partners.

Physical disease

For those people leading a sexually active life, any one of the wide variety of physical diseases is likely to be accompanied by a temporary loss of interest in sex. Should the disease be acute and temporary in nature it is highly likely that libido will be restored as the illness subsides and the patient's previous sex life will be able to continue at its previous level.

But there are diseases, like those affecting the heart, which are associated in patients' minds with sexual difficulties even although this is frequently unjustified and due simply to lack of knowledge. Other diseases, for example diabetes, can affect body function in such a way that sexual function becomes impaired. Disorders, such as incontinence, can have similar effects. And, understandably, patients undergoing surgery or treatment related to the sex organs may anticipate encountering sexual difficulties. These are some examples of perceived and actual difficulty associated with physical disease and they have been selected for discussion here.

Difficulties associated with heart disease

Most people are aware that intercourse makes considerable demands on the cardiopulmonary system and so patients who have suffered a heart attack or have a chronic cardiac condition such as hypertension (high blood pressure), not surprisingly are fearful about the possible harmful effects of resuming normal sexual relations. It is true that sexual intercourse involves considerable activity and exertion. The pulse rate may rise from around 70 to as high as 180 beats per minute, the blood pressure from 120 to over 250, and the respiratory rate from 16 to more than 40 per minute.

However, there is general agreement among cardiologists that sexual activity is compatible with heart disease as long as the patients know how to assess their ability and identify warning signs of heart strain. Puksta (1979) provides guidelines about the kind of advice which nurses could give to a male postcoronary patient, although they are equally applicable to females. Intercourse can usually be resumed within a few weeks, readiness for this assessed on the patient's ability to perform exercises of comparable physical exertion. For example, the 'stair-climbing test' (two flights of stairs at a brisk rate) is a good form of assessment. The patient needs to be advised of warning signs of heart strain: a rapid pulse and respiration rate persisting 30 minutes after intercourse; palpitations 15 minutes after; chest pain during or after; exhaustion following intercourse or extreme fatigue on the next day. Advice on when to avoid sexual relations can also be given and abstinence recommended: soon after a large meal or drinking alcohol; in extremely hot or cold environments; in an anxiety-provoking situation; and if strenuous activity is anticipated after intercourse.

Nurses and doctors see fit to give heart patients every sort of advice — from dietary needs to whether gardening will be too strenuous for a while — but advice about sex is given less frequently. This is probably thought to be the least of the patient's many concerns; and the patient probably feels too embarrassed to ask, thinking it trivial if the subject has not been raised for him. Much of this misunderstanding and anxiety could be avoided if advice and discussion about sexual activity were given to patients as routinely as other subjects concerning rehabilitation and this is becoming more common, particularly in coronary care units.

Difficulties associated with chronic respiratory disease

A person suffering from a chronic respiratory disease such as emphysema (alveolar distension resulting in oxygen insufficiency) is likely to experience difficulty with sexual intercourse due to dyspnoea (p. 138). It is not easy to alleviate this problem due to destruction of the lung tissue and the person may be advised to consider finding alternative ways of obtaining sexual satisfaction which do not involve physical exertion with which the cardiopulmonary system cannot cope.

Difficulties arising from diabetes

Men who have had diabetes for a number of years, particularly those whose condition has not been kept well stabilised, may experience impairment of sexual function. The precise incidence of impotence in diabetic men is uncertain, with reports giving varying figures as Morrison (1988) mentions. The causes are both psychological and physical, the former tending to be of sudden onset whereas the latter begins insidiously. Poor or absent erectile capacity is indicative of physical causes. Erection is particularly affected because the diabetic condition affects the autonomic nerves, especially the parasympathetic supply. There is no cure, as such, for physical diabetic impotence but psychosexual therapy, penile implants and drug therapy can be employed to combat the problem.

Less is known about the degree to which female diabetics experience a loss of sexual interest or strength of orgasm. Achieving better control of the diabetic condition may prevent or overcome these difficulties.

Difficulties associated with incontinence

Urinary incontinence is a common problem, particularly in women, and appears to have a profound effect on sexual function (Cardozo, 1988). Cardozo mentions a study of 103 women attending an incontinence clinic; 46% reported that their urinary disorder had adversely affected sexual relations. Incontinence during sexual intercourse was reported by 24% of women referred to a gynaecological urology clinic in another study. Cardozo recommends that more attention should be paid to the subject of 'sex and the bladder' so that people with bladder problems can be helped to enjoy their sex lives despite their disability.

Difficulties anticipated after surgery/treatment to sex organs

Not uncommonly men in the middle and older age groups require to have a prostatectomy (removal of the prostate gland) and it is not surprising that many of them have anxieties about the effect on sexual functioning. Patients can be reassured that impotence is rare in men who were previously sexually active.

For younger men, a more likely reason for treatment involving the sex organs is testicular cancer. Although relatively uncommon, naturally it is a distressing disease but treatment at an early stage can be successful and without long-term impairment of sexual function or fertility. For that reason, early detection is now emphasised and it is recommended that men should practise testicular self-examination; for further details see Stanford (1986) and/or Schäufele (1988).

Savage (1982) brings together some of the little information that is available on the effects of gynaecological treatments on female sexuality. In the article there is a good description of females' sexuality in general, and the possible conveyance of nurses' non-verbal messages which discourage patients from raising problems concerning sexuality. In a more recent article, Wallace (1987) considers how more sensitive nursing care could have helped a patient with sexual dysfunction following treatment for cancer of the vulva. She recommends that consideration of her sexual needs should begin right from the preoperative phase of nursing care.

Sexual self-image can be influenced in a negative way by post-radiation changes. Fear of damage to skin which is red and scaling may lead to avoidance of sexual intercourse. Savage points out that because gastrointestinal mucosa is especially sensitive to radiation there may be limitation on oral-genital or oral-anal sexual activity. Loss of vaginal elasticity can shorten and narrow the vagina, and together with pelvic fibrosis make male penetration painful. Patients can be helped to avoid this by being advised to either resume sexual activity or mechanically dilate the vagina and insert oestrogen cream.

Research quoted by Savage (1982) should remove any doubt about women needing help, advice and information regarding what to expect after surgery/radiation to sex organs. In one study 22 out of 28 patients presented with major vaginal alterations and impairment of sexual function after treatment with deep X-ray for cervical cancer. Fear of recurrence was given by four women as a reason for sexual abstinence. Three male partners reported that they had stopped having intercourse because they no longer found it satisfying, while 10 spoke of changes, although they were unable to describe them. In preparation for allocation to a gynaecology ward, nurses would benefit from reading the article.

Female circumcision is an example of another form of gynaecological procedure which has considerable consequences; it is practised in many countries, mainly in Africa and the Middle East. There is usually excision of the clitoris, the labia minora and majora but the extent of cutting varies from country to country. In Sudan the resulting wound is stitched up and only a small opening is left for the passage of urine and menstrual fluid — so-called 'infibulation'. It prevents male penetration, but the woman is 'opened up' ready for the wedding night and traditionally friends do this.

In Britain there are ethnic groups who advocate female circumcision. Midwives, in particular, will come across circumcised women who need extensive episiotomies before delivery — sometimes laterally as well as horizontally — and afterwards some wish to be re-stitched as they would not feel 'feminine' if this were not done. Circumcised women can also be admitted to the wards suffering from urinary tract infections, urinary retention, vaginal infections, bleeding, labial cysts and vaginal calculi (Graham, 1984), all of which can cause difficulties with the AL of expressing sexuality.

For many women, hysterectomy (removal of the uterus) may mark a positive turning point in sexual function with relief from problems such as heavy bleeding and the final removal of fear of pregnancy. Some women however experience symptoms known as the 'posthysterectomy syndrome' even when the ovaries have been conserved. The ovaries have an endocrine function and among other substances secrete androgen which is thought to be the basic hormone of libido. The symptoms are similar to those of the menopause and they can cause difficulty with some aspects of expressing sexuality. Nurses should be especially observant for any signs of undue fatigue and depression in women recovering from a hysterectomy. If the patient reports loss of libido and dyspareunia it should be reported to the doctor. Couch-Hockedy (1989) recommends that counselling should be offered to women undergoing hysterectomy, and to their partners, so that they are informed about problems which may arise and what might be done about them.

Physical disfigurement

Being and feeling physically attractive is a fundamental feature of any person's sexuality and an important aspect of sexual relationships. Western society places great emphasis on beauty and physical perfection. Indeed, numerous studies have demonstrated that physically attractive people fare better in all sorts of ways than those who are less attractive; and Darbyshire (1986) draws attention to the need for nurses to be aware of this since interactions with patients will be affected.

Altered body image of any kind inevitably affects self-image. Any disfigurement such as a facial birth mark, burn, operation scar, physical malformation or loss of a limb, alters a person's sexual self-image. This may cause a man or woman to fear that they may be unable to attract a partner, be regarded by others as sexually unattractive or even be rejected by their spouse. Price (1986) outlines some ways in which nurses can help patients to cope with such problems resulting from disfigurement and altered body image.

Difficulties after stoma surgery

Stoma surgery (p. 195) results in a form of permanent physical disfigurement. There is usually no physical reason to cause a loss of interest in sex or in the capacity to enjoy sexual intercourse. However, difficulty in accepting the stoma may lead to psychological difficulties about sex and even to impotence. Couples may simply need reassurance that sexual relations can be resumed without harming the stoma or they may need very practical advice on how to conceal the bag, prevent leakage and odour, and perhaps an alternative position for intercourse. Conception, pregnancy and childbirth are, as Black (1985) explains, all possible for women who have had stoma surgery, but good counselling support is essential.

Difficulties after breast removal

Mastectomy (the removal of a breast) is an example of a physical disfigurement which causes tremendous anxiety to a woman. The procedure is usually performed as treatment for cancer and fear about this adds to the patient's anxieties. Breast cancer manifests as a lump in the breast; if found in its early stages it is more amenable to successful treatment. For this reason women are encouraged to examine the breasts routinely. Self-examination of the breasts (Fig. 15.1) should be carried out once a month immediately after menstruation. Any lump, change in shape, puckering of the skin or change of skin colour should be reported to the doctor immediately.

Harwood (1983) reports an evaluation of teaching 50 female staff in a hospital and 50 nurses to examine the breasts monthly. During the course of 1 year, 10 women returned to the occupational health department having detected a change in the breast, and of these, two were confirmed as cancer. At the end of the year 50% of the non-nursing staff continued to examine the breasts monthly whereas only 20% of the nurses did so. There is obviously room for improvement related to nurses examining their breasts each month — Figure 15.1 illustrates how this can be done.

The question of whether or not self-examination of the breast is beneficial is still a subject of debate (Holmes, 1987). Evidence of the benefits is presented by Hill et al (1988) on the basis of a meta-analysis (i.e. analysis of results from several studies); in this case 12 studies involving 8118 patients. The authors conclude that the evidence in favour of regular breast self-examination for early detection of breast cancer is both more favourable and more consistent than is commonly accepted.

In the Southampton breast study (Nichols, 1983), 2% of those who developed cancer were under 45 years of age; 22% were 45–64 and 61% were in the 65+ group. Based on this information it is evident that monthly examination of the breasts needs to be a lifelong preventive activity. Breast cancer screening by mammography is now being introduced in the UK since it is thought to provide the best means of early detection; the planned programme aims to have 100 screening centres operational by 1990 for women aged between 50 and 64 (Sadler, 1987). The earlier breast cancer is treated, the better the outlook.

Radical mastectomy, involving removal of the whole breast and the axillary lymph nodes, is a mutilating operation sometimes followed by gross lymphoedema of the arm. It is thought that this might deter women from seeking help in the early stages of any change in the breast. Currently there is increasing interest in local removal of the tumour (lumpectomy) followed 2–3 weeks later by irradiation then by iridium wires threaded into the base of the breast for 2–3 days. It is hoped that this less mutilating operation which leaves the majority of breast tissue intact will encourage women to report any change in the breast immediately. There is also increasing recognition of the importance of involving women themselves in the choice

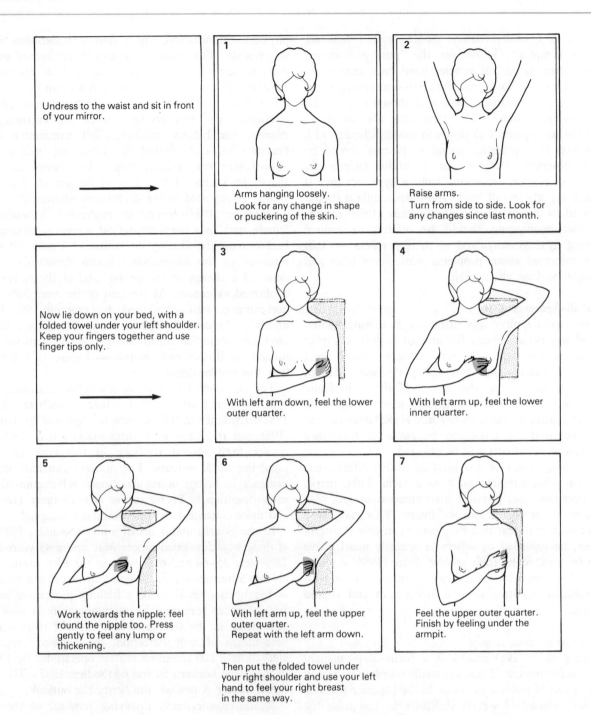

Fig. 15.1 Self-examination of the breasts (based on an illustration kindly supplied by the Family Planning Association, 27/35 Mortimer Street, London W1A 4QW)

of treatment for breast cancer. Wilson et al (1988) support this move and mention that women do not automatically choose to retain the breast.

The chairman of the Mastectomy Association (Westgate, 1981) — now renamed the Breast Care and Mastectomy Association (Swaffield, 1988) — gives excellent advice about what mastectomees can do to help patients come to terms with loss of a breast and what can be done in the

way of expressing sexuality for example, mastectomy does not preclude wearing pretty nightdresses and attractive swim suits and nurses should encourage patients to seek satisfaction by these apparently simple activities.

Although being without a breast does not have a direct effect on the mode of sexual functioning, it alters the woman's feelings about her sexuality. The breasts are a recognised sexual characteristic of the female body and after a mastectomy a woman may feel she has lost some of her sexual attractiveness and, indeed, may fear that her husband will be repulsed by the ugly scar. Wearing a breast prosthesis helps to restore the woman's appearance and confidence in public and, coming to terms with her new body image, helps her to cope with her sexual anxieties. In a stable and loving relationship the operation is unlikely to cause any long lasting impediment to shared sexual enjoyment. But, as Faulkner (1985) explains, full physical and emotional recovery after mastectomy takes time and counselling may be helpful in aiding this process. There is some research evidence in support of this view, one study demonstrating that patients given even limited counselling by specialist nurses suffered less depression and anxiety than others not offered this additional support (Wilkinson et al, 1988).

CHANGE OF DEPENDENCE/INDEPENDENCE STATUS FOR EXPRESSIMG SEXUALITY

With an AL which has as many dimensions as expressing sexuality there are many different ways in which there can be a change in a person's dependence/independence status, and it is important to remember that the change can be in either direction.

For those born disabled or handicapped the objective is for them to achieve their optimum 'independence' in the AL of expressing sexuality. Some of the ways in which this can be encouraged have been discussed already in relation to mentally handicapped people (p. 305).

Then there are those who, after developing independence in the AL of expressing sexuality, lose this to a greater or lesser extent as a result of injury or disease. The problems arising from physical disability, physical disease and physical disfigurement have already been discussed. These sorts of difficulties, although physical in origin, frequently cause psychological distress as well and so result in emotional as well as physical dependence.

SOME SPECIFIC PROBLEMS ASSOCIATED WITH EXPRESSING SEXUALITY

Dysmenorrhoea

This is pain associated with menstruation, either coinciding with the onset of a period (primary dysmenorrhoea) or persisting throughout it (secondary dysmenorrhoea). Until relatively recently, dysmenorrhoea was largely ignored as a medical problem, being considered as mainly psychological and simply 'the woman's lot' (O'Brien, 1988). A greater understanding of the pathophysiological mechanisms of dysmenorrhoea now means that more effective treatment can be offered, and medical advice should be sought in the case of severe and persistent difficulties.

For milder symptoms, women may find relief from resting or taking a hot bath; analgesics may be required as well.

Premenstrual syndrome

Some women experience before each period a feeling of tiredness and irritability. The increased secretion of the ovarian hormones causes an increased blood supply to the pelvic organs and this causes a feeling of weight and distension. Often there is also water retention throughout the body, causing an overall increase in body weight. It is not uncommon for premenstrual tension to be so severe as to cause depression, loss of concentration, accident proneness, outbursts of irrational and possibly violent behaviour.

Women who experience this syndrome can be advised to restrict fluid and salt intake and increase potassium intake by perhaps something as simple as eating one or two bananas. Nurses can advise adequate dietary fibre to avoid constipation; and that taking small meals at more frequent intervals prevents a low blood sugar which can worsen the condition. Relaxation classes and deep breathing exercises can also be suggested.

A great deal has been discovered about the syndrome in the last decade and a few special clinics have been established. Hanna (1980) describes the work of one Premenstrual Syndrome Clinic. She advises that the relatives of those women who become turbulent and possibly violent need help and support in understanding the behaviour until an individual plan can be worked out and evaluated as to its effectiveness in controlling that particular woman's condition.

As always, an individual plan is developed on the basis of information from assessment. Gath & Iles (1988) recommend the use of diaries (a daily diary of symptoms for 2–3 months) for this purpose, also noting that it is important to discover how far physical and psychological causes separately contribute to the premenstrual syndrome.

Menorrhagia

This is heavy and/or prolonged bleeding during menstruation. According to Lui (1988), bleeding in excess of 80 ml is considered heavy, and prolonged as more than 7 days. Some women suffer this discomfort habitually but, for others, menorrhagia may be a sign of physical disease. The excessive blood loss may cause anaemia and patients should be advised to include adequate amounts of iron-containing foods (red meat, eggs, green vegetables) in their diet. One of the problems caused by anaemia is lethargy, such that it may make the woman feel less attractive, and she may have to contend with loss of libido. There can be problems with the partner if either or both, for any reason, do not agree to sexual intercourse during menstruation. Treatment of menorrhagia can be classified as general, medical or surgical; hysterectomy should be regarded as a last resort (Lui, 1988).

Itchiness

Pruritus vulvae (vulval itchiness) is distressing and embarrassing and can be severe enough to interfere with sleep: the resultant tiredness can interfere with several aspects of expressing sexuality. The nurse could suggest to the patient avoiding tight clothing such as tight trousers, and wearing stockings instead of tights. Frequent washing of the genital area, using only bland soap, should be undertaken. Itching can be associated with diabetes, genital herpes or an abnormal urethral or vaginal discharge and the discomfort should always be medically investigated.

Abnormal discharges

Normally there is a discharge of clear or white mucus from the vagina and this thickens and increases in amount just before and after a period and throughout pregnancy. However, there may develop an excessive discharge which causes the woman's underclothes to be permanently wet or one which, when it dries, leaves a green or brown stain. Sometimes the discharge may have an offensive smell. An abnormal discharge may result from infection or perhaps from the presence of a foreign body, such as an unremoved tampon. A discharge which contains blood may indicate a more serious condition, such as cancer in the reproductive tract.

A discharge from the penis may indicate infection and the possibility of venereal disease must be considered. As these are usually contracted during intercourse with an already infected person, they are referred to nowadays as 'sexually transmitted diseases'. Gonorrhoea is common in the UK but syphilis is relatively rare. A white or yellow discharge from the urethra, accompanied by an increased frequency of micturition and dysuria, is characteristic of gonorrhoea in the male. Immediate treatment is essential and it is necessary for contacts to be traced and treated in order to prevent spread of the infection.

Dysuria

Sexual intercourse may aggravate dysuria associated with recurrent urinary tract infection (p. 197) and, in addition, the woman's persistent discomfort may be worsened by the act of intercourse. Either reason may mean she is unable to maintain an enjoyable sexual relationship and, indeed, the discomfort may be sufficiently severe as to cause her to abstain from sexual activity altogether.

In addition to advice mentioned previously, the woman should be advised that she and her partner should both wash the genital area prior to intercourse and apply a lubricant jelly before penetration. After intercourse the woman should empty her bladder to help flush away any pathogens in the area of the urinary orifice and take a drink to assist further flushing of the bladder thereafter.

Dyspareunia

This is pain actually during sexual intercourse, felt either on penetration or during subsequent movement of the penis in the vagina. The former problem may occur at first intercourse because the hymen has to be completely ruptured to permit entry of the penis or it may be due to soreness from tissue scarring following an episiotomy performed at childbirth, or from tightness of the vagina resulting from inadequate relaxation or dryness due to insufficient lubrication.

Pain felt during intercourse usually means that nearby tissue is receiving pressure, directly or indirectly, and this may occur if the uterus is misplaced (retroverted uterus), or an ovary is enlarged or the rectum distended.

People suffering from dyspareunia should seek medical advice because most of its causes are amenable to medical or psychological treatment, thus enabling the person to resume enjoyable intercourse.

Drug-induced decrease in libido

There are many reasons for concern about impaired libido but nurses should be aware of the fact that certain drugs, whether prescribed or illegal, can have this effect and that patients should be alerted to the possibility of sexual difficulty. Durie (1987) explains the effects of some commonly prescribed drugs (including beta-blockers, tranquillisers and antidepressives), noting that opiates and excessive alcohol and cigarette-smoking also lower libido and sexual performance.

Intravenous drug use and the risk of AIDS

Also in relation to the subject of drugs, mention should be made of the particular risk of contracting HIV and AIDS which arises from intravenous drug abuse. The key advice to this group at risk is to avoid ever sharing needles (or other injecting equipment), always to clean equipment and always to dispose of it properly. More detail on this issue is contained in articles by Gafoor (1988) and Carr & Dalton (1988).

The special problems of people with HIV and AIDS

Before closing this final section of the chapter which has been concerned with a variety of specific problems associated with the AL of expressing sexuality, note requires to be made of the very special problems of people who are HIV seropositive or who have AIDS or who, quite simply, are worried about this new and frightening epidemic. This book is not the place for a detailed discussion of the many problems which confront these people. Indeed, despite the short life of 'the AIDS problem', many books solely concerned with this topic have been published already and a couple of these are listed at the end of the chapter as recommended further reading.

Much has been said in this chapter about HIV and AIDS. Most of that has been about the nature and extent of the infection and disease and, importantly, about strategies for its prevention. Comparatively little has been mentioned about the effects of HIV and AIDS on the individual affected or about the nursing needs of those individuals. Yet, assuming the infection continues to spread and the number of people with AIDS continues to rise, the implications for nursing will be considerable.

The clinical features of HIV infection are complex and include opportunistic diseases (such as infections and parasitic diseases which the body's damaged immune defence cannot fight) as well as those caused directly by the virus itself. The progress of HIV infection may be thought of as in four stages — an acute phase, an asymptomatic stage, the stage known as ARC (AIDS-related complex) and then AIDS itself. These stages are identified and described in an extremely helpful booklet, published in 1988 by WHO under the title 'Guidelines for nursing management of people infected with human immunodeficiency virus (HIV)'. It should be noted, however, that any publication on HIV and AIDS which is recommended now is likely to be out of date before long since knowledge and understanding of the disease process are increasing all the time. It is unlikely, however, that what the booklet refers to as 'the basic principles of good nursing practice' will alter with time. These, in summary, concern the responsibility of nurses to contribute to efforts aimed at preventing the spread of HIV and AIDS, and to care for those infected in a way 'that respects the dignity of the individual'.

Individualising nursing

The first part of this chapter reflects the Roper, Logan and Tierney model for nursing — the nature of the AL of expressing sexuality; the relationship of the lifespan to the AL; the effect of the individual's dependence/independence status; the influence of physical, psychological, sociocultural, environmental and politicoeconomic factors on the AL. In the second part of the chapter, a selection of problems and discomforts which are experienced by people in relation to the AL have been described. With this background of *general* knowledge about the AL, it should be possible to incorporate such information in an individualised nursing plan when such information is relevant to the person's current circumstances.

While describing the Roper, Logan and Tierney model for nursing, *general* information was provided about Individualising nursing (p. 51) which in fact is synonymous with the concept of the nursing process.

Out of this background of *general* knowledge about the AL of expressing sexuality and about Individualising nursing, it should then be possible to extract the issues which are relevant to an individual's current circumstances (whether in a health or an illness setting), i.e. to make an

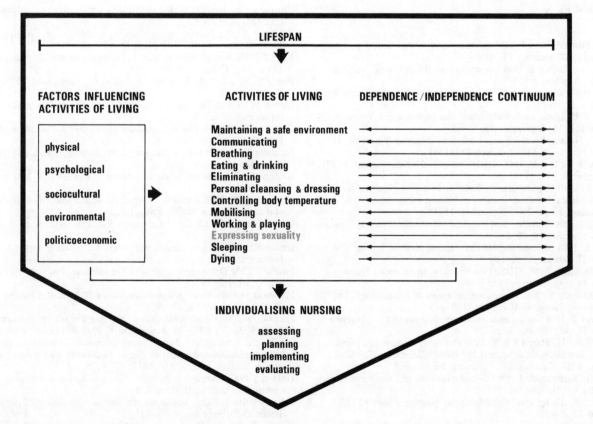

Fig. 15.2   The AL of expressing sexuality within the model for nursing

assessment of relevant issues according to the individual's stage on the lifespan; according to current level of dependence/independence; and take into account the relevant physical. psychological, sociocultural (including ethical, spiritual and religious), environmental and politicoeconomic (including legal) factors. Collectively, this information would provide a profile of the person's individuality in relation to this AL.

This assessment would be achieved by various means such as observing the person; acquiring information about the individual's usual habits in relation to this AL partly by asking appropriate questions, partly by listening to the patient and/or relatives, and using relevant information from available records including medical records. The collected information could then be examined to identify any actual problems being experienced with the AL and these could be arranged in some order of priority. The nurse might also recognise some potential problems — not all possible potential problems but those which are relevant. Realistic goals, mutually agreed with the patient when this is possible, could then be set to prevent potential problems from becoming actual ones; to alleviate or solve the actual problems; or to help the person cope with those which cannot be alleviated or solved.

Keeping in mind what the person can and cannot do unaided, the nursing interventions to achieve the mutually set goals could then be selected according to local circumstances and available resources.

Following implementation of the interventions, their effects could be evaluated in relation to the goals set, and if goals were not reached, they would then be revised or re-scheduled, or even discarded. It is worth repeating here that although discussed in four phases — assessing, planning, implementing and evaluating — individualising nursing is not a linear progression; it assumes a built-in responsiveness to feedback at any of the phases, with ample allowance for change within the overall framework.

This chapter has been concerned with the AL of expressing sexuality. However, as stated previously, it is only for the purpose of discussion that any AL can be considered on its own; in reality the various activities are so closely related and do not have distinct boundaries. Figure 15.2 is a reminder that the AL of expressing sexuality is related to the other ALs and also to the various components of the model for nursing. However, it must be repeated that it may not be relevant to consider this particular AL for every patient in every circumstance. Professional judgement is required to assess its relevance to any one patient.

REFERENCES

Behi R, Edwards-Behi E 1987 Sexuality and mental handicap. Nursing Times 83 (43) October 28: 50–53

Beischer N, Mackay E 1986 Obstetrics and the newborn. Bailliére Tindall, London, p 530

Black P 1984 Who stops smoking in pregnancy? Nursing Times 80 (19) May 9: 59–61

Black P 1985 Stoma care: body image and reproduction. Nursing Mirror 161 (13) September 25: 32–33

Bozett F, Hanson S 1986 Focus on fathers. Nursing Times 82 (11) March 12: 38–40, 82 (12) March 19: 41–44

Bradshaw P L, Issa M 1981 Gender surgery. Nursing Times 77 (37) September 9: 1595–1597

Bunyan S, Clark N, Herranz A, Kaur S, Morley S, Morgan K, Owen S 1986 Mental handicap: human rights and relationships. The Professional Nurse 2 (2) November: 41–43

Campling J 1980 Sexuality and the disabled woman. Nursing Times Supplement August 28: 14

Cardozo L 1988 Sex and the bladder. British Medical Journal 296 (6622) 27 February: 587–588

Carr J, Dalton S 1988 AIDS: Less morality, more sense. Nursing Times 84 (39) September 28: 30–32

Couch-Hockedy S 1989 Women's experiences of gynaecology. The Professional Nurse 4 (4) January: 173–175

Darbyshire P 1986 Body image: when the face doesn't fit. Nursing Times 82 (40) October 1: 28–30

Day S, Ward H, Harris J R W 1988 Prostitute women and public health. British Medical Journal 297 (6663) December 17: 1585

Deakin G 1988 Male sexuality. Nursing 26: 961–962

Deakin G, Kirkpatrick L 1987 Sexual problems and their treatment. Nursing 3 (19): 709–714

Durie B 1987 Drugs and sexual function. Nursing Times 83 (32) August 12: 34–35

Ellis H 1981 Time is of the essence. Nursing Mirror 152 (26) June 24: 43–44

Ernsberger R, Jones E 1988 Femshield (a female condom). Newsweek CX1 (22) May 30: 3

Faulkner A 1985 Mastectomy: reclaiming a body image. Nursing Times Community Outlook May: 11–13

Fong R 1978 Sexual abnormalities 1. Harmless variations. Nursing Times 74 (24) June 15: 1015–1016

Fraser J, Ross C 1986 Time of the month. Nursing Times 82 (30) July 23: 56–58

Gafoor M 1988 AIDS: Drug abuse and HIV. Nursing Times 84 (39) September 28: 29–30

Gath D, Iles S 1988 The premenstrual syndrome. British Medical Journal 297 (6643): 237–238

Glenister H 1988 A programme for AIDS. Nursing Times 84 (18) May 4: 31–32

Graham S 1984 The unkindest cut. Nursing Times 80 (3) January 18: 8–10

Greengross W 1976 Entitled to love: the sexual and emotional needs of the handicapped. Malaby Press, London

Greenwood J 1988 Or die of ignorance. Editorial. Edinburgh Medicine 52: 3

Griffiths E 1988 No sex please, we're over 60. Nursing Times 84 (1) January 6: 34–35

Hanna J 1980 Defeating the curse of the calendar. Nursing Mirror 151 (14) October 2: 36–37

Harwood D 1983 Breast self-examination by NHS staff. Nursing Times 79 (50) December 14: 27–29

Hicks C 1987 AIDS: Innocent victims. Nursing Times 83(6) February 18: 19

Hill D, White V, Jolley D, Mapperson K 1988 Self-examination of the breast: is it beneficial? Meta-analysis of studies investigating breast self-examination and extent of disease in patients with breast cancer. British Medical Journal 297 (6643): 271–275

Holden J 1987 Postnatal depression: 'She just listened'. Nursing Times Community Outlook July: 6–7, 10

Holmes P 1985 AIDS: 'Isolate the disease, not the patient'. Nursing Times 81 (6) February 6: 14–15

Holmes P 1986 It's OK to say no (Child abuse). Nursing Times 82 (3) January 15: 18

Holmes P 1987 Examining the evidence (breast self-examination). Nursing Times 83 (31) August 5: 28–30

Jones R 1988 With respect to lesbians. Nursing Times 84 (20) May 18: 48–49

Jourard S M 1966 An exploratory study of body accessibility. British Journal of Social and Clinical Psychology 5: 221–231

Kay K 1988 AIDS — A global concern. Paper presented to the 3rd International Intensive Care Nursing Conference, Montreal, Canada (31.8.88). Unpublished

Kenn C, Goorney B 1988 Changes in sexual attitudes and behaviour in the light of increased awareness of AIDS. British Journal of Sexual Medicine 15 (5) May: 162–165

Lemonick 1988 It's a boy, and here's why. Time 131 (1) January 4: 45

Linken A, Marshall P, Thorpe D 1980 Sexual attitudes factor. Nursing Focus 1 (9) May: 358–360

Llewelyn S, Fielding G 1983 Sex: more than the facts. Nursing Mirror 156 (11) March 16: 38–39

Lowery M 1987 Adult survivors of childhood incest. Journal of Psychosocial Nursing 25 (1): 27–31

Lui D 1988 Management approaches in menorrhagia. British Journal of Sexual Medicine July: 10–13

Masling J 1988 Menopause: a change for the better? Nursing Times 84 (39) September 28: 35–38

Masters W H, Johnson V E 1966 Human sexual response. Little Brown, Boston

Masters W H, Johnson V E 1970 Human sexual inadequacy. Little Brown, Boston

McAree J 1987 Child abuse: A family affair. Nursing Times April 22: 26–30

Milligan A 1987 Lifting the curse. Nursing Times 83 (18) May 6: 50–51

Moore J 1985 Rape: the double victim. Nursing Times 81 (19) May 8: 24–25

Morrison H 1988 Diabetic impotence. Nursing Times 84 (32) August 10: 35–37

Moyes B 1977 A doctor is a doctor. New Society November 10: 289–291

Neill K 1988 Working with AIDS patients. Nursing Times 84 (16) April 20: 62–63

Nichols S 1983 The Southampton breast study — implications for nurses. Nursing Times 79 (50) December 14: 24–27

Nursing Times 1988 Clinical Update — 'Patch hormone contraceptive suits over-35s'. Nursing Times 84 (43) October 26: 10

O'Brien P M S 1988 Management approaches in dysmenorrhoea. British Journal of Sexual Medicine July: 6–10

Orr J 1988 The porn brokers. Nursing Times 84 (20) May 18: 22

Panja S K 1988 Behavioural profile of females attending sexually transmitted diseases (STD) clinics. British Journal of Sexual Medicine 15 (2) February: 50–52

Parker S 1988 AIDS: soothing away the anxieties. Nursing Times 84 (39) September 28: 26–28

Pernoll M, Benson R (eds) 1987 Current obstetric and gynecologic diagnosis and treatment. Appleton & Lange, Norwalk, Connecticut, p 233

Phillips K 1986 Neonatal drug addicts. Nursing Times 82 (12) March 19: 36–38

Power D 1981 Children in danger. Nursing Mirror 152 (5) January 29: 29–32

Pownall M 1987 'It's only the change of life.' Nursing Times 83 (50) December 16/23: 36–37

Price B 1986 Body image: keeping up appearances. Nursing Times 82 (40) October 1: 58–61

Puksta NS 1979 All about sex . . . after a coronary. American Journal of Nursing 77 (4) April: 602–605

Sadler C 1984 Last resort contraceptive. Nursing Mirror 158 (20) May 16: 14

Sadler C 1987 The breast report. Nursing Times 83(40) October 7: 31–32

Savage J 1982 No sex please, Mrs Smith. Nursing Mirror 154 (7) February 17: 28–32

Schäufele B 1988 Teaching testicular self-examination. The Professional Nurse 3 (10) July: 409–411

Shapiro R 1984 Putting the sex back into contraception. Nursing Times Community Outlook April 11: 123–131

Shapiro R 1986 Fertility rights (Sterilisation). Nursing Times 82 (5) January 29: 24–26

Snell J 1988 AIDS and the risk to infants. Nursing Times 84 (9) March 2:20

Spencer B 1986 If the cap fits . . . Nursing Times 82 (5) January 29: 22–24

Stanford J 1986 Testicular self-examination. The Professional Nurse 1 (5) February: 132-133

Stanford J 1988 Knowledge and attitudes to AIDS. Nursing Times Occasional Paper (6) 84 (24): 47–50

Swaffield L 1988 Mastectomy — and more . . . Nursing Standard 2 April 30: 36

Thomson V 1987 Sexuality in pregnancy. Nursing Times 83 (7) February 18: 63

Torrance C, Milligan S 1986 How safe is the 'safe' period? Nursing Times 82 (26) June 25: 37–38

Vousden M 1987 Child abuse: behind closed doors. Nursing Times April 22: 24–26

Wallace L 1987 Sexual adjustment after radical genital surgery. Nursing Times 83 (51) December 30: 41–43

Warden J 1987 The politics of AIDS. British Medical Journal 294 (6569): 455

Webb C 1985 Teaching sexuality in the curriculum. Senior Nurse 3 (5) November: 10–12

Webb C 1986 Sexuality, nursing and health. John Wiley, Bristol

Wells R 1982 The lover. Nursing Times Supplement August 4: 8–9

Westgate B 1981 Facts and figures. Nursing Mirror 152 (1) January 1: 30–32

WHO 1987 Sexology for health professionals: aspects of sexuality and family planning (Module 3). World Health Organization Regional Office for Europe, Denmark (and BLAT Centre for Health and Medical Education, BMA House, London)

WHO 1988 Guidelines for nursing management of people infected with human immunodeficiency virus (HIV). WHO AIDS Series 3. World Health Organization, Geneva

Wigington S 1981 Depo-Provera: an injectable contraceptive. Nursing Times 77 (42) October 14: 1794–1798

Wilkinson S, Maguire P, Tait A 1988 Life after breast cancer. Nursing Times 84 (40) October 5: 34–37

Williams J 1986 Not just the baby blues. Nursing Times 82 (20) May 14: 38–40

Wilson R G, Hart A, Dawes P J D K 1988 Mastectomy or conservation: the patient's choice. British Medical Journal 297 (6657) November 5: 1167–1169

Wright J 1986 Fetal alcohol syndrome. Nursing Times 82 (13) March 26: 34–35

Yates A 1987 Sexuality: And baby makes three . . . Nursing Times 83 (32) August 12: 31–33

Young M 1981 Incest victims and offenders: myths and realities. Journal of Psychosocial Nursing 9(10) October: 37–39

ADDITIONAL READING

Bullard D G, Knight S E (eds) 1982 Sexuality and physical disability, personal perspectives. Mosby, St Louis

Hogan R M 1980 Human sexuality in nursing process perspective. Appleton Century Crofts, New York

Lennox G I 1987 Overview of human sexuality. Nursing 3 (19): 700–705

Manchester J 1987 Human sexuality: an introduction. Nursing 3 (19): 696–698

McMullen R 1988 Living with HIV in self and others. GMP Publishers, London

Pratt R 1987 AIDS: A strategy for nursing care 2nd. edn. Edward Arnold, London

Salvage J 1988 Nurses, gender and sexuality. Heinemann, London

Webb C 1986 Sexuality, nursing and health. John Wiley, Bristol

16
Sleeping

The activity of sleeping

All parents can testify to their children asking endlessly 'Why have we to go to bed'? Most parents believe that because children are growing, they need relatively more sleep than adults. Scientists have now produced evidence to support this idea and have unravelled many other mysteries about sleep, although some still remain. Adults vary considerably in the amount of sleep they require but, on average, spend about one-quarter to one-third of their lives sleeping. In terms of time alone then, it is for everyone an important Activity of Living.

It appears that all living creatures have periods of activity alternating with periods of inactivity and these are governed by the sleep-wakefulness cycle controlled largely by the hypothalamus. Human beings do not seem to be born with a 24-hour rhythm of sleeping and waking. The recurrence of sleep every 24 hours constitutes a rhythm which the human body has 'learned' through experience. The word circadian describes this learned rhythm, and the term 'biological clock' refers to the mechanism which produces the rhythm. The previous idea that all babies slept for most of the 24 hours is now refuted; each baby is different. In acquiring their rhythm most babies sleep for about 16 hours, at first spread round the clock but by the time they are 3 months old the amount of night sleep has usually doubled.

To include sleeping as an 'activity' is not paradoxical, for although sleep provides the greatest degree of rest, the body systems are still functioning albeit at a reduced level. Sleep has been described as a recurrent state of inertia and unresponsiveness; a state in which a person does not respond overtly to what is going on in the surrounding environment. Although consciousness is lost temporarily, a

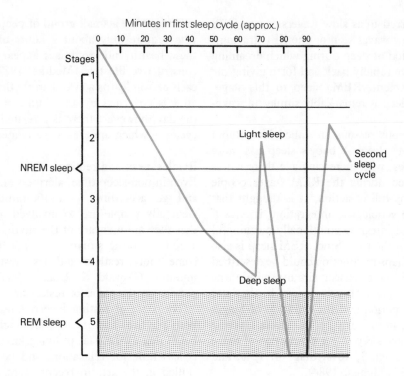

Minutes in first sleep cycle (approx.)

Stages

NREM sleep

REM sleep

Light sleep

Deep sleep

Second sleep cycle

Fig. 16.1 A sleep cycle

sufficient new stimulus as from an alarm clock will rouse the person. In this respect sleeping differs from the states of coma and anaesthesia which are also discussed in this chapter.

THE NATURE OF SLEEPING

How does one know that a person is asleep? Most people sleep with closed eyes; they lie still for part of the time but they move at intervals throughout the sleep periods; sometimes there is relaxation in the muscles of the face and neck so that the jaw is unsupported and the mouth open; breathing is slower and usually deeper; flaccid muscles in the upper respiratory tract are thought to be responsible for snoring. But what is the nature of this phenomenon called sleep?

In recent years, this very question has been exercising the minds of experts in various parts of the world who are conducting research on sleep, and some of the mystery still remains. The writings of a number of researchers are mentioned in this chapter, but many of the references are based on findings from the Sleep Research Laboratory at the University of Edinburgh headed by Professor Ian Oswald who is renowned in this field of enquiry. Although complete answers cannot yet be given to all the queries about sleep, a great deal of information has been collected by recording tracings of the electrical waves from the brains of people who are sleeping — electroencephalograms

(EEGs). The information revealed, particularly about sleep occurring in cycles, has helped in understanding the nature of sleeping.

The sleep cycle

Each sleep cycle is approximately 90–100 minutes in duration and there are usually four to six cycles in a person's normal sleep period (Oswald & Adam, 1983). Each sleep cycle can be described as having five stages which were defined by Rechtshaffen & Kales in 1968. The pattern which these stages tend to follow in young healthy adults in shown in Figure 16.1.

Stage 1. The sleeper has just 'dropped off'. There is a general relaxation; there are fleeting thoughts, and the sleeper can be wakened by any slight stimulus. If awakened, the state is remembered merely as one of drowsiness; it is not described as sleep. But if not interrupted, the next stage is entered after about 15 minutes.

Stage 2. There is greater relaxation, and thoughts have a dream-like quality. The sleeper is unmistakedly asleep but can be wakened easily.

Stage 3. This stage usually occurs after 30 minutes of sleep. There is complete relaxation and the pulse rate slows as do most other bodily functions. Familiar noises such as a flushing toilet do not usually waken the sleeper. If undisturbed, the next stage follows.

Stage 4. The sleeper is relaxed, rarely moves, is difficult to waken, and is in a 'deep sleep'. If sleep-walking occurs, or if there is enuresis, it occurs at this stage. (Sometimes

Stages 3 and 4 are referred to as slow wave sleep or SWS because of the large, slow waves seen on the EEG tracing.)

Stage 5. This is a period of sleep during which dreaming occurs and the eyes move rapidly back and forth giving the name Rapid Eye Movement (REM) sleep to this stage. Physiologically, REM sleep is remarkably similar to wakefulness.

Stages 1 to 4 for obvious reasons are called Non Rapid Eye Movement (NREM) sleep. A baby's sleep has more REM than NREM stages; with increasing age there is less REM sleep. If awakened during the REM stages people may report vivid dreams full of action. It is thought that dreams may promote psychological integration; it is as if they update memory and integrate emotionally meaningful experiences with those of the past. Since REM sleep is also observed in fetuses, perhaps its function could be described more simply as organising electrical circuits within the brain. The REM stages are relatively longer in the later cycles of any one sleep period and the duration of Stages 3 and 4 relatively longer in the early cycles. Overall, young healthy adults tend to have sleep in the proportion of Stage 1, 4%; Stage 2, 50%; Stage 3, 10%; Stage 4, 13%; and Stage 5 — REM — 23% (Johns, 1984).

Although everyone has those sleep cycles, there is considerable variation in the length of time which people will spend sleeping and in what is considered sufficient sleep.

The sufficiency of sleep
It is difficult to say what constitutes sufficient sleep; according to Johns (1984), the range of normal for adults is 3–12 hours, with an average sleep time of 7.25 hours per night. It would seem, however, that a sleep debt can be built up over time which can be compensated by a longer than usual sleep period. After deprivation, Stages 3 and 4 deficit is made up before REM sleep deficit, and for this reason some writers refer to NREM sleep as 'obligatory'.

In one study, in an attempt to discover the effects of sleep loss, experimental volunteers were kept awake for over a week at a time. As well as having difficulty in performing certain tasks it was found that they had a strong tendency to fall asleep yet seemed to be able to maintain semi-automatic activity such as walking while they slept; a point which highlights the danger of continuing to work while short of sleep at jobs which carry risk for the worker and for others. In some instances bizarre hallucinations also occurred after extreme sleep deprivation. It would seem, however, that the 'effects of sleep loss are not only evident after extreme deficits; fine effects can be detected after as little as 2 hours deprivation' (Wedderburn & Smith, 1980). To go to the other extreme, 'extra' sleep has not been shown to improve performance. A researcher, quoted by Wedderburn & Smith, gave people extra sleep after they already had a long night's sleep, and found that their performance on some tasks was worse after 'excessive' sleep.

It is difficult to say what 'lack of sleep' and 'extra sleep'

mean because a small group of people have been identified who require only about 2 hours of sleep each night and these healthy non-somniacs appear to enjoy a happy and constructive lifestyle (Meddis, 1977). It would seem that each person learns a circadian rhythm of sleep which thereafter is governed by an inbuilt 'biological clock'. During the day, however, there is a related cycle — the ultradian cycle — which appears to be related to restlessness.

Restlessness and resting
Even in non-sleep time, alertness and drowsiness can come and go according to a 100-minute ultradian rhythm. Generally people are so involved in what they are doing that they are unaware of the rhythm; but on their own, in a dull or boring situation, it appears that individuals 'become more restless and less restless about every 100 minutes' (Oswald & Adam, 1983). It is interesting to ponder on the states of restlessness and resting.

The state of resting incorporates the art of relaxation, both physical and mental, although it is now a common belief that as the pace of living has greatly increased, there is less time for relaxation, and people have become less skilled in the art. In recent years, a growing interest in, for example, yoga and transcendental meditation may be indicative of a renewed public awareness of the value of relaxation and rest. Often the term relaxation is used to describe pleasurable activities such as sport or reading or art usually as a change from the daily work routine but sometimes involving a great deal of activity. The relaxation of yoga however is claimed to be not a change but a resting period, a cessation of activity, a complete 'letting go' permitting refreshment of body and mind. Authorities on yoga believe that 20 minutes of yoga can bring greater benefits than hours of sleep (Lathlean, 1980).

So, the benefits of long, sound sleep are not entirely clear and even sleep researchers are by no means in agreement about the purpose of sleeping. Oswald & Adam (1983) support the restorative theory, that sleep promotes the restoration and growth of all body cells. It is slow wave sleep (Stages 3 and 4) which appears to be crucial in this regard and, being associated with recovery of the cerebrum (and possibly other tissues), it is the most indispensable part of our sleep. The function of REM sleep is still poorly understood.

The restorative theory of sleep is based on the knowledge that the adrenal gland releases adrenaline, noradrenaline and corticosteroids in large amounts during wakefulness but only in small quantities during sleep and among other things, these hormones inhibit the formation of new protein in tissues. When asleep, the relative absence of adrenocorticosteroids, and the presence of other hormones, especially the growth hormone and testosterone, promote renewal of body tissue. Of course these activities are only part of a complex chemical and enzymatic system controlling the body's renewal and restoration. The processes involved, however, are not yet fully understood and it could even be that these restorative processes occur simply because the body is resting, rather than that the person is actually sleeping.

There are, however, a number of other theories about sleep. Some writers consider that the function of sleep might simply be energy conservation. The decreasing amount of sleep taken in old age might therefore be due to the decreasing metabolic rate and energy usage associated with advancing years (Canavan, 1984). Horne (1983) suggests that only specific portions of sleep (Stage 4 and about 50% of REM) are obligatory. Further, he suggests that this portion of sleep is essential only to brain functioning, while the rest of the body needs only physical rest and feeding for restoration to take place.

Another theorist has suggested that sleep is merely an instinct or a genetic hangover from an earlier era when secluded inactivity at night alternated with daytime activity as part of a survival strategy (Meddis, 1977).

LIFESPAN: EFFECT ON SLEEPING

The component of the model called the lifespan is certainly relevant when considering sleeping. This AL is affected by age both in terms of duration and quality. The 'chronology of sleep', showing shifts in sleep patterns over the course of a lifetime, is outlined in an article by Wardle (1986).

Not only do the young require more sleep than adults, as already stated, but their sleep has relatively more Stages 3 and 4 sleep in which the growth hormones are secreted, and this is not surprising in view of their rapid physical growth. They also have relatively more REM sleep presumably because of the vast amount of brain development and learning in the early years of life.

The sleep of the neonate is composed of almost equal amounts of REM and NREM sleep. Babies sleep for about 16 hours each day split into 6 to 8 sleep periods but gradually there are longer periods of sleep, mostly at night, and longer periods awake. By the age of 4, the average child sleeps for 11 hours each night, perhaps with an additional short day-time nap. However, although babies and toddlers seem to spend quite a lot of time asleep, waking problems in young children are not uncommon. Richman (1983) found that about 20% of children in their second year waken regularly at night. The wakefulness can be related to factors within the child, or stress and tension within the family, but sometimes it is due to parental over-responsiveness to wakefulness which in fact, reinforces the pattern. A useful discussion of the problems of sleeping difficulties among young children, and ways in which parents can prevent them, is provided by Keys (1988) on the basis of her experience as a health visitor in Scotland.

By the age of 15 years, most people have a sleep period which, on average, is of 7–8 hours' duration. From ado-lescence onwards, REM averages about 20% of the time spent asleep, though the absolute amount of time spent sleeping tends to gradually diminish with age. Healthy adolescents and young adults usually sleep so well that little will disturb them. However as these same sound sleepers become middle-aged they may complain of insufficient or broken sleep, especially the women (Oswald, 1980).

In general, the older person, according to Adam (1980) sleeps for a shorter period than the young and it is more broken by periods of wakefulness; it also contains relatively less REM sleep. She describes an interesting study of 212 healthy people aged 65–93, carried out in the USA, which found that by the age of 75, the older person (and no difference was found between males and females) spends more time in bed, though not necessarily asleep, and had more naps than younger people; and that by age 85, there was an increasing use of sedatives probably indicating more difficulty in falling asleep. In this study, 92% of these healthy elderly people believed that they got the right amount of sleep.

DEPENDENCE/INDEPENDENCE IN SLEEPING

Unlike some of the other ALs already discussed, each individual is independent for the actual activity of sleeping. Unlike the majority of the other ALs too, this component does not have a direct relationship with the lifespan component. Babies, although helpless for many ALs, spend most of their time sleeping; and the elderly, at the opposite end of the lifespan and sometimes dependent for other ALs, also spend more time in bed, although not necessarily asleep, than younger adults. However, while the activity itself is independent, the environmental conditions for sleep are not necessarily so. The infant is dependent on others for maintaining a suitable temperature conducive to sleep, at least by use of clothing if not by control of atmospheric temperature. The safety of the environment is also controlled by others and there can be accidents, for example, because a baby has rolled out of a high bed when asleep, or has smothered in a pillow, or has been harmed by a domestic pet.

Children and adolescents can also be dependent on others for sleep. If there is prolonged stress or tension in the family they may develop disturbed sleeping patterns (Richman, 1983) and when there is noise, for whatever reason, there may be difficulty in getting to sleep and the problem of getting back to sleep, once wakened.

The sleep of adults may also be dependent on others, especially in relation to disturbance by excessive noise and particularly if on shiftwork. Perhaps the major concern about dependence in adulthood, however, is related to the use of sleeping pills. A considerable number of people, especially in industrialised countries, are anxious about difficulties with falling asleep and staying asleep for what they believe to be an appropriate period, and they resort to drugs to enhance their own capacity for this AL. The widespread use and abuse of drugs has created considerable problems not only in terms of cost to the taxpayer (if there is a national health service where they are free or heavily subsidised) but also in terms of creating dependence on drugs. All hypnotics, anyway, become less effective with regular use; studies of people who have taken sleep medications for months or years indicate few beneficial effects in terms of either falling asleep or staying asleep (Canavan, 1984). So it would seem that long-term dependence on sleeping pills is not a satisfactory solution to a person's sleep problem, whatever its nature.

FACTORS INFLUENCING SLEEPING

Like all other ALs sleeping is influenced by a variety of factors. In keeping with the relevant component of the model, these are described under the following headings — physical, psychological, sociocultural, environmental and politicoeconomic factors.

Physical factors

Some physiological functions are closely related to sleeping. As far as circadian rhythms are concerned it appears that the 24-hourly cycle is one to which most species synchronise their bodily rhythms. During a 24-hour period there is a cycle of many physiological functions such as heart rate, metabolic rate, respiratory rate and body temperature all tending to reach maximum values during the late afternoon and early evening, and minimum values in the early hours of the morning (Hawkins & Armstrong-Esther, 1978). Perhaps this would be expected. Most people are active during the day and asleep at night. There is evidence that these internally controlled rhythms are timed to synchronise with external cues and when the harmony is upset for example by travelling rapidly across time zones, there is desynchronisation which manifests itself as fatigue, malaise, lassitude and inability to make effective decisions — the syndrome known as jet-lag. The period varies with the individual, but it usually takes about 3 to 7 days to correct jet-lag and get body time and sleep time back in harmony (Smith & Wedderburn, 1980).

Physical exercise may affect sleep. Children enjoy a great deal of exercise during their waking hours, and although overstimulation may, on occasion, prevent them from falling asleep quickly, exercise can raise body temperature which, in turn, may contribute to their sleep having relatively longer periods of Stages 3 and 4 sleep when the growth hormones are secreted in large amounts. It has been shown too that after exercise, athletes have more Stages 3 and 4 sleep, and even adults taking more exercise than usual will secrete more growth hormone from the pituitary gland during the succeeding sleep period, thus facilitating

maximal protein synthesis and restoration of the body cells (Oswald & Adam, 1983).

Eating certain foods and drinking certain beverages is also said to affect sleep. There is a popular belief, for example, that cheese and coffee cause disturbed sleep. Although there does not seem to be much evidence about cheese perhaps there is some justification for advocating decaffeinated coffee. Two cupfuls of coffee (300 mg caffeine) have been found to cause disturbed sleep in old people whereas a group of researchers found that a milk and cereal drink, Horlicks, led to less wakefulness when compared with nights when a placebo pill was taken (Brezinova & Oswald 1972). However Oswald & Adam subsequently concluded (1983) that although milk and proprietary food drinks, being easily digestible sources of nourishment, probably are helpful in inducing sleep their effect should not be exaggerated. The effect of a change in usual food and fluid intake at bedtime is more important than the actual type of food/drink taken.

Some people consider that alcohol helps them to sleep. This belief may be true if taken in moderation especially if related to a pattern of fluid intake as a bedtime beverage but it has been shown that alcohol produces a lighter sleep pattern with more awakenings (Whitfield, 1982). There is certainly evidence of disturbed sleep, and indeed bad dreams, when there is withdrawal from alcohol dependence. When calorie intake affects weight, it has been found that the change in weight affects sleep. As obese people lose weight, they sleep less; and when patients with anorexia nervosa are regaining weight, they sleep longer and REM sleep is increased (Adam, 1980).

Snoring may affect sleep, although it is the listener who is kept awake. Snoring may be indicative of a number of pathological conditions so should not be dismissed lightly but it may have no known cause or cure. Usually any mention of snoring is greeted with hilarity but in fact it can disrupt a sleeping partnership and become a justification for divorce in the USA (Felstein, 1979). Recent research suggests that one type of snoring — sleep apnoea — can also be dangerous as Dopson (1988) explains. In sleep apnoea, there is loud snoring and 'breathing pauses'. In view of the potential danger, it is recommended that the condition should be recognised and treated, and suggested that night nurses are in a position to diagnose the condition and should let the doctor know if a patient snores loudly or has breathing difficulties at night.

Psychological factors

The individual's psychological status is linked to sleeping. Mood can be considered as a continuum with excitement at one pole and depression at the other. Transient insomnia caused by excitement has been experienced by most people and may not cause undue distress. The sleeplessness associated with depression may however be severe, and continue over a period of weeks. The depressed person can lie awake for hours dwelling on unhappy themes of hopelessness, and when sleep does come, is easily wakened, only to resume thoughts of rejection and failure, or even suicide. However the primary characteristic of sleep change in depression is early morning wakening; indeed, it is a major diagnostic feature.

Perhaps worry and anxiety rather than excitement and depression are the most common disturbers of sleep. It would seem that people who are worried or dissatisfied with their day-time lives are often worried and dissatisfied with their sleep. Almost everyone has had periods of anxiety and apprehension at some point in their lives even over such episodes as examinations or employment interviews. However Oswald (1980) considers that the individual should be 'protected from over-treatment'. After all, a certain amount of anxiety is inevitable in the process of living.

Dreams are believed by some people to have enormous psychological significance (Hearne 1986). Dreams certainly have a strange fascination for man. At one time it was thought that the soul departed from the body during sleep in order to mingle with supernatural beings who would provide guidance about the future. The possible symbolism of dreams has also been given considerable credence and reinforced by writers such as Freud and Jung. Cohen (1979) maintains that 'the heart (and soul) of classic sleep research was to attempt to . . . establish correlations between specific physiological events and dream characteristics.'

It is now known that dreaming occurs mainly, although not exclusively, during REM sleep. The researchers assure us that everyone dreams but most are not remembered. The rate of forgetting is remarkably fast. Subjects in the Sleep Research Laboratory in Edinburgh who were wakened during REM sleep recalled a dream in about 80% of cases; wakened 5 minutes after REM sleep, there was only fragmentary recall; aroused 10 minutes later, there was scarcely any recall. So anyone who wakens up recalling a vivid dream, has probably surfaced out of REM sleep. Dreams themselves can be frightening, some are bizarre, some are amusing; most are interesting to recount; indeed not uncommonly, dreams are the substance of art, music, drama, and literature.

Whatever the quantity or quality of sleep, the psychological effect of wakening up refreshed or unrefreshed determines a person's belief about being a good or bad sleeper; in other words, assessment of sleep is largely subjective.

Sociocultural factors

Sociocultural factors also influence sleeping. For example they will determine where a person sleeps and with whom. In Western cultures, it is usual to sleep in a bed which is raised up from the floor but in Japan, the bedroll on the floor is traditional; and in some nomadic, ethnic groups it is usual to sleep on the ground in the open, or in a tent or in a hammock.

In Western cultures, it is usual for a husband and wife or a co-habiting couple to sleep together in one bed, but most other people sleep alone. However in other cultures it is not uncommon for several members of the family (or extended family) to sleep in the same 'sleeping-space' and if they do sleep singly or in couples, it may not be in a segregated personal bedroom; it could be in a room common to the entire family.

Cultural differences can also be identified with regard to what is worn for sleeping. Nomadic Eskimos, for example, wear the same clothes during the day and at night; in other cultures, nightdresses or pyjamas are worn, and for some people are a means of expressing sexuality; for other people the accepted norm is to sleep in the nude.

Some of these sociocultural characteristics related to sleeping may seem strange but with the ease of international travel and the popularity of television-viewing, most people now know much more about the effect that social and cultural characteristics have on the AL of sleeping.

Environmental factors

Sleep can be affected by a number of environmental factors. Sleep tends to come more easily in a familiar environment — a cool, quiet dark room in surroundings which are well known, with personal belongings at hand and so on. The safety of the environment is also important. A high bed, where there is difficulty getting in and out and anxiety of falling, may disturb the sleep of an elderly or disabled person; and the sleep of parents temporarily may be affected when a child changes from sleeping in a cot to sleeping in a bed. People who know they are sleep-walkers may not be able to fall asleep unless they are reassured that windows have been closed, and that objects which potentially could cause accidents have been removed from the immediate environment; indeed some sleep-walkers find some means of attaching themselves to the bed so that they will wake up rather than sleep walk. People affected by unfamiliar surroundings, such as a hotel or hospital ward, may have to reassure themselves by checking the fire precautions and the siting of fire escape doors.

Environmental noise may or may not affect sleep. Again familiarity with the environment allows many people to sleep despite, for example, the noise of a nearby factory or a busy thoroughfare or an aircraft flight path. Yet these same people may have difficulty falling asleep in a strange environment perhaps because of the sound of the waves on a beach or even by the excessive quietness of a rural setting. Night shift workers may have major complaints about noise when they are attempting to sleep during the day; although if habitually on night shift, many seem to learn to ignore the noise.

Room temperature may affect the ability to fall asleep and to remain asleep. The body temperature actually falls during sleep; there is a slight normal lowering between the hours of 0200 and 0600 which is not surprising because during sleep, there is minimal functioning of the various body systems. However, any further lowering of temperature usually wakens the sleeper, as indeed does any increase. Perhaps to be expected, the climate has an influence, and where there are extremes of climate, attempts are made to control and modify the indoor temperature. In hot climates bedrooms increasingly are equipped with air-conditioning systems; some are sophisticated and expensive; others primitive, although sometimes amazingly effective. Likewise in cold climates, insulation and central heating systems are used or some other means of providing heat and warmth. The physiological control of body temperature is less efficient in children and the elderly so it is recommended in the UK, for example, that bedroom temperatures should not fall below 18°C during the night. For elderly people who cannot afford to heat a bedroom during winter, having the bed moved into the heated livingroom is suggested; wearing socks and a hat in bed is further advice given to the elderly in order to prevent hypothermia (Professional Nurse, 1986).

It is interesting that latitude does not seem to alter sleeping. Within the Arctic Circle, the inhabitants sleep similar hours to us despite experiencing unending daylight in the summer and months of darkness during the winter. In countries where an afternoon siesta is the norm, the people sleep again at night.

The effect of space and weightlessness on sleep is still being researched. During the last two decades there have been spectacular advances in space exploration and data are being collected about the effect of this somewhat novel environment on human sleeping patterns.

Politicoeconomic factors

It may not strike one immediately that the AL of sleeping is influenced by politicoeconomic factors. However any consideration of where people sleep will usually involve housing or a shelter of some kind and certainly in Western culture, this will be related to economic status. The size of the house will influence whether family members have their own bedroom or a shared one, their own bed or a shared one. Some people, however, because of low earning power (for whatever reason), may have to cope with a living space which is grossly overcrowded and the family may have to sleep in the room in which they have lived and cooked all day; there is no choice. For others who would be considered as vagrants it may be necessary, even in a cold climate, to sleep 'rough', exposed to unfavourable weather conditions which endanger health and are certainly not conducive to satisfactory sleep. In some countries the government or voluntary agencies will make provision for such people, usually in the form of communal sleeping accommodation at low cost.

Type of work of course is closely related to politicoeconomic factors, and during the last few decades, there have been a number of studies about shift work and its effect on sleep. As a rule the 24-hour biological clock makes man fall asleep at night and awaken in the morning, and this reflects the individual's normal body rhythms, with their characteristic low level of arousal at night and higher level during the day. However night shift removes sleeping from the night sequence and out of harmony with body time. Much of the early research on sleep and nightshift work concluded that the body clock would gradually be reset over a period of about 7 nights, and then following a spell of night work, there would be a delayed return to normal. However results of later studies quoted in Smith & Wedderburn (1980) and covering a wide range of variables (including deep body temperature, potassium excretion, adrenalin excretion, blood pressure and reaction time) all show that experienced shift workers demonstrate a flatter than normal night shift curve of these readings on the first night, and that this is retained without much deviation over subsequent consecutive night shifts. It is replaced by a typical day curve on the first full day without night work. So the body clocks of shift workers remain set to 'real' time. Smith & Wedderburn suggest that these findings were made possible because the researchers were able to collect more data; instead of using one or two readings each night, as in the older studies, they used body-borne microchip recorders which collected continuous readings of several variables. They conclude that although shift workers get used to night work, this is because they 'become better at handling the contradiction of being biologically geared to day activity while being required to work at night, and not because they reset their body clocks!' Typically the duration of day-time sleeps after night shifts are short and often, although feeling fatigued, it is difficult to fall asleep. So a sleep debt builds up.

The problem of shift work in nursing continues to be an issue of concern and controversy. Brown (1988) examines various shift patterns in nursing. She notes recommendations made by an Australian scientist who, on the basis of research which revealed a high error and accident rate among people who worked an early morning shift which followed a late afternoon/evening shift, considers this combination should be avoided and, instead, the shift rotas should move forwards (i.e. earlies, lates, nights, off) in sympathy with the body's 'running clock'.

The problems of shift work, long hours and interruptions of sleep are also of concern to doctors. In a study of young hospital doctors in Cambridge, UK and New York, and reported by Oswald & Adam (1983), it was shown that sleep loss caused them to be more easily irritated; they could not react to complexity and could only think of one thing at a time: such impairment of functioning can affect the safety of patients as well as the doctors themselves. Recently, this issue has become a matter of public as well as professional debate in the UK. Junior hospital doctors are pressing for a reduction in working hours and, at the time of writing, the Government has indicated that this will happen. There is concern, however, that a reduction even to 72 hours per week, although substantial, will not be adequate. A recent newspaper article (Wilkie, 1989) reports that, although junior doctors in the United States only work 36-hour shifts, a leading sleep researcher considers this to be overlong for safety. He emphasises the need for reduction in the length of time continuously without sleep, rather than overall hours' reduction. Such rules apply to pilots as Durnford (1988) outlines, arguing that the reasoning pertains to the situation of doctors. Like pilots, there are certain occupational groups — another example being long-distance lorry drivers — which have to comply with rules and regulations which limit working hours. The International Labour Organisation has recommendations regarding working hours, but they are not always implemented and clearly this is an opportunity for improvement on the basis of new knowledge which has been provided through sleep research.

INDIVIDUALITY IN SLEEPING

Individuality is the final component of the model. From the foregoing discussion, it is evident that there are many dimensions in each component of the model which help one to describe how a particular person develops individuality in the AL of sleeping. Below is a résumé of the main points discussed.

Lifespan: effect on sleeping
- Length/frequency/type of sleep
  - in infancy and childhood
  - in adolescence and adulthood
  - in old age

Dependence/independence in sleeping
- Provision of conditions conducive to sleep
- Use of sleeping pills

Factors influencing sleeping
- Physical
  - circadian rhythms
  - physical exercise
  - pre-sleep routines
  - effect of food/drink
  - snoring
- Psychological
  - mood (especially anxiety/depression)
  - dreams
  - knowledge about sleep
  - attitude towards sleep
  - beliefs about quantity/quality of sleep
- Sociocultural
  - sleeping space
  - type of bed/bedding
  - own/shared bed
  - night attire
- Environmental
  - hot/cold atmosphere
  - ventilation
  - noise/quietness
  - safety aspects
- Politicoeconomic
  - income/type of housing
  - own/shared room
  - type of work (incl. shift work)

Sleeping: patients' problems and related nursing

Sleeping is such a complex activity and highly sensitive to disturbance, so perhaps it is to be expected that when a person is ill, some problems will be encountered, even transiently, in relation to this AL. However, as refreshing sleep is considered to be therapeutic, it is important for the nurse to know about the person's usual habits in relation to sleeping so that this knowledge can be used to devise an individualised plan of nursing and everything possible done to promote normal sleep. As Carter (1985) comments, 'assisting patients to fulfil their individual sleep requirements would seem to be an important aspect of patient care for nurses'.

In order to individualise nursing, it is necessary to assess the activity of sleeping in so far as it is relevant to the particular person. Assessing involves observing the patient; acquiring information about the patient's sleeping habits (partly by asking appropriate questions, partly by listening to the patient and/or relatives); and using relevant material from available records such as medical records. The nurse would be seeking answers to the following questions:

- when does the individual usually sleep?
- where does the individual sleep?
- what factors influence the individual's AL of sleeping?
- what does the individual know about sleeping?
- what is the individual's attitude to sleeping?
- how well does the individual sleep?
- has the individual any long-standing difficulties with sleeping and if so, how have these been coped with?

• what problems, if any, does the individual have at present with sleeping or seem likely to develop?

Of course, the nurse does not necessarily ask these actual questions because much of the information can be acquired in the course of discussing other topics included in an assessment interview and, later, in a less formal way by conversing with the patient. However it is achieved, Manian (1988) advocates proper assessment of a patient's sleep within the framework of the nursing process. There may be benefits in incorporating a 'sleep history' since, as Clapin-French (1986) points out in relation to long-term elderly patients, this tends to be a neglected aspect of history-taking in nursing assessment.

The collected information can then be examined to identify any problems being experienced with the AL and these can be arranged in some order of priority. The nurse may recognise potential problems which can also be discussed with the patient. Realistic goals can then be set in conjunction with the patient to prevent potential problems from becoming actual ones; to alleviate or solve the actual problems; or to help the patient cope with those which cannot be alleviated or solved.

Keeping in mind what the patient can and cannot do for himself, the nursing interventions to achieve the set goals can then be selected according to circumstances and available resources. These interventions should be written on the nursing plan along with the date on which evaluation will be carried out, in order to discern whether or not the stated goals are achieved. Of course, other professional groups such as doctors, physiotherapists and dietitians are usually involved in the care programme and it is important to ensure that the total care of the patient is discussed and mutually agreed. On the Nursing Plan proforma suggested by Roper, Logan and Tierney (p. 58) there is a page for appropriate entries of this type in order to indicate the relationship between nursing interventions derived from medical/other prescription and nurse-initiated interventions. In relation to the AL of sleeping, one area of medically-prescribed nursing intervention relates to the administration of hypnotic drugs, if prescribed by the doctor.

However, before thinking in terms of individualised nursing, a general idea of the conditions which can be responsible for, or can change, the dependence/independence status for the AL of sleeping and which can be experienced by the person as a problem in carrying out the AL will be provided. The remainder of this section is a general discussion of the types of patients' problems related to sleeping and associated nursing activities. Patients' problems with this AL are grouped under the following headings:

- Change of environment and routine
- Change of dependence/independence status
- Some specific problems associated with sleeping
- Altered consciousness.

CHANGE OF ENVIRONMENT AND ROUTINE

There are many reasons for a newly-admitted patient experiencing sleep problems. One major reason may be the strange environment of a hospital ward. Whatever their previous sleeping arrangements, the majority of patients in the UK are admitted into an open Nightingale type of ward; some into two-, four- or six-bedded bays, recesses or rooms; and only a minority have single rooms. In many instances a patient has no choice about sleeping in the presence of others.

The hospital bed. The bed itself may be very different. All patients are admitted into a single bed, yet many will have been used to sleeping in a double bed. The majority of hospital beds are higher than the divan type of bed used in most homes although new models can be mechanically adjusted. If the height cannot be adjusted, this can be anxiety-producing for those who are accustomed to getting up to go to the toilet during the night; the nurse can help by establishing whether the patient would prefer to summon assistance or to have at hand a commode/bedpan/urinal. This information would be written in the nursing plan so that all staff would be informed. Where adjustable height beds are in use, it is important for nurses to remember to lower them before the patient goes to sleep.

Some beds are specially designed. One for example is adjustable so that the sitting position can be maintained during sleep. If it is necessary for the patient to adopt this position because of severe dyspnoea, it is often a relief to be so well supported, and although not a natural position for sleeping, the patient usually adapts reasonably well. Other special beds which may be used by patients include: air, low air loss, water, sand, fluidised sand, mud, bead, net suspension, Ko-Ro, Stryker and flotation beds. Sleeping on these types of beds is 'different' and initially there is a period of adaptation until the patient becomes gradually used to the change. The objective in using them is dispersal of body weight over a greater surface area for the prevention of pressure sores (p. 218). The patient needs to understand why such a bed is necessary and should be encouraged to report any problems with it.

Most people's concept of a bed includes careful selection of a mattress and the choice can be very personal. Hospital mattresses can be sufficiently different to interfere with sleep, particularly on the first few nights. Horsehair mattresses were found to be a particular cause of sleep disturbance in a recent study of patients' sleep on surgical wards (Closs, 1988). Plastic covers on mattresses and/or pillows were also a source of complaint; Closs recommends that consideration be given to the waterproof, but vapour-permeable, materials which are now available. This study's findings about patients' dissatisfaction with hospital beds, however, are not novel; a Royal Commission on the National Health Service (1978) reported that one in eight patients found their hospital beds uncomfortable.

Apart from the bed itself, hospital bedding can differ from that used at home and patients who experience such a difference may require some time for adjustment. Nowadays many people favour one single covering article for ease of bed-making such as a quilt or a downie. However some people like to feel the weight of bedclothes and therefore choose to use conventional sheets and blankets. Wherever possible, arrangements should be made to interfere as little as possible with patients' preferences and thereby provide the greatest possibility of continuance of good sleeping habits. To this end an increasing number of hospitals offer patients the choice between a quilt and conventional bedding.

Wearing night attire provided by the hospital is much less common than previously, but just as day clothes are personal and important to one's self-image, so are night clothes and any difference can therefore interfere with sleep. In some cases where night clothes might become soiled with excreta or vomit, it is preferable for the patient to wear hospital gowns. In the interests of maintaining morale, it is important that they are attractive as well as comfortable.

Pre-sleep routine. Each patient has been socialised into a pre-sleep routine with an individualised sequence which is necessary for comfort and conducive to relaxation. Many patients continue to be capable of carrying out that routine while in hospital and they should be encouraged to do so. Information from dependent patients, or their relatives if patients are not able to give it, will help nurses develop a nursing plan which includes pre-sleep routines along lines with which the patient is familiar. Obviously, in a hospital ward, the routines of individual patients have to be compatible with communal living and care requirements but, sometimes perhaps, nursing routines unnecessarily compromise those of importance to patients. The inevitable hospital routine which dictates that patients retire early to bed (and wake up earlier) does seem to have detrimental consequences, in particular contributing to the increased time which patients take to get to sleep in hospital compared with home (Closs, 1988).

Posture. Depending on the cause for admission to hospital, and the patient's treatment, a changed posture may be necessary, and help may be required to adapt to the change. For example, in the absence of a special bed when a patient has to be nursed sitting up it may be more comfortable to use an adjustable height bed-table with a pillow on it, on which to rest with flexed arms, thus ensuring the best conditions for breathing and sleeping. Lying supine over a length of time for any reason can cause a feeling of fullness in the abdomen; this can be due to the upper abdominal organs resting against the diaphragm, so slight raising of the head of the bed may allow the organs to slide down a little, relieving the pressure and permitting sleep. Patients with a lower limb on traction are usually nursed in a high bed with the bedclothes arranged in two sections around the elevated limb; such patients may feel more comfortable if a pillow is placed close to each side of the body on which they can rest their arms. Research has shown that both snoring and sleep apnoea (temporary cessation of breathing during sleep) occur more commonly among people who sleep flat on their backs (Koskenvuo et al, 1985). Nurses could help alleviate these problems by encouraging patients to adopt alternative positions in bed.

Whatever recommendation is made regarding posture during sleep, it should be written in the nursing plan so that all staff are informed of these measures.

Temperature. People who have sleeping problems are often highly sensitive to the environmental temperature. Sometimes however, it is difficult for the nurse to exert any control over local conditions. For example for safety reasons, in high-rise hospitals, the windows on the upper floors may not be able to be opened, so natural ventilation is not possible. Also the heating or cooling system is often controlled centrally and not all radiators have individual heat control mechanisms. In such circumstances, an immediate solution is to make adjustments to night attire and to bedding if patients feel they are too hot or too cold; or to use cooling fans, or adequately covered hot water bottles or an electric blanket.

Fever also leads to disturbed sleep. Active management of pyrexial patients, perhaps by administering an antipyrexial agent, might assist in promoting sleep along with other temperature-reducing interventions (p. 237).

Noise. In the last few decades, almost everyone has had to become more tolerant to an increase in the noise level from a variety of environmental sources; the term 'noise pollution' is now used and discussed in Chapter 7 in relation to maintaining a safe environment. But even people who appear to enjoy bombardment by noise when well, can rarely tolerate it when they are ill. The night nurse's work can be pre-planned so that noisy trolleys are not needed in the ward after patients have settled for the night, and any procedures which must be performed during the night should be carried out as quietly as possible. Empty beds for possible new admissions can be near the ward entrance so that their occupation will cause as little disturbance to as few patients as possible. The same applies if the death of a patient is expected during the night. These are just some of the feasible ways in which nurses can attempt to minimise noise at night in the interests of patients' sleep. Certainly, nurses should be aware of the fact that noise is one of the most important causes of sleep disturbance, a fact recently reinforced by the findings of the research study conducted by Closs (1988); noise emerged as the most frequent of all causes of night-time awakening in patients' reports of sleep problems in hospital.

When a patient becomes disorientated at night removal to a single room may be helpful where adequate lighting simulates daytime and lessens shadows which may be the cause of distress; staff can speak normally, as opposed to whispering which is thought to increase the patient's confusion. On the other hand, the patient may be more confused by the move, in which case re-orientation in the ward may be more practical; a short period of disturbance there being preferable for all concerned to a longer one in a sideward.

Light. Many people are very sensitive to and disturbed by even a low intensity of light for sleeping. Night lighting in the newer hospitals is well dimmed and arranged near floor level so that it is below the eye level of patients in bed. If a nurse decides to help a patient to sleep by shading a nearby light, fire safety factors should be complied with; otherwise drawing bed curtains or using a mobile screen may help to intercept the disturbing light.

Disturbance of circadian rhythm. It it useful to remember that there are a few people admitted to hospital who have been working on night shift and they may have problems with sleeping because of their altered sleeping pattern. Also travellers who have passed through time zones can become ill or have an accident and may arrive in hospital with altered circadian rhythms. A study done by Armstrong-Esther & Hawkins (1982) tentatively suggests that some elderly people may have lost their physical responsiveness to light and dark and come to rely more on social synchronisers. Once these are disturbed by admission to hospital, the elderly patient may have no reliable cues and goes into a state of internal desynchronisation. This state in which the body's rhythms are out of synchrony may be the cause of sleep disturbance, as well as confusion and incontinence, which indeed is often observed in the elderly after admission to hospital. Nurses should be alert to these possible variants when gathering information about a patient's sleeping habits.

CHANGE OF DEPENDENCE/INDEPENDENCE STATUS

Apart from environmental factors, people who would normally be considered 'good' sleepers, may require some assistance to sleep when in hospital. Before interfering with a person's independence in this AL however, it is important that the nurse identifies the patient's usual sleeping pattern. After all there are people whom Meddis (1977) labels nonsomniacs, some of them requiring as little as 2 hours of sleep per night, and they are not upset by wakefulness. Nevertheless, most people expect to sleep at night and three broad categories of insomnia have come to be recognised.

Sleeplessness

Inability to get to sleep. Some people report that it takes them as long as 90 minutes to get to sleep and they are likely to continue this pattern during their stay in hospital. Provided the nurse has ascertained that they are not unduly anxious about it and that it is not interfering with their health, there is no need for treatment. But should such patients remain wakeful for an even longer period, they may need help from the nurse. Among the 'delayed onset' sleepers are a group who could be termed 'worriers'; having ensured that they are physically comfortable, an opportunity to talk about the cause of the worry may leave them feeling less anxious which can encourage sleep. Whenever possible this group could be left to sleep until they awaken naturally in the morning.

Excessive wakefulness. There are those who fall asleep quickly but report that they waken frequently and stay awake for longer or shorter periods. When this information appears on the nursing assessment, the night nurse should be alerted to observing the patient frequently throughout the night in an attempt to record the sleep pattern. It is well-known that a few minutes awake during the night can seem much longer. It should also be recognised that, for elderly people, an increase in the number and amount of wake times after sleep onset is a normal phenomenon (Hayter, 1983), and perhaps they simply require reassurance that this is so. The patient who stays awake for longer periods may fall asleep again quite naturally after voiding and having a hot drink. Being punitive to patients who state that they have had a poor night, but to the nurse appear to have been asleep, is unrealistic; if the patient feels that he has had a poor night, then the quality of sleep has not been sufficient to produce a feeling of refreshment. Sleep researchers acknowledge that the EEG does not record the 'quality' of sleep. A sympathetic understanding of these patients' problem, expressed by attending to their pre-sleep routine, can help them to relax and fall into a refreshing sleep. The nurse should attempt to identify any change in the patient's daytime activities and note if, because of lack of sleep, they are more easily fatigued. Appetite should also be observed; tired people seldom eat well.

People who suffer from depression may be troubled by excessive wakefulness and in the long periods when they are awake are helped by having someone to whom they can talk about their problems. Depression is an illness which can now be treated successfully and if patients have not already sought medical help, they can be encouraged to do so.

Early morning waking. Depression can also be characterised by early morning waking, but the age group most commonly reporting early waking, as early as 0500 hours, is the elderly. If patients awaken early feeling refreshed, they can be offered a morning beverage; those in single rooms may wish to read or occupy themselves in some way; those in large wards can be encouraged to continue resting in bed to avoid disturbing the other patients.

Restlessness

Restlessness is a feature found in many patients with insomnia. After an extensive literature survey and many observations of restlessness in patients, Norris (1975) wrote:

Restlessness is a universal, discontinuous, animal behaviour evidenced by nonspecific, repetitive, unorganised, diffuse, apparently nonpurposeful motor activity that is subject to limited control.

It is not always possible to identify the cause but careful documentation of restless behaviour exhibited by many different patients will provide a data bank base from which should come a better understanding of this form of interference with sleep. Nowadays, records and tape-recordings are available which teach pre-sleep relaxation, the intention being to reduce restlessness and promote sleep and some people find them effective. The use of rhythmic sound on tape recordings has also proved helpful, such as the noise of waves on a seashore, but more research would be required before making generalisations about the desirability of nurses introducing such methods of reducing restlessness and thus inducing sleep.

Although certain forms of restlessness may be nonspecific the nurse must realise that some drugs prescribed for purposes other than sleeping, are disturbers of sleep and promote restlessness. A commonly used medication in this category is the diuretic group. As well as relieving oedema for example, they promote frequent elimination of urine, and although these drugs are normally administered in the early part of the day to preclude disturbance of sleep, their effect may persist into the night. Drugs given to relieve constipation may also cause minor abdominal discomfort and disturbed sleep, or even promote defaecation during the night unless administered at a time which will produce the desired effect during the day. Some antidepressant drugs may cause not only disturbance of sleep but actually induce wakefulness because they act in a manner similar to caffeine. When assessing a patient's sleeping pattern, it is therefore important that the nurse is aware of the effect of other currently prescribed drugs which may in fact be the cause of restlessness.

It is worth noting too, that restlessness may occur because some people admitted to hospital do not mention, initially, that they have been accustomed to taking sedatives at home. After all, in a survey of over 2000 people it was found that 15% of men and 25% of women (Whitfield, 1982) who go to see the family doctor attend because of insomnia, and any sleep difficulties will probably be exacerbated by admission to hospital.

Drug dependence

Apart from people who have been on sedation at home there are some patients who, in spite of all general comfort measures, fail to sleep and require to have sleeping pills which are prescribed by the doctor and given by the nurse. When hypnotic drugs have been ordered to induce sleep, they should be given a few minutes before lights are turned out. If analgesics are also required to relieve pain they should be administered sufficiently early for them to take effect before the hypnotic is given thus enhancing the effect of the hypnotic. The name of the drug, and the dose and time at which it is given are recorded, and also the time at which the patient fell asleep, the time of waking, and mood on waking.

Almost paradoxically, sleeping drugs, although given to induce sleep, can have a detrimental effect on the individual's sleeping pattern due to the development of tolerance. Following many experiments carried out at the Edinburgh Sleep Research Laboratory, it was found that after taking sleeping pills for several nights, the person slept badly when the pills were discontinued; indeed, return to a natural sleeping pattern could take up to 6–8 weeks (Oswald & Adam, 1983). It is important that the nurse should be aware of this and ensure that the patient who has had hypnotics in hospital is informed of this effect (and also relatives) when being discharged from hospital. The patient can be reassured that normal sleeping patterns will return even if there are difficulties during the initial period at home following withdrawal of hypnotics.

In general, the use of hypnotics to treat sleep problems is usually unsatisfactory and knowing this should encourage nurses to exploit non-pharmacological methods of promoting sleep for patients, whether in hospital or home. Gournay (1988) explains how a drug-free strategy can work by reporting on the management of two patients.

SOME SPECIFIC PROBLEMS ASSOCIATED WITH SLEEPING

Sleeping is such a sensitive and highly individualised activity that all sorts of circumstances may interfere with a person's ability to rest and sleep, as has been discussed so far in this chapter. One specific problem which has not been commented on at any length is that of *pain* as a particular source of sleep disturbance. Closs (1988) found, in her study of sleep in surgical wards, that pain was cited along with noise as being the main factors perceived as disturbing to sleep in hospital. Pain was mentioned by 127 patients of the 200 questioned, with a further 45 who reported other kinds of discomfort (such as cramp, nausea and indigestion). Closs recommends that closer attention should be paid to night-time pain management, both in terms of administration of analgesia as well as the use of non-medical methods of pain control and sleep promotion.

One type of pain which, rightly or wrongly, is sometimes associated with sleep is cramp. The patient wakens during a sleep period complaining of intense pain in the foot or calf. The surrounding muscles are tense and rigid and when the foot is affected there is inability to move, usually the big toe. It is thought to be due to interference with the blood supply; alternate raising of the leg above the level of the bed, and letting it dangle at the side below the level of the bed helps to drain the blood from, and take fresh blood into the area giving relief. Some people find that pressing the foot on a cold surface relieves the spasm but there does not appear to be any documented evidence that this is so. It is best for the nurse to find out whether or not the patient has had cramp previously and if so, how he coped with it. Medical management of night cramps may include prescription of oral quinine.

Other discomforts have been described in earlier chapters which interfere with the relevant AL and often also interfere with sleep. All aspects of promoting comfort, rest and sleep are priority items especially with ill patients, for whom rest and sleep are essential components of therapy. Many patients are aware of the sources of their discomfort and if given the opportunity will make them known so the nurse who takes time to listen can frequently identify the cause and take steps to alleviate or remove the discomfort. There are, of course, other avenues of expression. The patient who is uncomfortable may appear pale, tense, restless; or may lie rigidly in bed; or may be perspiring profusely. The nurse must be aware of these cues so that she can minimise the effect of, or eliminate the causes, and do everything possible to increase comfort and promote optimal resting and sleeping.

Clearly sleep is a state of altered consciousness but it is a normal Activity of Living. Other altered states of consciousness are found in a range of disease conditions which must be differentiated from sleep.

ALTERED CONSCIOUSNESS

In an article discussing altered states of consciousness, Findley (1984) first of all suggests a pragmatic definition of consciousness as 'a state of wakefulness, alertness and awareness of personal identity and environmental events, that is awareness of self and surroudings'. Consciousness refers to both arousal (requiring intact functioning of the ascending reticular formation of the brain stem) and the content of consciousness (requiring the intact functioning of the cerebral hemispheres). Altered consciousness, then, can be considered in terms of a gradual change from a normal conscious level through impaired attention, loss of alertness, drowsiness, sleep, stupor and finally coma. Clearly drowsiness and sleep are normal phenomena whereas stupor and coma are abnormal states.

Coma

The ability to assess accurately a patient's level of consciousness is one of the responsibilities of the nurse. The Glasgow Coma Scale (Fig. 16.2) is a standardised tool which is detailed enough to detect changes in conscious-

Eye opening *Score*	Motor response *Score*	Verbal response *Score*
high score	**6** If command such as 'lift up your hands' is obeyed	
	5 If purposeful movement to remove painful stimulus such as pressure over eyebrow	**5** If oriented to person, place and time
4 If eyes open spontaneously to approach of nurse to bedside	**4** If finger withdrawn after application of painful stimulus to it	**4** If conversation confused
3 If eyes open in response to speech	**3** If painful stimulation at finger tip flexes the elbow	**3** If inappropriate words are used
2 If eyes open in response to pain at finger tip	**2** If the patient's arms are flexed and finger tip stimulation results in extension of elbow	**2** If only incomprehensible sounds are uttered
low score **1** If eyes do not open in response to pain at finger tip	**1** If there is no detectable response to repeated and various stimuli	**1** If no verbal response

A normal person would score 15 on the scale; the lowest possible score is 3 which is compatible with, but does not necessarily indicate, brain death. A score of 7 is used as a definition of coma.

Fig. 16.2 Glasgow coma scale

ness, or 'responsiveness' as some practitioners prefer to call it. It assesses three modes of behaviour:

- eye opening
- motor response
- verbal response

and is incorporated in an observation record chart (Teasdale et al, 1975; Allan, 1984) which includes recording of other vital signs namely temperature, pulse, respiration and blood pressure. Each of the three behaviours is assessed independently.

Eye opening

Spontaneous eye opening. When the patient's eyes open on the approach of someone to his bedside, it is recorded as spontaneous. This observation will not be expected when the patient is asleep but nurses should be alert to the fact that in some brain-damaged patients the diurnal rhythm is reversed. Observation must therefore be made for any patient who can respond with spontaneous eye opening during the night and not during the day.

Eye opening to speech. If the patient's eyes do not open spontaneously he should be addressed in a normal voice by name and asked to open his eyes. If he does not do so repetition in a loud voice is used, avoiding a commanding tone because it is response to stimulation by sound which is being tested.

Eye opening to pain. Lack of response to verbal stimulation is followed by testing for response to physical stimulation, such as exerting pressure on the patient's finger nail-bed as shown in Figure 16.3.

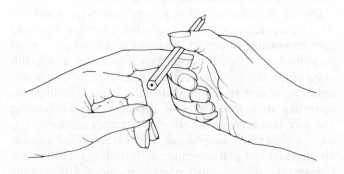

Fig. 16.3 Pressure on finger nail-bed (Teasdale et al, 1975)

Best motor response

Obeys commands. The patient is required to perform the specific movements requested. Should the relatives have informed the nurse (in the initial assessment phase) that the patient was deaf before the brain damage, then the request will be made by gesture or even in writing. It is preferable to ask the patient to raise an arm or a leg rather than to sequeeze the tester's fingers which can trigger off a reflex contraction; if the latter test is used, it is wise to

test that the patient will also release and squeeze again several times before recording this score.

Localises pain. Pressure applied over say the eyebrows (supra-orbital ridge) should stimulate the patient to move his arm thus showing that he has located the pain and is attempting to remove the stimulus.

Withdraws from painful stimulus. Pressure as in Figure 16.3 causes withdrawal of the finger.

Flexion response. Painful stimulation at the finger tip (Fig. 16.3) flexes the elbow but the patient does not achieve a localising response when stimulus is applied at other sites.

Extension response. The patient's arms are flexed and finger tip stimulation (Fig. 16.3) produces straightening at the elbow.

No response to pain. This is scored when there is no detectable response to repeated and various stimuli.

Verbal response

Orientated. After arousal, the patient is asked who he is, where he is and what year and month it is; he is not expected to give the exact day of the month. If accurate answers are given it is recorded that he is orientated.

Confused conversation. A patient can sometimes produce language, even phrases, but if he cannot give the correct answers to questions about orientation then it is recorded that his conversation is confused.

Inappropriate words. When a patient only utters one or two words, more often in response to physical stimulation than to speech, it is recorded that he is using inappropriate words.

Incomprehensible sounds. The utterance of groans, moans or indistinct mumbling without any intelligible words is recorded on this score.

No verbal response. If prolonged and repeated stimulation does not produce phonation then the nil score is recorded.

Use of some type of chart for factual information renders obsolete such terms as deeply unconscious, and semi-conscious; deeply comatose, and semi-comatose — all terms which can mean different things to different people. The chart can be marked and kept at the bedside so that any member of the team caring for the patient can see by glancing at the chart whether or not there has been any change on any item in the scale. When using this scale it should be remembered that the score obtained could be affected when the patient cannot speak due to the presence of an endotracheal tube, or if the patient is deaf or speaks a different language.

The Glasgow Coma Scale provides an indication of overall brain dysfunction and can be scored out of 15. The Scale is quick and easy to use and allows data to be documented in a logical manner.

As well as assessing responsiveness level it will be necessary for members of the caring team to accept responsibility for managing several of the unresponding comatose patient's other activities of living. These are breathing, eating and drinking, eliminating, personal cleansing and dressing (prevention of pressure sores), controlling body temperature, mobilising passively and maintaining a safe environment. All procedures associated with these ALs should be carried out by the nurse in such a way that not only life is maintained but also the patient's dignity is safeguarded. The unconscious patient is usually nursed in the semiprone position.

Convulsions (fits)

A form of transient unconsciousness sometimes occurs as a feature of what is termed a convulsion. When a baby has a convulsion or seizure it often heralds a febrile illness. In other age groups, there may be a variety of causes, including cerebral anoxaemia, hypoglycaemia, disturbance of calcium balance, electrolyte imbalance, excessive hydration, the injection of certain drugs and poisons, infections which produce high temperature elevations, and a number of metabolic disorders. Convulsions are also a feature of epilepsy but nowadays, good control, and indeed prevention of seizures, is achieved by means of anticonvulsant drugs (Oxley, 1981). Nevertheless, coping with epilepsy is not easy; some of the difficulties and stresses are described in an article called 'Facing up to my epilepsy', written by a district nurse who suffers from the condition (Cobell, 1989).

Anaesthesia

Convulsions or seizures may occur without much warning but it is possible to alter deliberately the level of human consciousness. This occurs when a patient is given a general anaesthetic. The anaesthetised person appears to be in a state of induced unconsciousness although there is increasing evidence that appearances are misleading; the patient on the operating table may actually hear what is being said and may be 'aware' of the inability to move. These findings certainly have implications for staff in the operating suite both prior to surgery and in the recovery room. Nowadays, for many operations, light anaesthetics are used so patients recover consciousness quite quickly after surgery. Stephens & Boaler (1977) maintain that deliberately wakening patients is undesirable; they should be given time to regain consciousness at their own pace.

In circumstances where there is altered consciousness — coma, convulsions, general anaesthetic — the skill and adaptability of the nurse are of paramount importance. In these states, even when transient in nature, the person is dependent for all Activities of Living, indeed for survival. Like sleep, as might be expected, these states of altered consciousness are characterised by changes in the electrical activity of the cerebral cortex when recorded by EEG. Every advance in the research centres provides more information about the 'how' and 'why' of altered consciousness, including sleep. Perhaps in the not too distant future, it will be possible to refute Dr Johnson's observation some decades ago:

no searcher . . . can tell by what power the mind and body are thus chained down in irresistible stupefaction . . . the witty and the dull, the clamerous and the silent, the busy and the idle, are all overpowered by the gentle tyrant, and all lie down in the equality of sleep.

Individualising nursing

The first part of this chapter reflects the Roper, Logan and Tierney model for nursing — the nature of the AL of sleeping; the relationship of the lifespan to the AL; the effect of the individual's dependence/independence status; the influence of physical, psychological, sociocultural, environmental and politicoeconomic factors on the AL. In the second part of the chapter, a selection of problems and discomforts which are experienced by people in relation to the AL have been described. With this background of *general* knowledge about the AL, it should be possible to incorporate such information in an individualised nursing plan when such information is relevant to the person's current circumstances.

While describing the Roper, Logan and Tierney model for nursing, *general* information was provided about Individualising nursing (p. 51) which in fact is synonymous with the concept of the process of nursing.

Out of this background of *general* knowledge about the AL of sleeping and about Individualising nursing, it should then be possible to extract the issues which are relevant to an individual's current circumstances (whether in a health or an illness setting), i.e. to make an assessment of relevant issues according to the individual's stage on the lifespan; according to current level of dependence/independence; and take into account the relevant physical, psychological, sociocultural (including ethical, spiritual and religious), environmental and politicoeconomic (including legal) factors. Collectively, this information would provide a profile of the person's individuality in relation to this AL.

As indicated earlier in the text, this assessment would be achieved by various means such as observing the person; acquiring information about the individual's usual habits in relation to this AL partly by asking appropriate questions, partly by listening to the patient and/or relatives, and using relevant information from available records including medical records. The collected information could then be examined to identify any actual problems being experienced with the AL and these could be arranged in some order of priority. The nurse might also recognise some potential problems — not all possible potential

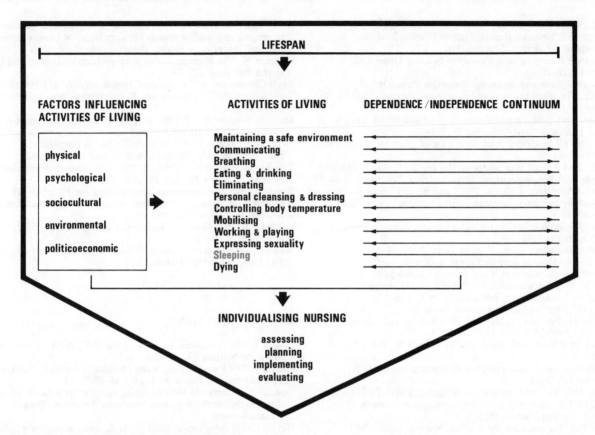

LIFESPAN

FACTORS INFLUENCING ACTIVITIES OF LIVING	ACTIVITIES OF LIVING	DEPENDENCE/INDEPENDENCE CONTINUUM

physical

psychological

sociocultural

environmental

politicoeconomic

Maintaining a safe environment
Communicating
Breathing
Eating & drinking
Eliminating
Personal cleansing & dressing
Controlling body temperature
Mobilising
Working & playing
Expressing sexuality
Sleeping
Dying

INDIVIDUALISING NURSING

assessing
planning
implementing
evaluating

Fig. 16.4 The AL of sleeping within the model for nursing

problems but those which are relevant. Realistic goals, mutually agreed with the patient when this is possible, could then be set to prevent potential problems from becoming actual ones; to alleviate or solve the actual problems; or to help the person cope with those which cannot be alleviated or solved.

Keeping in mind what the person can and cannot do unaided, the nursing interventions to achieve the mutually set goals could then be selected according to local circumstances and available resources.

Following implementation of the interventions, their effects could be evaluated in relation to the goals set, and if goals were not reached, they would then be revised or rescheduled, or even discarded. It is worth repeating here that although discussed in four phases — assessing, planning, implementing and evaluating — individualising nursing is not a linear progression; it assumes a built-in responsiveness to feedback at any of the phases, with ample allowance for change within the overall framework.

This chapter has been concerned with the AL of sleeping. However, as stated previously it is only for the purpose of discussion that any AL can be considered on its own; in reality the various activities are so closely related and do not have distinct boundaries. Figure 16.4 is a reminder that the AL of sleeping is related to the other ALs and also to the various components of the model for nursing. However, it must be repeated that it may not be relevant to consider this particular AL for every patient in every circumstance. Professional judgement is required to assess its relevance to any one patient.

Acknowledgement

Thanks are extended to Jose Close of the Nursing Research Unit, Department of Nursing Studies, University of Edinburgh for her helpful suggestions towards the revision of this chapter.

REFERENCES

Adam K 1980 A time for rest and a time for play. Nursing Mirror 150(10) March 6: 17–18
Allan D 1984 Glasgow coma scale. Nursing Mirror 158(23) June 13: 32–34
Armstrong-Esther C, Hawkins L 1982 Day for night: circadian rhythms in the elderly. Nursing Times 78(30) July 28: 1263–1265
Brezinova V, Oswald I 1972 Sleep after a bedtime beverage. British Medical Journal 2 May 20: 431–433
Brown P 1988 Shift work: punching the body clock. Nursing Times 84(44) November 2: 26–28
Canavan T 1984 The psychobiology of sleep. Nursing 2(23) March: 682–683
Carter D 1985 In need of a good night's sleep. Nursing Times 81(46): 24–26
Clapin-French E 1986 Sleep patterns of aged persons in long-term care facilities. Journal of Advanced Nursing 11: 57–66

Closs S J 1988 A nursing study of sleep on surgical wards. Nursing Research Unit Research Report, Dept of Nursing Studies, University of Edinburgh, Scotland, UK

Cobell R 1989 Facing up to my epilepsy. Nursing Times 85(2) January 11: 27–29

Cohen D 1979 Sleep and dreaming. Pergamon Press, Oxford

Dopson L 1988 When the snoring has to stop. Nursing Times 84(42) October 19: 22–23

Durnford S 1988 Junior hospital doctors: tired and tested. British Medical Journal 297(6654) October 15: 931–932

Felstein I 1979 The sufferer who doesn't suffer. Nursing Mirror 146 April 12: 42–43

Findley L 1984 Altered consciousness. Nursing 2(23) March: 663–666

Gournay K 1988 Sleeping without drugs. Nursing Times 84(11): 46–49

Hawkins L, Armstrong-Esther C 1978 Circadian rhythms and night shift working in nurses. Nursing Times Occasional Paper 74(13) May 4: 49–52

Hayter J 1983 Sleep behaviours of older persons. Nursing Research 32(4) July/August: 242–246

Hearne K 1986 Dream sense. Nursing Times 1(82): 28–31

Horne J A 1983 Human sleep and tissue restitution: some qualifications and doubts. Clinical Science 65: 569–578

Johns M W 1984 Normal sleep. In: Priest R G (ed) Sleep: an international monograph, Update Books ch 1, p 13–17

Keys M 1988 Silent nights. Professional Nurse 3(9): 353–357

Koskenvuo M, Partinen M, Kaprio J 1985 Snoring and disease. Annals of Clinical Research 17(5): 247–251

Lathlean J 1980 Relaxation using yoga. Nursing 1(20) December: 882–884

Manian R 1988 Can I sleep now, nurse? Nursing Standard 12(3) December 17: 22–23

Meddis R 1977 The sleep instinct. Routledge & Kegan Paul, London

Norris C 1975 Restlessness: a nursing phenomenon in search of a meaning. Nursing Outlook 23: 103–107

Oswald I 1980 No peace for the worried. Nursing Times 150(11) March 13: 34–35

Oswald I, Adam K 1983 Get a better night's sleep. Martin Dunitz, London

Oxley J 1981 Fitting the symptoms. Nursing Mirror Clinical Forum Supplement 12, December 9

Professional Nurse 1986 Hypothermia nursing intervention — practice check. Professional Nurse 1(5): 136–138

Rechtshaffen A, Kales A 1968 A manual of standardised terminology, techniques and scoring system for sleep stages of human subjects. National Institutes of Health, Bethesda, Maryland, USA

Richman N 1983 Management of sleep problems. Maternal and Child Health 8(6) June: 227–233

Royal Commission on the National Health Service 1978 Patients' attitudes to the hospital service. Research paper No. 5. HMSO, London

Smith P, Wedderburn Z 1980 Sleep, body rhythms and night-work. Nursing 1(20) December: 889–892

Stephens D, Boaler J 1977 The nurse's role in immediate post-operative care. British Medical Journal 1: 1199–1202

Teasdale G, Galbraith S, Clarke K 1975 Observation record chart. Nursing Times 71(25) June 19: 972–973

Wardle J 1986 The chronology of sleep. Nursing 3(9): 325–326

Wedderburn Z, Smith P 1980 Sleep: its function and measurement. Nursing 1(20) December: 852–855

Whitfield W 1982 Breaking the habit. Nursing Mirror 155(10) September 8: 59–60

Wilkie T 1989 Doctors working 36-hour shifts in US 'error-prone'. The Independent 709 January 18: 7

ADDITIONAL READING

Closs S J 1988 Assessment of sleep in hospital patients. Journal of Advanced Nursing 13: 501–510

Closs S J 1988 Patients' sleep-wake rhythms in hospital. Nursing Times Occasional Papers 84(1 & 2): 48–50 54–55

Douglas J, Richman N 1984 My child won't sleep: a handbook of sleep management for parents of preschool children. Penguin, Harmondsworth

Hayter J 1986 Advances in sleep research: implications for nursing practice. In: Tierney A J (ed) Advances in clinical nursing practice. Churchill Livingstone, Edinburgh, ch 1, p 21–46

Horne J 1988 Why we sleep. Oxford University Press, New York

Morgan K 1987 Sleep and ageing. Croom Helm, London

Turpin G 1986 Psychophysiology of sleep. Nursing 3(9): 313–320

Webster R A Thompson D R 1986 Sleep in hospital. Journal of Advanced Nursing 11(4): 447–457

17
Dying

The activity of dying

Dying is the final act of living. Death is what marks the end of life on earth, just as the event of birth marks its beginning. The only certain thing in our lives is that we will one day die; but there are many uncertainties as to why, when, where and how.

It is probably these uncertainties about dying which provoke uneasy feelings when people think about the prospect of their own death and the death of those they love. Life would not be worth living if death became a preoccupation but, if the subject is ignored, how can people develop the resources needed to comfort the bereaved, bear the sorrow of grieving and face death with dignity?

THE NATURE OF DYING

Most people try to avoid thinking about death. Currently in Western cultures, death is not a popular subject of discussion — and continues to be unacceptable in front of the dying and bereaved. This was not always so. At the beginning of the 20th century when infant and child mortality was high and life expectancy short; when family size was large; and when the mass of the population lived in small, overcrowded houses, there was ample opportunity for all age groups to be constantly reminded of death. Likewise today, in many developing countries, even small children are in frequent contact with the dead and dying.

Death and dying
To die suddenly from natural causes, in old age, and without loss of dignity is what most people would regard

as a 'good death'. It may be sudden as occurs for example following a massive coronary attack or a major accident; or it may be preceded by a process of dying. Accompanying an acute terminal illness or surgery, dying may take only a few days or a few weeks. On the other hand, when there is chronic illness with a poor prognosis, the process of dying may span several months.

Some people die suddenly not from natural causes but in quite violent circumstances. In most countries of the Western world, road accidents are a major cause of death in young adults, normally a particularly healthy group; international publicity is given to serious aircraft accidents which, although rare, almost always have a high mortality rate; industrial accidents for example in mines often cause mass deaths in large numbers; and in areas of the world where natural disasters such as floods, earthquakes, and hurricanes occur with relative frequency, there may be a heavy death toll. Every country has its major tragedies when whole families or even communities can be wiped out by such events.

Sudden violent death may not be accidental, however, but deliberate. Murder is not common but the incidence is rising in most industrialised nations. Most countries are aware of the increasing violence and terrorism in the modern world and of the corresponding need to protect individuals from undesirable and preventable acts of homicide. For many obvious reasons, the relatives' grief may be complicated by feelings of lust for revenge and fear for their own personal safety, and such circumstances may precipitate yet more deaths.

Violent death on a large scale as a result of war seems to be a constant feature in modern society; and in response to apparently unwarranted aggression perhaps war is inevitable as a means of national self-defence. However, following the Second World War, when the waste of human life on an international scale was recognised, the United Nations Organization was created to provide a forum for discussion about disputes in order to preclude the waging of war. Unfortunately this option is not always accepted and the death toll among armed forces and civilians continues in the countries still at war. The possibility of a nuclear holocaust adds considerably to the horror with the prospect of mass annihilation or, in its aftermath, the painful process of dying from the effects of radiation; although attempts are being made internationally to reduce the nuclear threat.

Most people, even those with a strong religious faith about an afterlife, are afraid of death and dying. However there are some individuals who, for a variety of reasons, want to die and intentionally take their own lives by committing suicide. Ritual suicide was once practised, for example, when a Hindu woman perished on the funeral pyre of her husband (Suttie); or when a Japanese Samurai, who for some reason felt dishonoured, committed Hari-Kari with a ceremonial sword. Nowadays these practices are rarely used, indeed Suttie is now illegal. Self-poisoning (Moore, 1986) is the most frequently used method and attempted suicide (parasuicide) is currently a common emergency in the casualty department of any busy hospital in most industrialised countries (Brooking & Minghella, 1987). Suicide is no longer a crime in the UK and has not been since the Suicide Act in 1961, but there is still a stigma attached to suicide which may serve to increase the already great amount of distress and guilt suffered by the relatives.

Although not suicidal in intent, there is another group of people who, when they are dying, want to die quickly; and there are some people attending a dying person, who want to 'help' them to die quickly. 'Bringing about an easy death' is the actual meaning of the term euthanasia, although mercy killing is a phrase often used as a synonym. It is a topic which evokes strong emotions and heated debate. Those with particular religious or personal convictions argue that it is morally wrong to end life deliberately (active euthanasia). Others consider that euthanasia is not a deliberate act of killing but merely allows death to occur for example by withholding antibiotics at the onset of a respiratory infection in an old, incapacitated person although providing care and comfort in every other way (passive euthanasia).

The subject of euthanasia has provoked lengthy debate about the 'right to die' in balance with the 'right to live'. The question is asked 'do we prolong life or prolong suffering?' And making the point, a letter to the editor of *Newsweek* in 1988 comments 'I am not asking you to transfer (a human) from life to death but from dying to death'. The debate is not new and history records examples of group euthanasia practices in the Greek island of Cos in the 1st century BC. It has gone on down through the centuries but has currently re-emerged with some force because of procedures made possible by recent technological advances; although often life-saving and often appropriate to use, they do raise ethical problems. Saunders (1986) writing about some of these problems maintains:

As often happens, we discover *how* to do something and only later *when* to do it. No treatment . . . carries with it the automatic commitment to use it just because it is technically feasible.

In a number of countries, proponents of euthanasia have formed societies — the first was in the UK in 1935 — to discuss and propagate their beliefs, and to provide information to people who wish assistance in reducing the distress of dying. In some instances, an even more positive stance has been taken and attempts have been made to introduce legislation making voluntary euthanasia possible.

It is difficult to discuss the nature of death and dying without considering the nature of grieving and bereavement. Most adults have some experience of these emotions following the death of a relative or friend; indeed grieving and bereavement are a part of the process of living although related to the process of dying and death.

Bereavement and grieving

Following the death of someone significant to them, those who are left behind almost inevitably suffer a deep sense of desolation. Grief is the emotional reaction which follows and is one of the most intense emotional experiences. Murray Parkes (1972) in his book, *Bereavement*, maintains that grief is 'the cost of commitment' in our lives.

It is not necessarily only husbands, wives or children who are bereaved, although one's immediate reaction is to think of these close relatives. Many others may be affected by a death, such as friends, colleagues, neighbours, co-patients, doctors and nurses. Gyulay (1975) identifies, in the case of a child's death, the 'forgotten grievers' as the father, siblings, grandparents, peers and friends, neighbours and teachers, and Capper (1982) makes the same point in relation to stillbirth although in this instance, the baby has not been known to those others as an individual with a separate identity.

It may seem surprising to include the father in this list until one remembers that in Western culture men are not expected to reveal deep emotion and so there has been the assumption that men do not feel grief so deeply as women. So intense is the emotion of grief that it affects even those sometimes wrongly assumed to be untouched by loss: the very young and the very old, the mentally ill and the mentally handicapped. 'The bereaved' are, by definition, those who suffer loss and grief in response to a death; those who were, in some important way, committed to the person who died.

Although feelings of loss and grief are almost universal responses in bereavement, many other reactions can occur. Shock, disbelief, anger, denial, shame, guilt, resentment, anxiety, fear, depression and despair are among the emotional reactions which may be experienced by the bereaved to a varying degree and at different times throughout the grieving process. However, sometimes a death brings relief to those left behind and this may be the case, for example, if the family has had to watch suffering in someone they love, and bear the burden of care during a prolonged terminal illness.

Initially there is usually a short period of intense grief when the bereaved person suffers profound despair and sorrow and openly mourns. Shock and total disbelief can be experienced at this time, especially in the case of sudden death, and the experience may seem unreal. Then there is a long period of sadness. Pining for the dead person is common, indeed normal, and often this takes the form of 'searching behaviour' involving attachment to places and objects associated with the dead person's life and their relationship.

While grieving, a sense of the persisting presence of the dead person appears to be a comforting phenomenon and illusions, hallucinations and dreams may occur. Such events seem to help to compensate for the reality of the loss, and the loneliness felt. Sometimes the bereaved person experiences intense anxieties for the future and feels totally incapable of taking decisions and coping with everyday demands.

Depression is not uncommon and, even long after the death, episodes of intense grief and despair may return. Restitution from bereavement involves adaptation to a new life as the death of a significant person inevitably alters the role and function of the bereaved; a widow is no longer a wife and a son may now be the head of the household. The old identity must be given up and a new one evolved. Usually, the new life is moulded gradually and some significant milestones include events such as returning to work, moving house and making new friends.

Bereavement can be a long, painful and lonely process. Although it is probably true that time heals, a person seldom remains unaffected by a bereavement even after a long time lapse. It is not that they forget the dead person but perhaps time gives them practice in adapting to living in changed circumstances.

All of the Activities of Living discussed so far can be seen to have a clear purpose. Some, such as breathing, are performed for survival; others like eating and drinking not only for survival but also for comfort and enjoyment; and yet others, the ALs of communicating and expressing sexuality, have as their purpose the interaction of human beings with one another in the process of living. In the same kind of way, is it possible to discern a purpose of dying?

Many people have some kind of personal belief about the meaning of death and often this is based on the philosophy of a particular religion. Most religions have some strong belief about the fate of man's spirit and soul after death. For example Christianity purports that there is life after death; Roman Catholics, Protestants and Jews believe that death marks the beginning of an afterlife with God, some being convinced that this existence is everlasting and will hold greater joy and peace than life on earth. Within such a philosophy then, the purpose of dying is to allow progression from life on earth to the afterlife. Some religious and ideological groups believe that one can triumph over death by giving up life when and how one chooses, for example in highjacking episodes or war activities for ideological causes; meaning is given to death by the meaningfulness of the cause. Such people willingly sacrifice their lives for the 'idea', and may believe it stands them in good stead for the afterlife. For those who do not hold such religious or ideological beliefs, dying may be seen to have no purpose other than to bring an inevitable end to living; a coming to terms with the finiteness of life. So, for some, death is a beginning; for some a transition; and for others, an end. And perhaps, albeit subconsciously, some of the grieving is a form of grief for oneself; another's death is a reminder of one's own death, a reminder of the transience of life and living.

For many people it may not be easy to see a meaning in the death of somebody who is loved; there is, however, a purpose in grieving. It is normal to grieve after the loss of a significant person in one's life. It allows the person to come to terms with the irreparable loss and draw to a close that part of life which was shared. Lake (1984) discussing *Living with Grief* goes so far as to say that grief renews the purpose of our lives because it forces the bereaved to take stock, adapt to a different set of circumstances, and make significant choices about future activities, although this may not all happen immediately. He considers that the dead person does not want the bereaved 'to be forever miserable'. The person who mourns may believe this intellectually, but may still find it difficult to differentiate between sorrow at the loss of the person and sorrow for self; the emptiness of being left to struggle alone. And some bereaved people can acknowledge, retrospectively, that their sorrow was tinged with self-pity. Grief is obviously not simply a matter of being unhappy — a patch of misery — it is a process with certain tasks to be undertaken, and there may be many moments of despair before life seems to be worth living again.

LIFESPAN: EFFECT ON DYING

The model of living includes the lifespan as one of its components; birth is the lifespan's starting point and death is its endpoint. However death can occur at any age and when it comes, it determines the length of an individual's lifespan. When the lifespan of groups of individuals is investigated, it is possible to detect trends in death rates within and between the groups and as most countries maintain population statistics, international comparisons can be made about average age of death and life expectancy. A century ago in most industrialised countries the life expectancy was around 40 years, slightly higher for females; nowadays, it is around 70–75 years.

The stages of the lifespan were discussed as a component of the model in an earlier part of the book and here the effect of death and dying will be reviewed in relation to the different age groups.

Prenatal period. Death can occur during early uterine existence which may be associated with a spontaneous abortion, when the products of conception are expelled or may have to be removed. Or the fetus may die at a late stage in pregnancy and the mother knows that the period of labour will produce only a dead child. Or some babies may die during the process of birth. It is not possible to know the 'reaction' of the fetus in these circumstances, but it is possible to observe the desolation experienced by parents who, in these instances, are the most directly af-

fected. The sense of loss and despair and even failure is the very antithesis of all their expectations, and alien to the usual atmosphere of a maternity ward if the mother is delivered in hospital; it is probably the hardest place in which to mourn a lost baby. Richardson (1980) quotes a mother describing the experience of stillbirth as 'the loneliest of losses; you are the only one who has had a relationship with the baby'. There have been a number of articles recently (Negus, 1987; Mallinson, 1989) about the importance of allowing the parents to see and even hold their stillborn baby and in some instances a photograph is taken. Despite the obvious distress, it is an important event in their lives and is thought to help with the grieving process.

Infancy. Some babies die during the early weeks of life or during the first 12 months of life sometimes in inexplicable, so-called 'cot deaths' — the sudden infant death syndrome. There are various theories about, for example, overwhelming stress; functional or anatomical defects; maturation failure; and critical phases of development, but the reason for these distressing sudden deaths in apparently thriving babies is not often detectable (Barker, 1987; Milner, 1987). However it has been shown in a small study in Portsmouth that the incidence of cot deaths fell by 30% when health visitors had identified babies at risk on a 'birth score' (based on factors such as low birth weight, smoking during pregnancy, young or single motherhood, unemployment and multiple birth) and had made structured extra visits (Pope, 1988). It is an unresolved problem and in some Western countries, as deaths from other conditions, particularly infections, have fallen, this syndrome is becoming one of the major causes of infant mortality. But in industrialised countries, if infants survive the first year, they have a good life expectancy.

Childhood. During the early decades of this century, childhood deaths were relatively common, often associated with infectious disease. Now in industrialised countries, deaths during childhood are rare, for example in the UK, they account for less than 1% of all deaths and the most common cause is accidents; theoretically accidents are preventable, a topic which is discussed on page 68 in Chapter 6, Maintaining a Safe Environment. Children do become aware of death and dying at quite an early age and it is interesting to note the findings of studies which have been conducted to ascertain what young children think about death. One of the earlier studies was carried out by Nagy in Hungary following the Second World War. A group of 378 children aged 3–10 years from different socioeconomic backgrounds and religions, and of varying intellectual ability were asked to express death-related thoughts verbally, in drawing and in writing. Nagy categorised the findings in three stages. In Stage I (3–5 years) there was no clear distinction between living and lifeless. The dead person was 'less alive' or asleep or had gone away and would return. In Stage II (5–6 years) death was personified as a death-man or skeleton who carried away living people and there was no return. In Stage III (9–10 years) death was inevitable and permanent; it was a termination of life.

In more recent studies mentioned by Boston & Trezise (1987) the distinctions made by under-5s and those in the age group 5–9 years seem to be similar. Even although children seem to enjoy the 'experience' of death through war games and fantasies, and inevitably nowadays see it depicted on television often associated with violence and accidents, the reality can be bewildering. The death of a pet may cause considerable distress but for the child it can be grossly disturbing when a parent is dying, yet Lovell (1987) argues that children should not be protected from the reality. Allowing them to share in the sorrow helps them with the grieving process she maintains, and avoids emotional problems later in life.

Boston and Trezise (1987) wholeheartedly agree with this approach and deplore the use of euphemisms. To say to the child, for example, that the person has 'gone away' provokes alarm when mother goes away shopping and father goes away to work. Children may also worry that their behaviour has caused the person to go away, and feel deep guilt. To say that the person has 'gone to sleep' is equally confusing as the child may be afraid to go to sleep, yet is encouraged each night to do so. Boston & Trezise maintain that far from being protective, the use of euphemisms can destroy the certainties and securities of the child's world.

And if, for some reason, a sibling dies, it is important to talk with children about their feelings and reactions. They can be angry — or even feel guilty — with a brother for dying and leaving them; Vas Dias (1987) mentions a 7-year-old after his brother's death, asking 'Mummy do you think Adam knew I loved him even if I didn't like him being ill?'

Adolescence. Although the teenager understands intellectually about the finality of life, time is a sort of insulation between the adolescent and eventual death. So the dying adolescent who is just beginning to enjoy independence and self-confidence does not want to end what has just begun, and in the confusion and distress and often anger, may feel isolated from both parents and peers.

The death of an adolescent is devastating especially to parents. In industrialised countries, parents do not expect to outlive their offspring and it is very difficult to comfort them after such a loss. Such premature death may be greatly resented. They have been cheated of time together which they had the right to expect; the dead person had so much to give and so much to live for. Hopes and faith about life are dealt a severe blow which can have a lifelong effect on the family. However many bereaved parents consider that although the loss leaves a permanent scar, it is possible to grow because of the experience and help others in similar circumstances.

It is a sad indictment on modern, industrialised society that the suicide rate in this age group has been steadily increasing over the past 20 years in the USA and in all European countries with the exception of West Germany and Greece, which have unusually high and low rates respectively. In their book *Suicide in Adolescence*, Dickstria & Hawton (1987) discuss the epidemiology of adolescent suicide and highlight some of the possible causes. They emphasise unemployment, above average intelligence, and loss of a parent through death or marital separation as important factors in the context of a society which lacks social cohesiveness, and which values material and technological possessions at the expense of the individual's emotional wellbeing.

Adulthood. During early adulthood, people are considered to be in the 'prime of life' and a consideration of personal death and dying is almost totally alien, at least in industrialised countries where life expectancy is high. Sudden death, therefore, perhaps as a result of a road accident, comes as a shock to the family. There has been no time to contemplate the event and no opportunity to begin the process of grieving in anticipation of death. There has been no chance to say goodbye, and often there is an aura of unreality in the immediate post-death period. For the bereaved family there may also be an untimely change in status; perhaps a young family bereft of a parent and spouse, perhaps a sudden termination of a promising career.

In later adulthood the physical and other changes associated with ageing probably serve to remind the individual of man's mortality; and an increasing incidence of disease in this age group, either personally or observed in friends and colleagues, make the possibility of death and the process of dying a reality. For a spouse who is bereaved at this stage in life it can mean intense loneliness despite the support of family and friends; and for the young adults of the family, it may mean the loss of a supportive parent and perhaps taking on increasing responsibility for the remaining parent.

The elderly. For the elderly there is the realisation that they are approaching the end of the lifespan and they are made aware of this by an increasing number of deaths in their peer group. The majority of elderly people are healthy and retain their independence and may die suddenly or have a very short terminal illness. For some however, if they are ill and dependent, death may be welcomed as a release from pain and discomfort; for a few, the process of dying can be a long, courageously endured struggle to cherish their dignity and self-esteem despite a frail body.

A long terminal illness may cause great difficulties for relations also. Although able to prepare themselves for the bereavement they have, in addition to their anxieties and fears, the burden of care at home, or hospital visiting, over a long period of time. For those who are bereaved by the death of an elderly person, it may mean the loss of a spouse with whom they have spent a lifetime, and for the younger generation it may mean the loss of a much-loved parent or grandparent.

Human death is never really absent from our personal lives or from the community in general; indeed there is truth in the popular philosophy that we are 'dying from the moment we are born'.

DEPENDENCE/INDEPENDENCE IN DYING

Death is universal and inevitable, and apart perhaps from suicide, there is little personal independence about the time of death although there are some who maintain that individuals 'have turned their face to the wall' and willed themselves to die.

In the presence of general weakness and disease, the dying person is often aware that with the passing of each day, there is some slight erosion of independence in the physical aspects of ALs. However at home and in hospital, as well as in a hospice, the care providers may be sufficiently empathetic to encourage the person to continue making choices for as long as possible and remain in control of pain relief (if pain is present), in control of his quality of living, and in control of the immediate environment. Self-esteem can remain intact and even with increasing physical dependence, there can be independence of spirit. So while preserving the right to live independently to the optimum for these circumstances, the care providers have to help the dying person to balance the degree of personal dependence/independence in the Activities of Living up until the time of death.

For the family of the dying person, there will probably be varying degrees of dependence on others during the period prior to death when family, friends, neighbours and colleagues often offer to assist with, for example, family transport and shopping as well as visiting the dying person. In the period of grieving, the presence and thoughtfulness of others can be comforting and supportive although the bereaved person knows that this is a transient phase until physical and emotional strength is renewed, and the support can be withdrawn.

FACTORS INFLUENCING DYING

Apart from the differences associated with the various stages of the lifespan, a number of factors influence death and dying. The various factors are discussed, using the categories which appear in the model, under the headings physical, psychological, sociocultural, environmental and politicoeconomic factors.

Physical factors
In old age, it is normal for all systems of the body to become less efficient and to undergo a gradual process of degeneration. Physically, the process of dying is not dis-

similar except that the progressive decline is brought about by disease, and the nature of the particular pathology involved determines the course and speed of the irreversible degeneration of biological functioning. It is therefore difficult to diagnose the onset of 'dying' as a physical process related to any specific body system, but it may be helpful to say it begins when medical treatment cannot halt the course of a disease, and can only alleviate the symptoms of the fatal illness. In many instances a considerable length of time may elapse between the medical diagnosis of fatal illness and the onset of rapid physical decline in the terminal stages of the illness which precede the event of death. In relation to the model for nursing, therefore, no specific body system is juxtaposed with the AL of dying.

Dying as a physical process, is a very complicated phenomenon and it is important to appreciate that it is seldom possible for doctors to diagnose the exact time of its onset or to give a precise prognosis of when death will occur.

In contrast, it is usually possible to determine with accuracy the time at which death ultimately occurs. For most purposes it can be assumed that death has occurred when a person's pulse and respiration have ceased. But sometimes a much more elaborate diagnosis of death is required especially if there has been admission to hospital and sophisticated, artificial, 'life-support systems' are being used to maintain vital body functions. Although not spelled out in legal terms, there is medical agreement about tests ascertaining complete and irreversible brain death, requiring confirmation by at least two experienced doctors. The criteria include fixation of pupils, absence of corneal and of vestibulo-ocular reflexes; absence of response within the cranial nerve distribution to sensory stimuli; no response to bronchial stimulation when a catheter is passed into the trachea; no spontaneous breathing movement when the patient is disconnected from a mechanical ventilator (Allan, 1987; Simpson, 1987). Agreed criteria for the definition of death are essential when removal of organs for transplant surgery is being considered, and they are strictly applied by a medical team quite separate from the transplant team. A report produced by the Health Departments of Great Britain and Northern Ireland ('Cadaveric Organs for Transplantation' 1983) provides a code of practice and deals with the various physical and ethical issues in detail. To cope with the many ethical problems surrounding the criteria, the concepts of 'clinical death' (death of the person), 'biological death' (death of the tissues) and 'brain death' (irreversible brain damage) have been introduced and recognised by a number of countries.

Most Activities of Living are affected by the physical changes which occur in the process of dying, and all cease when life ends — when the event of death occurs. After death, the body cools, the tissues and muscles lose their tone and rigor mortis (stiffening of the body) sets in after 2 or 3 hours.

There are also physical factors which are relevant in relation to bereavement. For those who are bereaved, there is usually extreme physical exhaustion. Unless the death is sudden and unexpected, there will probably have been a period of time prior to the death when it was necessary either to pay frequent visits to the hospital or to provide 24-hour care at home. Perhaps also there is a young family to be supervised in the usual Activities of Living, or full-time employment to be carried on during the dying period of the family member and immediately after, and inevitably there is accompanying physical stress.

The bereaved seem to be more susceptible to physical illness. It has been recognised for some years that the bereaved spouse is admitted to hospital more frequently than married persons of the same age, and that elderly bereaved are more likely to become physically ill than those in a younger age group. The elderly person is often in a precarious physical state anyway, and the stress of the death of a spouse may exacerbate physical weakness. Some writers do not hesitate to refer to the 'broken heart syndrome' and Pike (1983) quotes a reference which showed that 12% of surviving spouses die within a year of their wives' or husbands' dying, while mortality in a non-bereaved control group was only 1.2% for the same period. A number of writers maintain that the intensity of the trauma of grief has a direct effect on the body's physical function. The immune system is affected so the response to infection and neoplastic disorders is suppressed and as a consequence physical disease processes become evident; and this leads to further stress. Lake (1984) talks about the retreat into illness which must be taken seriously for its possible medical significance. The pain will be real pain but in a grieving person is also a frequently encountered and justifiable cry for help. The trouble is, he goes on, that the dysfunction is so often seen only in strictly medical terms. Obviously there is a close link between physical and psychological factors.

Psychological factors

It is much less easy to describe psychological aspects of the dying process because no individuals respond in the same way and because any one person's reaction to dying is influenced by his personality, personal beliefs and total life experience. Whether or not the person suspects or knows for certain that he is dying is also an important factor. It is no virtue in itself that all people should be told they are dying, or discover the fact for themselves. However, the person's understanding of his prognosis will affect his attitude, mood and behaviour. Those with experience of caring for dying people tend to agree that they usually *are* aware, without needing to be told, of their fatal prognosis. After all, the person is able to feel and see the symptoms and signs of the disease and to realise that he does not seem to be getting any better; he is able to consider the possibilities and probabilities of whether or not he will recover;

and most of all, he becomes aware of the altered way in which those around him begin to behave towards him. His increasing awareness of his situation is discernible in the way his own behaviour begins to change.

For some people, awareness of impending death may be accompanied by intense fear. Fear of death has been a source of speculation in both personality theory and psychotherapeutic clinic work but in two studies done in the USA and quoted in McCarthy (1980) the amount of education and level of intelligence have no direct influence on fear of death, nor does there seem to be a significant relationship between death, anxiety and age.

Of course, the psychological changes which take place are not the same for any two individuals but it appears that there are certain kinds of reactions which commonly occur in the dying person. Some of these have been described by Kubler-Ross (1982) following her interviews in North America with dying patients.

She says that, on realising what is happening, most people pass through a phase of '*denial and isolation*' in which they refuse to accept that they are dying. As denial lessens, the common reaction is one of '*anger*' and the person will ask 'Why me?' . . . 'What have I done to deserve this?' Sometimes attempts to cope with the situation then involve a stage of '*bargaining*'. The person tries to find ways of believing that a miracle recovery will happen or that he might be given more time and he makes 'bargains' with the doctor or with God. When these fail and the imminent loss of life and loved ones becomes a reality, '*depression*' is experienced and this is an almost universal feature of the dying process. There is profound regret over missed opportunities and failures of the past and an overwhelming sadness engulfs the dying person. With sensitive care the person can be helped through this by being reminded of the achievements of his life, by being shown that he is respected and loved, and reassured that he will be looked after to the end and that what is important is to cope with each day at a time, to make the most of what is left. It should be realised, however, that these phases are not necessarily a linear progression; there is overlap and movement back and forth. Nevertheless it is useful to identify the various reactions so that the person can be helped to deal with these powerful emotions; and each individual has a unique way of dealing with them.

It does seem that dying need not be the terrible nightmare which many people fear so much. There can be serenity and composure in dying and many people die peacefully in their sleep with no apparent struggle or distress. Indeed McCarthy (1980) describes the prospect of death as representing 'not only the end of growth, pleasure, thought, consciousness, accomplishment, striving . . . it constitutes a final opportunity to experience the self, maintain self-esteem, relate to others, care for loved ones.' And in an article by Jones (1987a) the patient who was enabled to live out his last days at home, free of pain and spared the suffering of an isolated, agonising demise maintained, 'I want my dying to be not all doom and gloom, but a celebration of my life.'

The immediate family and friends of the dying person are often under great stress, concerned about the discomforts and pain of a loved one and also about the impending loss of someone who is significant to them. When the death occurs, there is inevitably emotional upset reflecting the sense of desolation and loss. As memories flood back, those who are grieving may find it difficult to concentrate on other activities, often there is tearfulness, and there may be loss of appetite and loss of weight. These are expected symptoms of grief and are usually relatively transient; the person usually uses coping mechanisms to resume at least a semblance of normal activities of living. However there may be more prolonged psychological dysfunction related to grief.

Occasionally, the feelings of helplessness and hopelessness prove too much and the grief reaction is so intense and prolonged that the bereaved person suffers a mental breakdown which requires specialised medical treatment. This is more likely to happen to women than to men, to those of unstable personality, and to those bereaved by a sudden death, the death of a child or death as a result of suicide.

Sociocultural factors

In societies where care of the dying is still very much a family responsibility, the social customs which surround death tend to be elaborate. The various rituals and the ceremonies performed are designed to encourage the bereaved to mourn openly and to seek the sympathy and support of members of their community. Each society has its own way of treating death according to its culture.

Social customs throughout the world vary markedly. In the Middle East some funeral rituals involve prolonged and public exhibition of grief; and in some African societies mourners gather together to 'drown their sorrows' publicly in drinking ceremonies. Although the rituals differ, the common element is the emphasis on the importance and necessity of communal and overt mourning.

In Western societies elaborate ritual surrounding death is fast disappearing. In Victorian times, funerals were grand occasions and the whole community engaged in mourning. Death was a problem to be shared. Families were large but close-knit units; they wore black and withdrew to the confines of their home, ceasing for a while to participate in any social activities and centring life around opportunities to share their sorrow and grief and show respect to the dead. Probably what was especially helpful was the presence of people, although in fact it was less easy in those days anyway to be 'alone' for death — as it was for birth. Nowadays, with small nuclear families, often scattered over a wide geographical area or indeed overseas and with everyone 'in a hurry', sadness almost gets in the way of our busy lives. Moreover, death has become almost a taboo subject and people feel they must mourn discreetly and 'get over it' quickly. Norbert (1985) makes the comment that 'dying has been removed so hygienically behind the scenes of social life . . . and expedited . . . with technical perfection from deathbed to grave!'

Cremation is now much more popular than burial; the cremation service is brief and there is not even a grave to remind the community of the death and allow the bereaved to maintain some kind of visible, physical contact with the memory of the dead person. Of course although in Western culture the choice of cremation may seem to sever the final link, for other cultures it is the norm. The Navajo Indians for example, after elaborate mourning rituals, *must* burn the body in a special house or 'hogan'. Hindus and Sikhs must also be cremated, although they consider that children who are stillbirths or under the age of 4 years should be buried — 'they cannot stand the heat of cremation and have no awareness of their past actions'. Muslims, on the other hand, must be buried, and although they have no special formalities for babies and small children it should be noted that 'for 40 days after the delivery, the mother is considered unclean and may not touch a dead body' (Black, 1987).

Many of the social customs surrounding death have their origin in religion and involve a ceremonial which ensures proper disposal of the dead body. For the Muslim there are strict religious practices. Every Muslim believes that the time of his death is predetermined and nobody can do anything to alter it. While dying, the family and friends recite parts of the Koran so that these are the last words heard. After death, perfumes are applied to the body, it is wrapped in a special cloth, then placed in a grave facing Mecca. In the Islamic view, a Muslim is not the owner of his own body; it is held in trust from God. Suicide is therefore forbidden; a post-mortem removal of organs for transplant is not allowed, and cremation is not permitted (Walker, 1982). The practice of Orthodox Jews also requires that a dying person has a fellow Jew in attendance to read scriptures and recite prayers during his last hours. There is also a special way of laying out the corpse and similarly, mutilation of the body is forbidden. The ritual purification is a reflection of the belief that death is not the end, but the beginning of an afterlife with the Almighty. For the Hindu, too, death is not an end. Their faith is centred on the transmigration of souls with indefinite reincarnation, and the form of the new body depends on the type of life the person has led (Green, 1989); and the Dayak tribe of Borneo (Kastenbaum, 1981) believe the soul stays in heaven for a period of seven generations then is reborn on earth.

The beliefs held by the individual obviously affect his view of himself and of life and Neuberger (1987) provides some interesting examples from different religions. Someone who believes that life after death exists is less likely to fear death and more likely to see within the sorrow, an element of joy. In contrast, a person who believes that death is the end of everything may fear dying, and find only despair and loss in bereavement.

Environmental factors

In urbanised, industrialised countries there has been a clear trend towards death in *institutions* rather than at home as once was the case. Now in the UK, $\frac{1}{2}-\frac{2}{3}$ of deaths take place in hospitals and hospices and the rate is even higher among the elderly population.

Providing care for the dying person at home, although often desirable, is not always possible even with the help of community staff and Macmillan nurses who, in the UK, are specially prepared to nurse dying people and give support to their families/partners. The carer may be elderly or frail; children may be too young or may be unable to combine the care with employment and a career; the family may be unwilling to undertake the responsibility; or the procedures needed and/or the emotional burden may be beyond the skills of the family. Hospital care, on the other hand, is often considered to be undesirable, partly because appropriate facilities are not usually available in busy general wards.

Apart from the unsuitable environment and pace of a general ward, almost all writers on the subject do not hesitate to point out that ours is a death-denying, death-defying culture and it is not surprising that staff who are educated with an explicit commitment to life, find it difficult to feel positive about the care of those who cannot live. Many doctors still do feel powerless when cure is out of the question, and it is certainly only in recent years that explicit discussion of death and dying has been introduced to the nursing and medical curriculum.

Because of the difficulties inherent in both home and institutional care for the dying, a new development has emerged — the hospice movement. The idea itself is not really new. Boston & Trezise (1987) record that in the mid-19th century Mary Aikenhead founded in Dublin an order of nuns, one of whose duties was to care for the dying; and some decades later the order inaugurated a similar service in London. The hospice movement as we know it today, however, was really started in the 1950s. There were two main originators. One was an organisation, the Marie Curie Foundation, which raised funds to establish special residential homes for cancer sufferers. As well as providing skilled nursing it was intended to 'save much mental suffering, stress and strain for the relatives'. The other was an individual, Cicely Saunders, who eventually opened St Christopher's in 1967, the first hospice 'planned on an academic model of care, research and teaching' and involving not only the patient but the family. Hospices are designed as small, homely places to care for people during the final stages of terminal illness, and to save them from the rigours of aggressive therapy. Patients are encouraged to maintain their normal lifestyle for as long as possible and enjoy living to the optimum level for them according to their abilities, with effective symptom control, and with maximum family cooperation. Additional bedrooms are available to accommodate family members if necessary; daytime visitors are encouraged; children are made welcome.

The hospice movement in the UK now boasts about 100 institutions and the idea has been used abroad to the extent that there is now an International Hospice Institute. But, despite worldwide acclaim, Dame Cicely Saunders (1986) maintains:

> There is a constant challenge to evaluate and improve so that all hospice teams will continue to give to those they serve, the fullest potential for living until they die. This is offered to all who come; the obstinate loner, the devoted elderly couple, and the young parent desperately facing the unfulfilled responsibilities of a growing family . . .

Undoubtedly, hospices are places of excellence but most deaths still occur in hospital, and the importance of hospice skills is now being widely disseminated especially to hospitals which care for the elderly and short-stay hospitals so that all dying patients can benefit (Hockley et al, 1988).

The decision of where a person should be looked after in his terminal illness depends on many factors. Consideration must be given to the individual's particular needs and to his own wishes as well as those of the family. Although a terminal illness is not necessarily protracted, the majority of deaths do not happen quickly.

In societies where hospitals are a scarce resource, particularly in developing countries, the decision is less complicated. Care of the dying is accepted as a family responsibility and in such circumstances the dying person is to able to remain at home, to end his life in the care and company of close relatives.

For the bereaved, particularly following the death of a spouse, there is an obvious change in the immediate environment of the house; all around are constant reminders of previous routines in everyday activity of living which are no longer shared. The painfulness of the memories may be assuaged by packing or giving away the dead person's clothes and belongings, perhaps to family members, yet this in itself is a stressful activity. In some instances there may be an enforced change of environment, perhaps to a smaller house in a strange neighbourhood, because the death has caused a major change in economic circumstances. Where it is not economically imperative, many people would urge caution about making drastic changes too soon after bereavement because it is recognised that the mourner's decision-making capacities are often impaired in the initial stages of grief.

Politicoeconomic factors

In Western society, the commemoration of death is often

an occasion when economic distinctions are emphasised. The type of funeral, the type of ceremony, whether or not there are commemorative plaques or headstones are activities which may reflect the economic status of the dead person's family.

The economic status of a country is reflected in the cause of death and the life expectancy of the population. The most important causes of death in industrialised countries today are heart disease, cancer and stroke. Taken together in the UK, for example, these diseases account for two-thirds of all mortality in the late adulthood and old age stages of the lifespan, and some of these fatal diseases can be caused or aggravated by factors such as overindulgence in food or alcohol or smoking. In industrialised countries, life expectancy is around 70 years of age, slightly higher for women than for men, and mortality rates among the young are very low indeed. Even so there are social class differences; the less good mortality rates in the lower social classes are highlighted in a UK Report 'Inequalities in health' (Black, 1980) and these have persisted into the 1980s (Whitehead, 1987). The legislature usually determines how the death is recorded, and politicoeconomic factors influence the provision made by the state for funeral costs and financial assistance to dependants in the form of death grants, widow's pensions, widowed mother's allowances, or their equivalents, and this ready cash certainly helps the bereaved. The economic status of a country is also reflected in the availability of schemes for private insurance cover against death, although in fact, government employers and large multinational companies may provide compensation to families following major disasters where the employee is killed or severely injured, irrespective of the employee's private insurance arrangements. Money does not solve the problems of grief but poverty can certainly make them worse.

In many developing countries, however, the picture is quite different and reflects the lower economic status; infant mortality rates are high, preventable infectious diseases claim many lives, people still die from starvation and even those who manage to remain relatively healthy have a much shorter life expectancy than in the Western world. The economic status of a country to some extent influences what can be done to prevent the circumstances which lead to avoidable early deaths but the political decisions determine how much of the national budget can be relegated for health services. Political decisions also determine how much will be spent on costly hospital life-saving procedures which reach such a small percentage of the population, and how much will be used in the community rectifying the conditions which are the cause of so many deaths. In many instances, no financial provision is made by the state for dependants and in a number of these countries, it is not yet a legal requirement to record the death.

INDIVIDUALITY IN DYING

Each individual has personal beliefs about life, and about death and dying. The experience of death is unique to each person, and using the components of the model already discussed, it is possible to identify not only the problems related to dying but also the wishes of the individual during this terminal activity. Below is a résumé of the main points of the preceding discussion.

Lifespan: effect on dying
- Age group of dying person and family/friends

Dependence/independence in dying
- Status in relation to all ALs
- Suicide/other causes of death
- Status during grieving and bereavement

Factors influencing dying
- Physical
  - terminal illness/cause of death
  - diagnosis of death
  - physical effects on other ALs
  - physical effect on family/friends

- Psychological
  - personality and temperament
  - fears and anxieties about dying and death
  - awareness of approaching death
  - whether or not significant others know of prognosis
  - behaviour of others towards the dying person
  - effect of grieving and bereavement on family/friends

- Sociocultural
  - past life experience
  - personal beliefs about dying and death
  - religious/cultural rituals surrounding death and bereavement

- Environmental
  - selection of home/hospital/hospice
  - change of environment for family

- Politicoeconomic
  - home/family/financial circumstances
  - effect on cause of death and life expectancy
  - availability of health and support services for the dying and the bereaved

Dying: patients' problems and related nursing

The dying person and the family are faced with many problems and emotional demands of a highly complex nature. Not all dying people require, or even wish, the help of a nurse but for many people at the endpoint of the lifespan, some of their problems can at least be alleviated with skilled and sensitive nursing. Individualised nursing can only be carried out if the nurse knows about the patient's (and family's) problems, and about personal wishes (and those of the family) related to this last Activity of Living. While observing and while conversing with the patient and the family, the nurse would be seeking answers to the following questions:

- when is the individual likely to die?
- what factors influence the way the individual is dying?
- what does the individual (and family) know about the prognosis?
- what are the individual's beliefs about dying and death?
- what problems does the individual have at present or seem likely to develop?
- what effect does the dying process have on the family and how does this affect the individual?
- what do the patient and family want the nurse to do when the death occurs?
- if the patient has an organ donor card, do the family know, and what is the family's attitude?
- what effect will bereavement have on the family?

The information collected should then be examined to identify any problems being experienced in the process of dying. Potential problems should be identified and prevented when possible; and actual problems should be solved or alleviated; or the patient should be helped to cope with them. When possible, the patient and family should be involved in the process of assessment and should help to set realistic goals.

The nursing interventions (and what the patient agrees to do) to achieve the set goals should be selected according to local circumstances and available resources; these are then written on the nursing plan. In many instances, evaluation will have to be done daily because although, in the process of dying, there is often a gradual erosion of independence in all ALs, this may fluctuate from day to day, and the person who is dying should be helped to live to the optimum for that day. Cure is not the objective so palliative medicine is the appropriate approach; comfort and well-being are of paramount importance.

Of course, a multidisciplinary team may often be involved in the care of a dying person and it is important that the individualised nursing plan is congruent with the team's mutually agreed objectives, so that the patient can be helped to be as comfortable as possible for as long as possible, and can die with dignity.

In order to provide individualised nursing, the nurse needs to have a background knowledge of the general conditions which can be responsible for, or can change the individual's dependence/independence status, and which can be experienced by the person as problems. Against the background of the general discussion in the first half of this chapter, some specific problem areas are discussed under the following headings:

- change of environment and routine
- physical problems associated with dying
- psychological and sociocultural problems associated with dying
- the family's problems.

CHANGE OF ENVIRONMENT AND ROUTINE

When dying people are nursed in their own home setting, at least they are surrounded by family, friends, neighbours, and many of their personal possessions are in view or can be brought to them. The individual at least has a semblance of control over the immediate environment. Currently however, in many industrialised countries, people are transferred to hospital or hospice to die, totally removed from familiar surroundings. So following hospitalisation there comes a moment when they realise that they will not again see their own home and their worldly possessions. This very final environmental separation must be coped with as well as the other fears and anxieties and physical discomforts.

Most of the points about anxiety arising from a change of environment which were made when discussing the preceding 11 ALs, are augmented when the person appreciates that his own death will take place within the restricted personal living space of the hospital. Certainly initially the person is concerned that hospital routines will be unfamiliar, especially those associated with washing and toileting; that privacy will be threatened; that eating and drinking likes and dislikes may not be given much consideration, and the type of food may be alien to personal taste; that ward temperature and humidity may be uncomfortable; that noise levels and the presence of other people will disturb periods of sleep; that if bedfast, the capacity to mobilise will be out of personal control; that there will be difficulty communicating with staff and other patients who are all strangers. All of these potential problems are exacerbated if the person comes from a different cultural group, especially if there are strict religious/cultural practices associated with dying and death, some of which may not be feasible to countenance in an institutional setting.

In Western culture, because hospitals and a lot of their equipment and procedures are so geared to 'cure' — and lack of ability to cure is often seen as professional failure — it is not surprising that the prospect of dying and death in a hospital environment can create such problems for the patient and family. Hospitals may be lonely places in which to die, yet paradoxically it is rare for relatives to have the facilities to be alone with the dying person, free from potential interruptions.

It is, in fact, a sad reflection on our lack of preparation and provision for care of the dying that it was seen to be necessary to create what has become known as the hospice movement. It is undeniable that, in a hospice, there is expertise in terminal care; that there are calm, relaxed surroundings where care and concern for the wishes of the patient are paramount, and this permeates the environment. Indeed there is almost dismay that they have acquired an aura of élitism, an idea of excellence in practice which seem difficult to achieve. In hospices such an environment is deliberately created, and in the person's own home, it is perhaps not too difficult to provide such an environment where the individual is surrounded by personal belongings, and where community nursing staff, family and helpers can collaborate to provide support and respond to the individual's wishes. However, despite the general criticism which is still levelled about the care of dying people in hospital, some nursing staff do manage to create an environment of calmness and caring, and the patients themselves feel that they receive individualised attention even in the midst of a busy general hospital.

PHYSICAL PROBLEMS ASSOCIATED WITH DYING

The dying person is also a living person, and for each remaining day, the quality of life is important. In 1973, Cartwright et al did a nationwide survey in the UK of the quality of life before death and among other things, recommended that hospice skills should be disseminated to care of the elderly and short-stay wards so that all dying patients could benefit. Yet in a project by Hockley et al (1988) it was apparent that in the hospitals under study, there is still a need for a more effective multidisciplinary team to guide symptom control and provide supportive care. Physical discomforts can be so insistent. The psychological, sociocultural, environmental and economic factors relevant to each individual must of course be considered by the nurse but more time and effort can be given to those less tangible aspects of nursing if the dying person

can be helped to be physically comfortable. The person who is overwhelmed by distressing physical symptoms does not have the energy to enter into relationships or benefit from the support they can offer. Hockley et al included 26 terminally ill patients in their study and the range of discomforts reported by the patients to the researcher is given in Table 17.1. Almost all are physical discomforts.

Table 17.1 Discomforts suffered by terminally ill patients (from Hockley et al 1988 British Medical Journal 296 June 18: 1715–1717 reproduced by kind permission of the authors and editor of the British Medical Journal)

Symptoms	No. patients (n = 26)	Symptoms	No. patients (n = 26)
Anorexia	24	Pressure sores	16
Insomnia	23	Constipation	14
Immobility	23	Nausea	14
Malaise	23	Oedema	11
Sore mouth	21	Confusion	9
Cough	20	Incontinence	8
Dyspnoea	18	Vomiting	7
Pain	18	Malodorous wounds	2

In order to identify whether or not a patient is experiencing any of these problems, or may be likely to, the nurse needs to carry out an assessment of all the ALs so that relevant nursing interventions can be planned. Some of the nursing interventions which can alleviate physical problems are mentioned below, and to reduce excessive repetition, cross references are given to more detailed, earlier discussions of these topics.

Pain (p. 121–125) is probably what people fear most about the process of dying, and although it is experienced at other times throughout life, it can be of particular distress to dying people. As long ago as 1972, Hinton was reporting that about one in eight people suffered pain during terminal illness; and these findings are corroborated in more recent studies such as Hockley et al (1988). Table 17.1 shows that 18 out of 26 patients reported pain.

For a long time it seemed to be assumed that the pain of dying could not be controlled and had to be endured. The work of Dr Cicely Saunders and others has radically altered medical thinking about this and it is now quite clear that with prudent use of analgesic drugs, control of terminal pain can and should be achieved. The basic principle of management is that sufficiently potent analgesics are given *regularly* so that pain is not only relieved, but prevented and if pain does occur, then the dose should be increased or the drug changed (Regnard & Davies, 1986).

The prescribing of drugs is of course a medical responsibility but it is one which relies on competent nursing assessment of pain (p. 123) and regular evaluation of the effectiveness of the pain control methods employed. Very often nurses do patients a disservice by being reluctant to give analgesics unless the patient's pain is obvious and debilitating, thinking that the drugs may not be effective if given too often or too early in the terminal phase. In fact, routine administration of drugs can be effective for months in the majority of cases and in some instances is now administered via infusion to provide a regulated and constant level in the blood (p. 124). Other innovatory ideas include preparing the patient and/or family to self-administer drugs, thus providing a much appreciated opportunity for the person to remain at home, and even at work during a protracted period of dying (Harris, 1988a).

For children, too, improved methods of pain relief are being used effectively and Fradd (1988) cites the use of Entonox, epidural anaesthesia, continuous morphine infusions and lignocaine cream (EMLA). For children, too, terminal care need not be available only in the hospital; it may be available at home, hospice, hostel, school or residential home. If at home, and the child is suffering from a progressively fatal condition which worsens over several months or years, it may be important to offer respite care if the family are to retain the energy and strength to continue to care for the child in the family setting (Burne, 1988).

In addition to pain caused by the terminal illness, the patient may suffer from other types of pain too. If confined to bed pain may be experienced due to pressure or lack of movement. Joint pains and muscular tension can be alleviated with careful positioning, massage and the application of local heat (p. 265).

Anorexia, nausea and vomiting (p. 171, 172). When someone has a lengthy, terminal illness, one of the most distressing aspects is watching them almost literally fade away and this is particularly common in people who have certain types of cancer. Along with obvious weight loss, there is muscle wasting, skin breakdown, impaired wound healing, decreased immunocompetence; and the general debility, weakness and malaise lead to a further lack of interest in food and a further decline in nutritional status (Holmes, 1988). Some would say that in terminal illness nutritional support is not necessary; and clearly at some point in the process of dying, nutrition is not the paramount concern. But while the individual can enjoy meals — and food has a social function as well as the obviously physical one — everything should be done to provide small, easily digested meals which are appetising; and this is achieved in some units, even in large, busy general hospitals. Such people should be encouraged and helped if necessary, to clean their teeth or dentures, in the hope that it will be refreshing and encourage the inclination to eat. A coated tongue reduces any enjoyment of food flavour and a frank thrush infection may be painful, so mouth care (p. 218) every 2–4 hours may be required perhaps along with antifungal agents if thrush is present. Pineapple contains a proteolytic enzyme, ananase, which helps to clean the mouth and, if the patient enjoys the flavour, sucking a pineapple chunk, may be a welcome adjunct to organised mouth care. Iced tonic water to suck

has a similar effect as do iced lemon and glycerine Q-tips which are commercially produced. Persistent nausea can be relieved by the use of antiemetic drugs, although in a recent research project involving 105 patients who were on cytotoxic therapy, the use of acupuncture on the inner forearm (known as the Neugian P6) achieved beneficial antiemetic results (Dundee, 1988); and in a small study, Stannard (1989) reported that acupressure wrist bands were effective.

Difficulty in swallowing, and dehydration (p. 171, 165) Swallowing can be difficult if there is any obstruction in the upper alimentary tract such as a malignant growth, or pressure on the tract from growths or inflammation in neighbouring tissues. It may also occur when radiotherapy is prescribed in the upper trunk area, for example for lung cancer. Dysphagia makes eating and drinking uncomfortable so a local anaesthetic in gel form given before food, or food given in semi-solid form may ease the patient's difficulty. Ice to suck, covered in gauze, sometimes helps to reduce the fear of choking, and can be soothing and refreshing, as well as helping to keep buccal mucosa moist. In addition in order to prevent dehydration, frequent small drinks of the patient's choice should be made available and help may be needed if the patient is weak or unable to sit up. Adequate hydration is by far the best way of preventing a 'dirty' mouth (p. 218). The nurse may find, however, that it is fear of urinary incontinence which causes the patient to reduce fluid intake.

Difficulty with eliminating. The dying person can be extremely distressed by urinary incontinence (p. 183), and it is necessary for the nurse to approach this problem with sympathy and tact. Despite its hazards, catheterisation may be the best solution in these circumstances.

Faecal incontinence (p. 189) may be equally distressing, although constipation (p. 185) is more likely especially when opioid drugs are being used to provide analgesia. Irrespective of drugs, the lack of exercise, and reduced fluid and food intake also contribute to constipation and prophylactic treatment using laxatives may be necessary to prevent the potential problem of faecal impaction.

Pressure sores (p. 218). General debility, reduced movement, reduced food intake and lack of vitamin C, and impaired sensation may cause pressure sores to develop more readily in the dying person, and Crow (1988) gives a review of literature on the care of pressure sores. Regular turning to relieve prolonged pressure on any one part may be carried out, but if this is too disturbing, bed appliances alone should be used. Although prevention of pressure sores is important, it is more important to allow the dying person as much comfort and peace as possible in the absolutely final stages of life. Dying patients often seem to become very sensitive to pressure, such as from bedclothes, and great patience and skill may be needed to help the patient to remain comfortable in bed.

Difficulty in breathing, coughing (p. 138). The patient

and the visitors can be very distressed by dyspnoea. Chemotherapy can be prescribed to reduce inflammation of the bronchial mucosa and relieve laboured breathing but administration of oxygen is seldom helpful because use of the mask often merely increases the feeling of suffocation. Ventilating the room, placing the bed near a window even if only for the psychological effect, and being with the patient may ease the sense of panic and fear. The very noisy breathing known as the 'death rattle' can be subdued by using drugs which dry up the excessive secretions in the respiratory tract.

Any dyspnoea will be exacerbated by a persistent cough (p. 145) which may be dry (for example caused by mechanical irritation of the respiratory tract or diaphragm) or moist (for example caused by infection, chronic obstructive airways disease, asthma or heart failure). Cough may be treated by providing a simple linctus or humidifying the air to provide peripheral suppression of the cause of the cough. When such measures are unsuccessful it may be possible to alleviate the cough by using drugs which have either a peripheral or central suppression action.

Eye care. In the final stages of terminal illness, the person may be fully alert, or may have long, drowsy periods or may be drifting in and out of consciousness. Whatever the circumstances, it is usually soothing to bathe the eyes to prevent encrustation and inflammation around the eyelids.

Unpleasant odour. Unless the nurses are meticulous in carrying out nursing activities related to such conditions as incontinence or discharging wounds, an unpleasant smell can result and it is distressing to all concerned. Hormones or other drugs can be used to reduce the smell from a fungating lesion, such as may occur in advanced cancer of the breast. Good ventilation of the room and discreet use of deodorisers can be helpful and the patients will appreciate any attempt to minimise what for them is also a distressing problem.

Nursing activities aimed to promote physical comfort for the dying are not substantially different from those applicable to problems already described in each of the AL chapters and cross-referenced above. However, greater skill and patience are often demanded of the nurse because 'minor' discomforts can assume major proportions as the patient's independence and strength diminish. Patients can be encouraged to participate in their care when they feel able to do so, and nursing routines should be flexible enough to allow attention to be given at times when the patient can cope with the disturbance involved, and when pain control is at its optimum. Regnard & Davies (1986) provide information about specific drugs and techniques which have proved to be particularly helpful to dying people for the relief of a variety of symptoms.

As mentioned earlier, when physical discomforts receive adequate attention, more time and energy can be devoted to increasing the quality of life before death and there is increasing interest in achieving this by the use of massage and therapeutic touch (Bypass, 1988).

Children who are dying can be helped to tolerate physical procedures through the medium of play (Williams, 1987) and even in hospital this can be interesting and exciting says Fradd (1986). As far as possible, however, patients are helped to care for their dying child at home and in some hospitals, family therapy sisters assist parents in learning to give intravenous drugs and parenteral nutrition, working in close collaboration with a community paediatric nurse (Fradd, 1988).

PSYCHOLOGICAL AND SOCIOCULTURAL PROBLEMS ASSOCIATED WITH DYING

Each dying patient and those close to him will react to the approaching death in a very individual way. The emotional reactions will vary as will the nature of the problems experienced. Likewise, cultural influences (including ethical, spiritual and religious) will vary. There will be differences too according to whether the dying person is cared for at home or in hospital; and whether either or both parties are aware of the prognosis and the likely course of the terminal illness.

Fear and anxiety. Almost universally, dying people experienced. Likewise, cultural influences (including ethical, are reactions to any illness but are particularly intense in terminal illness because there is no prospect of recovery. There are so many things about which the dying person may feel apprehensive and afraid for example, fear of death, fear of pain, fear of the process of dying, fear of loss of control and dignity, and fear of being alone or of being rejected. And the type of communication which might help allay such fears is often lacking.

The knowledge that death will mean parting from family and friends obviously is a source of great sadness to the dying person and often there is considerable anxiety about their future and about how they will cope with their bereavement. The onset of depression, described earlier as a common feature of the dying process, is sometimes mistaken as a physical symptom but probably is more often caused by the dying person's feelings of sadness (Andrews et al, 1985), fear and regret.

In gaining strength and courage to face death without fear many people find their religious beliefs an invaluable resource. For some patients who die in hospital the chaplain becomes an important source of comfort and companionship. The hospital chaplain (or the representative of any faith) who is a welcome visitor for the patient should be made to feel welcome in the ward by the nursing staff. They are, after all, members of the multiprofessional health care team with a special role and function. With their religious knowledge and ability to give spiritual guidance, chaplains have a particular contribution to make to the care of the dying patient. Often they become the people in whom the patient confides inner-most fears and anxieties; sometimes the chaplain helps the dying patient to understand the significance of death and to accept it with dignity and without fear.

Whether or not there is a declared religious conviction the anxiety about maintaining dignity and control may have influenced the person to support the idea of euthanasia. In North America there is a document in use called a Living Will. It is a statement signed by the patient, perhaps some time before terminal illness, and witnessed by the family, indicating that if the person becomes so ill that there is no reasonable expectation of recovery from physical or mental disability, he or she be allowed to die and not kept alive by artificial means. Apparently it works so well in the USA that some doctors have been sued for persevering with active treatment **against** the patient's wishes (Buckman, 1988).

In a recent UK publication which reviews the policy of the British Medical Association on the subject — the Euthanasia Report 1988 — it is agreed that doctors should take 'living wills' into account but cautions that they are not binding in law. The Report rejects legislation favouring euthanasia and declares that the active intervention by anybody to terminate another person's life should remain illegal. The concept of patient autonomy is a crucial aspect of sensitive and informed patient care, the Report maintains, but autonomy works both ways; patients have the right to decline treatment, but do not have the right to demand treatment which the doctor cannot, in conscience, provide.

In Holland, the situation is somewhat different. Killing as such remains illegal but if a doctor, after consulting his colleagues, openly practises euthanasia, and then reports the act to the authorities, he is unlikely to be prosecuted. It is maintained that about 6000 patients choose euthanasia every year (Brewer, 1988) — a lethal drug is administered intentionally (active euthanasia) to a terminally ill patient who has asked to be relieved of suffering. It is interesting that at a recent international conference, an Indian doctor reminded delegates that 'voluntary euthanasia should not be thought of as just another Western luxury since in poor countries with poor health services, terminal illness can bankrupt a family much more comprehensively than in the West' (Brewer, 1988).

Loneliness. According to Kastenbaum (1981) and Norbert (1985) one of the greatest concerns among people who are dying is that they will be left alone. People who die in hospital sometimes can experience an overwhelming sense of loneliness; although they are not 'alone', they are without close companionship. The contact which the nurse has with the patient who is dying is frequent and, if allowed, can become the basis of a trusting relationship which will help to reduce loneliness and isolation. There is probably no patient who is more in need of tender loving care than the patient who is nearing death yet Norbert (1985) goes so far as to say that while still alive, the dying are physically deserted. On the other hand, the person may be surrounded by professionals and still *feel* alone, and deserted. The medical team's ability to defer the moment of death can cause even attentive staff to be so intent on gadgetry that they lose sight of the need for the human personal touch which is so precious to the patient.

Difficulty in facing the truth. The terminally ill person may not find it easy to seek a supportive relationship with the nurse, and the nurse may not find it easy to offer; often nurses seem to avoid involvement. Sometimes this is because they do not understand that reactions such as anger and depression are 'normal' in the process of dying. Often it is because they are afraid of being faced with the question 'Am I dying?' In fact, this direct question is not often asked but, if it is, it means the patient wants to talk about his fears and uncertainties. Nevertheless, there are people who continue to use denial, and they should not be assaulted with truths they are unwilling, or not yet ready, to face. In many instances, however, dying patients *are* aware of their prognosis. Even though the patient has not been told explicitly there are many subtle ways in which the information may be transmitted to him by doctors and nurses. Sometimes both the patient and family choose not to admit openly that they know the prognosis; in other cases the knowledge is frankly shared. Whether or not dying patients should be told of their prognosis is a complex and delicate question.

Writing about 'Breaking bad news' to a dying patient in a community setting, Harris (1988b) maintains that nurses often rationalise being 'economical with the truth' as sparing patients unnecessary distress. And there is also the opinion (sometimes reinforced by the family) that the person will not be able to cope with the truth but, Harris goes on, this implies that the patient is unable to exercise self-control and denies them responsible adult status. Such an attitude also denies the patient the opportunity to anticipate and make provision for the future.

There are good reasons on practical, psychological and spiritual grounds for adopting a policy in favour of telling the truth, and supporting the patient in the search for coping strategies. But equally, on occasions, there may be reasons for withholding this information, indeed Neuberger (1987) maintains that in some religions, it is anathema to tell patients they are dying. In practice, the decision should not be difficult if dying patients are given time and opportunity, with someone they can talk to and trust, to explore their fear and suspicions and to indicate what they want (and don't want) to know. What is important is for the nurse to be sensitive to the patient's own awareness of the situation and to know what has already been said by the doctor and relatives.

This of course means that the nurse must assess the patient's situation and the most important source of information is the patient. The nurse will learn what she needs to know by listening carefully, observing astutely and communicating effectively. Once she knows what the patient feels and understands about the situation, she can gain confidence to form a close relationship and show the patient that she is willing to listen. A dying patient, feeling lonely and afraid, will gain comfort from companionship and closeness. Spending time with him, talking or sharing in his silence, and taking care over physical needs can restore tranquillity to an existence which in so many ways is in turmoil. Showing sympathy and compassion are important aspects of nursing a dying patient and essential if the nurse is to help with the various psychological and spiritual problems which may arise in the dying process.

However, responding to the dying patient's feelings with unerring sensitivity is not at all easy, indeed it can cause considerable stress and strain. Part of the nurse's stress may be that inadequate preparation is provided about ways of discussing death with dying people and Conboy-Hill (1987) suggests the 'busy nurse' image may be reinforced by the nurses to deter patients from asking questions — a form of 'distancing' behaviour. On the other hand, it is sometimes overlooked that nursing a 'brain-dead' person (and there may be more than one, for example, in a neurological ward) who makes no apparent response to constant care and attention, is emotionally traumatic for the nurse. However, whatever the circumstance, before nursing staff can give support to patients and families, they must come to terms with their own attitudes about death and dying (Neuberger, 1987) and most nursing programmes now provide opportunities for students to explore this important aspect of professional preparation and practice.

THE FAMILY'S PROBLEMS

The patient's family too may feel afraid and anxious, and it is useful here to reiterate that the word 'family' has a wide interpretation and can include relatives, friends or partners, especially topical because of the current AIDS epidemic. They find it hard to watch if their loved one is suffering and find it difficult to understand the fluctuating moods, and sometimes unpredictable reactions. They may fear their own ability to cope with the event of death, to control their emotions and to face the future alone.

If the person is being looked after in hospital, the family may feel cut off and unable to find ways of expressing their love and concern; and in the publicity of an open ward they may find that maintaining their close relationship becomes difficult. In caring for a dying person at home the family faces other stresses arising from the total involvement of that situation. Their ability to cope emotionally may be eroded by the exhaustion of providing for all the needs of the dying person in the last stages of illness.

The positive value of establishing a supportive and humane relationship with the relatives of a dying patient was emphasised by one of the early writers on the subject, McNulty (1974) when she says:

Nurses have a lot to answer for in their apparent insensitivity to the needs of relatives . . . I think that we are sometimes afraid to stop for fear we might not be able to answer the questions asked; afraid because we cannot give the so much wanted good news; afraid because we might have to say 'I don't know'. If only we could realise that just by stopping for a moment and sharing our presence, we may have to some degree lightened the family's burden.

Being accessible is the essential point. The relatives should be encouraged to see the nurse or doctor in charge, and at visiting times, nurses must be available and able to make such arrangements. Yet Bond (1982) in a series of articles called 'Relatively Speaking' found that despite a great deal of literature about the need for communication, nurses still do not seem to make themselves available. Practical advice about when and how often to visit can be helpful to the family, because financial and social resources may be drained over a period yet the family want to help. Often, too, allowing close relatives to help in the care, for example by helping the patient to wash or have a meal, may be greatly appreciated as this gives a purpose to visits and provides the opportunity for affection and concern to be expressed.

It is particularly distressing when the patient is 'brain-dead' and no matter what the family do and how often they visit, there is no obvious sign from the patient that there is any response. Distress may be heightened if, for example, organ-transplantation is envisaged although paradoxically, the family may be somewhat comforted to know that the transplant will help some needy person. For the 'brain-dead' person, the goal of nursing is to facilitate dignified dying and a dignified death. It is perhaps the ultimate example of total dependence on nursing staff and demands the highest possible standards of nursing with an ongoing evaluation to deal with changing priorities. Included is care of the family during this emotionally traumatic experience and being sensitive to the needs of a visitor who sits constantly at the bedside perhaps to the neglect of other family members, not to mention personal health.

One of the most stressful of nursing duties is breaking the news of the actual event of death to the patient's next-of-kin and this is a task which must be done as sensitively and compassionately as possible. The nurse can do little to ease the relative's distress; what is important is that she is prepared for the fact that reactions cannot be predicted. The relative may appear totally inconsolable or almost unconcerned; sometimes anger is directed at the nurse or doctor. If the death is sudden (the family member recently saw them alive and well) the reaction is disbelief. If the death is in strange surroundings such as overseas or on holiday; or in dramatic circumstances such as following a fire, car or drowning accident, the family members (particularly if they are survivors of the accident) are shocked and numb, and often cannot even remember familiar phone numbers or addresses to seek help from relatives and friends. After certain sudden deaths, too, a postmortem is obligatory in many countries, and this heightens distress. Whatever the family's reaction — and the nurse is also emotionally affected by death and grief — the nurse must remain calm and kind. In most instances, requests by the family to see the body should be allowed as this can be important in confirming the reality and allowing the saying of a final farewell; and it is thought to help in the grieving process (Cathcart, 1988).

Dealing kindly with the practicalities will be appreciated. It is important that the next-of-kin understands what is written on the death certificate given by the doctor and knows that this has to be taken within a certain time to the office of the Registrar of Births, Deaths and Marriages in the district in which the hospital is situated (not the district of the deceased person's home). The Registrar provides the certificate which authorises an undertaker to arrange the funeral. Usually the nurse also returns the deceased person's effects to the next-of-kin and this should be done sympathetically, making sure that the person has some means of transport home. The way in which nurses deal with the family at this final contact with the hospital is very important. Kindness and practical help will be remembered with gratitude whereas a casual approach may well contribute to a lingering bad memory of the patient's time in hospital. The importance of providing practical comfort and support at the time of death is now recognised to be of such benefit that in some hospitals a specially designated liaison nurse is appointed to guide relatives through the immediate ordeal of mourning.

Following the death, there are many problems which may face bereaved people as they attempt to accept and cope with the loss. There are emotional problems of grief, the difficulties of social adjustment and sometimes there are economic strains too, if the deceased person was the family breadwinner. In the immediate bereavement period there may be death grants and widow's pensions to claim; insurance policies to negotiate; the children's future to be markedly altered; mortgage payments to reconsider; a re-routing of financial resources. Often quite crucial decisions have to be made at a time when the chief mourners are least able to cope.

The early stage of acute grief is particularly distressing and sometimes involves feelings of self-criticism and guilt, the person wondering if the death could have been prevented. Acute reactive depression and even suicidal thoughts may occur. Sometimes the problem is that the grief reaction may be delayed, particularly if the bereaved had much to do with the practicalities of the funeral or if the death was very sudden or totally unexpected in the illness. Then they may wonder why they do not feel shocked and sad, only later having to cope with these intense feelings. Some people find it distressing to mourn openly and find the funeral traumatic; others may be worried by the intensity of their emotions when alone and wonder if they might be on the verge of a complete mental breakdown. Most people appear to be surprised by just how long their feelings of loss and sadness last and begin to wonder if they will ever readjust and resume a normal life again. Bereavement is probably the most devastating experience which is faced in life and disrupts every activity of living. It is difficult for the person concerned to accept that it is a recognised process and a normal reaction to the loss of someone precious to them.

The most helpful contribution the nurse can make is to help the bereaved persons to face up to and work through the emotional difficulties. This means that they must be given time: time to grieve, time to talk, to reminisce, to express openly fears and worries and to begin to plan a new future. The community nurse is in an ideal position to assess the needs and problems of a bereaved person. An elderly man now on his own could be helped to cope with the domestic tasks previously done by his wife. A mother left to bring up young children might be given help to consider what to tell the children and how to support them in their grief.

In fact helping bereaved people is a communal responsibility; a basic human concern which can be shared by both professionals and the public. Bereavement is not an illness but a life event with which most people need the help of others. Giving help to the bereaved needs to begin before the death if this is possible, so that grief can be anticipated and preparations made for readjustment.

Grief cannot be cured, but it can be shared. Showing compassion to bereaved people will be a reminder that, despite their loss and feelings of intense loneliness, they are not entirely alone and that there is some reason to renew their sources of faith and hope, and have the courage to begin again; that there is the possibility of being and feeling happy again without being disrespectful to the person who has died.

Some bereaved people find it helpful to attend organised groups which have been created to provide an opportunity to share and talk through feelings of grief and thereby derive consolation, and in some instances, practical help from, for example, The Bereaved Parents Helpline; The Compassionate Friends; Cruse; The National Organisation for the Widowed and Their Children; Age Concern; The Gay Bereavement Project. After national disasters, a multiprofessional counselling team is sometimes used to assist bereaved families both in the immediate aftermath and with follow-up services over a period of time.

Caring for the dying and bereaved is an important aspect of nursing. The emphasis of all nursing is on helping people to cope with the activities of living; dealing with death is no different. Caring for the dying is concerned with life before death and helping the bereaved is about life after death.

The role of the nurse in caring for the dying was mentioned in Virgina Henderson's famous definition of the function of nursing (p. 13). She wrote: 'Nursing is primarily assisting the individual (sick or well) in the performance of those activities contributing to health, or its recovery (*or to a peaceful death*) that he would perform unaided if he had the necessary strength, will or knowledge . . .'

Nursing is concerned with helping people, both in living and in dying.

Individualising nursing

The first part of this chapter reflects the Roper, Logan and Tierney model — the nature of the AL of dying; the relationship of the lifespan to the AL; the effect of an individual's dependence/independence status; and the influence of physical, psychological, sociocultural, environmental and politicoeconomic factors on the AL. Examples of potential problems have been given and what might be done to prevent them from becoming actual problems. And a selection of actual problems and discomforts which can be experienced by people who are dying have been described. This provides a background of general knowledge about the AL as such.

While describing the Roper, Logan and Tierney model for nursing, general information was provided about individualising nursing (p. 51) which, in fact, is synonymous with the concept of the process of nursing.

Out of this background of general knowledge about the AL of dying, and about individualising nursing, it should then be possible to extract the issues which are relevant to one individual's current circumstances, i.e. make an assessment of relevant issues according to the individual's stage on the lifespan; according to current level of dependence/independence; and take into account the relevant physical, psychological, sociocultural, environmental and politicoeconomic factors. Collectively, this information would provide a profile of the person's individuality and therefore guides the nurse in devising a plan for individualising nursing.

As indicated earlier in the text, this assessment would be achieved by various means such as observing the person;

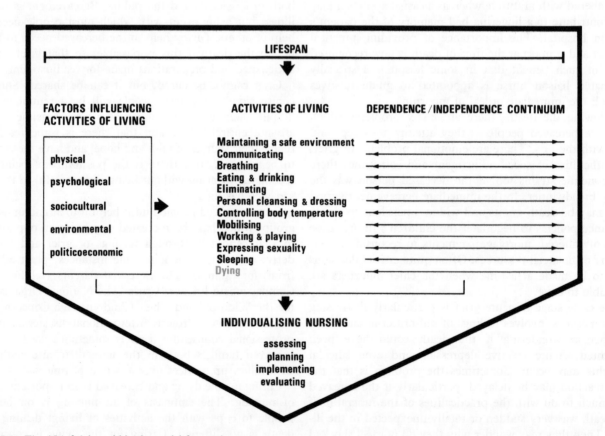

Fig. 17.1   The AL of dying within the model for nursing

acquiring information about the person's usual habits partly by asking appropriate questions, partly by listening to the patient and/or relatives; and using relevant information from available records, including medical records. The collected information could then be examined to identify any actual problems being experienced and these could be arranged in some order of priority. The nurse might also recognise some potential problems — not all possible potential problems but those which are relevant. Realistic goals, mutually agreed with the patient when this is possible, could then be set to prevent potential problems from becoming actual ones; to alleviate or solve the actual problems; or to help the person cope with those which cannot be alleviated or solved; and to help the person to die with dignity. Of course, some of the problems, although identified from the nursing assessment, may well be outwith the scope of nursing intervention. In such instances, after discussion with the patient when appropriate, these problems may be referred to other members of the health care team such as medical staff, dietitians or spiritual/religious advisers.

Keeping in mind what the person can and cannot do unaided, the nursing interventions to achieve the mutually set goals could then be selected according to local circumstances and available resources.

Following implementation of the interventions, their effects could be evaluated in relation to the goals set, and if goals were not reached, they could be revised or rescheduled, or even discarded.

It is worth repeating here that although discussed in four phases (assessing, planning, implementing and evaluating) individualising nursing is not a linear progression; it assumes a built-in responsiveness to feedback at any of the phases, giving ample allowance for change within the overall framework.

This chapter has been concerned with the AL of dying. However as stated previously, it is only for the purposes of discussion that any AL can be considered on its own; in reality, the various activities are closely related and do not have distinct boundaries. Figure 17.1 is a reminder that the AL of dying is related to the other ALs and also to the other components of the model for nursing.

REFERENCES

Andrews R, Jenkins J, Sugden J 1985 Origins of sadness as a response. Add-on Journal of Clinical Nursing 2 (34) February: 995–998
Allan D 1987 Criteria for brain stem death. The Professional Nurse 2 (11) August: 357–359
Barker W 1987 Close encounters of a preventive kind. Senior Nurse 7 (1) July: 13–15
Black D 1980 Working group on inequalities in health. HMSO, London
Black J 1987 Broaden your mind about death and bereavement in certain ethnic groups in Britain. British Medical Journal 295 August 29: 536–539
Bond S 1982 Communicating with families of cancer patients. Nursing Times 78 (24) June 16: 1027–1029
Boston S, Trezise R 1987 Merely mortal: coping with dying, death and bereavement. Methuen, London
Brewer C 1988 An option on death. Nursing Times 84 (11) March 16: 22
British Medical Association 1988 The Euthanasia Report. BMA, London
Brooking J, Minghella E 1987 Parasuicide. Nursing Times 83 (21) May 27: 40–43
Buckman R 1988 Patients who give up the will to live. Daily Telegraph May 3: 15
Burne R 1988 Terminal care in children. Journal of Family Medicine 13 (10) October: 284–287
Bypass R 1988 Soothing body and soul. Nursing Times 84 (24) June 15: 39–41
Capper E 1982 Stillbirth. Add-on Journal of Clinical Nursing 34 (February): 1490
Cartwright A, Hockley L, Anderson J 1973 Life before death. Routledge and Kegan Paul, London
Cathcart F 1988 Seeing the body after death. British Medical Journal 297 (6655) October 22: 997–998
Conboy-Hill S 1987 Dying people — how do nurses feel and what training do they want? Paper presented to British Psychology Society (London) Conference
Crow R 1988 The challenge of pressure sores. Nursing Times 84 (38) September 21: 68–73

Dickstria R, Hawton K (ed) 1987 Suicide in adolescence. Dordrecht, Nijhoff. Distributed by MTP Press
Dundee J 1988 Acupressure as an anti-emetic. Acupuncture in Medicine V (1): 22–24
Fradd E 1986 It's child's play. Nursing Times 82 (41) October 8: 40–42
Fradd E 1988 Tug of love. Nursing Times 84 (41) October 12: 32–35
Green J 1989 Death with dignity: Hinduism. Nursing Times 85 (6) February 8: 50–51
Gyulay J 1975 The forgotten grievers. American Journal of Nursing 75 (9) September: 1476–1479
Harris L 1988a Something to live for. Nursing Times 84 (32) August 10: 25–28
Harris L 1988b Breaking bad news. Community Outlook in Nursing Times 84 (30) July 27: 15–17
Health Departments of Great Britain and Northern Ireland 1983 Cadaveric organs for transplantation. HMSO, London
Hinton J 1972 Dying. Penguin, Harmondsworth
Hockley J, Dunlop R, Davies R 1988 Survey of distressing symptoms in dying patients and their families in hospital and the response to a symptom control team. British Medical Journal 296 (6638) June 18: 1715–1717
Holmes S 1988 Nourishing with care. Community Outlook in Nursing Times 84 (30) July 27: 24–28
Jones I 1987a A dignified death. Nursing Times 83 (20) May 20: 50–52
Jones I 1987b Living after loss. Nursing Times 83 (33) August 19: 45–46
Kastenbaum R 1981 Death, society and human experience. Mosby, St Louis
Kubler Ross E 1982 On death and dying. Tavistock, London
Lake T 1984 Living with grief. Sheldon Press, London
Lovell B 1987 Sharing the death of a parent. Nursing Times 83 (42) October 21: 36–39
McCarthy J 1980 Death, anxiety and loss of self. Gardner Press, New York
McNulty B 1974 The nurse's contribution in terminal care. Nursing Mirror 139 (15) October 10: 59–61
Mallinson G 1989 When a baby dies. Nursing Times 85 (9) March 1: 31–34
Milner A 1987 Recent theories on the cause of cot death. British Medical Journal 295 (6610) November 28: 1366–1368
Moore I 1986 Ending it all. Nursing Times 82 (7) February 12: 48–49

Murray Parkes C 1972 Bereavement: studies of grief in adult life. Penguin, Harmondsworth

Negus J 1987 Part of the family. Nursing Times 83 (15) April 15: 31–32

Neuberger J 1987 Caring for dying people of different faiths. Lisa Sainsbury Foundation, London

Newsweek 1988 Correspondence on 'A right to die!' Newsweek CX1 (15) April 11: 5

Norbert E 1985 The loneliness of dying. Blackwell, Oxford, p 23, 85

Pike C 1983 The broken heart symptoms and the elderly patient. Nursing Times 79 (19) March 2: 50–53

Pope N 1988 New hope on cot deaths? Nursing Times 84 (33) August 17: 21

Regnard C, Davies A 1986 A guide to symptom relief in advanced cancer. Haigh and Hockland, Manchester

Richardson R 1980 Losses: talking about bereavement. Open Books, Somerset

Saunders C 1986 The last refuge. Nursing Times 82 (43) October 22: 28–30

Simpson A 1987 Brain stem death. Nursing Times 83 (8) February 25: 41–42

Stannard D 1989 Pressure prevents nausea. Nursing Times 85 (4) January 25: 33–34

Vas Dias S 1987 Psychotherapy in special care baby units. Nursing Times 83 (23) June 10: 50–52

Walker C 1982 Attitudes to death and bereavement among cultural minority groups. Nursing Times 78 (50) December 15: 2106–2109

Whitehead M 1987 The health divide: inequalities in health in the 1980s. Health Education Council, London

Williams J 1987 Managing paediatric pain. Nursing Times 83 (36) September 9: 36–39

ADDITIONAL READING

Humphrey D, Wickett A 1987 The right to die. The Bodley Head, London

Jones A 1988 Nothing gay about bereavement. Nursing Times 84 (23) June 8: 55–57

Lugton J 1989 Relatives: communicating in the hospice. Nursing Times 85 (16) April 19: 28–30 and related articles in two subsequent issues

Melia K 1988 An easy death? Nursing Times 84 (8) February 24: 46–48

O'Neill P 1989 Services for the dying (a survey of nurses' awareness of services available to the dying). Nursing Times 85 (9) March 1: 36–37

Richards J 1987 Organ transplants: coping mechanisms. Nursing Times 83 (8) February 25: 43–44

Ruark J, Raffin T 1988 Stamford University Medical Center Committee on Ethics. Initiating and withdrawing life support: principles and practice in adult medicine. New England Journal of Medicine 318: 25–30

Saunders C, Baines M 1989 Living with dying: the management of terminal disease. Oxford University Press, Oxford

Simpson K 1989 Understanding mourning. Nursing Times 85 (4) January 25: 43–45

Tiffany R 1987 A growing concern (cancer and the developing world). Nursing Times 83 (9) March 4: 44–46

Index